Transient Ischemic Attack and Stroke

Transient Ischemic Attack and Stroke

Diagnosis, Investigation and Management

Sarah T. Pendlebury
Matthew F. Giles
Peter M. Rothwell

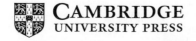

CAMBRIDGE UNIVERSITY PRESS
Cambridge, New York, Melbourne, Madrid, Cape Town, Singapore,
São Paulo, Delhi

Cambridge University Press
The Edinburgh Building, Cambridge CB2 8RU, UK

Published in the United States of America by Cambridge University
Press, New York

www.cambridge.org
Information on this title: www.cambridge.org/9780521735124

First published 2009

Printed in the United Kingdom at the University Press, Cambridge

A catalogue record for this publication is available from the British Library

Library of Congress Cataloging-in-Publication Data

Pendlebury, Sarah T.
    Transient ischemic attack and stroke : diagnosis, investigation,
and management / Sarah T. Pendlebury, Matthew F. Giles, Peter
M. Rothwell.
        p. ; cm.
    Includes bibliographical references and index.
    ISBN 978-0-521-73512-4 (pbk.)
1. Transient ischemic attack. 2. Cerebrovascular disease.   I. Giles,
Matthew F., 1970–   II. Rothwell, Peter M.   III. Title.
    [DNLM: 1. Ischemic Attack, Transient–diagnosis.   2. Stroke–
diagnosis.   3. Ischemic Attack, Transient–therapy.   4. Stroke–therapy.
WL 355 P398t 2009]
    RC388.5.P46 2009
    616.8′1–dc22

                                                                2008043638
ISBN 978-0-521-73512-4 paperback

Contents

Section 5–Secondary prevention

Section 6–Miscellaneous disorders

The color plates appear between pages 216 and 217.

Foreword

The provenance of this book on stroke goes back to the 1990s when Peter Rothwell joined our stroke research group in Edinburgh. It moves to Oxford where he married and works with Sarah Pendlebury, who is a geriatrician, and continues with Matthew Giles – the third author – who was a research fellow on Peter's Oxford Vascular Study (OXVASC), which he based on the earlier Oxfordshire Community Stroke Project (OCSP) which I ran in the 1980s. A 30 year cycle. During that time, the management of stroke has changed completely. We have sharpened up, we are faster, and governments, certainly in the UK, now make stroke one of their top priorities. We have stroke units staffed by stroke specialists. All people with strokes coming to hospital get CT scanned, more and more have MR scanning – not some time in the next few weeks, but within hours. Thirty years ago, we didn't know that aspirin was an effective drug for stroke secondary prevention, statins were somewhere over the horizon, blood pressure lowering long term after stroke was controversial, carotid surgery was out of control, vascular dementia was a minority interest, and there were no coils to occlude intracranial aneurysms. Everything has changed, and it is all somewhere in this book. Indeed, the authors' practice-based research has been responsible for a lot of these changes. Well perhaps not quite everything has changed; some things are much the same. Clinical skills are still needed, and clinical common sense, which is embedded in what we would now call clinical epidemiology, a rather special interest of the authors which should be obvious even to the casual reader. It is impossible to imagine what stroke medicine will look like in another 30 years, but in the meantime this is what it looks like now.

Professor Charles Warlow

Epidemiology, risk factors, pathophysiology and causes of transient ischemic attacks and stroke
Epidemiology

In order to understand the clinical management of transient ischemic attacks (TIAs) and stroke, to plan clinical services or to design randomized controlled trials, and to measure the overall impact of treatments, it is important to understand the epidemiology of stroke.

Definitions of transient ischemic attack and stroke

A stroke is defined as rapidly developing clinical symptoms and/or signs of focal, and at times global (applied to patients in deep coma and to those with subarachnoid hemorrhage), loss of brain function, with symptoms lasting more than 24-hours or leading to death, with no apparent cause other than that of vascular origin (Hatano 1976). Conventionally, a TIA is distinguished from stroke on the basis of an arbitrary 24-hour cut-off for resolution of symptoms Box 1.1. Hence a TIA is defined as an acute loss of focal brain or monocular function with symptoms lasting less than 24-hours and which is thought to be caused by inadequate cerebral or ocular blood supply as a result of arterial thrombosis, low flow or embolism associated with arterial, cardiac or hematological disease (Hatano 1976).

Since the early part of the twentieth century, a variety of definitions of TIA have been used (Table 1.1). However, the definition given in Box 1.1 has recently been challenged since the 24-hour time limit is arbitrary, rather than being based on clinical, imaging or pathological criteria. The 24-hour cut-off does not reflect the fact that the majority of TIAs last for less than 60 minutes, nor does it indicate a lack of infarction on brain imaging. Some TIAs are associated with radiological evidence of cerebral infarction, but there is poor correlation between clinical and imaging findings (Table 1.2). An alternative, but controversial (Easton *et al.* 2004), definition for TIA has been proposed as comprising a transient episode of neurological dysfunction caused by focal brain or retinal ischemia without evidence of acute infarction on brain imaging (Albers *et al.* 2002). The proposed new definition for TIA has the problem that brain imaging does not correlate particularly well with pathological infarction: brain imaging may be normal in clinically definite stroke,

---

Box 1.1. Definitions of transient ischemic attack and stroke as used in this book

Transient ischemic attack. An acute loss of focal brain or monocular function with symptoms lasting less than 24-hours and which is thought to be caused by inadequate cerebral or ocular blood supply as a result of arterial thrombosis, low flow or embolism associated with arterial, cardiac or hematological disease (Hatano 1976).

Stroke. Rapidly developing clinical symptoms and/or signs of focal, and at times global (applied to patients in deep coma and to those with subarachnoid hemorrhage), loss of brain function, with symptoms lasting more than 24-hours or leading to death, with no apparent cause other than that of vascular origin (Hatano 1976).

Table 1.1. History of the definition of transient ischemic attack

Year	Description
1914 Hunt (1914)	Characterized "the role of the carotid arteries in the causation of vascular lesions of the brain" and described "attacks of threatened hemiplegia and cerebral intermittent claudication"
1954; CM Fisher at the *First and Second Conferences on Cerebral Vascular Diseases*, Princeton, USA	Described "transient ischemic attacks . . . which may last from a few seconds up to several hours, the most common duration being a few seconds up to 5 or 10 minutes"
1961; CM Fisher at the *Third Conference on Cerebral Vascular Diseases*	TIA described as "the occurrence of single or multiple episodes of cerebral dysfunction lasting no longer than one hour and clearing without significant residuum"
1964 Acheson and Hutchinson (1964)	Series of patients with "transient cerebral ischemia" defined as "duration of attack less than an hour"
1964 Marshall (1964)	Series of 180 patients with TIAs defined as "of less than 24-hours duration"
1975 Advisory Council for National Institute of Neurological and Communicative Disorders and Stroke (1975)	TIA defined as lasting "no longer than a day (24-hours)", although typically lasting from 2 to 15 minutes
1976 World Health Organization bulletin (Hatano 1976)	TIA defined as lasting less than 24-hours
2002 For the TIA Working Group (Albers *et al.* 2002)	TIA definition proposed based on absence of infarction on brain scanning and a 1 hour time window

Note:
TIA, transient ischemic attack.

silent infarction may occur and imaging sensitivity is highly dependent on both imaging method and area of the brain being examined. Moreover, there is uncertainty regarding the pathological correlates of imaging changes such as diffusion-weighted magnetic resonance imaging (DWI) hyperintensity (Chs. 10 and 11) and leukoaraiosis, and, as imaging technology advances, what is defined as TIA will change. The definition of TIA used throughout this book is, therefore, the conventional one based on symptoms or signs lasting less than 24-hours.

Anything that causes a TIA may, if more severe or prolonged, cause a stroke (Sempere *et al.* 1998). There are many non-vascular conditions that may cause symptoms suggestive of TIA or stroke, and these are referred to in this book as "TIA mimics" or "stroke mimics." The separation of TIA from stroke on the basis of a 24-hour time limit is useful since the differential diagnosis of the two syndromes is different to some extent (i.e. the spectrum of TIA mimics differs from that of stroke mimics).

Given the common mechanisms underlying TIA and stroke, the investigation of patients with these syndromes is similar. However, in TIA and minor stroke, the emphasis is on rapid identification and treatment of the underlying cause in order to prevent a recurrent and possibly more severe event, whereas in severe stroke, the initial emphasis of investigation is on targeting treatment to minimize subsequent deficit. Therefore, in this book, we have considered TIA and minor stroke separately from severe stroke to reflect the difference in clinical approach to minor versus more severe cerebrovascular events.

There is no accepted definition for what constitutes "minor" stroke. This distinction between minor and major stroke is sometimes based on an a score on the National

Table 1.2. Advantages and disadvantages of conventional and imaging-based definitions of transient ischemic attack

Definition	Advantages	Disadvantages
Conventional definition	Diagnosis can be made at assessment (provided that symptoms have resolved) either prior to imaging or in centers where imaging is unavailable	Diagnosis based on an arbitrary cut-point of no physiological or prognostic significance
	Comparisons with previous studies using conventional definition possible	Diagnosis based on patient recall, which may vary with time
		Diagnosis cannot be made with certainty within 24-hours in a patient with resolving (but persistent) symptoms
Imaging-based definition	Based on pathophysiological endpoint and emphasizes prognostic importance of cerebral infarction	Diagnosis based on interpretation of imaging, which is likely to vary between individuals and centers; also, sensitivity of imaging techniques is likely to increase with time with developments in computed tomography and magnetic resonance technology
	Majority of transient ischemic attacks last less than 60 minutes	Pathophysiological significance of changes on new imaging techniques not fully understood
	Encourages use of neurodiagnostic investigations	Classification of events lasting >1 hour without infarction unclear
	Consistent with the distinction between unstable angina and myocardial infarction	Diagnosis cannot be made in centers where no imaging is available

Institutes of Health Stroke Scale (NIHSS) at assessment of ≤ 3 (Wityk *et al.* 1994) or a score of ≤ 2 on the modified Rankin Scale (mRS) at 1 month. Such distinctions are problematic because the NIHSS score will vary with time after the stroke and the mRS at 1 month may increase if a minor stroke is followed by a major stroke. We take the pragmatic view that minor stroke includes those strokes mild enough for patients to be seen in an emergency outpatient setting or to be sent home after initial assessment and treatment in hospital.

Approximately 85% of all first-ever strokes are ischemic; 10% are caused by primary intracerebral hemorrhage and approximately 5% are from subarachnoid hemorrhage (Rothwell *et al.* 2004). Within ischemic stroke, 25% are caused by large artery disease, 25% by small vessel disease, 20% by cardiac embolism, 5% by other rarer causes, and the remaining 25% are of undetermined etiology. Ischemic stroke may also be classified by anatomical location using simple clinical features as total anterior circulation stroke, partial anterior circulation stroke, lacunar stroke and posterior circulation stroke. This is of some help in identifying the likely underlying pathology and gives information as to prognosis (Ch. 9).

The burden of transient ischemic attack and stroke

Each year there are about one million strokes in the European Union (Sudlow and Warlow 1997), making it by far the most common neurological disorder (MacDonald *et al.* 2000) (Table 1.3). Approximately 25% of men and 20% of women can expect to suffer a stroke if they live to be 85 years old (Bonita 1992) and stroke is the second most common cause of death worldwide (Murray and Lopez 1996). However, mortality data underestimate the true burden of stroke since, in contrast to coronary heart disease and cancer, the major burden

Table 1.3. Comparative incidence and prevalence rates of common neurological conditions measured in a population-based study of approximately 100 000 people registered with 13 general practices in London, UK, and conducted between 1995 and 1996

Condition	Incidence rate (95% CI)[a]	Prevalence rate (95% CI)[a]
First TIA or stroke[b]	2.05 (1.83–2.30)	
Second TIA or stroke[b]	0.42 (0.33–0.55)	
Intracranial hemorrhage	0.10 (0.05–0.17)	0.5 (0.2–0.8)
Any stroke		9 (8–11)
Epilepsy[c]	0.46 (0.36–0.60)	4 (4–5)
First seizure	0.11 (0.07–0.18)	
Primary CNS tumor	0.10 (0.05–0.18)	
Parkinson's disease	0.09 (0.12–0.27)	2 (1–3)
Shingles	1.40 (1.04–1.84)	
Bacterial infection of CNS	0.07 (0.04–0.13)	1 (0.8–2.0)
Multiple sclerosis	0.07 (0.04–0.11)	2 (2–3)
Myaesthenia gravis	0.03 (0.008–0.070)	
Guillame–Barré	0.03 (0.01–0.06)	
Motor neurone disease	0.02 (0.003–0.050)	0.1 (0.01–0.30)

Notes:
CI, confidence interval; TIA, transient ischemic attack.
[a]Age- and sex-adjusted rates per 1000 population.
[b]Includes ischemic and hemorrhagic stroke.
[c]Two or more unprovoked seizures.
Source: From MacDonald *et al.* (2000).

of stroke is chronic disability rather than death (Wolfe 2000). Brain diseases, of which stroke forms a large proportion, cause 23% of healthy years lost and around 50% of years of life lived with disability in Europe (Olesen and Leonardi 2003).

Approximately a third of stroke survivors are functionally dependent at one year and stroke is the commonest cause of neurological disability in the developed world (Murray and Lopez 1996; MacDonald *et al.* 2000). Stroke also causes secondary medical problems, including dementia, depression, epilepsy, falls and fractures. In the UK, the costs of stroke are estimated to be nearly twice those of coronary heart disease (British Heart Foundation Statistics Database 1998; Rothwell 2001), accounting for about 6% of total National Health Service (NHS) and Social Services expenditure (Rothwell 2001). As the population ages over the coming two decades, the total stroke rate will probably increase unless there are substantial decreases in age- and sex-specific incidence (Rothwell *et al.* 2004a). Stroke deaths are projected to increase from 4.5 million worldwide in 1990 to 7.7 million in 2020, when stroke will account for 6.2% of the total burden of illness (Bonita 1992; Sudlow and Warlow 1997; Menken *et al.* 2000).

Additionally, TIAs are also common, and it is estimated that 54 000 TIAs occur each year in England (Giles and Rothwell 2007). By definition, TIA causes transient symptoms only and, therefore, has no long-term sequelae per se. However, the importance of TIA lies in the high early risk of stroke and the longer-term risk of other vascular disease. Indeed, it has been estimated that approximately 20% of strokes are preceded by TIA (Rothwell and Warlow 2005).

Understanding of the epidemiology of stroke has lagged behind that of coronary heart disease because of a lack of research funding for stroke (Rothwell 2001; Pendlebury *et al.* 2004; Pendlebury 2007) and because stroke is a much more heterogeneous disorder. Separate assessment of the different stroke subtypes should ideally be made in epidemiological studies of stroke. Stroke subtype identification was often not possible in early studies because of a lack of brain and vascular imaging and it remains problematic today because of the frequent difficulty in ascribing a cause for a given stroke even when imaging is available. The epidemiology of TIA is more challenging even than stroke since patients with TIAs are more heterogeneous and present to a variety of different clinical services, if they present to medical attention at all. Furthermore, reliable diagnosis of TIA requires early and expert clinical assessment (there is no diagnostic test for TIA), making epidemiological studies labor intensive and costly.

Mortality

Stroke mortality rises rapidly with age (Rothwell *et al.* 2005). The increase in mortality in the elderly is mainly a result of the steep rise in the incidence of stroke with age, but also, to a lesser extent, reflects the increase in case fatality in older patients. In other words, older people are more likely to have a stroke (incidence) and, if they do have one, it is more likely to be fatal (case fatality).

The age-standardized death rate attributed to stroke varies six-fold between developed countries while very little is known about the developing world (Inzitari *et al.* 1995; Connor *et al.* 2007). Particularly high reported rates of stroke occur in eastern Europe and Japan, and particularly low rates in certain parts of North America and some western European countries (Feigin *et al.* 2003). The reasons for these differences are unclear but one possibility is that the stroke subtypes more likely to be fatal, particularly intracranial hemorrhage or cardioembolic stroke, are more frequent in countries with high stroke mortality.

Incidence, prevalence and time trends

The incidence of new cases of first-ever TIA or stroke can only be reliably assessed in prospective population-based studies (Sudlow and Warlow 1996; Feigin *et al.* 2003; Rothwell *et al.* 2004) since hospital-based studies are subject to referral bias (Table 1.4). One of the most comprehensive population-based studies of stroke and TIA incidence is the Oxford Vascular Study, OXVASC, which has near-complete case ascertainment of all patients, irrespective of age, in a population of 91 000 defined by registration with nine general practices in Oxfordshire, UK (Coull *et al.* 2004). This is in contrast to previous studies, such as the MONICA project and the Framingham study, which had an age cut-off at 65 or 75 years or relied on voluntary participation.

The OXVASC study showed that the annual incidence of stroke in the UK in the first few years of this century, including subarachnoid hemorrhage, was 2.3/1000 and the incidence of TIA was 0.5/1000 (Rothwell *et al.* 2005), with about a quarter of events occurring in those under the age of 65 and about a half in those above the age of 75 (Fig. 1.1). The incidence of cerebrovascular events in OXVASC was similar to that of acute coronary vascular events in the same population during the same period (Fig. 1.2), with a similar age distribution (Rothwell *et al.* 2005). Incidence rates, however, measure first-ever-in-a-lifetime definite events only and exclude possible, recurrent and suspected events, so do not represent the true burden of a condition. This is especially true for TIA, where a significant proportion of cases referred to a TIA service have alternative, non-vascular

Table 1.4. Population- and hospital-based incidence studies

Study type	Description	Advantages	Disadvantages
Population based	Multiple overlapping, prospective methods of case ascertainment used to identify all individuals with condition of interest from a predefined population; includes searches of both primary and secondary care and databases of diagnostic tests and death certification/mortality statistics	More accurate measurement of incidence through minimizing referral bias; individuals who are not managed in hospital are included, particularly elderly, those with mild condition and fatal events occurring outside hospital	Time consuming and resource intensive
		Results of studies conducted in different populations and over different time periods can be directly compared (after statistical adjustment for age and sex)	Patients with the condition but who do not seek medical attention or who are misdiagnosed in primary care not included
		Representative of the requirements of an entire population	Mortality statistics are not collected reliably
Hospital based	Methods of case ascertainment used to identify all cases that are referred, admitted, managed or discharged from hospital setting from a predefined population	Less time consuming and less resource intensive	Prone to referral bias; outpatient attendance variably included and events managed only in the community not included
	Typically, hospital-based databases only searched.	Representative of the requirements for hospital services	Liable to inaccuracies of diagnostic coding
			Patients transferred between departments or hospitals either not identified or double counted
			Referral rates to hospital vary geographically and over time; comparison between studies, therefore, less reliable

conditions. Thus consequently, although the annual incidence of definite, first-ever-in-a-lifetime TIA in OXVASC was 0.5/1000, the rate of definite or possible, incident or recurrent TIA was 1.1/1000, and the rate of all referrals to a TIA clinic including all TIAs, suspected events with non-vascular causes and minor strokes was 3.0/1000 (Giles and Rothwell 2007) (Table 1.5).

Stroke prevalence is the total number of people with stroke in a population at a given time and is usually measured by cross-sectional surveys (Box 1.2). It is a function of stroke incidence and survival and, therefore, varies over time and between populations with differing age and sex structures. In the UK, stroke prevalence is approximately 5/1000 population and in 65 to 74 year olds is approximately 50/1000 in men and 25/1000 in

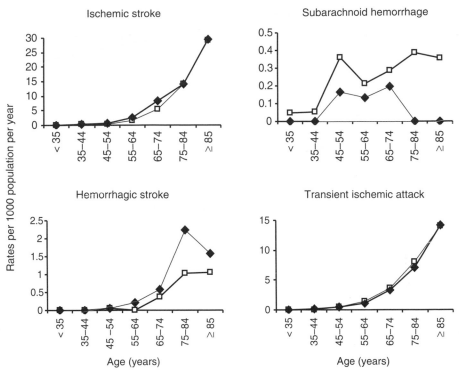

Fig. 1.1. Age-specific rates of all events for different types of acute cerebrovascular event in men (diamonds) and women (open squares) in Oxfordshire from 2002 to 2005 (Rothwell *et al.* 2005).

women (Wyller *et al.* 1994; Geddes *et al.* 1996; Bots *et al.* 1996). Measuring TIA prevalence is methodologically more challenging because it is difficult to confirm, without direct patient assessment, whether transient neurological symptoms reported in a population survey are of vascular origin. Accurate data are, therefore, lacking, but a large telephone survey of randomly selected households in the USA reported a prevalence of physician-diagnosed TIA of 23/1000 while a further 32/1000 recalled symptoms consistent with TIA that had not been reported to medical attention (Johnston *et al.* 2003).

A reduction in stroke and TIA incidence since the late 1980s would be expected, given that randomized trials have shown several interventions to be effective in the primary and secondary prevention of stroke. Indeed, it has been estimated that full implementation of currently available preventive strategies could reduce stroke incidence by as much as 50–80% (Murray *et al.* 2003; Wald and Law 2003). Stroke mortality rates certainly declined from the 1950s to the 1980s in North America and western Europe (Bonita *et al.* 1990; Thom 1993), but this decline has since levelled off. Although apparent trends in stroke mortality are very difficult to interpret because of changes over time in death certification practices and case-fatality, stroke incidence also appeared to decline in the 1960s and 1970s in the USA, Asia and Europe (McGowern *et al.* 1992; Kodama 1993; Tunstall-Pedoe *et al.* 1994; Numminen *et al.* 1996). However, the majority of subsequent studies during the 1980s and 1990s, when effective preventive treatments had become more widely available, have shown either no change (Wolf *et al.* 1992; Bonita *et al.* 1993; Stegmayr *et al.* 1994) or, more commonly, an increase in age- and sex-adjusted incidence (Johansson *et al.* 2000; Medin *et al.* 2004).

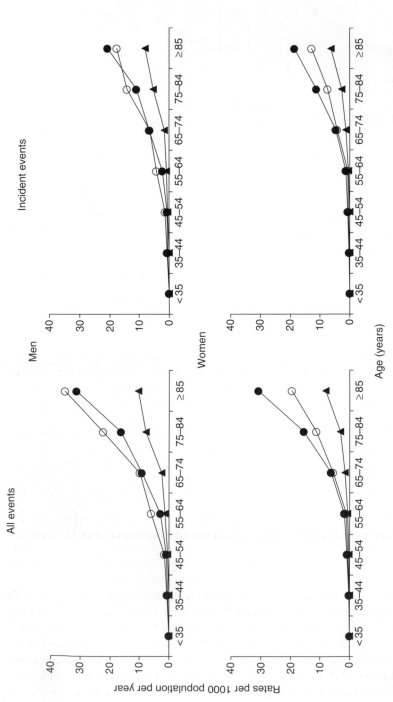

Fig. 1.2. Age-specific rates of all events and of incident events for stroke (i.e. not including transient ischemic attack; closed circles), myocardial infarction and sudden cardiac death combined (i.e. not including unstable angina; open circles), and acute peripheral vascular events (triangles) in men and women in Oxfordshire from 2002 to 2005 (Rothwell et al. 2005).

Table 1.5. Incidence rates of transient ischemic attack and stroke according to stringency of definition applied and previous cerebrovascular disease measured in OXVASC (2002–2005)

Category of event	Incidence rate (95% CI)[a]
TIA, incident only	
Definite	0.47 (0.39–0.56)
Definite and probable[b]	0.59 (0.5–0.68)
TIA, incident and recurrent	
Definite	0.82 (0.72–0.94)
Definite and probable[b]	0.95 (0.84–1.07)
All definite, probable and suspected TIA (including all referrals to a TIA service with an eventual non-neurovascular diagnosis)	2.06 (1.89–2.23)
Stroke,[c] incident only	
Definite and probable	1.39 (1.25–1.54)
Stroke,[c] incident and recurrent	
Definite and probable	1.85 (1.70–2.02)
All definite, probable and suspected (including all referrals to hospital of suspected stroke with an eventual non-neurovascular diagnosis)	2.29 (1.89–2.23)

Notes:
CI, confidence interval; TIA, transient ischemic attack.
[a]unadjusted rate per 1000 population.
[b]Probable TIA defined as any transient symptoms lasting less than 24-hours of likely (but not certain) vascular etiology that was felt to justify secondary prevention treatment.
[c]Stroke includes ischemic and primary intracerebral hemorrhage but not subarachnoid hemorrhage.
Source: From Giles and Rothwell (2007).

Box 1.2. Definitions of incidence and prevalence

Incidence rate. The number of new cases of a condition per unit time per unit of population at risk. Usually expressed as the number of new cases per 1000 or 100 000 population at risk per year.

Adjusted/standardized incidence rates. Overall incidence rates depend critically on the age and sex structure of the population studied. For example, a relatively old population may have a higher mortality rate than a younger population even if, age for age, the rates are similar. Incidence rates from different populations are, therefore, often compared following adjustment or standardization by applying age- and sex-specific rates to a "standard" population.

Prevalence rate. The total number of cases of a condition per unit of population at risk at a given time. Usually expressed as a percentage or the total number of cases per 1000 or 100 000 population at risk.

The most recent studies of time trends in stroke incidence do suggest that age-specific incidence is now falling (Sarti *et al.* 2003; Rothwell *et al.* 2004; Anderson *et al.* 2005; Hardie *et al.* 2005). Between the periods 1981–1984 and 2002–2004, a 40% reduction in the incidence of fatal and disabling stroke was found in Oxfordshire, UK (Rothwell *et al.* 2004), although this reduction was less marked in the oldest old (Fig. 1.3). High-quality population-based studies of time trends in TIA and minor stroke are lacking. However, moderate rises in TIA incidence were reported in Oxfordshire, UK, between the periods

(a)

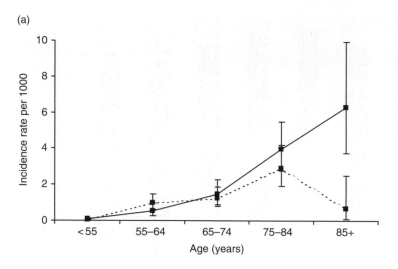

(b)

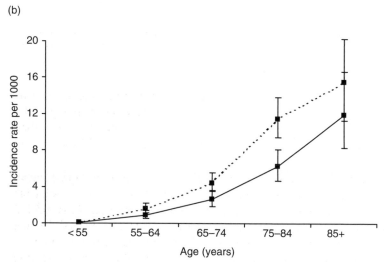

Fig. 1.3. The age-specific incidence of transient ischemic attack (a) and major disabling stroke (b) in Oxfordshire in 1981–1984 (the Oxford Community Stroke Project [OCSP], - - -) and 2002–2004 (the Oxford Vascular Study [OXVASC] —) (Rothwell *et al.* 2004).

1981–1984 and 2002–2004 (Fig. 1.3) (Rothwell *et al.* 2004) and in Novosibirsk, Russia, between the periods 1987–1988 and 1996–1997 (Feigin *et al.* 2000) but no significant change in TIA incidence was found in Dijon, France, between 1985 and 1994. It is difficult to find a single explanation for the decline in incidence of major stroke in recent years and a contemporaneous stabilization or increase in the rates of TIA. The former may be related to a decline in the prevalence of causative risk factors or to treatment of risk factors such as hypertension and elevated cholesterol, while the latter is likely to reflect changes in public health awareness and behavior, with people now being more likely to seek medical attention for transient neurological symptoms.

Racial and social factors

There are racial and social differences in susceptibility to stroke and TIA (Forouhi and Satter 2006) and in the incidence of the various stroke subtypes (Fig. 1.4). Some of these racial differences are partly caused by differences in risk factor prevalence: hypertension

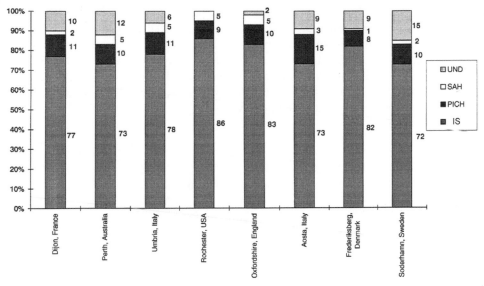

Fig. 1.4. The proportions of first-ever-in-a-lifetime strokes caused by ischemic stroke (IS), primary intracerebral hemorrhage (PICH), subarachnoid hemorrhage (SAH) and of undetermined cause (UND) in "ideal" incidence studies. Numbers indicate the percentage estimates (Sudlow and Warlow 1997).

and diabetes mellitus are more common in blacks and coronary heart disease is more common in whites, for example (Sacco 2001). Other differences are not properly understood, such as the much higher proportion of stroke caused by intracerebral hemorrhage in Southeast Asia and the Far East than in Western countries (Sudlow and Warlow 1996; Feigin *et al.* 2003).

Black populations. The burden of stroke is higher in blacks than whites for both ischemic, particularly small vessel stroke, and hemorrhagic stroke (Woo *et al.* 1999; Schneider *et al.* 2004; Pandey and Gorelick 2005; White *et al.* 2005; Wolfe *et al.* 2006a, b). This pattern may be related in part to a higher prevalence of hypertension and diabetes mellitus (Gillum 1999; Sacco 2001). Intracranial large artery occlusive vascular disease also appears to be more common in blacks than in whites (Sacco *et al.* 1995; Wityk *et al.* 1996; Lynch and Gorelick 2000). In the single relevant study, rates of TIA were found to be higher in blacks than whites (Kleindorfer *et al.* 2005).

Maori and Pacific Islands. People in New Zealand have a higher stroke incidence than Europeans, perhaps owing to differences in risk factors and health-related behaviors (Bonita *et al.* 1997; Feigin *et al.* 2006).

Japanese and Chinese populations. Stroke, particularly primary intracerebral hemorrhage, is more common in Japan and China than in Western countries (Huang *et al.* 1990) and this is accompanied by less extracranial but more intracranial arterial disease (Feldmann *et al.* 1990; Leung *et al.* 1993; Sacco *et al.* 1995; Wityk *et al.* 1996).

South Asian populations. People of South Asian origin in the UK have a high prevalence of coronary heart disease and stroke, central obesity (as evidenced by high waist-to-hip ratio), insulin resistance, non-insulin-dependent (type 2) diabetes and hypertension (Cappuccio 1997; Kain *et al.* 2002; Bhopal *et al.* 2005). This increase in vascular risk seems to be partly a result of genetic susceptibility, such as high serum lipoprotein A levels, and partly dietary- and lifestyle-induced changes in lipid levels.

Deprivation. In the UK, both stroke incidence and poor outcome after stroke are greater in areas of socioeconomic disadvantage (Kaplan and Keil 1993; Avendaño *et al.* 2004). This is partly because poverty is associated with adverse health behaviors and risk factors such as smoking (Hart *et al.* 2000a). There is also evidence that poor maternal and infant health is associated with increased mortality from stroke in later life (Barker 1995; Martyn *et al.* 1996). However, the adverse effect of socioeconomic deprivation also appears to be cumulative throughout life (Davey Smith *et al.* 1997; Hart *et al.* 2000b).

Seasonal and diurnal variation

In most studies, both stroke mortality and hospital admission rates are higher in winter than in summer (Douglas *et al.* 1991; Pan *et al.* 1995; Feigin and Weibers 1997). This seasonal variation might be explained by the complications of stroke being more likely to occur in the winter (e.g. pneumonia) and cannot simply be assumed to reflect stroke incidence. Where incidence has been measured in the community, there is little seasonal variation, at least in temperate climates, although primary intracerebral hemorrhage is somewhat more likely in the winter months and on cold days (Rothwell *et al.* 1996; Jakovljevic *et al.* 1996).

Stroke occurs most frequently in the hour or two after waking in the morning, but whether this applies to all subtypes of stroke is difficult to say because of the relatively small proportion of intracranial hemorrhages in most studies (Kelly-Hayes *et al.* 1995; Elliott 1998). Subarachnoid hemorrhage is very unlikely to occur during sleep and, in general, is most likely to occur during strenuous activities (Wroe *et al.* 1992). There are no equivalent data for TIA, although provisional results from OXVASC suggest that incidence also shows diurnal variation, and apparent TIA incidence falls slightly at the weekend, possibly because patients are less likely to present to medical attention (Giles *et al.* 2006).

References

Acheson J, Hutchinson EC (1964). Observations on the natural history of transient cerebral ischaemia. *Lancet* **ii**:871–874.

Advisory Council for the National Institute of Neurological and Communicative Disorders and Stroke (1975). C. II. *Stroke* **6**:564–616.

Albers GW, Caplan LR, Easton JD *et al.* (2002). Transient ischemic attack: proposal for a new definition. *New England Journal of Medicine* **347**:1713–1716

Anderson CS, Carter KN, Hackett ML *et al.* (2005). Study Group. Trends in stroke incidence in Auckland, New Zealand, during 1981 to 2003. *Stroke* **36**:2087–2093

Avendaño M, Kunst AE, Huisman M *et al.* (2004). Educational level and stroke mortality. A comparison of 10 European populations during the 1990s. *Stroke* **35**:432–437

Barker DJP (1995). Fetal origins of coronary heart disease. *British Medical Journal* **311**:171–174

Bhopal R, Fischbacher C, Vartiainen E *et al.* (2005). Predicted and observed cardiovascular disease in South Asians: application of FINRISK, Framingham and SCORE models to Newcastle Heart Project data. *Journal of Public Health* **27**:93–100

Bonita R (1992). Epidemiology of stroke. *Lancet* **339**:342–344

Bonita R, Stewart A, Beaglehole R (1990). International trends in stroke mortality 1970–1985. *Stroke* **21**:989–992

Bonita R, Broad JB, Beaglehole R (1993). Changes in stroke incidence and case-fatality in Auckland New Zealand 1981–1991. *Lancet* **342**:1470–1473

Bonita R, Broad JB, Beaglehole R (1997). Ethnic differences in stroke incidence and case fatality in Auckland New Zealand. *Stroke* **28**:758–761

Bots ML, Looman SJ, Koudstaal PJ *et al.* (1996). Prevalence of stroke in the general population. The Rotterdam study. *Stroke* **27**:1499–1501

British Heart Foundation Statistics Database (1998). *Coronary Heart Disease Statistics 1998*. London: British Heart Foundation

Cappuccio FP (1997). Ethnicity and cardiovascular risk: variations in people of African ancestry and South Asian origin. *Journal of Human Hypertension* **11**:571–576

Connor MD, Walker R, Modi G *et al.* (2007). Burden of stroke in black populations in sub-Saharan Africa. *Lancet Neurology* **6**:269–278

Coull AJ, Lovett JK, Rothwell PM *et al.* (2004). Population based study of early risk of stroke after transient ischaemic attack or minor stroke: implications for public education and organisation of services. *British Medical Journal* **328**:326

Davey Smith G, Hart C, Blane D *et al.* (1997). Lifetime socioeconomic position and mortality: prospective observational study. *British Medical Journal* **314**:547–552

Douglas AS, Allan TM, Rawles JM (1991). Composition of seasonality of disease. *Scottish Medical Journal* **36**:76–82

Easton JD, Albers GW, Caplan LR *et al.* (2004). Discussion: Reconsideration of TIA terminology and definitions. *Neurology* **62**:S29–S34

Elliott WJ (1998). Circadian variation in the timing of stroke onset: a meta-analysis. *Stroke* **29**:992–996

Feigin VL, Wiebers DO (1997). Environmental factors and stroke: a selective review. *Journal of Stroke and Cerebrovascular Diseases* **6**:108–113

Feigin VL, Shishkin SV, Tzirkin GM *et al.* (2000). A population-based study of transient ischemic attack incidence in Novosibirsk, Russia, 1987–1988 and 1996–1997. *Stroke* **31**:9–13

Feigin VL, Shishkin SV, Tzirkin GM *et al.* (2003). A population-based study of transient ischemic attack incidence in Novosibirsk, Russia 1987–1988 and 1996–1997. *Stroke* **31**:9–13

Feigin VL, Carter K, Hackett M *et al.* (2006). Ethnic disparities in incidence of stroke subtypes: Auckland Regional Community Stroke Study 2002–2003. *Lancet Neurology* **5**:130–139

Feldmann E, Dancault N, Kwan E *et al.* (1990). Chinese–white differences in the distribution of occlusive cerebrovascular disease. *Neurology* **40**:1541–1545

Forouhi NG, Sattar N (2006). CVD risk factors and ethnicity: a homogeneous relationship? *Atherosclerosis Supplement* **7**:11–19

Geddes JML, Fear J, Tennant A *et al.* (1996). Prevalence of self reported stroke in a population in northern England. *Journal of Epidemiology and Community Health* **50**:140–143

Giles MF, Rothwell PM (2007). Substantial underestimation of the need for outpatient services for TIA and minor stroke. *Age Ageing* **36**:676–680

Giles MF, Flossman E, Rothwell PM (2006). Patient behaviour immediately after transient ischemic attack according to clinical characteristics, perception of the event, and predicted risk of stroke. *Stroke* **37**:1254–1260

Gillum RF (1999). Risk factors for stroke in blacks: a critical review. *American Journal of Epidemiology* **150**:1266–1274

Hardie K, Jamrozik K, Hankey GJ *et al.* (2005). Trends in five-year survival and risk of recurrent stroke after first-ever stroke in the Perth Community Stroke Study. *Cerebrovascular Diseases* **19**:179–185

Hart CL, Hole DJ, Davey Smith G (2000a). Influence of socioeconomic circumstances in early and later life on stroke risk among men in a Scottish cohort study. *Stroke* **31**:2093–2097

Hart CL, Hole DJ, Davey Smith G (2000b). The contribution of risk factors to stroke differentials by socioeconomic position in adulthood: the Renfrew/Paisley study. *American Journal of Public Health* **90**:1788–1791

Hatano S (1976). Experience from a multicentre stroke register: a preliminary report. *Bulletin WHO* **54**:541–553

Huang CY, Chan FL, Yu YL *et al.* (1990). Cerebrovascular disease in Hong Kong Chinese. *Stroke* **21**:230–235

Hunt, J.R. (1914). The role of the carotid arteries in the causation of vascular lesions of the brain, with remarks on certain special features of symptomatology. *American Journal of Medical Science* **147**:704

Inzitari D, Lamassa M, Amaducci L (1995). Stroke epidemiology in Europe. *European Journal of Neurology* **2**:75–81

Jakovljevic D, Salomaa V, Sivenius J *et al.* (1996). Seasonal variation in the occurrence of stroke in a Finnish adult population. The FINMONICA Stroke Register. *Stroke* **27**:1774–1779

Johansson B, Norrving B, Lindgren A (2000). Increased stroke incidence in Lund-Orup, Sweden between 1983 to 1985 and 1993 to 1995. *Stroke* **31**:481–486

Johnston SC, Fayad PB, Gorelick PB *et al.* (2003). Prevalence and knowledge of transient ischemic attack among US adults. *Neurology* **60**:1429–1434

Kain K, Catto AJ, Young J *et al.* (2002). Increased fibrinogen, von Willebrand factor and tissue plasminogen activator levels in insulin resistant South Asian patients with ischaemic stroke. *Atherosclerosis* **163**:371–376

Kaplan GA, Keil JE (1993). Socioeconomic factors and cardiovascular disease: a review of the literature. *Circulation* **88**:1973–1998

Kelly-Hayes M, Wolf PA, Kase CS *et al.* (1995). Tempotal patterns of stroke onset. The Framingham Study. *Stroke* **26**:1343–1347

Kleindorfer D, Panagos P, Pancioli A *et al.* (2005). Incidence and short-term prognosis of transient ischemic attack in a population-based study. *Stroke* **36**:720–723

Kodama K (1993). Stroke trends in Japan. *Annals of Epidemiology* **3**:524–528

Lemesle M, Milan C, Faivre J *et al.* (1999). Incidence trends of ischemic stroke and transient ischemic attacks in a well-defined French population from 1985 through 1994. *Stroke* **30**:371–377

Leung SY, Ng THK, Yuen ST *et al.* (1993). Pattern of cerebral atherosclerosis in Hong Kong Chinese: severity in intracranial and extracranial vessels. *Stroke* **24**:779–786

Lynch GF, Gorelick PB (2000). Stroke in African Americans. *Neurology Clinic* **18**:273–290

MacDonald BK, Cockerell OC, Sander JWAS *et al.* (2000). The incidence and lifetime prevalence of neurological disorders in a prospective community-based study in the UK. *Brain* **123**:665–676

Marshall J (1964). The natural history of transient ischaemic cerebro-vascular attacks. *Quarterly Journal of Medicine* **33**:309–324.

McGowern PG, Burke GL, Sprafka JM *et al.* (1992). Trends in mortality, morbidity and risk factor levels for stroke from 1960–1990: the Minnesota Heart Survey. *Journal of the American Medical Association* **268**:753–759

Martyn CN, Barker DJP, Osmond C (1996). Mothers' pelvic size, fetal growth and death from stroke and coronary heart disease in men in the UK. *Lancet* **348**:1264–1268

Medin J, Nordlund A, Ekberg K (2004). Increasing stroke incidence in Sweden between 1989 and 2000 among persons aged 30 to 65 years: evidence from the Swedish Hospital Discharge Register. *Stroke* **35**:1047–1051

Menken M, Munsat TL, Toole JF (2000). The Global Burden of Disease Study, implications for neurology. *Archives of Neurology* **57**:418–420

Murray CJL, Lopez AD (1996). *The Global Burden of Disease: A Comprehensive Assessment of Mortality and Disability from Diseases, Injuries and Risk Factors in 1990 and Projected to 2020.* Boston, MA: Harvard University Press

Murray CJL, Lauer JA, Hutubessy RCW *et al.* (2003). Effectiveness and costs on interventions to lower systolic blood pressure: a global and regional analysis on reduction of cardiovascular risk. *Lancet* **361**:717–725

Numminen H, Kotila M, Waltimo O *et al.* (1996). Declining incidence and mortality rates of stroke in Finland from 1972 to 1991: results of 3 population-based stroke registers. *Stroke* **27**:1487–1491

Olesen J, Leonardi M (2003). The burden of brain diseases in Europe. *European Journal of Neurology* **10**:471–477

Pan WH, Li LA, Tsai MJ (1995). Temperature extremes and mortality from coronary heart disease and cerebral infarction in elderly Chinese. *Lancet* **345**:353–355

Pandey DK, Gorelick PB (2005). Epidemiology of stroke in African Americans and Hispanic Americans. *Medical Clinics of North America* **89**:739–752

Pendlebury ST (2007). Worldwide under-funding of stroke research. *International Journal of Stroke* **2**:80–84

Pendlebury ST, Rothwell PM, Algra A *et al.* (2004). Underfunding of stroke research: a Europe-wide problem. *Stroke* **35**:2368–2371

Rothwell PM (2001). The high cost of not funding stroke research: a comparison with heart disease and cancer. *Lancet* **19**:1612–1616

Rothwell PM (2005). Prevention of stroke in patients with diabetes mellitus and the metabolic syndrome. *Cerebrovascular Diseases* **1**:24–34

Rothwell PM, Warlow CP (2005). Timing of transient ischaemic attacks preceding ischaemic stroke. *Neurology* **64**:817–820

Rothwell PM, Wroe SJ, Slattery J *et al.* (1996). Is stroke incidence related to season or temperature? *Lancet* **347**:934–936

Rothwell PM, Coull AJ, Giles MF *et al.* (2004). Change in stroke incidence, mortality, case-fatality, severity and risk factors in Oxfordshire, UK from 1981 to 2004 (Oxford Vascular Study). *Lancet* **363**:1925–1933

Rothwell PM, Coull AJ, Silver LE *et al.* (2005). Population-based study of event-rate, incidence, case fatality and mortality for all acute vascular events in all arterial territories (Oxford Vascular Study). *Lancet* **366**:1773–1783

Sacco RL (2001). Newer risk factors for stroke. *Neurology* **57**:S31–S34

Sacco RL, Kargman DE, Gu Q *et al.* (1995). Race-ethnicity and determinants of intracranial atherosclerotic cerebral infarction. The Northern Manhattan Stroke Study. *Stroke* **26**:14–20

Sarti C, Stegmayr B, Tolonen H *et al.* (2003). Are changes in mortality from stroke caused by changes in stroke event rates or case fatality? Results from the WHO MONICA Project. *Stroke* **34**:1833–1840

Schneider AT, Kissela B, Woo D *et al.* (2004). Ischemic stroke subtypes: a population-based study of incidence rates among blacks and whites. *Stroke* **35**:1552–1556

Sempere AP, Duarte J, Cabezas C *et al.* (1998). Aetiopathogenesis of transient ischaemic attacks and minor ischaemic strokes: a community-based study in Segovia, Spain. *Stroke* **29**:40–45

Stegmayr B, Asplund K, Wester PO (1994). Trends in incidence, case fatality rate, and severity of stroke in Northern Sweden, 1985–1991. *Stroke* **25**:1738–1745

Sudlow CLM, Warlow CP (1996). Comparing stroke incidence worldwide. What makes studies comparable? *Stroke* **27**:550–558

Sudlow CLM, Warlow CP (1997). Comparable studies of the incidence of stroke and its pathological types. Results from an international collaboration. *Stroke* **28**:491–499

Thom JT (1993). Stroke mortality trends: an international perspective. *Annals of Epidemiology* **3**:509–518

Tunstall-Pedoe H, Kuulasmaa K, Amouyel P *et al.* (1994). Myocardial infarction and coronary deaths in the World Health Organization MONICA Project. Registration procedures, event rates and case-fatality rates in 38 populations from 21 countries in four continents. *Circulation* **90**:583–612

Wald NJ, Law MR (2003). A strategy to reduce cardiovascular disease by more than 80%. *British Medical Journal* **326**:1419

White H, Boden-Albala B, Wang C *et al.* (2005). Ischemic stroke subtype incidence among whites, blacks and Hispanics: the Northern Manhattan Study. *Circulation* **111**:1327–1331

Wityk RJ, Pessin MS, Kaplan RF *et al.* (1994). Serial assessment of acute stroke using the NIH Stroke Scale. *Stroke* **25**:362–365.

Wityk RJ, Lehman D, Klag M *et al.* (1996). Race and sex differences in the distribution of cerebral atherosclerosis. *Stroke* **27**:1974–1980

Wolf PA, D'Agostino RB, O'Neal MA *et al.* (1992). Secular trends in stroke incidence and mortality: the Framingham Study. *Stroke* **23**:1551–1555

Wolfe CDA (2000). The impact of stroke. *British Medical Bulletin* **56**:275–286

Wolfe CD, Corbin DO, Smeeton NC *et al.* (2006a). Estimation of the risk of stroke in black populations in Barbados and South London. *Stroke* **37**:1986–1990

Wolfe CD, Corbin DO, Smeeton NC *et al.* (2006b). Poststroke survival for black-Caribbean populations in Barbados and South London. *Stroke* **37**:1991–1996

Woo D, Gebel J, Miller R *et al.* (1999). Incidence rates of first-ever ischemic stroke subtypes among blacks: a population-based study. *Stroke* **30**:2517–2522

Wroe SJ, Sandercock P, Bamford J *et al.* (1992). Diurnal variation in the incidence of stroke: the Oxfordshire Community Stroke Project. *British Medical Journal* **304**:155–157

Wyller TB, Bautz-Holter E, Holmen J (1994). Prevalence of stroke and stroke-related disability in North Trondelag County Norway. *Cerebrovascular Diseases* **4**:421–427

This chapter outlines the major known risk factors for TIA and stroke. Knowledge of these risk factors is necessary in order to understand the aetiology of TIA and stroke, to predict risk and to develop effective preventive strategies.

There are many more data on risk factors for acute coronary events than for ischemic stroke (Bhatia and Rothwell 2005) because of more intensive investigation in routine clinical practice and because heart disease receives much higher levels of research funding than stroke (Rothwell 2001; Pendlebury 2007).

The main risk factors for stroke are listed in Box 2.1. There are probably few qualitative differences between risk factors for ischemic stroke and coronary heart disease, but there are quantitative differences. Smoking, raised plasma cholesterol and male sex are stronger risk factors for myocardial infarction, while hypertension is a stronger risk factor for stroke. The tendency for epidemiologists to lump all types of stroke together might explain some of the quantitative differences between risk factors for stroke and coronary heart disease. For example, it is possible that strokes associated with large artery disease have a more similar risk factor profile to coronary heart disease than cardioembolic stroke. To date, differences in risk factor relationships with the different stroke subtypes are unclear (Schulz et al. 2004; Jackson and Sudlow 2005). The prevalence of various demographic and risk factors for different stroke subtypes are shown in Table 2.1.

Non-modifiable risk factors
Age
Age is the strongest risk factor for ischemic stroke of all subtypes and for primary intracerebral hemorrhage, but it is less important for subarachnoid hemorrhage (Bamford et al. 1990; Rothwell et al. 2005). Overall stroke incidence at age 75–84 is approximately 25 times higher than at age 45–54 (see Fig. 1.2).

Sex and sex hormones
Ischemic stroke is slightly more common in men than in women (see Fig. 1.2) although the male excess is less marked than in coronary heart disease and peripheral arterial disease (Rothwell et al. 2005). This excess of vascular events in men has been attributed to differences in endogenous sex hormones, although there is little direct evidence to support this hypothesis. Exogenous high-dose estrogen given to elderly men with prostatic cancer increases their risk of vascular death (Byar and Corle 1988) and use of hormone replacement therapy in women after the menopause is associated with an increased risk of acute coronary sydrome, stroke and venous thromboembolism (Farquhar et al. 2005; Gabriel et al. 2005). The equalization of vascular risk in elderly males and females is, therefore, probably not explained by the natural menopause, although bilateral oophorectomy

Box 2.1. Risk factors for ischemic stroke

Factors associated with an increased risk of vascular disease

Increasing age	Raised hematocrit
Male sex	Sex hormones
Hypertension	Excess alcohol consumption
Cigarette smoking	Obesity and diet[a]
Diabetes mellitus	Raised white blood cell count
Blood lipids	Recent infection[a]
Atrial fibrillation	Hyperhomocyst(e)inemia
Social deprivation	Snoring[a]
Family history of stroke	Corneal arcus[a]
Physical inactivity	Psychological factors[a]
Raised von Willebrand factor[a]	Low serum albumin[a]
Increasing plasma fibrinogen[a]	Diagonal earlobe crease[a]
Raised factor VII coagulant activity[a]	
Raised tissue plasminogen activator antigen[a]	
Low blood fibrinolytic activity[a]	

Evidence of pre-existing vascular disease

Transient ischemic attacks	Cardiac failure
Cervical arterial bruit and stenosis	Left ventricular hypertrophy
Myocardial infarction/angina	Peripheral vascular disease

Note:
[a]Possible association with stroke.

without estrogen replacement in premenopausal women doubles the risk of vascular events (van der Schouw *et al.* 1996). Oral contraceptives increase the risk of ischemic stroke (the risk is less for hemorrhagic stroke) but the increased risk is small for low-dose estrogen preparations unless there are associated factors such as migraine or cigarette smoking (Chang *et al.* 1999; Bousser and Kittner 2000; Donaghy *et al.* 2002).

Modifiable risk factors
Blood pressure
Increasing blood pressure is strongly associated with subsequent stroke risk (Gil-Nunez and Vivancos-Mora 2005; Goldstein and Hankey 2006). The relationship between usual diastolic blood pressure and stroke is "log–linear" throughout the normal range, with no evidence of a threshold below which the risk becomes stable (Rodgers *et al.* 1996). Stroke mortality rises steeply with increasing systolic blood pressure and this is more marked in the young than in the old (Kearney *et al.* 2005) (Fig. 2.1). Stroke incidence doubles with each 7.5 mmHg increase in usual diastolic blood pressure in Western populations and with each 5.0 mmHg in Japanese and Chinese populations (MacMahon *et al.* 1990; Eastern Stroke and Coronary Heart Disease Collaborative Research Group 1998; Lewington *et al.* 2002).

The strength of the association between blood pressure and stroke is attenuated with increasing age, although the absolute risk of stroke in the elderly is far higher than in the young (Lewington *et al.* 2002). Nevertheless, hypertension is still a risk factor in the very

Table 2.1. Demographics and risk factor prevalence in incident strokes in OXVASC

	Prevalence (%)		
	IS[a]	PICH[b]	SAH[b]
Mean age	74.9	75.3	54.8
Male (%)	48.6	50.0	30.3
Previous acute coronary syndrome	11.5	15.4	3.0
Previous acute peripheral vascular event	2.9	3.8	0.0
History of hypertension	56.3	59.6	24.2
Diabetes mellitus	10.1	0.0	3.0
Hypercholesterolemia	20.1	14.3	6.1
Atrial fibrillation	18.2	15.4	0.0
Current smoker	17.2	15.4	24.2

Notes:
IS, ischemic stroke; PICH, primary intracerebral hemorrhage; SAH, subarachnoid hemorrhage.
[a]Three year data from 2002–2005.
[b]Five year data from 2002–2007.
Sources: From Rothwell et al. (2004a) and Lovelock et al. (2007).

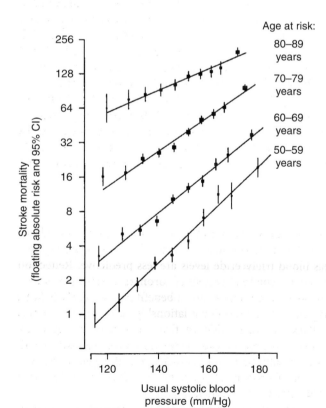

Age at risk:

80–89 years

70–79 years

60–69 years

50–59 years

Fig. 2.1. Stroke mortality by usual systolic blood pressure and age showing a steep rise in mortality with rising blood pressure and that the rate of risk increase with change in blood pressure is greater in the young than in the old (from Kearney et al. 2005). CI, confidence interval.

elderly, although it is weaker because stroke may be associated with low blood pressure owing to cardiac failure and other comorbid conditions (Birns *et al.* 2005). Moreover, in patients with bilateral severe carotid stenosis or occlusion, stroke risk is higher at low blood pressures, suggesting that aggressive blood pressure lowering may be harmful in this group (Rothwell *et al.* 2003). The relationship with systolic blood pressure is similar and possibly stronger than with diastolic blood pressure (Keli *et al.* 1992) and even 'isolated' systolic hypertension is associated with increased risk (Sagie *et al.* 1993; Petrovitch *et al.* 1995; Lewington *et al.* 2002). Hypertension is more common in stroke patients from black than from white populations (Sacco 2001).

Cigarette smoking

Cigarette smoking is associated with stroke, with a relative risk of approximately 1.5: there is a dose–response relationship; males and females are equally affected, and the association seems to become weaker in the elderly (Hankey 1999). The evidence for a link between cigarette smoking and primary intracerebral hemorrhage is less clear (Vessey *et al.* 2003). Smoking has been related to the extent of carotid disease on arterial angiography (Homer *et al.* 1991), on ultrasound (Fine-Edelstein *et al.* 1994; Howard *et al.* 1998) and in identical twins discordant for smoking (Haapanen *et al.* 1989).

Diabetes mellitus

Diabetes doubles the risk of ischemic stroke (Tuomilehto and Rastenyte 1999; Wannamethee *et al.* 1999; Rothwell 2005) and the risk of fatal stroke is higher in those with a higher glycosylated hemoglobin (HbA1c) at diagnosis (Stevens *et al.* 2004). There is a high prevalence of diabetes in stroke patients from black populations (Sacco 2001). It should be noted that any studies linking diabetes with stroke mortality data will exaggerate the association, because diabetics who have a stroke are more likely to die of it than non-diabetics (Jorgensen *et al.* 1994). Randomized trials have shown that diabetic treatment reduces the risk of microvascular complications of diabetes and decreases progression of carotid intima media thickness but it does not necessarily reduce the incidence of stroke and other macrovascular events (UK Prospective Diabetes Study (UKPDS) Group 1998; Diabetes Control and Complications Trial/Epidemiology of Diabetes Interventions and Complications Research Group 2003).

Blood lipids

Increasing levels of total plasma cholesterol and low density lipoprotein cholesterol, and to a lesser extent decreasing levels of high density lipoprotein cholesterol, are strong risk factors for coronary heart disease, whereas blood triglyceride levels are less predictive. Reduction of plasma cholesterol by 1 mmol/l reduces the relative risk of coronary events by at least a third (Lewington and Clarke 2005), with little diminution of benefit in the elderly (Clarke *et al.* 2002; Huxley *et al.* 2002; Baigent *et al.* 2005). The relationship between blood lipids and stroke is much weaker but there is some evidence that cholesterol is negatively associated with intracranial hemorrhage, which obscures the weak positive association with ischemic stroke in studies where stroke subtype is not characterized (Prospective Studies Collaboration 1995; Eastern Stroke and Coronary Heart Disease Collaborative Research Group 1998; Koren-Morag *et al.* 2002; Zhang *et al.* 2003).

Data from the Heart Protection Study of cholesterol lowering in patients with known vascular disease or diabetes have shown that such therapy reduces the risk of stroke on follow-up but it did not show a reduction in recurrent stroke (Heart Protection Study Collaborative Group 2002; Collins *et al.* 2004) possibly because of lack of differentiation of stroke subtype or the fact that patients were at low risk of stroke recurrence since the incident strokes occurred on average 4.6 years before the study onset. However, more recently, the Stroke Prevention by Aggressive Reduction in Cholesterol Levels (SPARCL) trial showed that atorvastatin in patients who had had a stroke or TIA within one to six months before study entry did reduce overall stroke risk (Amarenco *et al.* 2006), although there was a significant increase in risk of intracerebral hemorrhage on statin treatment (Ch. 24). Interestingly, the same trend had been found in the Heart Protection Study in the 3280 patients with previous stroke or TIA (Collins *et al.* 2004), in whom simvastatin 40 mg also increased the risk of hemorrhagic stroke. Thus, the randomized evidence does suggest that there is a causal association between plasma low density lipoprotein cholesterol and risk of ischemic stroke, but more work is required to determine the cause of the increase in risk of hemorrhagic stroke.

Atrial fibrillation

Non-rheumatic atrial fibrillation is by far the most common cause of cardioembolic stroke but cannot cause more than one-sixth of all ischemic strokes since it is present in this proportion of patients who have an ischemic stroke (Sandercock *et al.* 1992; Schulz and Rothwell 2003; Rothwell *et al.* 2004a); this excludes the very elderly, where its prevalence is highest (Wolf *et al.* 1991a). The average absolute risk of stroke in patients without prior stroke who have non-rheumatic atrial fibrillation and are not taking anticoagulation drugs is approximately 4% per year, five to six times greater than in those in sinus rhythm (Hart *et al.* 1999; Wolf *et al.* 1991b; Lip 2005); the risk is much higher again in patients with rheumatic atrial fibrillation.

The stroke risk associated with atrial fibrillation in an individual patient is higher in the presence of a previous embolic event, increasing age, hypertension, diabetes, left ventricular dysfunction or an enlarged left atrium (Stroke Prevention in Atrial Fibrillation Investigators 1992, 1995; Atrial Fibrillation Investigators 1994, 1998; Di Pasquale *et al.* 1995; Lip and Boos 2006). At least 10 similar stroke risk stratification schemes for atrial fibrillation have been published (Lip and Boos 2006; Nattel and Opie 2006). The best validated of these, the CHADS2 score, awards 1 point each for congestive heart failure, hypertension, age ≥ 75 years and diabetes mellitus and 2 points for prior stroke or TIA. Patients with a CHADS2 score of 0 have a stroke risk of 0.5% per year while those with a score of 6 have a yearly stroke risk of 15% or more (Ch. 14).

Paroxysmal atrial fibrillation carries the same stroke risk as persistent atrial fibrillation (Lip and Hee 2001; Saxonhouse and Curtis 2003) and should be treated similarly. There is no evidence that conversion to sinus rhythm followed by pharmacotherapy to try to maintain such rhythm is superior to rate control in terms of mortality and stroke risk (Segal *et al.* 2001; Blackshear and Safford 2003; Hart *et al.* 2003).

Some of the association between atrial fibrillation and stroke must be coincidental because atrial fibrillation can be caused by coronary and hypertensive heart disease, both of which may be associated with atheromatous disease or primary intracerebral hemorrhage. Although anticoagulation markedly reduces the risk of first or recurrent stroke, this is not necessarily evidence for causality because this treatment may be working in other ways, such as by inhibiting artery-to-artery embolism, although trials of warfarin in secondary prevention of stroke in sinus rhythm have shown no benefit over aspirin (Ch. 24).

Cardioembolism

Apart from atrial fibrillation, there are many other causes of cardioembolic stroke including prosthetic heart valves and patent foramen ovale (see Ch. 6).

Obesity and the metabolic syndrome

Any relationship between obesity and stroke is likely to be confounded by the positive association of obesity with hypertension, diabetes, hypercholesterolemia and lack of exercise, and the negative association with smoking and concurrent illness. Nevertheless, stroke is more common in the obese, and abdominal obesity appears to be an independent predictor of stroke (Suk *et al.* 2003). The constellation of metabolic abnormalities including central obesity, decreased high density lipoprotein, elevated triglycerides, elevated blood pressure and impaired glucose tolerance is known as the metabolic syndrome and is associated with a three-fold increase risk of type 2 diabetes and a two-fold increase in cardiovascular risk (Eckel *et al.* 2005; Grundy *et al.* 2005).

Metabolic syndrome is thought to be the main driver for the modern-day epidemic of diabetes and vascular disease. As well as primary prevention of acute vascular events in patients with the metabolic syndrome (Eckel *et al.* 2005; Grundy *et al.* 2005), an additional aim should be prevention of progression to frank diabetes. Both lifestyle modification with diet and exercise (Tuomilehto *et al.* 2001; Diabetes Prevention Program Research Group 2002) and treatment with angiotensin-converting enzyme inhibitors or angiotensin antagonists (Yusuf *et al.* 2000; Dahlof *et al.* 2002; Julius *et al.* 2004) have been shown to be effective in reducing progression to diabetes in patients with the metabolic syndrome.

Diet

Relating various dietary constituents to the risk of vascular disease is difficult since observational data are likely to be biased. As noted above, there is good evidence that dietary and lifestyle modification can improve vascular risk in patients with the metabolic syndrome, but randomized trials of dietary interventions, including fish oil supplementation and vitamin supplementation, have generally been disappointing (Steinberg 1995; Orencia *et al.* 1996; Stephens 1997; GISSI-Prevenzione Investigators 1999; Leppala *et al.* 2000; Yusuf *et al.* 2000; Heart Protection Study Collaborative Group 2002; Hooper *et al.* 2004, 2008).

Reduction in salt intake reduces blood pressure in both normotensive and hypertensive individuals (He and MacGregor 2004) and there is evidence that adding salt to food increases the risk of cerebral hemorrhage (Jamrozik *et al.* 1994). In contrast, a high intake of potassium may reduce stroke risk (Khaw and Barrett-Connor 1987; Whelton *et al.* 1997). It remains unclear whether reducing sodium intake lowers stroke risk.

Exercise

A systematic review of 23 studies found that moderate and high levels of physical activity are associated with reduced risk of all stroke (Lee *et al.* 2003). This reduced risk is thought to be related to lower body weight, blood pressure, blood viscosity, fibrinogen concentration and better lipid profiles.

Alcohol

A systematic review of 35 observational studies indicated that heavy (> 5 units/day) alcohol consumption increases the relative risk of stroke by 1.6 (95% confidence interval [CI], 1.4–1.9) particularly hemorrhagic stroke (relative risk, 2.18; 95% CI, 1.5–3.2) (Reynolds *et al.* 2003). Moderate consumption of alcohol appears to lower stroke risk by comparison with abstention (Reynolds *et al.* 2003; Elkind *et al.* 2006). Whether 'binge' drinking is associated with stroke is uncertain (Hillbom *et al.* 1999) but it is possible that irregular drinking carries a higher risk (Mazzaglia *et al.* 2001).

Hemostatic variables

Despite much effort, very few consistent associations have been found between coagulation parameters, fibrinolytic activity, platelet behavior and risk of stroke (Markus and Hambley 1998; Sacco 2001). Although there is a relationship between increasing plasma fibrinogen and stroke (Rothwell *et al.* 2004b; Danesh *et al.* 2005), it is attenuated by adjusting for cigarette smoking and other confounding variables such as infections and social class (Brunner *et al.* 1996; Lowe *et al.* 1997). Raised plasma factor VII coagulant activity, raised tissue plasminogen activator antigen, low blood fibrinolytic activity, and raised von Willebrand factor are risk factors for coronary heart disease and perhaps also for stroke (Meade *et al.* 1993; Qizilbash *et al.* 1997; Macko *et al.* 1999).

Hematocrit

Although cerebral blood flow is strongly related to hematocrit, any effect of increasing hematocrit on risk of stroke, or type of stroke, is weak and confounded by cigarette smoking, blood pressure and plasma fibrinogen (Welin *et al.* 1987). However, raised hematocrit does seem to be associated with an increased case-fatality in ischemic stroke (Allport *et al.* 2005).

Infections and inflammation

Both chronic and acute infection have been implicated in the development and stability of atheromatous plaques (Danesh *et al.* 1997). However, observational epidemiological studies of infections in general (Grau *et al.* 1998) and of chronic dental infection (Beck *et al.* 1996), together with serological evidence of specific infectious agents (e.g. *Chlamydia pneumoniae*, *Helicobacter pylori* and cytomegalovirus), have not shown convincing evidence of a relationship with stroke or coronary heart disease (Markus and Mendall 1998; Danesh *et al.* 1999, 2000; Fagerberg *et al.* 1999; Glader *et al.* 1999; Strachan *et al.* 1999; Danesh *et al.* 2003; Ngeh *et al.* 2003). An early randomized trial to eliminate chlamydia infection as a risk was far too small to be reliable (Gurfinkel *et al.* 1997) but further antibiotic intervention trials are ongoing (Danesh 2005; Jespersen *et al.* 2006).

Homocysteinemia

There is an association between the rare inborn recessive condition of homocystinemia and arterial and venous thrombosis, and observational data link coronary heart disease, stroke, and venous thromboembolism with increasing plasma homocysteine (Wald *et al.* 2002, 2004). This led to trials of folic acid and pyridoxine supplementation to lower homocysteine levels (Hankey 2002; Hankey and Eikelboom 2005). Results from such trials have so far been disappointing: the Vitamin Intervention for Stroke Prevention Study (VISP) and the Norwegian Vitamin Trial (NORVIT) (Toole *et al.* 2004; Bonaa *et al.* 2006) trials showed no treatment effect on recurrent stroke, coronary events or deaths. Preliminary results from the Study of Vitamins to Prevent Stroke (VITATOPS) trial have shown no evidence of reduced levels of inflammation, endothelial dysfunction, or the hypercoagulability postulated to be increased by elevated homocysteine levels in patients with previous TIA or stroke treated with folic acid, vitamin B_{12} and vitamin B_6

(Dusitanond *et al.* 2005). However, a recent systematic review of all randomized trials of homocysteine lowering does suggest a modest reduction in stroke risk (Wang *et al.* 2007).

Non-stroke vascular disease

Coronary heart disease is associated with ischemic stroke in postmortem (Stemmermann *et al.* 1984), twin (Brass *et al.* 1996), case–control (Feigin *et al.* 1998) and cohort studies (Harmsen *et al.* 1990; Shaper *et al.* 1991; Wolf *et al.* 1991b; Touzé *et al.* 2006) as are electrocardiographic abnormalities, cardiac failure, left ventricular hypertrophy, claudication and asymptomatic peripheral vascular disease (Leys *et al.* 2006).

Abdominal aortic aneurysms occur in about 10–20% of patients with cerebrovascular disease but it is not known if people with aneurysms have more stroke or other vascular events compared with people without aneurysms (Hollander *et al.* 2003; Leys *et al.* 2006).

Other possible associations

Innumerable other risk factors have been linked with coronary heart disease, and to a lesser extent stroke, but data are sparse and there is probably a lot of confounding.

References

Allport LE, Parsons MW, Butcher KS *et al.* (2005). Elevated hematocrit is associated with reduced reperfusion and tissue survival in acute stroke. *Neurology* **65**:1382–1387

Amarenco P, Bogousslavsky J, Callahan A III *et al.* (2006). High-dose atorvastatin after stroke or transient ischemic attack. *New England Journal of Medicine* **355**:549–559

Atrial Fibrillation Investigators (1994). Risk factors for stroke and efficacy of antithrombotic therapy in atrial fibrillation. *Archives of Internal Medicine* **154**:1449–1457

Atrial Fibrillation Investigators (1998). Echocardiographic predictors of stroke in patients with atrial fibrillation. *Archives of Internal Medicine* **158**:1316–1320

Baigent C, Keech A, Kearney PM *et al.* (2005). Efficacy and safety of cholesterol-lowering treatment: prospective meta-analysis of data from 90 056 participants in 14 randomized trials of statins. *Lancet* **66**:1267–1278

Bamford J, Sandercock PAG, Dennis M *et al.* (1990). A prospective study of acute cerebrovascular disease in the community: the Oxfordshire Community Stroke Project 1981–86. 2. Incidence, case fatality rates and overall outcome at one year of cerebral infarction, primary intracerebral and subarachnoid haemorrhage. *Journal of Neurology, Neurosurgery and Psychiatry* **53**:16–22

Beck J, Garcia R, Heiss G *et al.* (1996). Periodontal disease and cardiovascular disease. *Journal of Periodontology* **67**:1123–1137

Bhatia M, Rothwell PM (2005). A systematic comparison of the published data available on risk factors for stroke, compared with risk factors for coronary heart disease. *Cerebrovascular Diseases* **20**:180–186

Birns J, Markus H, Kalra L (2005). Blood pressure reduction for vascular risk: is there a price to be paid? *Stroke* **36**:1308–1313

Blackshear JL, Safford RE (2003). AFFIRM and RACE trials: implications for the management of atrial fibrillation. *Cardiology Electrophysiology Review* **7**:366–369

Bonaa KH, Njlstad I, Ueland PM *et al.* (2006). Homocysteine lowering and cardiovascular events after acute myocardial infarction. *New England Journal of Medicine* **354**:1578–1588

Bousser MG, Kittner SJ (2000). Oral contraceptives and stroke. *Cephalagia* **20**:183–189

Brass LM, Hartigan PM, Page WF *et al.* (1996). Importance of cerebrovascular disease in studies of myocardial infarction. *Stroke* **27**:1173–1176

Brunner E, Davey Smith G, Marmot M *et al.* (1996). Childhood social circumstances and psychosocial and behavioural factors as determinants of plasma fibrinogen. *Lancet* **347**.1008 1013

Byar DP, Corle DK (1988). Hormone therapy for prostate cancer: results of the Veterans Administration Cooperative Urological Research Group Studies. *NCI Monographs* 7:165–170

Chang CL, Donaghy M, Poulter N *et al.* (1999). Migraine and stroke in young women: case–control study. *British Medical Journal* 318:13–18

Clarke R, Lewington S, Youngman L *et al.* (2002). Underestimation of the importance of blood pressure and cholesterol for coronary heart disease mortality in old age. *European Heart Journal* 23:286–293

Collins R, Armitage J, Parish S *et al.* (2004). Effects of cholesterol-lowering with simvastatin on stroke and other major vascular events in 20 536 people with cerebrovascular disease or other high-risk conditions. *Lancet* 363:757–767

Dahlof B, Devereux RB, Kjeldsen SE *et al.* (2002). Cardiovascular morbidity and mortality in Losartan Intervention For End Point Reduction in Hypertension (LIFE) study: a randomized trial against atenolol. *Lancet* 359:995–1003

Danesh J (2005). Antibiotics in the prevention of heart attacks. *Lancet* 365:365–367

Danesh J, Collins R, Peto R (1997). Chronic infections and coronary heart disease: is there a link? *Lancet* 350:430–436

Danesh J, Youngman L, Clark S *et al.* (1999). *Helicobacter pylori* infection and early onset myocardial infarction: case–control and sibling pairs study. *British Medical Journal* 319:1157–1162

Danesh J, Whincup P, Walker M *et al.* (2000). *Chlamydia pneumoniae* IgG titres and coronary heart disease: prospective study and meta-analysis. *British Medical Journal* 321:208–213

Danesh J, Whincup P, Walker M (2003). *Chlamydia pneumoniae* IgA titres and coronary heart disease: prospective study and meta-analysis. *European Heart Journal* 24:881

Danesh J, Lewington S, Thompson SG *et al.* (2005). Plasma fibrinogen level and the risk of major cardiovascular diseases and non-vascular mortality: an individual participant meta-analysis. *Journal of American Medical Association* 294:1799–1809

Diabetes Control and Complications Trial/ Epidemiology of Diabetes Interventions and Complications Research Group (2003).

Intensive diabetes therapy and carotid intima-media thickness in type I diabetes mellitus. *New England Journal of Medicine* 346:393–403

Diabetes Prevention Program Research Group (2002). Reduction in the incidence of type 2 diabetes with lifestyle intervention or metformin. *New England Journal of Medicine* 346:393–403

di Pasquale G, Urbinati S, Pinelli G (1995). New echocardiographic markers of embolic risk in atrial fibrillation. *Cerebrovascular Diseases* 5:315–322

Donaghy M, Chang CL, Poulter N *et al.* (2002). European Collaborators of the World Health Organization Collaborative Study of Cardiovascular Disease and Steroid Hormone Contraception. Duration, frequency, recency, and type of migraine and the risk of ischemic stroke in women of childbearing age. *Journal of Neurology, Neurosurgery and Psychiatry* 73:747–750

Dusitanond P, Eikelboom JW, Hankey GJ *et al.* (2005). Homocysteine-lowering treatment with folic acid, cobalamin and pyridoxine does not reduce blood markers of inflammation, endothelial dysfunction or hypercoagulability in patients with previous transient ischemic attack or stroke: a randomized substudy of the VITATOPS trial. *Stroke* 36:144–146

Eastern Stroke and Coronary Heart Disease Collaborative Research Group (1998). Blood pressure, cholesterol and stroke in Eastern Asia. *Lancet* 352:1801–1807

Eckel RH, Grundy SM, Zimmet PZ (2005). The metabolic syndrome. *Lancet* 365:1415–1428

Elkind MS, Sciacca R, Boden-Albala B *et al.* (2006). Moderate alcohol consumption reduces risk of ischemic stroke: the Northern Manhattan Study. *Stroke* 37:13–19

Fagerberg B, Gnarpe J, Gnarpe H *et al.* (1999). *Chlamydia pneumoniae* but not cytomegalovirus antibodies are associated with future risk of stroke and cardiovascular disease: a prospective study in middle-aged to elderly men with treated hypertension. *Stroke* 30:299–305

Farquhar CM, Marjoribanks J, Lethaby A *et al.* (2005). Long term hormone therapy for perimenopausal and postmenopausal women. *Cochrane Database of Systematic Reviews* 3:CD004143

Feigin VL, Wiebers DO, Nikitin YP *et al.* (1998). Risk factors for ischemic stroke in a Russian community: a population-based case–control study. *Stroke* **29**:34–39

Fine-Edelstein JS, Wolf PA, O'Leary *et al.* (1994). Precursors of extracranial carotid atherosclerosis in the Framingham Study. *Neurology* **44**:1046–1050

Gabriel SR, Carmona L, Roque M *et al.* (2005). Hormone replacement therapy for preventing cardiovascular disease in post-menopausal women. *Cochrane Database Systems Review* **2**:CD002229

Gil-Nunez AC, Vivancos-Mora J (2005). Blood pressure as a risk factor for stroke and the impact of antihypertensive treatment. *Cerebrovascular Diseases* **20**:40–52

GISSI-Prevenzione Investigators (1999). Dietary supplementation with *n*-3 polyunsaturated fatty acids and vitamin E after myocardial infarction: results of the GISSI-Prevenzione trial. *Lancet* **354**:447–455

Glader CA, Stegmayr B, Boman J *et al.* (1999). *Chlamydia pneumoniae* antibodies and high lipoprotein (a) levels do not predict ischemic cerebral infarctions: results from a nested case–control study in northern Sweden. *Stroke* **30**:2013–2018

Goldstein LB, Hankey GJ (2006). Advances in primary stroke prevention. *Stroke* **37**:317–319

Grau AJ, Buggle F, Becher H *et al.* (1998). Recent bacterial and viral infection is a risk factor for cerebrovascular ischemia: clinical and biochemical studies. *Neurology* **50**:196–203

Grundy SM, Cleeman JI, Daniels SR *et al.* (2005). Diagnosis and management of the metabolic syndrome: an American Heart Association/National Heart Lung and Blood Institute Scientific Statement. *Circulation* **112**:2735–2752

Gurfinkel E, Bozovich G, Daroca A *et al.* (1997). Randomized trial of roxithromycin in non-Q-wave coronary syndromes: ROXIS Pilot Study. *Lancet* **350**:404–407

Haapanen A, Koskenvuo M, Kaprio J *et al.* (1989). Carotid arteriosclerosis in identical twins discordant for cigarette smoking. *Circulation* **80**:10–16

Hankey GJ (1999). Smoking and risk of stroke. *Journal of Vascular Risk* **6**:207–211

Hankey GJ (2002). Is homocysteine a causal and treatable risk factor for vascular diseases of the brain (cognitive impairment and stroke). *Annals of Neurology* **51**:279–281

Hankey GJ, Eikelboom JW (2005). Homocysteine and stroke. *Lancet* **365**:194–196

Harmsen P, Rosengren A, Tsipogiannia A *et al.* (1990). Risk factors for stroke in middle-aged men in Goteborg Sweden. *Stroke* **21**:223–229

Hart RG, Benavente O, McBride R *et al.* (1999). Antithrombotic therapy to prevent stroke in patients with atrial fibrillation: a meta-analysis. *Annals of Internal Medicine* **131**:492–501

Hart RG, Halperin JL, Pearce, LA *et al.* (2003). Lessons from the Stroke Prevention in Atrial Fibrillation trials. *Annals of Internal Medicine* **138**:831–838

He FJ, MacGregor GA (2004). The effect of longer-term modest salt reduction on blood pressure. *Cochrane Database of Systematic Reviews* **1**:CD004937

Heart Protection Study Collaborative Group (2002). MRC/BHF Heart Protection Study of cholesterol lowering with simvastatin in 20 536 high-risk individuals: a randomized placebo-controlled trial. *Lancet* **360**:7–22

Hillbom M, Numminen H, Juvela S (1999). Recent heavy drinking of alcohol and embolic stroke. *Stroke* **30**:2307–2312

Hollander M, Hak AE, Koudstaal PJ *et al.* (2003). Comparison between measures of atherosclerosis and risk of stroke: the Rotterdam Study. *Stroke* **34**:2367–2372

Homer D, Ingall TJ, Baker HL *et al.* (1991). Serum lipids and lipoproteins are less powerful predictors of extracranial carotid artery atherosclerosis than are cigarette smoking and hypertension. *Mayo Clinic Proceedings* **66**:259–267

Hooper L, Capps N, Clements G *et al.* (2004). Foods or supplements rich in omega-3 fatty acids for preventing cardiovascular disease in patients with ischemic heart disease. *Cochrane Database of Systematic Reviews* **4**:CD003177

Hooper L, Capps N, Clements G *et al.* (2008). Anti-oxidant foods or supplements for preventing cardiovascular disease. *Cochrane Database of Systematic Reviews* **3**:CD001558

Howard G, Wagenknecht LE, Burke GL *et al.* (1998). Cigarette smoking and progression of atherosclerosis: the Atherosclerosis Risk in

Communities (ARIC) Study. *Journal of the American Medical Association* **279**:119–124

Huxley R, Lewington S, Clarke R (2002). Cholesterol, coronary heart disease and stroke: a review of published evidence from observational studies and randomized controlled trials. *Seminars in Vascular Medicine* **2**:315–323

Jackson C, Sudlow C (2005). Are lacunar strokes really different? A systematic review of differences in risk factor profiles between lacunar and non-lacunar infarcts. *Stroke* **36**:891–901

Jamrozik K, Anderson CA, Stewart-Wynne EG (1994). The role of lifestyle factors in the etiology of stroke. A population-based case–control study in Perth Western Australia. *Stroke* **25**:51–59

Jespersen CM, Als-Nielsen B, Damgaard M *et al.* (2006). Randomized placebo controlled multicentre trial to assess short term clarithromycin for patients with stable coronary heart disease: CLARICOR trial. *British Medical Journal* **332**:22–27

Jorgensen HS, Nakayama H, Raaschou HO *et al.* (1994). Stroke in patients with diabetes. The Copenhagen Stroke Study. *Stroke* **25**:1977–1984

Julius S, Kjeldsen SE, Weber M *et al.* (2004). Outcomes in hypertensive patients at high cardiovascular risk, treated with regimens based on valsartan or amlodipine: the VALUE randomized trail. *Lancet* **363**:2022–2031

Kearney PM, Welton M, Reynolds K *et al.* (2005). Global burden of hypertension: analysis of worldwide data. *Lancet* **365**:217–223

Keli S, Bloemberg B, Kromhout D (1992). Predictive value of repeated systolic blood pressure measurements for stroke risk. The Zutphen Study. *Stroke* **23**:347–351

Khaw KT, Barrett-Connor E (1987). Dietary potassium and stroke-associated mortality. A 12-year prospective population study. *New England Journal of Medicine* **316**:235–240

Koren-Morag N, Tanne D, Graff E *et al.* (2002). Low and high density lipoprotein, cholesterol and ischemic cerebrovascular disease. The Bezafibrate Infarction Prevention Registry. *Archives of International Medicine* **162**:993–999

Lee CD, Folsom AR, Blair SN (2003). Physical activity and stroke risk. A meta-analysis. *Stroke* **34**:2475–2482

Leppala JM, Virtamo J, Fogelholm R *et al.* (2000). Controlled trial of alpha-tocopherol and beta-carotene supplements on stroke incidence and mortality in male smokers. *Arteriosclerosis, Thrombosis and Vascular Biology* **20**:230–235

Lewington S, Clarke R (2005). Combined effects of systolic blood pressure and total cholesterol on cardiovascular disease risk. *Circulation* **112**:3373–3374

Lewington S, Clarke R, Qizilbash N *et al.* (2002). Age-specific relevance of usual blood pressure to vascular mortality: a meta-analysis of individual data for one million adults in 61 prospective studies. *Lancet* **360**:1903–1913

Leys D, Woimant F, Ferrieres J *et al.* (2006). Detection and management of associated atherothrombotic locations in patients with a recent atherothrombotic ischemic stroke: results of the DETECT survey. *Cerebrovascular Diseases* **21**:60–66

Lip GY (2005). Atrial fibrillation (recent onset). *Clinical Evidence* **14**:71–89

Lip GY, Boos CJ (2006). Antithrombotic treatment in atrial fibrillation. *Heart* **92**:155–161

Lip GY, Hee FL (2001). Paroxysmal atrial fibrillation. *Quarterly Journal of Medicine* **94**:665–678

Lovelock CE, Molyneux AJ, Rothwell PM For the Oxford Vascular Study (2007). Change in incidence and aetiology of intracerebral haemorrhage in Oxfordshire, UK, between 1981 and 2006: a population-based study. *Lancet Neurology* **6**:487–493

Lowe GDO, Lee AJ, Rumley A *et al.* (1997). Blood viscosity and risk of cardiovascular events: the Edinburgh Artery Study. *British Journal of Haematology* **96**:168–173

MacMahon S, Peto R, Cutler J *et al.* (1990). Blood pressure, stroke and coronary heart disease. Part 1. Prolonged differences in blood pressure: prospective observational studies corrected for the regression dilution bias. *Lancet* **335**:765–774

Macko RF, Kittner SJ, Epstein A *et al.* (1999). Elevated tissue plasminogen activator, antigen and stroke risk. The Stroke Prevention in Young Women Study. *Stroke* **30**:7–11

Markus HS, Hambley H (1998). Neurology and the blood: haematological abnormalities in ischemic stroke. *Journal of Neurology, Neurosurgery and Psychiatry* **64**:150–159

Markus HS, Mendall MA (1998). *Helicobacter pylori* infection: a risk factor for ischemic cerebrovascular disease and carotid atheroma. *Journal of Neurology, Neurosurgery and Psychiatry* **64**:104–107

Mazzaglia G, Britton AR, Altmann DR *et al.* (2001). Exploring the relationship between alcohol consumption and non-fatal or fatal stroke: a systematic review. *Addiction* **96**:1743–1756

Meade TW, Ruddock V, Stirling Y *et al.* (1993). Fibrinolytic activity, clotting factors and long term incidence of ischemic heart disease in the Northwick Park Heart Study. *Lancet* **342**:1076–1079

Nattel S, Opie L (2006). Controversies in atrial fibrillation. *Lancet* **367**:262–272

Ngeh J, Gupta S, Goodbourn C *et al.* (2003). *Chlamydia pneumoniae* in elderly patients with stroke (C-PEPS): a case–control study on the seroprevalence of *Chlamydia pneumoniae* in elderly patients with acute cerebrovascular disease. *Cerebrovascular Diseases* **15**:11–16

Orencia AJ, Daviglus ML, Dyer AR *et al.* (1996). Fish consumption and stroke in men. 30-year findings of Chicago Western Electric Study. *Stroke* **27**:204–209

Pendlebury ST (2007). Worldwide under-funding of stroke research. *International Journal of Stroke* **2**:80–84

Petrovitch H, Curb D, Bloom-Marcus E (1995). Isolated systolic hypertension and risk of stroke in Japanese-American men. *Stroke* **26**:25–29

Prospective Studies Collaboration (1995). Cholesterol, diastolic blood pressure and stroke: 13 000 strokes in 450 000 people in 45 prospective cohorts. *Lancet* **346**:1647–1653

Qizilbash N, Duffy S, Prentice CRM *et al.* (1997). Von Willebrand factor and risk of ischemic stroke. *Neurology* **49**:1552–1556

Reynolds K, Lewis B, Nolen JD *et al.* (2003). Alcohol consumption and risk of stroke: a meta-analysis. *Journal of the American Medical Association* **289**:579–588

Rodgers A, MacMahon S, Gamble G *et al.* (1996). Blood pressure and risk of stroke in patients with cerebrovascular disease. *British Medical Journal* **313**:147

Rothwell PM (2001). The high cost of not funding stroke research: a comparison with heart disease and cancer. *Lancet* **19**:1612–1616

Rothwell PM (2005). Prevention of stroke in patients with diabetes mellitus and the metabolic syndrome. *Cerebrovascular Diseases* **1**:24–34

Rothwell PM, Howard SC, Spence D (2003). Relationship between blood pressure and stroke risk in patients with symptomatic carotid occlusive disease. *Stroke* **34**:2583–2590

Rothwell PM, Coull AJ, Giles MF *et al.* (2004a). Change in stroke incidence, mortality, case fatality, severity and risk factors in Oxfordshire, UK from 1981 to 2004 (Oxford Vascular Study). *Lancet* **363**:1925–1933

Rothwell PM, Howard SC, Power DA *et al.* (2004b). Fibrinogen and risk of ischemic stroke and coronary events in 5183 patients with transient ischemic attack and minor ischemic stroke. *Stroke* **35**:2300–2305

Rothwell PM, Coull AJ, Silver LE *et al.* (2005). Population-based study of event-rate, incidence, case fatality and mortality for all acute vascular events in all arterial territories (Oxford Vascular Study). *Lancet* **366**:1773–1783

Sacco RL (2001). Newer risk factors for stroke. *Neurology* **57**:S31–S34

Sagie A, Larson MG, Levy D (1993). The natural history of borderline isolated systolic hypertension. *New England Journal of Medicine* **329**:1912–1917

Sandercock PAG, Bamford J, Dennis M *et al.* (1992). Atrial fibrillation and stroke: frequency in different stroke types and influence on early and long term prognosis. The Oxfordshire Community Stroke Project. *British Medical Journal* **305**:1460–1465

Saxonhouse SJ, Curtis AB (2003). Risks and benefits of rate control versus maintenance of sinus rhythm. *American Journal of Cardiology* **91**:27D–32D

Schulz UG, Rothwell PM (2003). Differences in vascular risk factors between aetiological subtypes of ischemic stroke in population-based incidence studies. *Stroke* **34**:2050–2059

Schulz UG, Flossman E, Rothwell PM (2004). Heritability of ischemic stroke in relation to age, vascular risk factors and subtypes of incident stroke in population-based studies. *Stroke* 35:819–824

Segal JB, McNamara RL, Miller MR *et al.* (2001). Anticoagulants or antiplatelet therapy for non-rheumatic atrial fibrillation and flutter. *Cochrane Database Systematic Reviews* 1:CD001938

Shaper AG, Phillips AN, Pocock SJ *et al.* (1991). Risk factors for stroke in middle-aged British men. *British Medical Journal* 302:1111–1115

Steinberg D (1995). Clinical trials of antioxidants in atherosclerosis: are we doing the right thing? *Lancet* 346:36–38

Stemmermann GN, Hayashi T, Resch JA *et al.* (1984). Risk factors related to ischemic and hemorrhagic cerebrovascular disease at autopsy: the Honolulu Heart Study. *Stroke* 15:23–28

Stephens N (1997). Anti-oxidant therapy for ischemic heart disease: where do we stand? *Lancet* 349:1710–1711

Stevens RJ, Coleman RL, Adler AI *et al.* (2004). Risk factors for myocardial infarction, case fatality and stroke case fatality in type 2 diabetes: UKPDS 66. *Diabetes Care* 27:201–207

Strachan DP, Carrington D, Mendall MA *et al.* (1999). Relation of *Chlamydia pneumoniae* serology to mortality and incidence of ischemic heart disease over 13 years in the Caerphilly Prospective Heart Disease Study. *British Medical Journal* 318:1035–1039

Stroke Prevention in Atrial Fibrillation Investigators (1992). Predictors of thromboembolism in atrial fibrillation: II Echocardiographic features of patients at risk. *Annals of Internal Medicine* 116:6–12

Stroke Prevention in Atrial Fibrillation Investigators (1995). Risk factors for thromboembolism during aspirin therapy in patients with atrial fibrillation: the Stroke Prevention in Atrial Fibrillation Study. *Journal of Stroke and Cerebrovascular Disease* 5:147–157

Suk SH, Sacco RL, Boden-Albala B *et al.* (2003). Abdominal obesity and risk of ischemic stroke: the Northern Manhattan Stroke Study. *Stroke* 34:1586–1592

Toole JF, Malinow MR, Chambless LE *et al.* (2004). Lowering homocysteine in patients with ischemic stroke to prevent recurrent stroke, myocardial infarction and death: the Vitamin Intervention for Stroke Prevention (VISP) randomized controlled trial. *Journal of the American Medical Association* 291:565–575

Touzé E, Warlow CP, Rothwell PM (2006). Risk of coronary and other nonstroke vascular death in relation to the presence and extent of atherosclerotic disease at the carotid bifurcation. *Stroke* 37:2904–2909

Tuomilehto J, Rastenyte D (1999). Diabetes and glucose intolerance as risk factors for stroke. *Journal of Cardiovascular Risk* 6:241–249

Tuomilehto J, Lindstrom J, Erikkson JG *et al.* (2001). Prevention of type 2 diabetes mellitus by changes in lifestyle among subjects with impaired glucose tolerance. *New England Journal of Medicine* 344:1343–1350

UK Prospective Diabetes Study (UKPDS) Group (1998). Intensive blood-glucose control with sulphonylureas or insulin, compared with conventional treatment and risk of complications in patients with type 2 diabetes (UKPDS 33). *Lancet* 352:837–853

van der Schouw YT, van der Graaf Y, Steyerberg EW *et al.* (1996). Age at menopause as a risk factor for cardiovascular mortality. *Lancet* 347:714–718

Vessey M, Painter R, Yeates D (2003). Mortality in relation to oral contraceptive use and smoking. *Lancet* 362:185–191

Wald DS, Law M, Morris JK (2002). Homocysteine and cardiovascular disease: evidence on causality from a meta-analysis. *British Medical Journal* 325:1202–1206

Wald DS, Law M, Morris JK (2004). The dose–response relationship between serum homocysteine and cardiovascular disease: implications for treatment and screening. *European Journal of Cardiovascular Prevention and Rehabilitation* 11:250–253

Wang X, Qin X, Demirtas H *et al.* (2007). Efficacy of folic acid supplementation in stroke prevention: a meta-analysis. *Lancet* 369:1876–1882

Wannamethee SG, Perry IJ, Shaper AG (1999). Non-fasting serum glucose and insulin concentrations and the risk of stroke. *Stroke* 30:1780–1786

Welin L, Svardsudd K, Wilhelmsen L *et al.* (1987). Analysis of risk factors for stroke in a cohort of men born in 1913. *New England Journal of Medicine* 317:521–526

Whelton PK, He J, Cutler JA *et al.* (1997). Effects of oral potassium on blood pressure: meta-analysis of randomized controlled clinical trials. *Journal of the American Medical Association* **277**:1624–1632

Wolf PA, Abbott RD, Kannel WB (1991a). Atrial fibrillation as an independent risk factor for stroke: the Framingham Study. *Stroke* **22**:983–988

Wolf PA, D'Agostino RB, Belanger AJ *et al.* (1991b). Probability of stroke: a risk profile from the Framingham Study. *Stroke* **22**:312–318

Yusuf S, Phil D, Sleight DM *et al.* (2000). Effects of an angiotensin-coverting-enzyme inhibitor ramipril on cardiovascular events in high-risk patients. *New England Journal of Medicine* **342**:145–153

Zhang X, Patel A, Horibe H *et al.* (2003). Cholesterol coronary heart disease and stroke in the Asia Pacific region. *International Journal of Epidemiology* **32**:563–572

Chapter 3

Genetics

Advances in techniques of genetic investigation have allowed researchers to begin to understand the role of genetic factors in both sporadic stroke and in single gene disorders. Although genetic investigations still have a relatively limited role in routine clinical practice, it is important that clinicians are aware of the relevance of family history of vascular disease to the management of patients with TIA and stroke, and of the common hereditary forms of cerebrovascular disease.

Genetic risk factors for "sporadic" stroke

The contribution of genetic factors to stroke risk in populations has been difficult to establish, as is the case for coronary heart disease (Alberts 1991) and it is made more difficult by the facts that stroke is a heterogeneous clinical syndrome with numerous underlying pathologies and that many of the risk factors for stroke have strong genetic components. Reliable interpretation of published family history studies is undermined by major heterogeneity, insufficient detail and potential publication and reporting bias, with much stronger associations in smaller and less methodologically rigorous studies (Flossmann *et al.* 2004). Few studies consider the number of affected and unaffected relatives or phenotyped strokes in detail, and the majority of studies do not adjust associations for intermediate phenotypes (Flossmann *et al.* 2005). No twin study and only a minority of family history studies have differentiated between ischemic and hemorrhagic stroke in the proband. There are very few data on the influence of family history on stroke severity and no data on stroke recovery. Generally, genetic influences are stronger in patients with a relatively early age of stroke onset, and a family history of stroke confers a higher risk of stroke if onset was below 70 years of age (Schulz *et al.* 2004).

Based on the assumption that at least some of the risk of apparently sporadic stroke is genetic, large numbers of studies using different methodologies have been carried out in an attempt to identify the genes involved (Dichgans 2007) (Table 3.1). However, it seems likely that the genetic component of stroke risk is modest and that many, indeed probably hundreds, of genes are involved, each one contributing only a small increased risk. Studies so far have generally not been large enough to reliably detect the sort of small effects that might realistically be expected and have had other methodological limitations, including poor choice of controls in case–control studies, inadequate distinction between the different pathological types and subtypes of stroke for which genetic influences may differ, failure to replicate positive results in an independent and adequately sized study, and testing of multiple genetic or subgroup hypotheses with no adjustment of p values for declaring statistical significance (Dichgans and Markus 2005; Sudlow *et al.* 2006).

Candidate gene studies

Most genetic studies so far have been candidate gene studies, in which the frequency of different genotypes at a specific locus or loci within a gene or genes thought likely to be in

Table 3.1. Summary of different methods of identifying genetic risk factors for stroke

	Description	Advantages	Disadvantages
Candidate gene study	A molecular variant in a gene that is functionally relevant to the disease of interest is first identified. The role of the gene in conferring risk for that disease is then studied using a case–control or cohort method	Large number of potential genes available for study	Genes of interest must be identified a priori and novel genes are not identified. A positive association does not prove causation but represent close linkage between the gene of interest and a nearby disease-causing locus
Linkage study	Analysis of pedigree by the tracking of a gene through a family by following the inheritance of a (closely associated) gene or trait. If genes are linked by residing on the same chromosome, there would be a greater association than if the genes were not linked	Polygenic disorders can be studied	Because stroke is a disease of middle and old age, identification of living, affected relatives is difficult
Whole genome association study	Variations in many single nucleotide polymorphisms throughout the genome are analyzed and compared between individuals with and without a disease. Genetic variations that are more frequent in those with the disease are then considered pointers to the disease-causing locus	Huge numbers of genes can be studied at the same time	Multiple associations are identified, which invariably include many false positives

some way connected with stroke risk are compared between stroke cases and stroke-free controls. Candidate genes have generally been selected on the basis of their known or presumed involvement in the control of factors or pathways likely to influence stroke risk: blood pressure, lipid metabolism, inflammation, coagulation, homocysteine metabolism and so on (Hassan and Markus 2000; Casas *et al.* 2004). Rigorous meta-analyses of candidate gene studies, both in stroke and other vascular diseases such as coronary heart disease, have highlighted various methodological problems, particularly the inadequate size of studies (Keavney *et al.* 2000; Wheeler *et al.* 2004; Sudlow *et al.* 2006). Large numbers of candidate gene studies have together identified a handful of genes that, on the basis of results from meta-analyses, seem likely to influence risk of ischemic stroke modestly. These genes include those encoding factor V Leiden, methylenetetrahydrofolate reductase, prothrombin and angiotensin-converting enzyme (Casas *et al.* 2004, 2006).

Linkage studies

As yet, there have been far fewer stroke genetics studies that use more traditional genetic study designs, based on collecting information and DNA from related individuals with and without the disease of interest. This is at least partly because family members of stroke patients are often no longer alive, and so obtaining information and samples for DNA extraction from large enough numbers of relatives is challenging (Hassan *et al.* 2002). The Icelandic deCODE group identified two candidate genes for ischemic stroke, encoding the enzymes phosphodiesterase-4D and arachidonate 5-lipoxygenase-activating protein (ALOX5AP; Gulcher *et al.* 2005). There is still some debate, however, about their influence in non-Icelandic populations, since their effect on ischemic stroke risk has been confirmed in only a few replication studies (Gulcher *et al.* 2006; Rosand *et al.* 2006).

Whole genome association studies

The combination of technological developments allowing rapid genotyping at multiple loci, the attraction of non-hypothesis-driven genetic studies, and the recognized limitations of traditional linkage approaches have led to an increasing interest in genome-wide association studies, where multiple polymorphisms across the genome are genotyped and compared in cases and controls, looking for loci where significant differences may suggest genetic influences on disease risk. Only one small, uninformative preliminary study in stroke has been published so far (Matarín *et al.* 2007).

Association with intermediate phenotypes

Genetic studies have started to emerge of so-called intermediate phenotypes, markers of predisposition to stroke or other vascular diseases, which can be measured in large numbers of subjects both with and without vascular risk factors or disease. These intermediate phenotypes include carotid intima media thickness and leukoaraiosis as measured or graded on computed tomographic (CT) scans or magnetic resonance imaging (MRI) of the brain, and both linkage and candidate gene approaches have been used (Humphries and Morgan 2004; Dichgans and Markus 2005).

Inherited disorders

A few strokes are clearly 'familial' with a simple Mendelian pattern of inheritance of the underlying cause (Table 3.2). Some of these genetic causes of stroke are described below:

Cerebral autosomal dominant arteriopathy with subcortical infarcts and leukoencephalopathy

Cerebral autosomal dominant arteriopathy with subcortical infarcts and leukoencephalopathy (CADASIL) is an autosomal dominant syndrome characterized by recurrent small vessel ischemic stroke in middle age and subcortical dementia with pseudobulbar palsy, usually in the absence of vascular risk factors (Singhal *et al.* 2004). Mood disturbance and migraine with aura often precede the strokes but there is considerable phenotypic variation (Dichgans *et al.* 1998). Death usually occurs in the sixth or seventh decade. Brain MRI is always abnormal in symptomatic patients, and often in asymptomatic subjects too, and shows widespread focal, diffuse and confluent white matter changes (Fig. 3.1), particularly in the periventricular and subcortical regions (Chabriat *et al.* 1995, 1998; Hutchinson *et al.* 1995; Dichgans *et al.* 1998). Changes at the temporal poles, the external capsule and the corpus callosum are characteristic.

The disease has been reported from many parts of the world and there are now more than 500 families described. The prevalence of genetically proven disease in the west of Scotland has been reported to be 1.98 per 100 000 adults and the probable mutation prevalence was estimated to be 4.14 (95% CI, 3.04–5.53) per 100 000 adults (Razvi *et al.* 2005).

The underlying small vessel arteriopathy is distinct from arteriosclerotic and amyloid angiopathy and can be found in skin and muscle biopsies as well as in the leptomeningeal and perforating arteries of the brain (Jung *et al.* 1995). There is concentric thickening of the arterial walls with extensive deposition of eosinphilic granular material in the media and internal elastic membrane (Fig. 3.1).

The genetic locus is on chromosome 19q12 (Tournier-Lasserve *et al.* 1993). The deleterious mutations in the human equivalent of the mouse *Notch3* gene were found

Table 3.2. Causes of stroke (including intracranial venous thrombosis and intracranial hemorrhage) that may be familial

Type	Conditions
Vascular anomalies	Intracranial vascular malformation
	Hereditary hemorrhagic telangiectasia
	Saccular aneurysm
Hematological disorders	Hemophilia and other coagulation factor deficiencies
	Antithrombin III deficiency
	Protein C deficiency
	Activated protein C resistance
	Protein S deficiency
	Plasminogen abnormality/deficiency
	Dysfibrinogenemia
	Sickle cell disease/trait
Connective tissue disease	Marfan's syndrome
	Pseudoxanthoma elasticum
	Ehlers–Danlos syndrome
	Fibromuscular dysplasia
Other	Migraine
	Fabry's disease
	Polycystic kidney disease
	Cardiac myxoma
	Cardiomyopathy
	Von Hippel–Lindau disease
	Mitochondrial cytopathy
	Cerebral autosomal dominant arteriopathy with subcortical infarcts and leukoencephalopathy (CADASIL)

to be the causative for CADASIL (Dichgans *et al.* 1996; Joutel *et al.* 1996). The *Notch3* gene is involved in mediating signal transduction between neighboring cells. In contrast to other *Notch* genes, which are ubiquitously expressed, *Notch3* is mainly expressed in vascular smooth muscle cells. Arteries from transgenic mice show a diminished flow-induced dilatation, and the pressure-induced myogenic tone is significantly increased in their arteries compared with those in wild-type mice (Dubroca *et al.* 2005). Approximately 70% of the characterized mutations so far cluster in exons 3 and 4 (Joutel *et al.* 1997). At present, there appears to be no genotype–phenotype correlation. The vast majority of known patients are members of affected families, but de novo mutations have been reported and so CADASIL can affect patients without a family history (Joutel *et al.* 2000).

The diagnosis should be considered in patients under 70 years of age who present with symptoms of subcortical cerebrovascular disease especially if they occur without classical risk factors but with an appropriate family history. The characteristic changes on MRI, which is the most useful and sensitive screening tool, are apparent in all symptomatic and a large number of as yet asymptomatic patients. The diagnosis is confirmed in the majority of

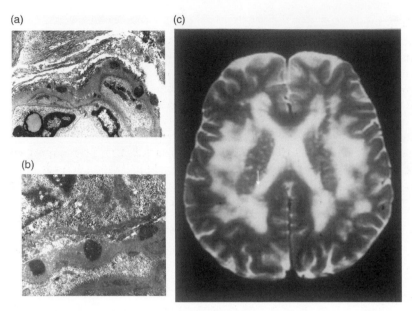

Fig. 3.1. Investigations from a patient with CADASIL (see text). Electron micrographs (a, b) of muscle shows thickening of the basal lamina of the small blood vessels and the presence of dense eosinophilic material; magnetic resonance brain imaging shows widespread leukoaraiosis (c).

patients by screening for mutations, particularly in exons 3 and 4. The search for rarer mutations, however, is very costly and not usually carried out except for research. A useful alternative is to search for granular osmiophilic material in skin biopsies, although this can also be normal (Ebke *et al.* 1997).

Hereditary dyslipidemias
Hereditary dyslipidemias such as familial hypercholesterolemia, type II and type IV hyperlipidemia and Tangiers' disease predispose to premature large vessel atherosclerosis and hence stroke (Meschia 2003; Hutter *et al.* 2004).

Connective tissue disease
Several inherited connective tissue disorders predispose to arterial dissection and other vascular abnormalities, including aneurysms and vasoocclusive disease.

Fabry's disease
Fabry's disease is an X-linked disorder causing deficiency of α-galactosidase, which leads to an accumulation of glycosphingolipids in vascular endothelial and other cells. The associated cerebrovascular disorders are mainly ischemic stroke, but intracerebral hemorrhage and subarachnoid hemorrhage can also occur. Approximately two-thirds of the infarcts involve the vertebrobasilar territory. Strokes usually occur from the third decade onward. Systemic non-vascular features of the phenotype include angiokeratomata, painful acroparesthesiae and renal failure. The frequency of previously unknown Fabry's disease in patients with cryptogenic stroke under the age of 55 has been reported to be up to 5% (Rolfs *et al.* 2005).

Cardiac disorders

Hypertrophic cardiomyopathy is frequently autosomal dominant with incomplete pene-trance. Mutations in several genes encoding structural muscle proteins have been found (Franz *et al.* 2001). Approximately 20% of those with dilated cardiomyopathy have familial disease, with autosomal dominant, recessive, X-linked and mitochondrial inheritance seen (Franz *et al.* 2001). Most cardiomyopathies predispose to arrhythmia but there are also a number of primary cardiac arrhythmias including the long QT syndromes of Jervell, Lange and Nielsen, which are autosomal recessive, and the Romano Ward, which is autosomal dominant. A variety of mutations in sodium and potassium channels have been implicated (Viskin and Long 1999). There are also reports of familial atrial fibrillation (Brugada *et al.* 1997). Atrial myxoma (Ch. 6) is associated with a high risk of embolization and stroke and can be familial, particularly in younger patents and in men (Carney 1985).

Mitochondrial disorders

Various mitochondrial disorders may be associated with stroke-like episodes and cardio-myopathy (Ch. 6).

Hematological disorders

Various genetic blood disorders including sickle cell anemia and familial thrombophilias (Ch. 2) are associated with stroke.

References

Alberts MJ (1991). Genetic aspects of cerebrovascular disease. *Stroke* 22:276–280

Brugada R, Tapscott T, Czernuszewicz GZ *et al.* (1997). Identification of a genetic locus for familial atrial fibrillation. *New England Journal of Medicine* 336:905–911

Carney JA (1985). Differences between nonfamilial and familial cardiac myxoma. *American Journal of Surgery and Pathology* 9:53–55

Casas JP, Hingorani AD, Bautista LE *et al.* (2004). Meta-analysis of genetic studies in ischemic stroke: thirty-two genes involving approximately 18 000 cases and 58 000 controls. *Archives of Neurology* 61:1652–1661

Casas JP, Cavalleri GL, Bautista LE *et al.* (2006). Endothelial nitric oxide synthase gene polymorphisms and cardiovascular disease: A HuGE review. *American Journal of Epidemiology* 164:921–935

Chabriat H, Vahedi K, Iba-Zizen MT *et al.* (1995). Clinical spectrum of CADASIL: a study of 7 families. *Lancet* 346:934–939

Chabriat H, Levy C, Taillia H, *et al.* (1998). Patterns of MRI lesions in CADASIL. *Neurology* 51:452–457

Dichgans M (2007). Genetics of ischaemic stroke. *Lancet Neurology* 6:149–161

Dichgans M, Markus HS (2005). Genetic association studies in stroke: methodological issues and proposed standard criteria. *Stroke* 36:2027–2031

Dichgans M, Mayer M, Müller-Myhsok B *et al.* (1996). Identification of a key recombinant narrows the CADASIL gene region to 8 cM and argues against allelism of CADASIL and familial hemiplegic migraine. *Genomics* 32:151–154

Dichgans M, Mayer M, Uttner I *et al.* (1998). The phenotypic spectrum of CADASIL: clinical findings in 102 cases. *Annals of Neurology* 44:731–739

Dubroca C, Lacombe P, Domenga V *et al.* (2005). Impaired vascular mechanotransduction in a transgenic mouse model of CADASIL arteriopathy. *Stroke* 36:113–117

Ebke M, Dichgans M, Bergmann M *et al.* (1997). CADASIL: skin biopsy allows diagnosis in early stages. *Acta Neurology Scandinavica* 95:351–357

Flossmann E, Schulz UG, Rothwell PM (2004). Systematic review of methods and results of studies of the genetic epidemiology of ischemic stroke. *Stroke* 35:212–227

Flossmann E, Schulz UG, Rothwell PM (2005). Potential confounding by intermediate phenotypes in studies of the genetics of ischaemic stroke. *Cerebrovascular Diseases* **19**:1–10

Franz WM, Muller OJ, Katus HA (2001). Cardiomyopathies: from genetics to the prospect of treatment. *Lancet* **358**:1627–1637

Gulcher JR, Gretarsdottir S, Helgadottir A *et al.* (2005). Genes contributing to risk for common forms of stroke. *Trends in Molecular Medicine* **11**:217–224

Gulcher JR, Kong A, Gretarsdottir S *et al.* (2006). Reply to "Many hypotheses but no replication for the association between PDE4D and stroke". *Nature Genetics* **38**:1092–1093

Hassan A, Markus HS (2000). Genetics and ischaemic stroke. *Brain* **123**:1784–1812

Hassan A, Sham PC, Markus HS (2002). Planning genetic studies in human stroke: sample size estimates based on family history data. *Neurology* **58**:1483–1488

Humphries SE, Morgan L (2004). Genetic risk factors for stroke and carotid atherosclerosis: insights into pathophysiology from candidate gene approaches. *Lancet Neurology* **3**:227–235

Hutchinson M, O'Riordan J, Javed M *et al.* (1995). Familial hemiplegic migraine and autosomal dominant ateriopathy with leukoencephalopathy (CADASIL). *Annals of Neurology* **38**:817–824

Hutter CM, Austin MA, Humphries SE (2004). Familial hypercholesterolemia, peripheral arterial disease and stroke: a HuGE minireview. *American Journal of Epidemiology* **160**:430–435

Joutel A, Corpechot C, Ducros A *et al.* (1996). *Notch3* mutations in CADASIL, a hereditary adult-onset condition causing stroke and dementia. *Nature* **383**:707–710

Joutel A, Vahedi K, Corpechot C *et al.* (1997). Strong clustering and stereotyped nature of *Notch3* mutations in CADASIL patients. *Lancet* **350**:1511–1515

Joutel A, Dodick DD, Parisi JE *et al.* (2000). De novo mutation in the *Notch3* gene causing CADASIL. *Annals of Neurology* **47**:388–391

Jung HH, Bassetti C, Tournier-Lasserve E *et al.* (1995). Cerebral autosomal dominant arteriopathy with subcortical infarcts and leukoencephalopathy: a clinicopathological and genetic study of a Swiss family. *Journal of Neurology, Neurosurgery and Psychiatry* **59**:138–143

Keavney B, McKenzie C, Parish S *et al.* (2000). Large-scale test of hypothesised associations between the angiotensin-converting-enzyme, insertion/deletion polymorphism and myocardial infarction in about 5000 cases and 6000 controls. International Studies of Infarct Survival (ISIS) Collaborators. *Lancet* **355**:434–442

Matarín M, Brown WM, Scholz S *et al.* (2007). A genome-wide genotyping study in patients with ischaemic stroke: initial analysis and data release. *Lancet Neurology* **6**:414–420

Meschia JF (2003). Familial hypercholesterolemia: stroke and the broader perspective. *Stroke* **34**:22–25

Razvi SS M, Davidson R, Bone I *et al.* (2005). The prevalence of cerebral autosomal dominant arteriopathy with subcortical infarcts and leucoencephalopathy (CADASIL) in the west of Scotland. *Journal of Neurology, Neurosurgery and Psychiatry* **76**:739–741

Rolfs A, Bottcher T, Zschiesche M *et al.* (2005). Prevalence of Fabry disease in patients with cryptogenic stroke: a prospective study. *Lancet* **366**:1794–1796

Rosand J, Bayley N, Rost N *et al.* (2006). Many hypotheses but no replication for the association between PDE4D and stroke. *Nature Genetics* **38**:1091–1092

Schulz UG, Flossman E, Rothwell PM (2004). Heritability of ischemic stroke in relation to age, vascular risk factors and subtypes of incident stroke in population-based studies. *Stroke* **35**:819–824

Singhal S, Bevan S, Barrick T *et al.* (2004). The influence of genetic and cardiovascular risk factors on the CADASIL phenotype. *Brain* **127**:2031–2038

Sudlow C, Martinez Gonzalez NA, Kim J *et al.* (2006). Does apolipoprotein E genotype influence the risk of ischemic stroke, intracerebral hemorrhage, or subarachnoid hemorrhage? Systematic review and meta-analyses of 31 studies among 5961 cases and 17 965 controls. *Stroke* **37**:364–370

Tournier-Lasserve E, Joutel A, Melki J *et al.* (1993). Cerebral autosomal dominant arteriopathy with subcortical infarcts and leukoencephalopathy maps to chromosome 19q12. *Nature Genetics* **3**:256–259

Viskin S, Long QT (1999). Syndromes and torsade de pointes. *Lancet* **354**:1625–1633

Wheeler JG, Keavney BD, Watkins H *et al.* (2004). Four paraoxonase gene polymorphisms in 11 212 cases of coronary heart disease and 12 786 controls: meta-analysis of 43 studies. *Lancet* **363**:689–695

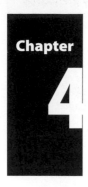

Anatomy and physiology

Knowledge of the anatomy of the blood supply of the brain is often helpful in understanding the etiology and mechanisms of TIA and stroke, which enable accurate targeting of acute treatment and secondary prevention. An awareness of the mechanisms underpinning the regulation of cerebral blood flow allows the clinician to identify patients at risk of stroke and assess the possible effects of treatments.

The anatomy of the cerebral circulation

The brain makes up only 2% of the total body weight, but when the body is at rest, it receives 20% of the cardiac output and consumes about 20% of the total inspired oxygen. The anterior two-thirds of the brain is supplied by the two internal carotid arteries, and the posterior third of the brain by the two vertebral arteries (Fig. 4.1). These four arteries anastomose at the base of the brain to form the circle of Willis (Fig. 4.2).

The detailed anatomy of the cerebral circulation is well described by Sheldon (1981). There is individual variation in arterial anatomy and thus in the territories of supply of the various major arteries, which can be asymmetrical and may change over time, depending on obstruction to vessel flow and the availability of functional collaterals (van der Zwan *et al.* 1992) (Fig. 4.3). Developmental anomalies of the major cerebral vessels include:

- inequality in size of the two vertebral arteries
- a combined origin of the left common carotid and innominate arteries
- the right common carotid artery arising from the aortic arch
- the left vertebral artery arising directly from the aorta
- hypoplasia or absence of the proximal part of one anterior cerebral artery so that blood flow to both anterior cerebral arteries comes from one internal carotid artery
- hypoplasia or absence of one or both posterior communicating artery(ies)
- hypoplasia or absence of the anterior communicating artery
- a persistent trigeminal artery joining the internal carotid artery to the basilar artery
- a paired or fenestrated basilar artery.

The **internal carotid artery** starts as the carotid sinus at the bifurcation of the **common carotid artery** at the level of the thyroid cartilage. It runs up the neck, without any branches, to the base of the skull where it passes through the foramen lacerum to enter the carotid canal of the petrous bone. It then runs through the cavernous sinus in an S-shaped curve (the carotid siphon) pierces the dura and exits just medial to the anterior clinoid process. It then bifurcates into the anterior cerebral artery and the larger middle cerebral artery.

The **external carotid artery** also starts at the bifurcation. Branches supply the jaw, face, scalp, neck and meninges via the superficial temporal, facial and occipital arteries.

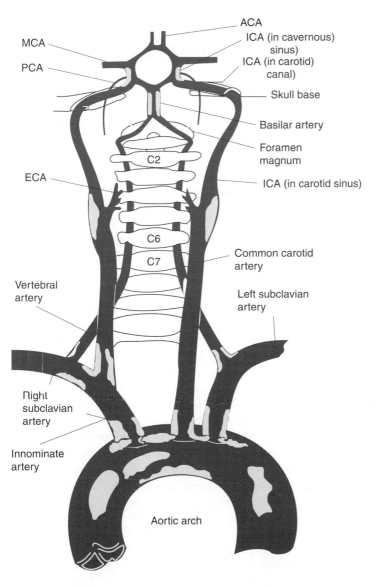

ACA
ICA (in cavernous) sinus)
ICA (in carotid) canal)
MCA
PCA
Skull base
Basilar artery
Foramen magnum
C2
ECA
ICA (in carotid sinus)
C6
C7
Common carotid artery
Left subclavian artery
Vertebral artery
Right subclavian artery
Innominate artery
Aortic arch

Fig. 4.1. The anatomy of the arterial circulation to the brain and eye. Gray indentations into the arterial lumen represent sites at which atherothrombosis is particularly common. ACA, anterior cerebral artery; ECA, external carotid artery; ICA, internal carotid artery; MCA, middle cerebral artery; PCA, posterior cerebral artery.

The **ophthalmic artery** is the first major branch of the internal carotid artery and arises in the cavernous sinus. It passes through the optic foramen to supply the eye and other structures in the orbit.

The **posterior communicating artery** is the next artery to arise from the internal carotid artery and passes back to join the first part of the posterior cerebral artery, so contributing to the circle of Willis. Tiny branches supply the adjacent optic chiasm, optic tract, hypo-thalamus, thalamus and midbrain.

The **anterior choroidal artery** arises from the last section of the internal carotid artery, just beyond the posterior communicating artery origin, and supplies the optic tract, internal capsule, medial parts of the basal ganglia, the medial part of the temporal lobe, thalamus, lateral geniculate body, proximal optic radiation and midbrain. Occasionally it arises from the proximal middle cerebral artery or posterior communicating artery. Minor twiglets

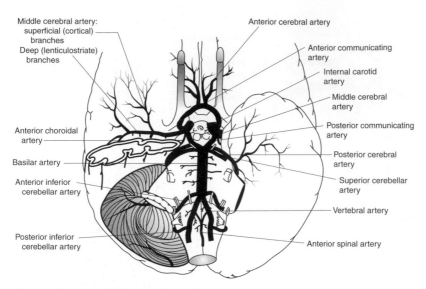

Fig. 4.2. The circle of Willis at the base of the brain as seen from below. There is considerable anatomical variation and this figure represents one of the more common arrangements.

from the distal internal carotid artery contribute blood to the pituitary gland, optic chiasm and nearby structures, including the meninges.

The **anterior cerebral artery** passes horizontally and medially to enter the interhemispheric fissure; it then anastomoses with its counterpart of the opposite side via the **anterior communicating artery**, curves up around the genu of the corpus callosum and supplies the anterior and medial parts of the cerebral hemisphere. Small branches also supply parts of the optic nerve and chiasm, hypothalamus, anterior basal ganglia and internal capsule.

The **middle cerebral artery** enters the Sylvian fissure and divides into two to four branches, which supply the lateral parts of the cerebral hemisphere. From its main trunk, a medial and lateral group of tiny lenticulostriate arteries and arterioles pass upwards to penetrate the base of the brain and supply the basal ganglia and internal capsule (Marinkovic *et al.* 1985). Some of these small penetrating vessels extend up into the white matter of the corona radiata in the centrum semiovale towards the small medullary perforating branches of the cortical arteries coming down from above.

The **vertebral artery** arises from the proximal subclavian artery and ascends to pass through the transverse foramina of the sixth to second cervical vertebrae, giving off small muscular branches on the way. It then passes posteriorly around the articular process of the atlas to enter the skull through the foramen magnum. It unites with the opposite vertebral artery on the ventral surface of the brainstem at the pontomedullary junction to form the basilar artery. Branches to the meninges arise at the foramen magnum. The vertebral artery gives rise to the anterior and posterior spinal arteries; the posterior inferior cerebellar artery, which supplies the inferior vermis and inferior and posterior surfaces of the cerebellar hemispheres and brainstem; and the small penetrating arteries to the medulla.

The **basilar artery** ascends ventral to the pons to the ponto–midbrain junction in the interpeduncular cistern, where it divides into the two posterior cerebral arteries. Numerous small branches penetrate the brainstem and cerebellum. The basilar artery also gives rise to the anterior inferior cerebellar artery, which supplies the rostral cerebellum, brainstem, inner ear, and the superior cerebellar artery, which supplies the brainstem, superior half of the cerebellar hemisphere, vermis and dentate nucleus.

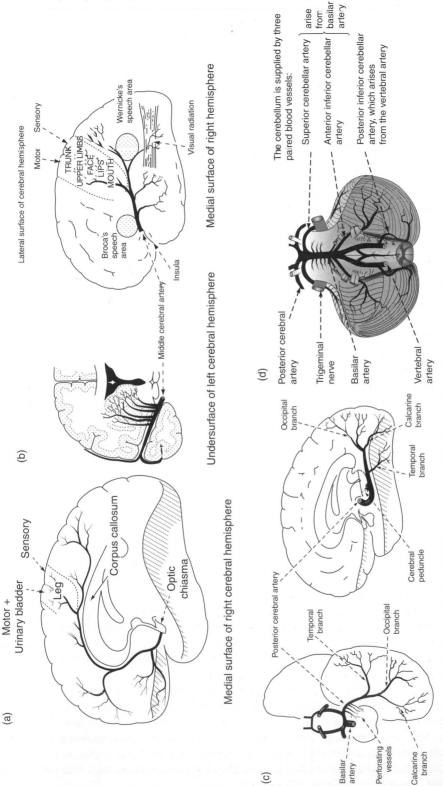

Fig. 4.3. Brain areas supplied by the anterior (a), middle (b) and posterior (c) cerebral arteries and the basilar artery (d).

(a)

Motor +
Urinary bladder

Sensory

Leg

Corpus callosum

Optic chiasma

Medial surface of right cerebral hemisphere

(b)

Lateral surface of cerebral hemisphere

Motor   Sensory

TRUNK
UPPER LIMBS
FACE
LIPS
MOUTH

Broca's
speech
area

Wernicke's
speech area

Visual radiation

Insula

Middle cerebral artery

Medial surface of right hemisphere

Undersurface of left cerebral hemisphere

(c)

Basilar
artery

Perforating
vessels

Calcarine
branch

Posterior cerebral artery

Temporal
branch

Occipital
branch

Occipital
branch

Calcarine
branch

Temporal
branch

Cerebral
peduncle

Posterior cerebral artery

(d)

The cerebellum is supplied by three
paired blood vessels:

Superior cerebellar artery } arise
from
basilar
artery

Anterior inferior cerebellar
artery

Posterior inferior cerebellar
artery, which arises
from the vertebral artery

Posterior cerebral
artery

Trigeminal
nerve

Basilar
artery

Vertebral
artery

The **posterior cerebral artery** encircles the midbrain close to the oculomotor nerve at the level of the tentorium and supplies the inferior part of the temporal lobe, and the occipital lobe (Marinkovic *et al.* 1987). Many small perforating arteries arise from the proximal portion of the posterior cerebral artery to supply the midbrain, thalamus, hypothalamus and geniculate bodies. Sometimes a single perforating artery supplies the medial part of each thalamus, or both sides of the midbrain. In approximately 15% of individuals, the posterior cerebral artery is a direct continuation of the posterior communicating artery, its main blood supply then coming from the internal carotid artery rather than the basilar artery.

The meninges are supplied by branches of the external carotid artery, internal carotid artery and vertebral arteries. The most prominent branches from the external carotid artery are the middle meningeal artery and tributaries of the ascending pharyngeal and occipital arteries. Most of the branches from the internal carotid artery arise near the cavernous sinus and from the ophthalmic artery in the orbit. Branches from the vertebral artery arise at the foramen magnum. There are numerous meningeal anastomoses between these small arteries.

The scalp is supplied by branches of the external carotid artery, particularly the superficial temporal, occipital and posterior auricular arteries. Above the orbit, there is a contribution from terminal branches of the ophthalmic artery. There is a rich anastomotic network between the various arteries of the scalp.

Collateral blood supply to the brain

The collateral blood supply to the brain is described by Liebeskind (2003). Common sites of collateral blood supply to and within the brain are:

- circle of Willis between anterior and posterior cerebral arteries
- leptomeningeal anastomoses between surface of brain and anterior, middle and posterior cerebral arteries
- muscular branches of the vertebral artery in the neck
- orbital anastomoses between branches of the external carotid and ophthalmic arteries
- dural anastomoses between meningeal and internal, external and vertebral arteries
- choroidal anastomoses between internal carotid and posterior cerebral arteries.

Normally, the internal carotid artery provides blood to the anterior two-thirds of the ipsilateral cerebral hemisphere and the posterior circulation is supplied by the vertebral, basilar and posterior cerebral arteries. Collateral channels may develop in response to occlusion of one or more of the intracerebral vessels, particularly if flow limitation is gradual rather than sudden. Unlike the normal cerebral blood supply, the functional capacity of the collateral blood supply to respond to changes in perfusion pressure is limited. Collateral blood flow may develop through various mechanisms in different areas.

> *The circle of Willis.* This is formed by the proximal part of the two anterior cerebral arteries connected by the anterior communicating artery, and the proximal part of the two posterior cerebral arteries, which are connected to the distal internal carotid arteries by the posterior communicating arteries. However, approximately 50% of circles have one or more hypoplastic or absent segments, usually one of the communicating arteries, and atheroma may limit the potential for collateral flow (Fig. 4.2).

Leptomeningeal anastomoses. These may develop on the surface of the brain between cortical branches of the anterior, middle and posterior cerebral arteries and, to a lesser extent, between pial branches of the cerebellar arteries.

Muscular branches of the vertebral artery in the neck. At positions distal to a vertebral obstruction, these muscular branches may receive blood retrogradely from occipital and ascending pharyngeal branches of the external carotid artery, or from the deep and ascending cervical arteries. In addition, anastomoses can develop between branches of the subclavian artery and external carotid artery when the common carotid artery is obstructed.

Around the orbit. Branches of the external carotid artery can anastomose with branches of the ophthalmic artery if the internal carotid artery is severely stenosed or obstructed. Collateral flow from the external carotid artery into the orbit then passes retrogradely through the ophthalmic artery to fill the carotid siphon, middle cerebral artery and anterior cerebral artery. Sometimes flow may even reach the posterior cerebral artery and vertebrobasilar system.

Dural anastomoses. These can develop between meningeal branches of the internal carotid artery, external carotid artery and vertebral arteries. Occasionally, small dural anastomoses develop between cortical, leptomeningeal and dural arteries.

Parenchymal anastomoses. These occasionally develop in the precapillary bed of the perforating arteries at the base of the brain supplying the basal ganglia.

The anterior choroidal artery. This branch of the internal carotid artery can anastomose with the posterior choroidal artery, a branch of the posterior cerebral artery.

Venous drainage

The venous anatomy is very variable. Venous blood flows centrally via the deep cerebral veins and peripherally via the superficial cerebral veins into the dural venous sinuses, which lie between the outer and meningeal inner layer of the dura and drain into the internal jugular veins (Stam 2005) (Fig. 4.4). The cerebral veins do not have valves and are thin walled, and the blood flow is often in the same direction as in neighboring arteries. There are numerous venous connections between the cerebral veins and the dural sinuses, the venous system of the meninges, skull, scalp, and nasal sinuses, allowing infection or thrombus to propagate between these vessels.

The regulation of cerebral blood flow

Knowledge of cerebral blood flow regulation, and the relationship between cerebral blood flow and cerebral metabolism, has had a major influence on the understanding of the pathophysiology of impaired perfusion reserve and acute ischemic stroke (Frackowiak 1986; Marchal *et al.* 1996; Baron 2001; Rutgers *et al.* 2004).

Cerebral blood flow in normal humans is approximately 50 ml/min per 100 g brain. Using positron emission tomography (PET) (Frackowiak *et al.* 1980), it has been shown that cerebral blood flow, cerebral blood volume and cerebral energy metabolism, measured as cerebral metabolic rate of oxygen ($CMRO_2$) or glucose (CMRglu) are all coupled, and higher in gray than in white matter. This means that the oxygen extraction fraction is similar (approximately one-third) throughout the brain (Leenders *et al.* 1990). Therefore, in normal resting human brain, cerebral blood volume is a reliable reflection of function or $CMRO_2$. There is a gradual fall of cerebral blood flow, cerebral blood volume, CMRglu and

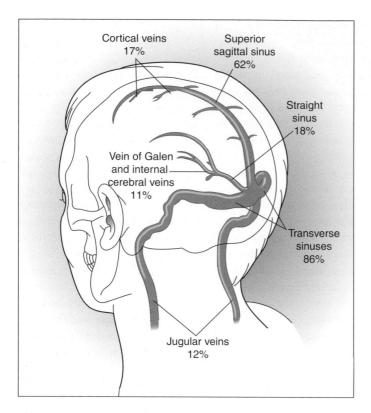

Fig. 4.4. Schematic diagram of the anatomy of the venous drainage of the brain. The frequencies of thrombosis in the various sinuses are given as percentages (see Ch. 29). In most patients, thrombosis occurs in more than one sinus.

CMRO$_2$ with age, but they remain coupled so that the oxygen extraction fraction remains more or less constant (Blesa *et al.* 1997).

Cerebral blood flow and blood gas tensions

Cerebral blood flow is very susceptible to small changes in arterial partial pressure of carbon dioxide (PaCO$_2$): an acute rise of 1 mmHg causes an immediate increase in cerebral blood flow of approximately 5% through dilatation of cerebral resistance vessels. In chronic respiratory failure, however, adaptation occurs so that cerebral blood flow is normal despite hypercapnia. Modest changes in arterial oxygen tension do not affect cerebral blood flow, but when the PaO$_2$ falls below about 50 mmHg, and oxygen saturation starts falling, there is a fall in cerebral vascular resistance and cerebral blood flow rises (Brown *et al.* 1985). Increasing PaO$_2$ above the normal level has little effect on cerebral blood flow.

Cerebral blood flow and brain function

Increasing regional functional activity of the brain, for instance in the motor cortex contralateral to voluntary hand movements, increases regional metabolic activity in the same area (Lassen *et al.* 1977; Geisler *et al.* 2006). The increasing CMRO$_2$ and CMRglu are achieved not by increasing oxygen extraction fraction or the glucose extraction fraction but by rapid (over seconds) local vasodilatation of the cerebral resistance vessels, increase in cerebral blood volume and, therefore, in cerebral blood flow. Conversely, low functional and metabolic demand, as occurs in a cerebral infarction, are associated with a low cerebral blood flow.

Cerebral blood flow, perfusion pressure and autoregulation

Cerebral blood flow depends on cerebral perfusion pressure and cerebrovascular resistance. The perfusion pressure is the difference between systemic arterial pressure at the base of the brain when in the recumbent position and the venous pressure at exit from the subarachnoid space, the latter being approximated by the intracranial pressure. Cerebral perfusion pressure divided by cerebral blood flow gives the cerebrovascular resistance. In normal humans, cerebral blood flow remains almost constant when the mean systemic blood pressure is between approximately 50 and 170 mmHg, which, under normal circumstances when the intracranial venous pressure is negligible, is the same as the cerebral perfusion pressure. This homeostatic mechanism to maintain a constant cerebral blood flow in the face of changes in cerebral perfusion pressure is known as autoregulation (Reed and Devous 1985; Powers 1993). Autoregulation is less effective in the elderly, and so postural hypotension is more likely to be symptomatic (Wollner et al. 1979; Parry et al. 2006).

Within the autoregulatory range, as cerebral perfusion pressure falls there is, within seconds, vasodilatation of the small cerebral resistance vessels, a fall in cerebrovascular resistance and a rise in cerebral blood volume; as a result, cerebral blood flow remains constant (Aaslid et al. 1989). If vasodilatation is maximal and cerebral perfusion pressure continues to fall owing to a drop in systemic blood pressure or an increase in intracranial pressure, cerebral blood flow starts to decline as the cerebral perfusion reserve is exhausted. However, metabolic activity is maintained by increasing oxygen extraction fraction: this is "misery" perfusion or oligemia. Eventually, the oxygen extraction fraction is maximal, and with further cerebral perfusion pressure reduction, metabolic activity is reduced, $CMRO_2$ starts to fall and metabolism becomes limited by perfusion. This is what is normally meant by ischemia; the perfusion reserve is exhausted and flow is inadequate to meet the metabolic demands of the tissues. At this point, the patient becomes symptomatic with non-focal neurological features such as faintness if the whole brain is involved or focal neurological features such as hemiparesis if only part of the brain is involved.

If the perfusion pressure rises above the autoregulatory range, where compensatory vasoconstriction and cerebral perfusion pressure are maximal, then hyperemia occurs followed by vasogenic edema, raised intracranial pressure and the clinical syndrome of hypertensive encephalopathy.

Cerebral perfusion reserve

It follows from the above that the ratio of cerebral blood flow to cerebral blood volume is a measure of cerebral perfusion reserve (Schumann et al. 1998). Below a ratio of approximately 6.0, even if cerebral blood flow is still normal, vasodilatation and cerebral blood volume are maximal and the reserve is exhausted, as shown by a rising oxygen extraction fraction on PET.

Chronically impaired perfusion reserve tends to occur when one or both internal carotid arteries are stenosed by at least 50% of the luminal diameter (Brice et al. 1964; DeWeese et al. 1970; Schroeder 1988), or are occluded, and the collateral circulation is inadequate (Powers et al. 1987; Kluytmans et al. 1999). In this situation, the brain is vulnerable to any further fall in cerebral perfusion pressure and cerebral metabolism is beginning to become impaired, with the appearance of structural abnormalities on MRI (van der Grond et al. 1996; Isaka et al. 1997; Derdeyn et al. 1999).

Indirect assessment of perfusion reserve can be achieved by using transcranial Doppler ultrasound, single-photon emission CT, PET, dynamic CT or functional MRI to measure cerebral blood flow response to hypercapnia during carbon dioxide inhalation, breath holding or after intravenous acetazolamide, a carbonic anhydrase inhibitor (Arigoni *et al.* 2000; Kikuchi *et al.* 2001; Shiogai *et al.* 2002, 2003; Shiino *et al.* 2003). However, there is uncertainty about how these various tests should be standardized and how to define "normality," given that a continuous variable is being measured. It should be noted that indirect methods of measuring perfusion reserve are inaccurate when the normal relationships between cerebral blood flow, cerebral blood volume, oxygen extraction fraction and vascular reactivity break down, as they may well do in newly ischemic or infarcted brain.

Impaired perfusion reserve is associated with an increased likelihood of recurrent stroke (Yamauchi *et al.* 1996), prior ischemic events in patients with carotid occlusion (Derdeyn *et al.* 1999, 2005), presence of silent brain infarction and increased likelihood of need for carotid shunting in carotid endarterectomy (Kim *et al.* 2000). Extracranial to intracranial bypass surgery has been shown to improve cerebral perfusion reserve in patients with large vessel occlusive disease and is currently being assessed (Adams *et al.* 2001; Grubb *et al.* 2003) as a treatment for secondary prevention of stroke in patients with carotid occlusion and reduced cerebral perfusion reserve in whom the risk of ipsilateral stroke on medical treatment is high (Grubb and Powers 2001). Medical treatment with angiotensin-converting enzyme inhibitors has also been shown to increase cerebral perfusion reserve in patients with previous minor stroke (Hatazawa *et al.* 2004).

Cerebral blood flow, hypertension and stroke

In chronically hypertensive patients, the autoregulatory range is shifted upwards so that cerebral blood flow starts falling and ischemic symptoms occur at a higher systemic blood pressure than normal (Strandgaard and Paulson 1992), but autoregulation appears otherwise to be maintained (Traon *et al.* 2002) except in malignant hypertension (Immink *et al.* 2004). The upward shift of autoregulation appears to return towards normal when hypertension is treated. Conversely, hypertensive encephalopathy is more likely to occur in acute hypertension when the upper limit of autoregulation is still normal, such as occurs in eclampsia.

Autoregulation is impaired, or abolished, in damaged areas of brain and then cerebral blood flow becomes "pressure passive" and follows perfusion pressure. Both static and dynamic cerebral autoregulation are impaired in patients with stroke (Strandgaard *et al.* 1992; Eames *et al.* 2002; Georgiadis *et al.* 2002; Novak *et al.* 2003) but treatment of hypertension with angiotensin-converting enzyme inhibitors and angiotensin II receptor antagonists subacutely after stroke appears to lower systemic pressure without compromising cerebral blood flow (Paulson and Waldemar 1990; Moriwaki *et al.* 2004; Nazir *et al.* 2004).

References

Aaslid R, Lindegaard KF, Sorteberg W *et al.* (1989). Cerebral autoregulation dynamics in humans. *Stroke* 20:45–52

Adams HP Jr., Powers WJ, Grubb RL Jr., (2001). Preview of a new trial of extracranial-to-intracranial arterial anastomosis: the carotid occlusion surgery study. *Neurosurgery Clinics of America* 12:613

Arigoni M, Kneifel S, Fandino J *et al.* (2000). Simplified quantitative determination of cerebral perfusion reserve with $H_2(15)O$ PET and acetazolamide. *European Journal of Nuclear Medicine* 27:1557–1563

Baron JC (2001). Perfusion thresholds in human cerebral ischemia: historical perspective and therapeutic implications. *Cerebrovascular Diseases* 11:2–8

Blesa R, Mohr E, Miletich RS *et al.* (1997). Changes in cerebral glucose metabolism with normal aging. *European Journal of Neurology* 4:8–14

Brice JG, Dowsett DJ, Lowe RD (1964). Haemodynamic effects of carotid artery stenosis. *British Medical Journal* **ii**:1363–1366

Brown MM, Wade JP, Marshall J (1985). Fundamental importance of arterial oxygen content in the regulation of cerebral blood flow in man. *Brain* **108**:81–93

Derdeyn CP, Grubb RL Jr., Powers WJ (1999). Cerebral hemodynamic impairment: methods of measurement and association with stroke risk. *Neurology* **53**:251–259

Derdeyn CP, Grubb RL Jr., Powers WJ (2005). Indications for cerebral revascularization for patients with atherosclerotic carotid occlusion. *Skull Base* **15**:7–14

DeWeese JA, May AG, Lipchik EO et al. (1970). Anatomic and haemodynamic correlations in carotid artery stenosis. *Stroke* **1**:149–157

Eames PJ, Blake MJ, Dawson SL et al. (2002). Dynamic cerebral autoregulation and beat to beat blood pressure control are impaired in acute ischaemic stroke. *Journal of Neurology, Neurosurgery and Psychiatry* **72**:467–472

Frackowiak RSJ (1986). PET scanning: can it help resolve management issues in cerebral ischaemic disease? *Stroke* **17**:803–807

Frackowiak RSJ, Jones T, Lenzi GL et al. (1980). Regional cerebral oxygen utilization and blood flow in normal man using oxygen-15 and positron emission tomography. *Acta Neurologica Scandinavica* **62**:336–344

Geisler BS, Brandhoff F, Fiehler J et al. (2006). Blood-oxygen-level-dependent MRI allows metabolic description of tissue at risk in acute stroke patients. *Stroke* **37**:1778–1784

Georgiadis D, Schwarz S, Cencetti S et al. (2002). Noninvasive monitoring of hypertensive breakthrough of cerebral autoregulation in a patient with acute ischemic stroke. *Cerebrovascular Diseases* **14**:129–132

Grubb RL Jr., Powers WJ (2001). Risks of stroke and current indications for cerebral revascularization in patients with carotid occlusion. *Neurosurgery Clinics of North America* **12**:473–487

Grubb RL Jr., Powers WJ, Derdeyn CP et al. (2003). The Carotid Occlusion Surgery Study. *Neurosurgery Focus* **14**:e9

Hatazawa J, Shimosegawa E, Osaki Y et al. (2004). Long-term angiotensin-converting enzyme inhibitor perindopril therapy improves cerebral perfusion reserve in patients with previous minor stroke. *Stroke* **35**:2117–2122

Immink RV, van den Born BJ, van Montfrans GA et al. (2004). Impaired cerebral autoregulation in patients with malignant hypertension. *Circulation* **110**:2241–2245

Isaka Y, Nagano K, Narita M et al. (1997). High signal intensity of T_2-weighted magnetic resonance imaging and cerebral hemodynamic reserve in carotid occlusive disease. *Stroke* **28**:354–357

Kikuchi K, Murase K, Miki H et al. (2001). Measurement of cerebral hemodynamics with perfusion-weighted MR imaging: comparison with pre- and post-acetazolamide ^{133}Xe-SPECT in occlusive carotid disease. *American Journal of Neuroradiology* **22**:248–254

Kim JS, Moon DH, Kim GE et al. (2000). Acetazolamide stress brain-perfusion SPECT predicts the need for carotid shunting during carotid endarterectomy. *Journal of Nuclear Medicine* **41**:1836–1841

Kluytmans M, van der Grond, KJ, van Everdingen KJ et al. (1999). Cerebral hemodynamics in relation to patterns of collateral flow. *Stroke* **30**:1432–1439

Lassen NA, Roland PE, Larsen B et al. (1977). Mapping of human cerebral functions: a study of the regional cerebral blood flow pattern during rest its reproducibility and the activations seen during basic sensory and motor functions. *Acta Neurology Scandinavica* **64**:262–263

Leenders KL, Perani D, Lammertsma AA et al. (1990). Cerebral blood flow, blood volume and oxygen utilisation. Normal values and effect of age. *Brain* **113**:27–47

Liebeskind DS (2003). Collateral circulation. *Stroke* **34**:2279–2284

Marchal G, Beaudouin V, Rioux P et al. (1996). Prolonged persistence of substantial volumes of potentially viable brain tissue after stroke. A correlative PET–CT study with voxel-based data analysis. *Stroke* **27**:599–606

Marinkovic SV, Milisavljevic MM, Kovacevic MS et al. (1985). Perforating branches of the middle cerebral artery. Micro-anatomy and clinical significance of their intracerebral segments. *Stroke* **16**:1022–1029

Marinkovic SV, Milisavljevic MM, Lolic-Draganic V et al. (1987). Distribution of the occipital branches of the posterior cerebral artery. Correlation with occipital lobe infarcts. *Stroke* **18**:728–732

Moriwaki H, Uno H, Nagakane Y *et al.* (2004). Losartan, an angiotensin II (AT1) receptor antagonist, preserves cerebral blood flow in hypertensive patients with a history of stroke. *Journal of Human Hypertension* **18**:693–699

Nazir FS, Overell JR, Bolster A *et al.* (2004). The effect of losartan on global and focal cerebral perfusion and on renal function in hypertensives in mild early ischaemic stroke. *Journal of Hypertension* **22**:989–995

Novak V, Chowdhary A, Farrar B *et al.* (2003). Altered cerebral vasoregulation in hypertension and stroke. *Neurology* **60**:1657–1663

Parry SW, Steen N, Baptist M *et al.* (2006). Cerebral autoregulation is impaired in cardioinhibitory carotid sinus syndrome. *Heart* **92**:792–797

Paulson OB, Waldemar G (1990). ACE inhibitors and cerebral blood flow. *Journal of Human Hypertension* **4**(Suppl 4):69–72

Powers WJ (1993). Acute hypertension after stroke: the scientific basis for treatment decisions. *Neurology* **43**:461–467

Powers WJ, Press GA, Grubb RL *et al.* (1987). The effect of haemodynamically significant carotid artery disease on the haemodynamic status of the cerebral circulation. *Annals of Internal Medicine* **106**:27–34

Reed G, Devous M (1985). South-western Internal Medicine Conference: cerebral blood flow autoregulation and hypertension. *American Journal of Medical Science* **289**:37–44

Rutgers DR, Klijn CJ, Kappelle LJ *et al.* (2004). Recurrent stroke in patients with symptomatic carotid artery occlusion is associated with high-volume flow to the brain and increased collateral circulation. *Stroke* **35**:1345–1349

Schroeder T (1988). Haemodynamic significance of internal carotid artery disease. *Acta Neurologica Scandinavica* **77**:353–372

Schumann P, Touzani O, Young AR *et al.* (1998). Evaluation of the ratio of cerebral blood flow to cerebral blood volume as an index of local cerebral perfusion pressure. *Brain* **121**:1369–1379

Sheldon JJ (1981). *Blood Vessels of the Scalp and Brain.* Oak Ridge, NJ: CIBA Pharmaceutical Corporation.

Shiino A, Morita Y, Tsuji A *et al.* (2003). Estimation of cerebral perfusion reserve by blood oxygenation level-dependent imaging: comparison with single-photon emission computed tomography. *Journal of Cerebral Blood Flow and Metabolism* **23**:121–135

Shiogai T, Uebo C, Makino M *et al.* (2002). Acetazolamide vasoreactivity in vascular dementia and persistent vegetative state evaluated by transcranial harmonic perfusion imaging and Doppler sonography. *Annals of the New York Academy of Sciences* **977**:445–453

Shiogai T, Koshimura M, Murata Y *et al.* (2003). Acetazolamide vasoreactivity evaluated by transcranial harmonic perfusion imaging: relationship with transcranial Doppler sonography and dynamic CT. *Acta Neurochirurgia Supplement* **86**:57–62

Stam J (2005). Thrombosis of the cerebral veins and sinuses. *New England Journal of Medicine* **352**:1791–1798

Strandgaard S, Paulson OB (1992). Regulation of cerebral blood flow in health and disease. *Journal of Cardiovascular Pharmacology* **19**: S89–S93

Traon AP, Costes-Salon MC, Galinier M *et al.* (2002). Dynamics of cerebral blood flow autoregulation in hypertensive patients. *Journal of Neurology Science* **195**:139–144

van der Grond J, Eikelboom BC, Mali WPThM (1996). Flow-related anaerobic metabolic changes in patients with severe stenosis of the internal carotid artery. *Stroke* **27**:2026–2032

van der Zwan A, Hillen B, Tulleken CAF *et al.* (1992). Variability of the territories of the major cerebral arteries. *Journal of Neurosurgery* **77**:927–940

Wollner L, McCarthy ST, Soper NDW *et al.* (1979). Failure of cerebral autoregulation as a cause of brain dysfunction in the elderly. *British Medical Journal* **1**:1117–1118

Yamauchi H, Fukuyama H, Nagahama Y *et al.* (1996). Evidence of misery perfusion and risk for recurrent stroke in major cerebral arterial occlusive diseases from PET. *Journal of Neurology, Neurosurgery and Psychiatry* **61**:18–25

Pathophysiology of acute cerebral ischemia

The brain normally derives its energy from the oxidative metabolism of glucose. Because there are negligible stores of glucose in the brain, when cerebral blood flow falls and the brain becomes ischemic, a series of neurophysiological and functional changes occur at various thresholds of flow before cell death (infarction). The degree of cell damage depends not only on the depth of ischemia but also its duration and the availability of collateral circulation (Liebeskind 2003; Zemke *et al.* 2004; Harukuni and Bhardwaj 2006). Different mechanisms are responsible for reversible loss of cellular function and for irreversible cell death, and there are also differences between the mechanisms that cause death of neurons, glia and endothelial cells, and perhaps between cells in white versus gray matter.

Mechanisms of cerebral ischemia

When cerebral blood flow falls below approximately 20 ml/min per 100 g brain, the oxygen extraction fraction becomes maximal and the cerebral metabolic rate of oxygen begins to fall, resulting in ischemia (Wise *et al.* 1983). The electroencephalograph readings flatten, evoked responses disappear and neurological signs appear. In fact, a high oxygen extraction fraction is only seen early after acute ischemic stroke, in the first day or so, and functional recovery is still possible if flow is restored. Although the exact cellular pathways of ischemia and infarction are not fully described in humans, four overlapping mechanisms are at work: excitotoxicity, depolarization, inflammation and apoptosis (Table 5.1). Excitotoxicity and depolarization are processes that occur within minutes and hours of an ischemic insult, while inflammation and apoptosis occur within hours and days. The clinical significance of these different mechanisms lies in the potential to design therapies that intervene at different levels in cellular pathways, thereby preventing or delaying damage to neuronal cells and increasing the potential for recovery (neuroprotection), although developments so far have been disappointing (Shuaib and Hussain 2008).

Excitotoxicity

Focal impairment of cerebral blood flow restricts the delivery of oxygen and glucose, with resultant disruption of cellular oxidative phosphorylation and energy production. Membranes become rapidly depolarized and extracellular glutamate accumulates by movement across electrical gradients, compounded by disturbance of synaptic reuptake processes. Extracellular glutamate binds to and activates various membrane receptors, most importantly NMDA (*N*-methyl-D-aspartate) and AMPA (α-amino-3-hydroxy-5-methyl-4-isooxazolepropionate), which open transmembrane channels permeable to cations including sodium, potassium, calcium and hydrogen. Water follows passively as the influx of sodium and chloride ions exceeds the efflux of potassium ions, and the resulting edema has deleterious effects locally and distantly through mass effect.

Table 5.1. Summary of the principle mechanisms of cerebral ischemic damage

Mechanisms	Events
Excitotoxicity	Membrane depolarization in response to disrupted cellular oxidative and energy production processes leading to damaging activity of secondary messengers
Depolarization	Local depolarization caused by focal hypoxia decompensates already threatened metabolism in penumbra and propagates ischemic damage
Inflammation	Injury mediated by enzymic (proteases and collagenases), cellular (neutrophils and macrophages) and vascular processes
Apoptosis	Programed or ordered cell death mediated by caspase enzymes

An intracellular increase in the secondary messenger calcium initiates a series of damaging cytoplasmic and nuclear events (Bano and Nicotera 2007). Proteolytic enzymes are activated, which degrade cytoskeleton proteins such as actin and spectrin. Free radical species are generated by activated cyclooxygenase and phospholipase enzymes and these overwhelm endogenous scavenging mechanisms and cause lipid peroxidation and membrane damage as well as triggering inflammation and apoptosis. These cellular pathways and resultant damage are particularly important in the mitochondria (Back *et al.* 2004; Warner *et al.* 2004; Zemke *et al.* 2004).

Depolarization

In the core of the ischemic region, cells undergo anoxic depolarization with the release of potassium ions and glutamate and never repolarize. However, depolarization can be induced in nearby neurons by the resultant increase in extracellular potassium and glutamate, and sometimes repolarization can occur at the expense of further energy consumption. Repetitive de- and repolarization around ischemic areas is thought to further decompensate metabolism in the penumbra and propagate local ischemia (Hossmann 2006).

Inflammation

Intracellular calcium ions and free radicals trigger the expression of a range of pro-inflammatory genes, leading to the production of inflammatory mediators such as interleukin-1β, tumor necrosis factor and platelet-activating factor, by injured brain cells. Adhesion molecules on endothelial cell surfaces are also induced, leading to the accumulation and movement of neutrophils into the brain parenchyma (Zheng and Yenari 2004). This process can cause further damage through processes in the vasculature (local vasoconstriction and platelet activation), at the cellular level (protease and collagenase production) and by initiation of cell signaling (macrophage recruitment and microglial activation).

Apoptosis

Apoptosis is programed cell death and differs from necrosis in that it results in minimal inflammation and release of genetic material. Although necrosis is the predominant process that follows acute ischemia, apoptosis is important after more minor injury, particularly within the ischemic penumbra. Apoptosis is executed by the production, activation and action of caspases, which are protein-cleaving enzymes that dismantle cytoskeleton proteins and enzymes responsible for cellular repair (Zhang *et al.* 2004). Neurons are particularly susceptible to caspase-mediated cell death after cerebral ischemia, as demonstrated by the reduction in infarct size by caspase inhibitors in experimental models.

The ischemic penumbra and the therapeutic time window

Around acutely infarcted brain, there is an ischemic penumbra (Astrup *et al.* 1981). Here the blood flow is low, function depressed and the oxygen extraction fraction high. In other words, there is viable tissue with misery perfusion where the needs of the tissue are not being met. The tissue may die or recover, depending on the speed and extent of restoration of blood flow. This concept opens up the possibility of a therapeutic time window during which restoration of flow or neuronal protection from ischemic damage might prevent both immediate cell death and the recruitment of neurons for apoptosis (see Ch. 21).

Recently PET studies in humans have demonstrated that about one-third of the ultimately infarcted tissue identified by late CT is in areas where, within hours of stroke onset, there had been potentially viable "penumbral" tissue (Marchal *et al.* 1996a). However, it is still not clear for how long this penumbral region persists in a potentially viable state, although time periods as long as 18 hours have been suggested and it appears that some recovery is possible if flow is restored (Lassen *et al.* 1991; Furlan *et al.* 1996). Accurate information about the ischemic penumbra, and any areas of luxury perfusion, requires PET, which is not practical in the routine management of acute ischemic stroke. More recently diffusion weighted and perfusion MRI (Baird *et al.* 1997; Barber *et al.* 1998a), and dynamic CT have been proposed to delineate the penumbra, but there is uncertainty over the exact interpretation of these techniques (Guadagno *et al.* 2004) (Ch. 11).

Recanalization and reperfusion

Spontaneous recanalization, at least of middle cerebral artery occlusion, occurs in up to two-thirds of patients within a week of stroke onset, many in the first 48 hours (Fieschi *et al.* 1989; Kaps *et al.* 1992; Zanette *et al.* 1995; Arnold *et al.* 2005). In general, the CT identified and functional outcomes are both better with recanalization and reperfusion, and even with early hyperperfusion, than if the middle cerebral artery remains occluded (Wardlaw *et al.* 1993; Marchal *et al.* 1996b; Barber *et al.* 1998b).

During or following a cerebrovascular event, some brain areas may show relative or absolute hyperemia owing to good collateral flow, reperfusion after an occluded artery has been reopened and/or inflammation and vasodilatation in response to hypercapnia. In hyperemic areas, oxygen extraction fraction is low and there is luxury perfusion, indicating that flow is in excess of metabolic requirements, perhaps because the tissue has been irreversibly damaged.

Ischemic cerebral edema

Cerebral ischemia causes not only reversible and then irreversible loss of brain function, but also cerebral edema (Symon *et al.* 1979; Hossman 1983). Ischemic edema is partly "cytotoxic" and partly "vasogenic." Cytotoxic edema starts early, within minutes of stroke onset, and affects the gray more than the white matter, where damaged cell membranes allow intracellular water to accumulate. Vasogenic edema, which starts rather later, within hours of stroke onset, affects the white matter more, where the damaged blood–brain barrier allows plasma constituents to enter the extracellular space. Ischemic cerebral edema reaches its maximum in two to four days and then subsides over a week or two.

Cerebral edema not only increases local hydrostatic pressure and compromises blood flow further but also causes mass effect, brain shift and eventually brain herniation (Fig. 5.1). Death in the first week after cerebral infarction is often a result of these mass effects.

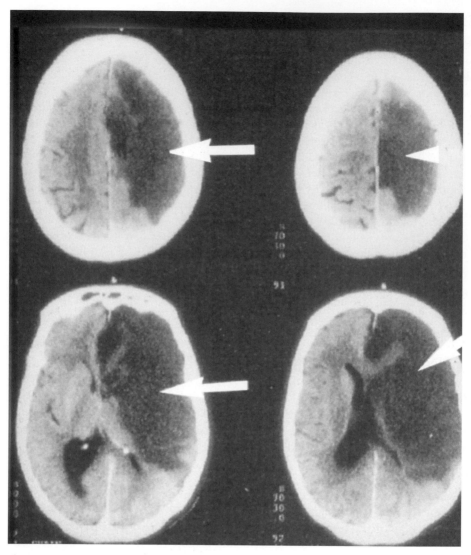

Fig. 5.1. Brain CT images showing a large hypodense (arrows) edematous cerebral infarct in the distribution of the middle cerebral artery, with midline shift. Such large infarcts cause herniation of the cingulate gyrus under the falx cerebri; of the ispsilateral uncus under the tentorium to compress the oculomotor nerve, posterior cerebral artery and brainstem; and of the contralateral cerebral peduncle to cause ipsilateral hemiparesis.

Diaschisis

Acute or chronic cerebral injury may cause effects in remote areas of brain (Meyer *et al.* 1993), so-called diaschisis, by reducing neuronal inputs and metabolic activity: in the contralateral cerebellum and ipsilateral internal capsule, thalamus and basal ganglia after cortical lesions; in the ipsilateral cortex following internal capsule and thalamic lesions; and in the contralateral hemisphere. The functional consequences of diaschisis are not clear (Bowler *et al.* 1995).

Pathophysiology of acute intracerebral hemorrhage

The events following intracerebral hemorrhage have been most intensively studied for the most common type: rupture of one or more deep perforating arteries. The extravasated blood causes disruption of white matter tracts and irreversible damage to neurones in the deep nuclei or the cortex. The resultant increase in intracranial pressure may threaten other parts of the brain, particularly when the intracranial pressure reaches levels of the same order of magnitude as the arterial pressure, bringing the cerebral perfusion pressure close to zero (Rosand et al. 2002). Direct mechanical compression of the brain tissue surrounding the hematoma and, to some extent, vasoconstrictor and pro-inflammatory substances in extravasated blood also lead to impaired blood supply (Castillo et al. 2002; Butcher et al. 2004). Cellular ischemia leads to further swelling from edema (Gebel et al. 2002; Siddique et al. 2002), which is initially cytotoxic and later vasogenic.

Hydrocephalus may be an additional space-occupying factor. This complication is especially likely to occur with cerebellar hematomas, but a large hematoma in the region of the basal ganglia may also cause enlargement of the ventricular system by rupture into the third ventricle or through dilatation of the opposite lateral ventricle, with midline shift and obstruction of the third ventricle, while the ipsilateral ventricle is compressed. The zone of ischemia around the hematoma may swell through systemic factors such as hypotension or hypoxia. Often there is also loss of cerebral autoregulation in the vasculature supplying the region of the hematoma. Some perifocal ischemic damage occurs at the time of bleeding and cannot be prevented, but it is uncertain whether the vicious cycle of ongoing ischemia causing steadily increasing pressure can be interrupted in its early stages.

References

Arnold M, Nedeltchev K, Remonda L et al. (2005). Recanalisation of middle cerebral artery occlusion after intra-arterial thrombolysis: different recanalisation grading systems and clinical functional outcome. Journal of Neurology, Neurosurgery Psychiatry 76:1373–1376

Astrup J, Siesjo BK, Symon L (1981). Thresholds in cerebral ischaemia. The ischaemic penumbra. Stroke 12:723–725

Back T, Hemmen T, Schuler OG (2004). Lesion evolution in cerebral ischemia. Journal of Neurology 251:388–397

Baird AE, Benfield A, Schlaug G et al. (1997). Enlargement of human cerebral ischaemic lesion volumes measured by diffusion-weighted magnetic resonance imaging. Annals of Neurology 41:581–589

Bano D, Nicotera P (2007). Ca^{2+} signals and neuronal death in brain ischemia. Stroke 38(Suppl 2):674–676

Barber PA, Darby DG, Desmond PM et al. (1998a). Prediction of stroke outcome with echoplanar perfusion- and diffusion-weighted MRI. Neurology 51:418–426

Barber PA, Davis SM, Infeld B et al. (1998b). Spontaneous reperfusion after ischaemic stroke is associated with improved outcome. Stroke 29:2522–2528

Bowler JV, Wade JP H, Jones BE et al. (1995). Contribution of diaschisis to the clinical deficit in human cerebral infarction. Stroke 26:1000–1006

Butcher KS, Baird T, MacGregor L et al. (2004). Perihematomal edema in primary intracerebral hemorrhage is plasma derived. Stroke 35:1879–1885

Castillo J, Dávalos A, Alvarez-Sabín J et al. (2002). Molecular signatures of brain injury after intracerebral hemorrhage. Neurology 58:624–629

Federico F, Simone IL, Lucivero V et al. (1998). Prognostic value of proton magnetic resonance spectroscopy in ischemic stroke. Arch Neurology 55:489–494

Fieschi C, Argentino C, Lenzi GL et al. (1989). Clinical and instrumental evaluation of patients with ischaemic stroke within the first six hours. Journal of Neurological Sciences 91:311–322

Furlan M, Marchal G, Viader F et al. (1996). Spontaneous neurological recovery after stroke and the fate of the ischaemic penumbra. *Annals of Neurology* **40**:216–226

Gebel JM Jr., Jauch EC, Brott TG *et al.* (2002). Natural history of perihematomal edema in patients with hyperacute spontaneous intracerebral hemorrhage. *Stroke* **33**:2631–2635

Graham GD, Kalvach P, Blamire AM *et al.* (1995). Clinical correlates of proton magnetic resonance spectroscopy findings after acute cerebral infarction. *Stroke* **26**:225–229

Guadagno JV, Donnan GA, Markus R *et al.* (2004). Imaging the ischaemic penumbra. *Current Opinions in Neurology* **17**:61–67

Harukuni I, Bhardwaj A (2006). Mechanisms of brain injury after global cerebral ischemia. *Neurology Clinic* **24**:1–21

Hossman KA (1983). Experimental aspects of stroke. In *Vascular Disease of the Central Nervous System*, Ross Russell, RW (ed.), pp. 73–100. Edinburgh: Churchill Livingstone.

Hossmann KA (2006). Pathophysiology and therapy of experimental stroke. *Cell and Molecular Neurobiology* **26**:1057–1083

Kaps M, Teschendorf U, Dorndorf W (1992). Haemodynamic studies in early stroke. *Journal of Neurology* **239**:138–142

Lassen NA, Fieschi C, Lenzi GL (1991). Ischaemic penumbra and neuronal death: comments on the therapeutic window in acute stroke with particular reference to thrombolytic therapy. *Cerebrovascular Diseases* **1**:32–35

Liebeskind DS (2003). Collateral circulation. *Stroke* **34**:2279–2284

Marchal G, Beaudouin V, Rioux P *et al.* (1996a). Prolonged persistence of substantial volumes of potentially viable brain tissue after stroke. A correlative PET–CT study with voxel-based data analysis. *Stroke* **27**:599–606

Marchal G, Furlan M, Beaudouin V *et al.* (1996b). Early spontaneous hyperperfusion after stroke. A marker of favourable tissue outcome? *Brain* **119**:409–419

Meyer JS, Obara K, Muramatsu K (1993). Diaschisis. *Neurology Research* **15**:362–366

Rosand J, Eskey C, Chang Y (2002). Dynamic single-section CT demonstrates reduced cerebral blood flow in acute intracerebral hemorrhage. *Cerebrovascular Diseases* **14**:214–220

Shuaib A, Hussain MS (2008). The past and future of neuroprotection in cerebral ischaemic stroke. *European Neurology* **59**:4–14

Siddique MS, Fernandes HM, Wooldridge TD *et al.* (2002). Reversible ischemia around intracerebral hemorrhage: a single-photon emission computerized tomography study. *Journal of Neurosurgery* **96**:736–741

Symon L, Branston NM, Chikovani O (1979). Ischemic brain edema following middle cerebral artery occlusion in baboons: relationship between regional cerebral water content and blood flow at 1 to 2 hours. *Stroke* **10**:184–191

Wardlaw JM, Dennis MS, Lindley RI *et al.* (1993). Does early reperfusion of a cerebral infarct influence cerebral infarct swelling in the acute stage or the final clinical outcome? *Cerebrovascular Diseases* **3**:86–93

Warner DS, Sheng H, Batinic-Haberle I (2004). Oxidants, antioxidants and the ischemic brain. *Journal of Experimental Biology* **207**:3221–3231

Wise RJ S, Bernardi S, Frackowiak RS J *et al.* (1983). Serial observations on the pathophysiology of acute stroke. The transition from ischaemia to infarction as reflected in regional oxygen extraction. *Brain* **106**:197–222

Zanette EM, Roberti C, Mancini G *et al.* (1995). Spontaneous middle cerebral artery reperfusion in ischaemic stroke. A follow-up study with transcranial Doppler. *Stroke* **26**:430–433

Zemke D, Smith JL, Reeves MJ *et al.* (2004). Ischemia and ischemic tolerance in the brain: an overview. *Neurotoxicology* **25**:895–904

Zhang F, Yin W, Chen J (2004). Apoptosis in cerebral ischemia: executional and regulatory signalling mechanisms. *Neurology Research* **26**:835–845

Zheng Z, Yenari MA (2004). Post-ischemic inflammation: molecular mechanisms and therapeutic implications. *Neurology Research* **26**:884–892

Chapter 6

Causes of transient ischemic attack and ischemic stroke

It is important that clinicians should have a thorough understanding of the causes of TIA and ischemic stroke (Table 6.1). Since there is no qualitative difference between TIA and stroke, anything that causes an ischemic stroke may also cause a TIA. The separation of TIA and stroke on the basis of an arbitrary time limit of 24-hours for resolution of symptoms in TIA is useful, not because there is any difference in the underlying causes of TIA and stroke, but because the differential diagnosis is not the same for short-lived as for longer focal neurological deficits (Chs. 8 and 9 for the differential diagnosis of TIA and stroke, respectively). Rare causes of TIA and stroke are proportionately more common in young compared with elderly patients, since degenerative arterial disease is unusual in the young. Venous infarction is discussed in Ch. 29.

Approximately 25% of ischemic strokes are caused by identifiable atherothromboembolism from large artery disease, 25% by small vessel disease, 20% by cardioembolism, approximately 5% by rarities, and the remainder are of undetermined etiology (Schulz and Rothwell 2003) (Table 6.2).

Large vessel disease and atherothromboembolism

Atheroma seems to be an almost inevitable accompaniment of ageing, at least in developed countries. Atherosclerosis is a multifocal disease affecting large and medium-sized arteries particularly where there is branching, tortuosity or confluence of vessels (see Fig. 4.1). Turbulence caused by changes in blood flow direction is thought to contribute to endothelial damage and ultimately to plaque formation. Atheroma begins in childhood as fatty streaks, possibly in response to endothelial injury, and over many years arterial smooth muscle cells proliferate, the intima is invaded by macrophages, fibrosis occurs and cholesterol is deposited to form fibrolipid plaques (Ross 1999; Goldshmidt-Clermont et al. 2005; Gotto 2005). Individuals with atheroma in one artery usually have widespread vascular disease, making them at high risk of ischemic heart disease, stroke and claudication (Mitchell and Schwartz 1962; Rothwell 2001), particularly among white males, who often have accompanying hypercholesterolemia. There appear to be important racial differences in the distribution of atheroma, and race is an independent predictor of lesion location. White males tend to develop atheroma in the extracranial cerebral vessels, aorta and coronary arteries, whereas intracranial large vessel disease appears to be relatively more common in black, Hispanic and Asian populations (Feldmann et al. 1990; Leung et al. 1993; Sacco et al. 1995; Wityk et al. 1996; White et al. 2005) and tends to affect younger patients and those with type 1 diabetes mellitus (Sacco et al. 1995). Some but not all, sources report that women have more intracranial disease than men.

Pathological, angiographic and ultrasonic studies show that the most common extracranial sites for atheroma are the aortic arch, the proximal subclavian arteries, the carotid

Table 6.1. Causes of cerebral ischemia

Types	Examples
Arterial wall disorders	Atherothromboembolism
	Intracranial small vessel disease
	Leukoaraiosis
	Dissection (Table 6.4)
	Fibromuscular dysplasia
	Congenital arterial anomalies
	Moyamoya syndrome
	Embolism from arterial aneurysms
	Inflammatory vascular diseases
	Irradiation
Cardioembolism (Table 6.3)	
Hematological disorders (Box 6.1)	
Miscellaneous conditions	Pregnancy/puerperium
	Migraine
	Oral contraceptives and other female sex hormones
	Perioperative
	Recreational drugs
	Cancer
	Chronic meningitis
	Inflammatory bowel disease
	Mitochondrial disease
	Fabry's disease
	Homocystinemia
	Hypoglycemia/hypercalcemia
	Fat embolism
	Fibrocartilaginous embolism
	Snake bite
	Epidermal naevus syndrome
	Susac's syndrome
	Cerebral autosomal dominant arteriopathy with subcortical infarcts and leukoencephalopathy (CADASIL)

bifurcation (Fig. 6.1) and the vertebral artery origins (Fig. 6.2). Plaques in the subclavian arteries frequently extend into the origin of the vertebral arteries, and similar plaques may occasionally occur at the origin of the innominate arteries. Frequently, the second portion of the vertebral artery as it passes through the transverse foramen is also affected, but the atheroma, which tends to form a ladder-like arrangement opposite cervical discs and osteophytes, does not normally restrict the lumen size significantly.

Table 6.2. Distribution of stroke etiology in four population-based studies

	OXVASC ($n = 102$)	OCSP ($n = 545$)	Rochester ($n = 454$)	Erlangen ($n = 531$)
Large vessel				
No.	17	77	74	71
% (95% CI)	16.7 (9.4–23.9)	14.1 (11.2–17.1)	16.3 (12.9–19.7)	13.4 (10.5–16.3)
Small vessel				
No.	20	119	72	120
% (95% CI)	19.6 (11.9–27.3)	21.8 (18.4–25.3)	15.9 (12.5–19.2)	22.6 (19.0–26.2)
Cardioembolic				
No.	19	127	132	143
% (95 % CI)	18.6 (11.1–26.2)	23.3 (19.8–26.9)	29.1 (24.9–33.3)	26.9 (23.2–30.7)
Other				
No.	3	33	12	9
% (95 % CI)	2.9 (0.06–8.4)	6.1 (4.2–8.4)	2.6 (1.4–4.6)	1.7 (0.8–3.2)
Not defined				
No.	43	189	164	188
% (95 % CI)	42.2 (32.6–51.7)	34.7 (30.7–38.7)	36.1 (31.7–40.5)	35.4 (31.3–39.5)

Notes:
OXVASC, Oxford Vascular Study; OCSP, Oxford Community Stroke Project; CI, confidence interval.
Source: From Schulz and Rothwell (2003).

Intracranial arteries are morphologically different from extracranial arteries in having no external elastic membrane, fewer elastic fibers in the media and adventitia and a thinner intimal layer. The major sites for atheroma formation in the anterior circulation are the carotid siphon, the proximal middle cerebral artery and the anterior cerebral artery around the anterior communicating artery origin. In the posterior circulation, the intracranial vertebral arteries are often affected just after they penetrate the dura (Fig. 6.3) and distally near the basilar artery origin. Plaques are also found in the proximal basilar artery and also prior to the origin of the posterior cerebral arteries. The mid-basilar segment may be affected around the origins of the cerebellar arteries (Fig. 6.4). Occlusion of a branch artery at its origin by disease in the parent vessel seems to occur more commonly in the posterior circulation, "basilar branch occlusion," than in the anterior circulation, where occlusion of the small perforating arteries is usually caused by intrinsic small vessel disease.

Atheromatous medium-sized arteries at the base of the brain, particularly the vertebral and basilar arteries, may become affected by dolichoectasia. The arteries are widened, tortuous and elongated and may be visualized on MRI or, if the walls are calcified, on CT. Dolichoectasia is usually found in elderly patients with hypertension and diabetes and it may cause stroke through embolization of thrombus or by occlusion of small branch arteries. In younger patients, it should raise the possibility of Fabry's disease.

Stroke mechanisms related to large artery atherosclerosis

There are four principal mechanisms by which atherosclerotic lesions may cause ischemic stroke.

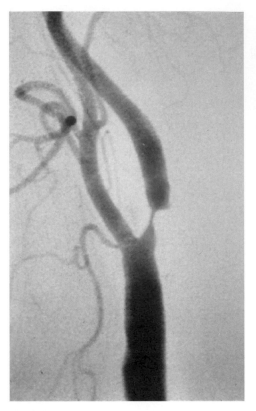

Fig. 6.1. Digitally subtracted arterial angiogram showing a severe stenosis of the internal carotid artery.

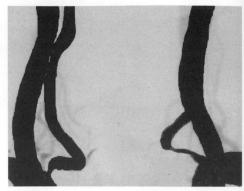

Fig. 6.2. Digitally subtracted arterial angiogram of the origins of both common carotid and vertebral arteries showing bilateral vertebral artery stenosis.

- Thrombi may form on lesions and cause local occlusion.
- Embolization of plaque debris or thrombus may block a more distal vessel. Emboli are usually the cause of obstruction of the anterior circulation intracranial vessels (Lhermitte *et al.* 1970; Ogata *et al.* 1994), at least in white males in whom intracranial disease is relatively rare. Since emboli follow the prevailing direction of flow in a vessel, most emboli from the internal carotid arteries will travel to the retina or the anterior two-thirds of the ipsilateral cerebral hemisphere. However, in patients with vascular disease, flow patterns may be abnormal owing to vessel occlusion and collateral flow. Infarction may occur ipsilateral to a chronically occluded internal carotid artery as emboli from the contralateral internal carotid pass via the anterior communicating artery.
- Small vessel origins may be occluded by growth of plaque in the parent vessel, such as in the basilar artery or proximal middle cerebral artery.
- Severe reduction in the diameter of the vessel lumen caused by plaque growth may lead to hypoperfusion and infarction of distal "borderzone" brain regions where blood supply is poorest.

Approximately 90% of atherothromboembolic strokes in whites are caused by atheroma in the extracranial vessels, whereas intracranial disease appears to be equally important in blacks and Hispanics (Sacco *et al.* 1995; Wityk *et al.* 1996). Atheromatous disease in the ascending aorta and the aortic arch is increasingly recognized as a source of cerebral emboli and an independent risk factor for ischemic stroke in vivo (Amarenco *et al.* 1994; Jones *et al.* 1995; Heinzlef *et al.* 1997; MacLeod *et al.* 2004).

Plaque activation and stroke risk

Atheromatous plaques are typically slow growing or quiescent for long periods but may suddenly develop fissures or ulcers (Fig. 6.5). Activated plaques trigger platelet aggregation,

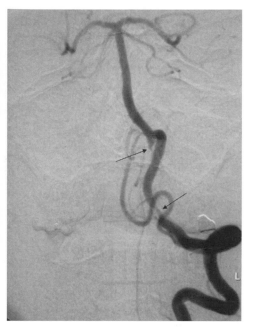

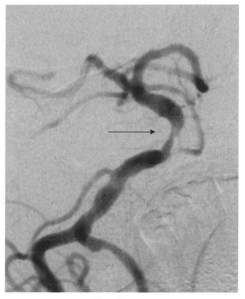

Fig. 6.4. Digitally subtracted arterial angiogram showing stenosis (arrow) of an ecstatic basilar artery.

Fig. 6.3. Digitally subtracted arterial angiogram showing occlusion of the distal right vertebral artery (top arrow) and a tight stenosis of the left vertebral artery (lower arrow).

(a)

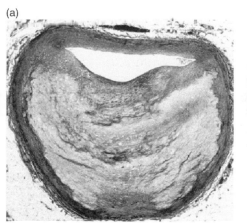

(b)

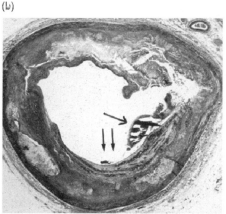

Fig. 6.5. Histological sections showing a quiescent plaque with a thick fibrous cap (a) and a ruptured plaque (b) with adherent thrombus (arrow).

thrombus formation (Viles-Gonzalez *et al.* 2004; Redgrave *et al.* 2006) and embolism. In keeping with the concept of acute intermittent activation of plaques, the likelihood of stroke in patients with cerebral atheromatous disease varies with time, being highest in the few days after a TIA or stroke (Coull *et al.* 2004; Rothwell and Warlow 2005) (Ch. 15). Strokes in large arteries are particularly likely to recur early (Lovett *et al.* 2004). Furthermore, emboli are more often detected with transcranial Doppler sonography if carotid stenosis is recently symptomatic (Dittrich *et al.* 2006; Markus 2006), and the rate of Doppler-detected emboli in the middle cerebral artery tends to decline with time after stroke (Kaposzta *et al.* 1999).

Plaque irregularity or ulceration, which is best visualized on catheter angiography (Fig. 6.6) but can sometimes be seen on contrast-enhanced MR angiography (Fig. 6.7), is independently associated with increased stroke risk. Irregularity of plaque as seen on radiological examination probably represents plaque ulceration and instability, with thrombosis, and so the likelihood of complicating embolism (Molloy and Markus 1999; Rothwell *et al.* 2000a, Lovett *et al.* 2004). There is also evidence to suggest that ulcerated carotid plaques are more likely than smooth plaques to be associated with vascular events in other territories, such as the coronary arteries (Rothwell *et al.* 2000b), suggesting that plaque activation is a systemic phenomenon. The trigger for activation is not known, but infective, inflammatory or genetic mechanisms have been proposed.

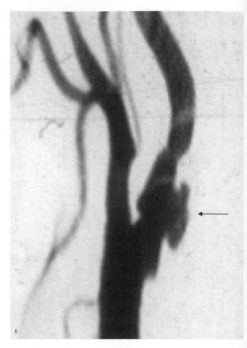

Fig. 6.6. Digitally subtracted arterial angiogram showing an ulcerated plaque at the carotid bifurcation, with contrast seen within the plaque (arrow).

Cholesterol embolization syndrome

Cholesterol embolization syndrome is a rare disorder that is thought to be caused by rupture of atheromatous plaques particularly in the abdominal aorta, either spontaneously or as a complication of instrumentation of large atheromatous arteries, anticoagulation or thrombolysis. Cholesterol debris is released and showers of emboli impact in the microcirculation of organs, including the stomach, skin, brain and spinal cord. Hours or days after instrumentation or surgery, a syndrome very similar to systemic vasculitis or infective endocarditis develops, with malaise, fever, abdominal pain, proteinuria and renal failure, stroke-like episodes, drowsiness, confusion, skin petechiae, splinter hemorrhages, livedo reticularis, cyanosis of fingers and toes, raised erythrocyte sedimentation rate, neutrophil leukocytosis and eosinophilia. The diagnosis is made by finding cholesterol debris in the microcirculation of biopsy material, usually from the kidney but sometimes from skin or muscle (Cross 1991; Rhodes 1996). The prognosis is poor, with a high mortality rate, and treatment is supportive.

Small vessel disease and leukoaraiosis
Small vessel disease
The small penetrating arteries of the brain, less than 0.5 mm in diameter, include the lenticulostriate branches of the middle cerebral artery, the thalamoperforating branches

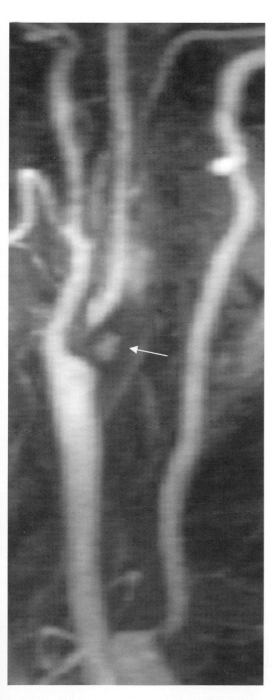

Fig. 6.7. Contrast-enhanced MR carotid angiogram showing a severe stenosis caused by an ulcerated plaque, with contrast seen within the plaque (arrow).

of the proximal posterior cerebral artery and the perforating arteries to the brainstem. Occlusion of one of these small vessels usually causes infarction, albeit in a small area of brain, since there is no significant collateral circulation. Such "lacunar" infarcts make up approximately one-quarter of first ischemic strokes (Bamford *et al.* 1987; Sempere *et al.* 1998; Schulz and Rothwell 2003) but case-fatality is low at around 1%. The few pathological data available suggest that these small arteries are much less likely to be occluded by emboli from the heart or from extracranial sites of atherothrombosis compared with the trunk or cortical branches of the middle cerebral artery (Tegeler *et al.* 1991; Boiten *et al.* 1996; Gan *et al.* 1997). In keeping with the pathological observations, ischemic lacunar strokes are less often associated with middle cerebral artery emboli detected with transcranial Doppler than are large artery strokes (Koennecke *et al.* 1998).

It is thought that the small perforating arteries of the brain are occluded by thrombus complicating a distinct small vessel arteriopathy – "hyaline arteriosclerosis" or "simple small vessel disease" (Lammie *et al.* 1997) – that differs from atheroma. Hyaline arteriosclerosis is an almost universal change in the small arteries and arterioles of the aged brain, particularly in the presence of hypertension or diabetes. The muscle and elastin in the arterial wall are replaced by collagen; there is subintimal hyalinization, the wall thickens, the lumen narrows and the vessel becomes tortuous. In complex small vessel disease, there is more aggressive disorganization of the small vessel walls, accompanied by foam cell infiltration. Whether simple and complex small vessel diseases are related is unclear.

The current view is that both complex small vessel disease and atheroma at or near the origin of the small perforating vessels arising from the major cerebral arteries cause most of the small deep infarcts responsible for lacunar ischemic strokes, which make up about one-quarter of symptomatic cerebral ischemic events (Bamford *et al.* 1987; Schulz and Rothwell 2003). However, this hypothesis is not universally accepted (Millikan and Futrell 1990) since there is little direct postmortem evidence of occlusion of these vessels leading to lacunar infarcts. Certainly, at least some small infarcts in the brainstem and internal capsule are caused by atheroma at the mouth of the small penetrating vessels spreading from atheroma of the larger parent artery (Fisher and Caplan 1971; Fisher 1979). It is also conceivable that this small vessel arteriopathy can lead to small, deep hemorrhages as well as lacunar infarcts (Labovitz *et al.* 2007); indeed, both types of stroke often coincide (Samuelsson *et al.* 1996; Kwa *et al.* 1998).

Leukoaraiosis

There are a number of alternative terms for leukoaraiosis, including Binswanger's disease, chronic progressive subcortical encephalopathy, subcortical arteriosclerotic encephalopathy and periventricular leukoencephalopathy. This reflects the confusion between the clinical, radiological and pathological literature (Munoz 2006). On CT, there is roughly symmetrical but irregular periventricular hypodensity, with or without ventricular dilatation and focal white matter hypodensities. This is better seen as high signal on T_2-weighted MR images (Fig. 6.8). This periventricular radiological appearance is caused by a variety of pathological changes, including demyelination, axonal loss and gliosis, which all are thought to occur as a consequence of diffuse rather than focal ischemia although the exact mechanism remains unclear. Vascular occlusion has not been seen (Caplan 1995; Pantoni and Garcia 1997).

Leuokoaraiosis is frequent in the normal elderly but is more marked in those with hypertension, dementia (Ch. 31) or stroke, but not increasing carotid stenosis (Bots *et al.* 1993; Adachi *et al.* 1997; Munoz 2006). It is also common in patients with cerebral amyloid angiopathy (Ch. 7). It is a risk factor for ischemic, particularly lacunar, and hemorrhagic stroke (Inzitari 2003) and is associated with increased bleeding risk with anticoagulants (Gorter 1999). It seems likely that the association between leukoariosis and stroke occurs because hypertension causes both pathological syndromes in the same individual rather than leukoaraiosis itself being the cause of the stroke.

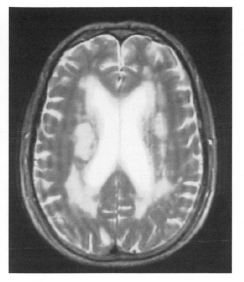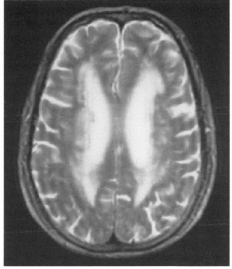

Fig. 6.8. Brain MRI scans showing the typical appearances of advanced periventricular leukoaraiosis.

Cardioembolism

Approximately 20% of ischemic stroke is cardioembolic. There are a large number of potential cardiac sources of embolism (Table 6.3) but it may be difficult to be certain whether an identified putative embolic source is the cause of a stroke, particularly if there are alternative causes such as coexistent large artery disease, or if the stroke is lacunar and unlikely to be caused by cardiac embolism.

Atrial fibrillation is discussed in Ch. 2.

Coronary artery disease

Overall, there is approximately a five-fold relative excess risk of stroke in the first few days and weeks after myocardial infarction, but the absolute risk of clinically evident systemic embolism is well under 5% (Dutta *et al.* 2006a). The risk of embolism is higher in anterior infarcts, large infarcts and the presence of a dyskinetic wall segment. Some postmyocardial infarction strokes may be caused by hypotension and boundary zone infarction, atrial fibrillation with left atrial thrombus, paradoxical embolism or coronary and aortic instrumentation (see below), while others are primarily hemorrhagic as a consequence of antithrombotic and thrombolytic drugs. Rarely, the same non-atheromatous disorder can cause both ischemic stroke and acute myocardial infarction: giant cell arteritis, aortic arch dissection or infective endocarditis. The long-term risk of stroke after acute myocardial infarction is approximately 1.5% per annum and 8% in five years (Martin *et al.* 1993; Loh *et al.* 1997).

Infective endocarditis

About one-fifth of patients with infective endocarditis have an ischemic stroke or TIA as a result of embolism of valvular vegetations. Cerebrovascular symptoms usually occur before the infection has been controlled and may be the presenting feature (Hart *et al.* 1990,

Table 6.3. Causes of cardioembolism

Area affected	Causes
Left atrium	Atrial fibrillation
	Sinoatrial disease
	Myxoma
	Interatrial septal aneurysm
Mitral valve	Infective endocarditis
	Non-bacterial thrombotic (marantic) endocarditis
	Rheumatic disease
	Prosthetic valve
	Mitral annulus calcification
	Libman–Sacks endocarditis
	Papillary fibroelastoma
Aortic valve	Infective endocarditis
	Non-bacterial thrombotic or marantic endocarditis
	Rheumatic disease
	Prosthetic valve
	Calcification and/or sclerosis
	Syphilis
Left ventricular mural thrombus	Myocardial infarction
	Left ventricular aneurysm
	Cardiomyopathy
	Myxoma
	Blunt chest injury
	Mechanical artificial heart
Paradoxical embolism from the venous system	Atrial septal defect
	Ventricular septal defect
	Patent foramen ovale
	Pulmonary arteriovenous fistula
Congenital cardiac disorders	Particularly with right to left shunt
Cardiac surgery	Catheterization, angioplasty
Others	Primary oxalosis, hydatid cyst

Salgado 1991). Hemorrhagic transformation of an infarct occurs in 20–40%. Primarily hemorrhagic strokes, intracerebral or, rarely, subarachnoid, are more commonly caused by pyogenic vasculitis and vessel wall necrosis than by mycotic aneurysms; these aneurysms can be single or multiple and most often affect the distal branches of the middle cerebral artery (Masuda *et al.* 1992; Krapf *et al.* 1999). They tend to resolve with time and cerebral angiography to detect unruptured aneurysms with a view to surgery is unnecessary (van der Meulen *et al.* 1992).

Early institution of the correct antibiotic therapy is the most effective way to prevent thromboembolism in infective endocarditis, the risks of which are highest in the first

24–48 hours after diagnosis. Anticoagulation should not be given to patients with native valve or bioprosthetic valve endocarditis because of the risk of intracerebral hemorrhage from mycotic aneurysms and arteritis and the reduction in embolism risk with antibiotic therapy. For patients with mechanical valves who are taking long-term anticoagulation at the time of developing infective endocarditis, the correct management is unclear. Other neurological complications of infective endocarditis include meningitis, diffuse encephalopathy, acute mononeuropathy, cerebral abscess, discitis and headache (Jones and Siekert 1989; Kanter and Hart 1991).

Fever, cardiac murmur and vegetations are not invariably present in patients with infective endocarditis, and blood cultures are indicated in unexplained stroke particularly if there is raised erythrocyte sedimentation rate, mild anemia, neutrophil leukocytosis or a history of intravenous drug abuse. The cerebrospinal fluid (CSF) can be normal, but $> 100 \times 10^6$ cells/l polymorphs is said to suggest endocarditis, although similar counts have been described in intracerebral hemorrhage and in hemorrhagic transformation of an infarct, but not in ischemic stroke (Powers 1986).

Non-bacterial thrombotic or marantic endocarditis

Small, friable and sterile vegetations made of fibrin and platelets can be found on the heart valves of patients with cancer, in the antiphospholipid antibody syndrome systemic lupus erythematosus and possibly in protein C deficiency. Thrombotic emboli from such vegetations can be demonstrated using trans-esophageal echocardiography and are frequently seen in patients with cancer and cerebral ischemia (Dutta *et al.* 2006b).

Prosthetic heart valves

Prosthetic valves, particularly mechanical ones, are associated with thrombosis and embolism, and infective endocarditis. The overall risk of clinically evident embolism is 1–2% per annum in those taking anticoagulants (Vongpatanasin *et al.* 1996), with mitral valve prostheses being the most prone to thrombosis.

Mitral leaflet prolapse

Mitral leaflet prolapse is a common incidental finding. It can be complicated by gross mitral regurgitation, infective endocarditis, atrial fibrillation and left atrial thrombus and thus embolism to the brain. However, there is no excess risk of first or recurrent stroke in patients with uncomplicated mitral leaflet prolapse (Orencia *et al.* 1995a, b).

Calcification of the aortic and mitral valves

Calcification, and possibly sclerosis, of the aortic and mitral valves may be a cause of embolism of calcific or complicating thrombotic material. However, these degenerative disorders of heart valves are so common, particularly in the elderly, that it has been very difficult to associate them causally with stroke (Boon *et al.* 1996).

Paradoxical embolism and patent foramen ovale

Autopsy examples have established that paradoxical embolism can occur from venous thrombi through the right to the left side of the heart. Emboli may pass through a patent foramen ovale, which is found in approximately one-quarter of healthy people, an atrial septal defect or a ventriculoseptal defect (Gautier *et al.* 1991; Jeanrenaud and Kappenberger 1991; Cabanes *et al.* 1993). There is an increased incidence of patent foramen ovale in patients with cryptogenic stroke (Mas *et al.* 2001; Lamy *et al.* 2002) but the risk of recurrent stroke in patients with a patent foramen ovale is low and so routine endovascular closure cannot be recommended (Amarenco 2005; Homma and Sacco 2005; Kizer and Devereux 2005; Messe *et al.* 2005; Mas 2003) particularly since there is evidence of a continuing risk of stroke after closure of patent foramen ovale (Wahl *et al.* 2001).

Atrial septal aneurysm

Atrial septal aneurysm is an echocardiographic finding in some normal people. The combination of atrial septal aneurysm and patent foramen ovale was thought to carry a higher stroke risk than patent foramen ovale alone (Mas *et al.* 2001; Lamy *et al.* 2002), with a reported risk of recurrent stroke in such patients as high as 15% (Mas *et al.* 2001), but more recent data from a larger study have cast doubt on this observation (CODICE Study Group 2006). Interestingly, there appears to be an association between patent foramen ovale and migraine, particularly migraine with aura, and this is particularly strong where there is coexistent atrial septal aneurysm. There are anecdotal reports of improvement in migraine symptoms following patent foramen ovale closure (Holmes 2004; Diener *et al.* 2005).

Cardiac myxomas

Cardiac myxomas are rare, occasionally familial, and arise in any heart chamber, but 75% are found in the left atrium. Tumor material, or complicating thrombus, may embolize and often there are features of intracardiac obstruction (dyspnea, cardiac failure, syncope) and constitutional upset (malaise, weight loss, fever, rash, arthralgia, myalgia, anemia, raised erythrocyte sedimentation rate, hypergammaglobulinemia) (Ekinci and Donnan 2004). Myxomatous emboli impacted in cerebral arteries may cause aneurysmal dilatation, with subsequent intracerebral or subarachnoid hemorrhage (Sabolek *et al.* 2005).

Dilating cardiomyopathies

Cardiomyopathies may be complicated by intracardiac thrombus but associated embolic stroke is rare.

Cardiac surgery

Cardiac surgery is complicated by stroke or retinal/optic nerve infarction in about 2% of cases, the risk being greater for valve than for coronary artery surgery (Newman *et al.* 2006). Postoperative confusion is much more common, and cognitive deficits may persist for some weeks (Newman *et al.* 2006). Possible mechanisms for postoperative confusion include embolization during or after surgery, hypotension, cholesterol embolization, simultaneous carotid endarterectomy, thrombosis associated with heparin-induced thrombocytopenia, and intracranial hemorrhage caused by anticoagulation or thrombocytopenia.

Sinoatrial disease

Sinoatrial disease or the sick sinus syndrome is associated with systemic embolism, particularly if there is bradycardia alternating with tachycardia, or atrial fibrillation (Bathen *et al.* 1978).

Instrumentation of the coronary arteries and aorta

Instrumental procedures in coronary arteries or the aorta may dislodge valvular or athero-matous debris causing neurological complications (Ayas and Wijdicks 1995) and cholesterol embolization.

Arterial dissection and trauma
Arterial dissection

Arterial dissection is a common cause of ischemic stroke and TIA in young adults and may also occur in older people. Sometimes there is a predisposing cause (Schievink 2001; Rubinstein *et al.* 2005) (Table 6.4) but often there is no explanation. The artery may become occluded by the wall hematoma itself; thrombosis and embolism may complicate occlusive or non-occlusive dissections, and aneurysmal bulging of the weakened wall may occur (O'Connell *et al.* 1985). Arterial rupture is unusual.

There are a number of characteristic features in the history and examination that point to cervical dissection:

- potential neck injury
- pain in the neck, side of the head, face or eye may accompany ipsilateral internal carotid artery dissection; pain at the back of the head and neck, usually unilaterally, may accompany vertebral dissection
- Horner's syndrome may arise as a result of damage to sympathetic nerves around the internal carotid artery; this occurs in up to 50%
- a self-audible bruit, which may be described as pulsatile tinnitus, caused by dissection adjacent to the base of the skull occurs in about 30%
- ipsilateral palsy of a cranial nerve occurs in about 10%, often affecting cranial nerve XII or another lower cranial nerve and rarely cranial nerve III
- cervical root lesions have been reported in association with vertebral artery dissections from pressure or ischemia.

The presence of cranial neuropathy may result in a misdiagnosis of brainstem stroke. Cranial nerve palsies may result from local pressure from the false internal carotid artery lumen, thromboembolism or hemodynamic compromise to the blood supply of the nerve. Cranial nerve III receives its blood supply from the ophthalmic artery, branches of the internal carotid or the posterior cerebral artery and, consequently, may rarely become ischemic after carotid dissection.

The features listed above may precede the onset of cerebral ischemia by hours or days, and relevant points in the history may, therefore, not be volunteered spontaneously by the patient. Alternatively, diagnostic pointers to dissection may be absent altogether and then the diagnosis becomes one of exclusion/confirmation on imaging. Cervical arterial dissection generally has a benign prognosis, with a 95% survival at 10 years, although the risk of stroke is high during the first few days and weeks. Secondary aneurysm formation can cause symptoms through local pressure but it does not appear to increase the risk of thromboembolism.

The incidence of diagnosed internal carotid artery dissection is approximately 1–4 per 100 000 per year. Vertebral dissection is a little less common. The actual incidence of dissections is likely to be considerably higher, but the diagnosis is often missed, particularly in older patients. Usually only one artery is involved but in about 10%, multiple arteries

67

Table 6.4. Causes of dissection of the extra- and intracranial arteries

Type		Causes
Traumatic		
	Penetrating injury	Catheter angiography
		Jugular vein cannulation
		Missile wounds
		Neck/oral injury or surgery
	Non-penetrating injury	Blow to the neck
		Neck injury: fracture, subluxation or dislocation
		Neck movements: whiplash injury, "head-banging," hairdresser visit, head injury, falls
		Yoga
		Chiropractic manipulation
		Labor
		Seizures
		Vomiting
		Bronchoscopy
		Atlanto-axial dislocation
		Occipito-atlantal instability
		Skull base fracture
		Cervical rib
		Fractured clavicle
		Carotid compression tests
		Attempted strangulation
Spontaneous		Marfan's syndrome
		Ehlers–Danlos syndrome
		Pseudoxanthoma elasticum
		Inflammatory arterial disease
		Infective arterial disease, e.g. syphilis
		Fibromuscular dysplasia
		Cystic medial necrosis

may be affected simultaneously or in close succession. Recurrence rates are low at approximately 1% per annum except in familial cases of arterial dissection or hereditary connective tissue disorder, where rates are higher (Leys *et al.* 1995).

On angiography, there is usually a long, tapered, narrow or occluded segment, perhaps with an intimal flap, double lumen or intraluminal thrombus, and sometimes an associated aneurysm. Intracranial arterial occlusion, presumably embolic, may be seen. Carotid dissection can often be strongly suspected on Duplex (Sturzenegger *et al.* 1993, 1995; Flis *et al.* 2007), but the most sensitive and specific imaging evidence of both carotid and vertebral dissection comes from a combination of axial MRI through the lesion, to show the acute hematoma in the arterial wall, with MR angiography (Auer *et al.* 1998, Flis *et al.* 2007) (Fig. 6.9).

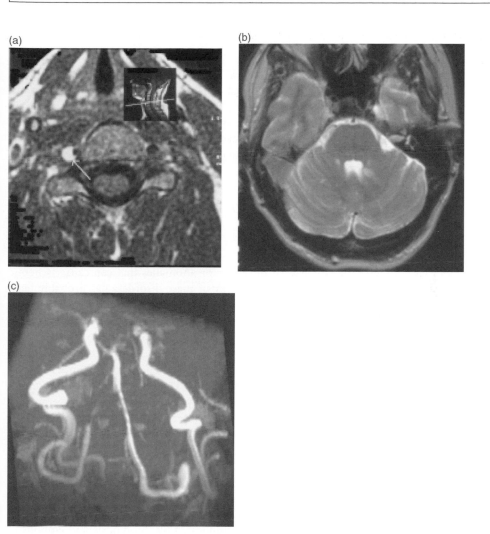

Fig. 6.9. (a) A T_2-weighted MRI scan showing high signal in the wall of the right internal carotid artery (arrow) indicating a recent dissection. (b) A T_2-weighted MRI scan showing several areas of cerebellar infarction. (c) An MR angiography showing absence of the right vertebral artery.

Intracranial arterial dissection

Intracranial dissection is much rarer. It may present with subarachnoid hemorrhage owing to rupture of a pseudo-aneurysm, as well as with ischemic stroke, and is less often diagnosed during life (Farrell *et al.* 1985; de Bray *et al.* 1997; Chaves *et al.* 2002).

Aortic arch dissection

Aortic arch dissection can cause profound hypotension, with global, and sometimes boundary zone, cerebral ischemia or focal cerebral ischemia if the dissection spreads up one of the neck arteries. Clues to this diagnosis are anterior chest or interscapular pain, along with diminished, unequal or absent arterial pulses in the arms or neck and a normal electrocardiogram, unlike acute myocardial infarction, acute aortic regurgitation and pericardial effusion.

Trauma

Penetrating and non-penetrating neck injuries are more likely to damage the carotid than the better protected vertebral artery. The vertebral artery appears to be more vulnerable to rotational and hyperextension injuries of the neck, particularly at the level of the atlas and axis. Laceration, dissection and intimal tears may be complicated by thrombosis and then embolism and, therefore, ischemic stroke at the time of the injury or some days or even weeks after the injury. Later stroke may be a consequence of the formation of a traumatic aneurysm, arteriovenous fistula or a fistula between the carotid and vertebral arteries (Davis and Zimmerman 1983).

The subclavian artery can be damaged by a fractured clavicle or a cervical rib, with later embolization up the vertebral arteries or even up the right common carotid artery (Prior et al. 1979).

Rare arterial disorders

There are a large number of rare arterial disorders or anomalies that can cause ischemic stroke (Tables 3.2 and 6.1). The frequency of many of these disorders has probably been underestimated because of under-investigation and lack of radiological imaging of the cerebral vasculature beyond the carotid bifurcation.

Fibromuscular dysplasia

Fibromuscular dysplasia is a rare segmental disorder with a female preponderance affecting small and medium-sized arteries (Slovut and Olin 2004). There is fibrosis and thickening of the arterial wall alternating with atrophy, giving the typical angiographic appearance of a "string of beads." It is most common in the renal arteries, resulting in hypertension. The mid-cervical portion of the internal carotid artery is the most frequently affected artery to the brain but the vertebral arteries at the level of the first two cervical vertebrae may also be involved. Intracranial pathology is exceptional (Arunodaya et al. 1997). Fibromuscular dysplasia is associated with intracranial saccular aneurysms and arteriovenous malformations and dissection. Since fibromuscular dysplasia of some arteries to the brain is found in up to 1% of routine autopsies, associations with cerebral ischemia or infarction may be coincidental. Occasionally, however, it may be complicated by thrombosis and embolism. The natural history is unknown.

Congenital arterial anomalies

Occasionally, the carotid arteries are hypoplastic or absent, and kinking, acute angulation, tortuosity and looping of the internal carotid artery may be seen on angiograms (Metz et al. 1961). Such appearances can be caused by atheroma, fibromuscular dysplasia or congenital abnormality. There is a tendency to regard anomalies in children and young adults as "congenital" and those in the middle aged and elderly as "atherosclerotic."

Congenital carotid loops

Carotid loops may be associated with aneurysm formation and rarely with embolism, endothelial damage and thrombosis; exceptionally there may be focal ischemia on head movement (Sarkari et al. 1970; Desai and Toole 1975). Rarely, these loops may cause hypoglossal nerve lesions or pulsatile tinnitus.

Some inherited disorders of connective tissue (Table 3.2) can present with, or be complicated by, arterial dissection or even rupture, intra- and extracranial aneurysm formation, caroticocavernous fistula and mitral leaflet prolapse for example Ehlers–Danlos syndrome (North *et al.* 1995), pseudoxanthoma elasticum (Mayer *et al.* 1994) and Marfan's syndrome (Bowen *et al.* 1987; Schievink *et al.* 1994).

Moyamoya syndrome

In Japanese, *moyamoya* means "puff of smoke" and describes the characteristic radiological appearance of the fine anastomotic collaterals that develop from the perforating and pial arteries at the base of the brain, the orbital and ethmoidal branches of the external carotid artery and the leptomeningeal and transdural vessels in response to severe stenosis or occlusion of one, or both, distal internal carotid arteries (Yonekawa and Khan 2003). The circle of Willis and the proximal cerebral and basilar arteries may also be involved.

Moyamoya seems to be mainly confined to the Japanese and other Asians, and in most cases the cause is unknown (Bruno *et al.* 1988; Chiu *et al.* 1998). Some cases are familial (Kitahara *et al.* 1979); others appear to be caused by a generalized fibrous disorder of arteries (Aoyagi *et al.* 1996), and a few may result from a congenital hypoplastic anomaly affecting arteries at the base of the brain, or associated with Down's syndrome (Cramer *et al.* 1996). The syndrome may present in infancy with recurrent episodes of cerebral ischemia and infarction, mental retardation, headache, epileptic seizures and, occasionally, involuntary movements. In adults, subarachnoid or primary intracerebral hemorrhage are also common owing to rupture of collateral vessels. There have also been a few reports of associated intracranial aneurysms (Iwama *et al.* 1997) and also of cerebral arteriovenous malformations.

Embolism from intra- and extracranial arterial aneurysms

Embolism from thrombus within the cavity of an aneurysm is rare and is difficult to prove in cases where there may be other potential sources of embolization. Intracranial aneurysms more commonly present with rupture and subarachnoid hemorrhage, whereas internal carotid artery aneurysms tend to cause pressure symptoms including a pulsatile and sometimes painful mass in the neck or pharynx, ipsilateral Horner's syndrome or compression of the lower cranial nerves. Extracranial vertebral artery aneurysms may cause pain in the neck and arm, a mass, spinal cord compression and upper limb ischemia (Catala *et al.* 1993).

Irradiation

Excessive irradiation of the head and neck can damage intra- and extracranial arteries, both large and small. Within the radiation field, a localized, stenotic, and sometimes apparently atheromatous, lesion may become symptomatic months or years later. There can be considerable fibrosis of the arterial wall and even aneurysm formation (Zuber *et al.* 1993; Bitzer and Topka 1995; Griewing *et al.* 1995; O'Connor and Mayberg 2000). The most common causes of this large artery variant are radiotherapy to the neck following laryngeal carcinoma, which leads to disease around the carotid bifurcation, and radiotherapy to pituitary tumors, which leads most commonly to disease in the basilar artery. Management is uncertain and the prognosis variable. Patients who have had radiotherapy for cerebral tumors more commonly develop a progressive small vessel vasculopathy.

Inflammatory vascular disease

There are a number of acute, subacute and chronic inflammatory "vasculitic" disorders of the arterial or venous wall (Box 6.1). These disorders may be associated with ischemic

71

Box 6.1. Inflammatory vascular diseases causing stroke

Giant cell arteritis	Relapsing polychondritis
Systematic lupus erythematosus	Progressive systemic sclerosis
Antiphospholipid antibody	Sarcoid angiitis
syndrome	Primary vasculitis of the central nervous system
Primary systematic vasculitis	Takayasu's disease
Rheumatoid disease	Buerger's disease
Sjögren's syndrome	Malignant atrophic papulosis
Behçet's disease	Acute posterior multifocal placoid pigment epitheliopathy

stroke, intracranial hemorrhage, intracranial venous thrombosis (Ch. 29) or a generalized encephalopathy. Angiographic appearances can be diagnostic, particularly in larger artery vasculitis, but angiography is not particularly sensitive and the abnormalities seen may be non-specific and so diagnosis is often made on the basis of the clinical syndrome. Contrast-enhanced high-resolution MRI can be useful in showing contrast uptake in the walls of thickened and inflamed large cerebral arteries.

Giant cell arteritis

Giant cell arteritis is the most common vasculitic cause of stroke and is associated particularly with posterior circulation ischemia (Nesher 2000; Ronthal *et al.* 2003; Eberhardt and Dhadly 2007). Medium and large arteries are affected, especially branches of the external carotid artery, the ophthalmic artery and the vertebral artery. The patients are elderly, with the diagnosis being rare under age 60 years. Malaise, polymyalgia and other systemic symptoms are frequently present. The erythrocyte sedimentation rate is usually raised, often to over 100 mm/h in the first hour.

Systemic lupus erythematosus

Systemic lupus erythematosus is more likely to cause a subacute or chronic generalized encephalopathy than symptomatic focal ischemia (Mills 1994; Moore 1997; Jennekens and Kater 2002a,b; D'Cruz *et al.* 2007). The underlying vascular pathology, where present, appears to be intimal proliferation rather than a vasculitis. The extracranial arteries are largely unaffected, but embolism from heart valve vegetations is quite common, particularly when there are circulating antiphospholipid antibodies (Mitsias and Levine 1994; Roldan *et al.* 1996). Intracranial venous thrombosis is rare (Vidailhet *et al.* 1990). In some patients with little clinical evidence of systemic lupus erythematosus, there is prominent livedo reticularis, which, when associated with stroke, is referred to as Sneddon's syndrome, in which antiphospholipid antibodies are particularly common (Stockhammer *et al.* 1993; Kalashnikova *et al.* 1994; Boesch *et al.* 2003; Hilton and Footitt 2003).

Antiphospholipid syndrome

Antiphospholipid syndrome is a constellation of various recurrent clinical events as well as specific immunological features: arterial and venous thrombosis, including recurrent ischemic stroke or TIA and intracranial venous thrombosis, migraine-like episodes, recurrent miscarriage, livedo reticularis, cardiac valvular vegetations, thrombocytopenia, false-positive syphilis serology and persistently raised circulating IgG anticardiolipin antibodies and/or the circulating lupus anticoagulant, usually detected by prolongation of the activated partial thromboplastin time (Katzav *et al.* 2003; Brey 2005; Sanna *et al.* 2005; Lim *et al.* 2006; Merrill 2007). Antiphospholipid antibodies are found in some normal people, and in systemic lupus erythematosus, hence an isolated finding of a raised antibody level in a patient with stroke is of uncertain significance. Antibodies are not uncommonly present after acute stroke, but only where they remain on retesting after six weeks should the diagnosis of antiphospholipid syndrome be made, particularly if other clinical features are lacking.

Primary systemic vasculitis

Primary systemic vasculitis is a group of related disorders including polyarteritis nodosa, Wegener's granulomatosis, the Churg–Strauss syndrome and various hypersensitivity vasculitides. Rarely, there is associated cerebrovascular disease, similar to that occurring in systemic lupus erythematosus (Futrell 1995; Savage *et al.* 1997; Ferro 1998). Stroke is usually lacunar (Reichhart *et al.* 2000) and there is often associated hematuria, eosinophilia, and circulating antineutrophil cytoplasmic antibodies.

Rheumatoid disease

Rheumatoid disease is rarely complicated by a systemic vasculitis, which can involve the brain (Genta *et al.* 2006). Occasionally atlanto-axial dislocation causes symptomatic vertebral artery compression (Howell and Molyneux 1988).

Sjögren's syndrome

Sjögren's syndrome is occasionally complicated by systemic vasculitis, causing focal cerebral ischemia, global encephalopathy and aseptic meningitis (Hietaharju *et al.* 1993; Bragoni *et al.* 1994; Delalande *et al.* 2004).

Behçet's disease

Neurological involvement in Behçet's disease may be subclassified into two major forms: a vascular–inflammatory process with focal or multifocal parenchymal involvement and a cerebral venous sinus thrombosis with intracranial hypertension. The vasculitis and meningitis may affect cerebral arteries, particularly in the posterior circulation, to cause ischemic stroke and possibly intracranial hemorrhage (Farah *et al.* 1998; Krespi *et al.* 2001; Siva *et al.* 2004; Borhani Haghighi *et al.* 2005).

Relapsing polychondritis

Relapsing polychondritis may be complicated by a generalized encephalopathy, stroke-like episodes and ischemic optic neuropathy as a result of systemic vasculitis (Stewart *et al.* 1988; Hsu *et al.* 2006).

Progressive systemic sclerosis

Progressive systemic sclerosis is hardly ever complicated directly by stroke, although a carotid and cerebral vasculopathy has been described (Heron *et al.* 1998; Lucivero *et al.* 2004).

Sarcoid angiitis

Sarcoid affects the cerebral vessels only rarely, usually causing a generalized encephalopathy rather than focal features owing to ischemia or hemorrhage (Zajicek 2000; Gullapalli and Phillips 2004; Spencer *et al.* 2005).

Primary vasculitis of the central nervous system

Primary vasculitis or isolated angiitis of the central nervous system (CNS) is a very rare disorder that affects leptomeningeal, cortical and sometimes spinal cord blood vessels. It is "isolated" in the sense that it is confined to the CNS. Histologically, it is similar to sarcoid angiitis and may occur in association with infections with herpes zoster, human immunodeficiency virus (HIV) and other pathogens. The course is subacute, often leading to death in weeks or months, with mental confusion and impairment, headache, vomiting, stroke-like episodes, and myelopathy. Systemic symptoms are very uncommon. Diagnosis is only really possible from meningeal/cortical biopsy (Hankey 1991; Vollmer *et al.* 1993; MacLaren *et al.* 2005).

Takayasu's disease

Takayasu's disease is a chronic vasculitis, histologically identical to giant cell arteritis but affecting only the aorta and large arteries arising from it; it occurs mainly in young Oriental women (Seko 2007). Systemic features are common, including malaise, weight loss, arthralgia and fever. Treatment is with immunosuppression, which may result in remission; occasionally surgery may be attempted (Liang and Hoffmann 2005). The neurological complications reflect progressive narrowing and eventual occlusion of the large arteries in the neck: claudication of the jaw muscles, ischemic oculopathy, syncope, seizures, confusion, boundary zone infarction and, rarely, focal ischemic stroke or TIAs (Hoffmann *et al.* 2000). In addition, there may be ischemia of the arms, and of the kidneys to cause hypertension, as well as ischemic necrosis of the lips, nasal septum and palate. Other causes of a similar aortic arch syndrome include advanced atheroma, giant cell arteritis, syphilis, subintimal fibrosis, arterial dissection, trauma and coarctation.

Buerger's disease

Buerger's disease or "thromboangiitis obliterans," is a rare inflammatory disorder of small and medium-sized arteries and veins, chiefly of the limbs and almost never of the cerebral circulation. It has a strong male preponderance and mainly affects smokers (Calguneri *et al.* 2004; Olin and Shih 2006).

Malignant atrophic papulosis

Malignant atrophic papulosis, or Dego's disease, is a very rare syndrome consisting of crops of painless pinkish papules on the trunk and limbs that heal as distinctive circular porcelain-white scars. It may be complicated by ischemic lesions in the gut, brain, spinal cord and nerve roots owing to endothelial proliferation in small arteries (Sotrel *et al.* 1983; Subbiah *et al.* 1996).

Acute posterior multifocal placoid pigment epitheliopathy

Acute posterior multifocal placoid pigment epitheliopathy is a rare and usually benign and self-limiting chorioretinal disorder, with rapidly deteriorating central vision. However, it can be complicated by systemic vasculitis, aseptic meningitis and stroke (Comu *et al.* 1996; de Vries *et al.* 2006).

Box 6.2. Hematological disorders causing ischemic stroke

Thrombophilia e.g. antithrombin III deficiency, protein C deficiency, factor V Leiden mutation,
    protein S deficiency, plasminogen abnormality or deficiency
Leukemia/lymphoma
Polycythemia
Essential thrombocythemia
Sickle cell disease/trait and other hemoglobinopathies
Iron-deficiency anemia
Paraproteinemias
Paroxysmal nocturnal hemoglobinuria
Thrombotic thrombocytopenic purpura
Disseminated intravascular coagulation

Hematological disorders

A number of hematological disorders may occasionally cause ischemic stroke and TIA
(Tatlisumak and Fisher 1996; Arboix and Besses 1997; Markus and Hambley 1998; Matijevic
and Wu 2006) (Box 6.2).

Thrombophilias

Thrombophilias and other causes of hypercoagulability are rare causes of stroke (Matijevic
and Wu 2006). Antithrombin III deficiency, protein C deficiency, activated protein C
resistance owing to factor V Leiden mutation, protein S deficiency and plasminogen
abnormality or deficiency can all cause peripheral and intracranial venous thrombosis.
Thrombosis is usually recurrent and there is often a family history. Thrombophilia may
cause arterial thrombosis, although the alternative diagnosis of paradoxical embolism
should always be considered in patients with these disorders. It should be noted that
deficiencies in any one of the factors associated with thrombophilia may be an incidental
finding and cannot necessarily be assumed to be the cause of stroke.

Leukemia and lymphoma

Leukemia and lymphoma may cause intracranial hemorrhage, particularly in acute myeloid
leukemia, most commonly through acute disseminated intravascular coagulation although
other hemostatic defects or CNS infiltration may be responsible (Rogers 2003; Glass 2006).
The hemorrhage is often fulminant, with bleeding usually occurring in the brain or
subdural compartment and occasionally in the subarachnoid space. Occasionally, cerebral
venous thrombosis or arterial occlusion may occur. **Malignant angioendotheliosis**, an
intravascular lymphoma, is a very rare cause of stroke-like episodes and progressive global
encephalopathy (Chapin *et al.* 1995; Zuckerman *et al.* 2006).

Polycythemia

Polycythemia is usually defined as a hematocrit above 0.50 in males and 0.47 in females.
Polycythemia rubra vera or primary polycythemia, a myeloproliferative disorder, may be
complicated by TIAs, ischemic stroke or intracranial venous thrombosis (Silverstein *et al.*
1962; Pearson and Wetherley-Mein 1978; Markus and Hambley 1998). Ischemic complications may occur because the platelet count is raised and platelet activity enhanced, or

because of increased whole-blood viscosity. Paradoxically, there may also be a hemostatic defect as a result of defective platelet function, resulting in intracranial hemorrhage. Increased stroke risk may also occur with secondary polycythemia caused by chronic hypoxia, smoking, congenital cyanotic heart disease, renal tumor or cerebellar hemangioblastoma.

Essential thrombocythemia

Essential thrombocythemia, or idiopathic primary thrombocytosis, is another myeloproliferative disorder in which the platelet count is raised, usually to over 1000×10^9 cells/l. Secondary thrombocytosis occurs in malignancy, splenectomy, hyposplenism, surgery, trauma, hemorrhage, iron deficiency, infections, polycythemia rubra vera, myelofibrosis and the leukemias. There is a tendency for arterial and venous thrombosis and, paradoxically, intracranial hemorrhage because the platelets are hemostatically defective (Arboix et al. 1995; Harrison et al. 1998; Mosso et al. 2004; Ogata et al. 2005).

Sickle cell disease and other hemoglobinopathies

Sickle cell disease and rarely other hemoglobinopathies may be complicated by ischemic stroke or intracranial hemorrhage (Razvi and Bone 2006; Switzer et al. 2006). Patients are usually children homozygous for the sickle gene, although sometimes a sickle cell crisis, provoked by hypoxia, may occur in an adult heterozygote. Small and large arteries, as well as veins, develop a fibrous vasculopathy and are occluded by thrombi as a result of the abnormally rigid red blood cells and raised whole blood viscosity, thrombocytosis and impaired fibrinolytic activity.

Iron-deficiency anemia

Severe iron-deficiency anemia causes non-specific neurological symptoms, which are presumably hypoxic in origin, including poor concentration, malaise, giddiness, fatigue and weakness. Occasionally, TIAs and ischemic strokes seem to be provoked by profound anemia in association with severe extracranial occlusive arterial disease or thrombocytosis (Akins et al. 1996; Keung and Owen 2004).

Paraproteinemias

Multiple myeloma and macroglobulinemia cause anemia through defective erythropoesis and thus produce non-specific neurological symptoms as described above. A hemostatic defect caused by reduced platelet number, and sometimes associated uremia, may cause intracranial hemorrhage. However, most of the "cerebral" features of these patients can be explained by the "hyperviscosity syndrome," which is characterized by headache, ataxia, diplopia, dysarthria, lethargy, drowsiness, poor concentration, visual blurring and deafness. The same syndrome can be seen in primary polycythemia or leukemia. Arterial or venous cerebral infarction may occur and at autopsy the microcirculation is occluded with acidophilic material thought to be precipitates of the abnormal proteins (Davies-Jones 1995). It is exceptional for patients with neurological involvement not to have a raised erythrocyte sedimentation rate.

Paroxysmal nocturnal hemoglobinuria

Paroxysmal nocturnal hemoglobinuria is a very rare acquired disorder in which hemopoietic stem cells become peculiarly sensitive to complement-mediated lysis. Venous and possibly arterial thrombosis occurs in the brain and elsewhere. Patients are nearly always anemic at neurological presentation and there may be a history of dark urine, evidence of hemolysis, and a low platelet and granulocyte count (Al-Hakim *et al.* 1993; Audebert *et al.* 2005).

Thrombotic thrombocytopenic purpura

Thrombotic thrombocytopenic purpura is a rare acute or subacute disease in adults, rather similar to the hemolytic uremic syndrome in children, in which there is systemic malaise, fever, skin purpura, renal failure, hematuria and proteinuria. Hemorrhagic infarcts caused by platelet microthrombi occur in many organs; in the brain they may cause stroke-like episodes (Matijevic and Wu 2006) although more commonly there is global encephalopathy. The blood film shows thrombocytopenia, hemolytic anemia and fragmented red cells. The differential diagnosis includes infective endocarditis, idiopathic thrombocytopenia, heparin-induced thrombocytopenia with thrombosis, systemic lupus erythematosus, non-bacterial thrombotic endocarditis and disseminated intravascular coagulation.

Disseminated intravascular coagulation

Widespread hemorrhagic brain infarcts and intracranial hemorrhages tend to cause an acute or subacute global encephalopathy rather than stroke-like episodes. The diagnosis is confirmed by a low platelet count, low plasma fibrinogen, and raised fibrin degradation products and D-dimer.

Miscellaneous rare causes

Other rare causes of cerebral ischemia or infarction include those listed in Table 6.1, some of which are discussed below.

Pregnancy and the puerperium

Pregnancy is complicated by stroke in approximately 10 per 100 000 deliveries in developed countries, about twice the background rate (Turan and Stern 2004; Helms and Kittner 2005; Hender *et al.* 2006). The risks of stroke are not increased during gestation except for an increased risk in the two days prior to birth. During the first six weeks and especially the first few days postpartum, there is an increased risk of ischemic stroke and intracerebral hemorrhage. The diagnostic and therapeutic approaches to stroke are similar during pregnancy and postpartum to those in non-pregnant patients except for consideration of the well-being of the fetus. There is a theoretical risk of MRI exposure during the first and second trimester, and the risk–benefit ratio should be considered in each case.

Causes of stroke particularly relevant to pregnancy include intracranial venous thrombosis, arterial dissection during labor, acute middle cerebral or other large artery occlusion, low-flow infarction and disseminated intravascular coagulation complicating eclampsia, vasoconstriction secondary to drugs, infective endocarditis, peripartum cardiomyopathy, sickle cell crisis and intracranial hemorrhage(s) caused by eclampsia, anticoagulants, rupture of a pre-existing aneurysm or vascular malformation. Paradoxical embolism via patent foramen ovale may possibly occur as the pregnant woman performs a Valsalva maneuver during labor. Metastases of choriocarcinoma can present with stroke-like episodes and on CT look remarkably like primary intracerebral hemorrhages. Many cases of pregnancy-associated stroke remain cryptogenic, and the risk of recurrent stroke in a future pregnancy is not known.

Migraine

Migraine increases the risk of stroke by approximately three-fold, and stroke may occur during a migraine attack or remote from it (Chang *et al.* 1999; Donaghy *et al.* 2002; Bousser and Welch 2005; Tietjen 2005). Cerebral ischemia can induce migrainous symptoms and, further, migraine aura may resemble TIA, causing diagnostic difficulty (Ch. 8). The term "migrainous stroke" should be reserved for a persisting focal neurological deficit that starts during a typical migrainous aura, with or without headache, and that mimics the symptomatology of previously experienced auras (Bousser *et al.* 1985). Such migrainous strokes usually cause a homonymous hemianopia or focal sensory deficit without persisting disability, and do not appear to recur very often (Hoekstra-van Dalen *et al.* 1996).

Sometimes arterial occlusion is demonstrated by angiography in migrainous stroke and the cause is hypothesized to be in-situ thrombosis complicating vasospasm. No provoking factors are known. Other possible causes of stroke in the context of headache must be considered: carotid dissection, mitochondrial cytopathy, ruptured vascular malformation, antiphospholipid antibody syndrome and CADASIL (cerebral autosomal dominant arteriopathy with subcortical infarcts and leukoencephalopathy). Migraine auras without headache may be confused with TIA (Ch. 8).

Epidemiological studies suggest the existence of close but complex relationships between estrogens, migraine and stroke in women before the menopause (Chang *et al.* 1999; Donaghy *et al.* 2002; Bousser 2004). Migraine, particularly without aura, is strongly influenced by estrogens, as illustrated by the frequency of onset at puberty, menstrual migraine and improvement during pregnancy. The risk of stroke with migraine is further increased by tobacco smoking and oral contraceptive use (Chang *et al.* 1999; Donaghy *et al.* 2002). The pathophysiological mechanism underlying these close relationships remains unknown. In practice, given the very low absolute risk of stroke in young women, there is no absolute contraindication to oral contraceptive use in young female migraineurs, but they should be advised strongly not to smoke and to use a form with a low estrogen content or progestogens, particularly if they experience migraine with aura. Elevated blood pressure, an important stroke risk factor, is less common in migraineurs.

Both ischemic stroke and migraine can be consequences of underlying vascular disorders. Hereditary conditions, including CADASIL, MELAS (mitochondrial myopathy, encephalopathy, lactic acidosis and stroke) and hereditary hemorrhagic telangiectasia, appear to predispose to both migraine and stroke. Acquired antiphospholipid antibodies, while not a cause of migraine per se, may increase the risk of infarction in migraineurs.

Possible mechanisms for migraine-associated stroke include:

- involvement of the vasculature, including vasospasm, arterial dissection and small vessel arteriopathy
- hypercoagulability, involving elevated von Willebrand factor, or platelet activation
- elevated risk of cardioembolism through patent foramen ovale, or from atrial septal aneurysm.

Triptans and ergotamines, used to treat acute migraine attacks, appear to be safe in low-risk populations but should be avoided in hemiplegic migraine, basilar migraine and in patients with prior cerebral or cardiac ischemia.

Cancer

Cancer may cause stroke (Rogers 2003) through:

- hemorrhage into primary tumors: malignant astrocytoma, oligodendroglioma, medulloblastoma, hemangioblastoma

- embolism of non-infected heart valve vegetations: non-bacterial thrombotic, or marantic, endocarditis
- infection: fungi, herpes zoster, bacterial endocarditis
- tumor emboli
- metastases: melanoma, germ cell tumors, choriocarcinoma, lung tumors, hypernephroma
- hemostatic failure: leukemias, with hyperviscosity syndrome or "hypercoagulability"
- disseminated intravascular coagulation
- intracranial venous thrombosis
- irradiation damage or neoplastic compression or invasion of neck arteries: may rarely cause ischemic stroke.

Perioperative stroke

Perioperative stroke complicates under 2% of non-cardiac surgical procedures. It can be caused by hypotension and boundary zone infarction, trauma to and dissection of neck arteries, paradoxical embolism, fat embolism, infective endocarditis, myocardial infarction, atrial fibrillation or a hemostatic defect caused by antithrombotic drugs or disseminated intravascular coagulation. It is more common in patients with previous strokes, other manifestations of vascular disease and chronic obstructive lung disease (Limburg *et al.* 1998). Simultaneous carotid endarterectomy and coronary bypass grafting (Ch. 27) is associated with 10–15% risk of death, stroke or myocardial infarction, and the risk is higher in those with bilateral as opposed to unilateral carotid disease (Naylor *et al.* 2003a, b).

Recreational drugs

The use of recreational drugs, including cocaine, amphetamines and opiates, shows a marked temporal association (often within minutes to an hour) with the onset of both hemorrhagic and ischemic stroke (Neimann *et al.* 2000; O'Connor *et al.* 2005). Possible mechanisms for drug-associated stroke include acute severe elevation of blood pressure, cardiac arrhythmia, cerebral vasospasm and embolization from foreign material injected with the diluents. Infective endocarditis, particularly associated with *Staphylococcus aureus*, is an important cause of stroke in intravenous drug users. Dilated cardiomyopathy may also occur. Rupture of aneurysms and arteriovenous malformations have been detected in up to half of the patients with hemorrhagic stroke caused by cocaine abuse. Amphetamines can cause a small vessel vasculopathy, leading to intracerebral hemorrhage or infarction (Heye and Hankey 1996). Other sympathomimetic drugs such as ephedrine, phenylpropanolamine, fenfluramine and phentermine may cause stroke by similar mechanisms, as can ecstasy (3,4-methylenedioxy-*N*-methylamphetamine) (Wen *et al.* 1997).

Chronic meningitis

Meningitis caused by tuberculous, syphilitic and fungal infections may involve the arteries at the base of the brain, or the perforating arteries, and so be complicated by ischemic stroke and intracranial hemorrhage. Very occasionally, acute local infections such as tonsillitis, pharyngitis or lymphadenitis can cause inflammation and secondary thrombosis in the carotid artery in the neck (Lemierre's syndrome). Otitis media or mastoiditis may cause dural sinus thrombosis. Cerebral arterial and venous thrombosis may result from bacterial meningitis, ophthalmic herpes zoster, chicken pox, leptospirosis, HIV infection, cat scratch disease, neurotrichinosis and possibly borreliosis.

Inflammatory bowel disease

Both ulcerative and Crohn's colitis may occasionally be complicated by intracranial venous thrombosis, arterial occlusion and intracerebral hemorrhage (Lossos *et al.* 1995). Mechanisms include thrombocytosis, hyper-coagulability, immobility and paradoxical embolism, vasculitis and dehydration. The bowel disease is not necessarily severe at the time of the stroke. Coeliac disease can also be complicated by a cerebral vasculitis but this often presents with an encephalopathy rather than a stroke (Mumford *et al.* 1996).

Mitochondrial cytopathy

Mitochondrial cytopathy may present with stroke-like episodes often complicated by epilepsy and encephalopathy, a particular example of which is MELAS. Scanning with CT may show hypodensities, particularly in the occipital regions, and calcification of the

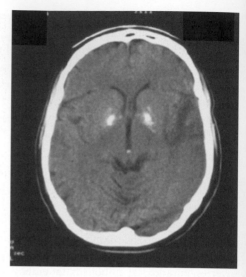

Fig. 6.10. A CT brain scan of a 40-year-old man with mitochondrial cytopathy, showing calcification of the basal ganglia and hypodensity in the left temporal lobe.

basal ganglia (Fig. 6.10). In MRI, there are T_2-weighted hyperintensities in the temporo-occipitoparietal regions that do not correspond to classical vascular territories (Fig. 6.11) and that may disappear on subsequent scans. Other clinical features often associated with mitochondrial disease include migraine, short stature, sensorineural deafness, diabetes and learning disability. The blood and CSF lactate are usually raised; most patients have an abnormal muscle biopsy, and diagnosis can often be made by detection of the relevant genetic mutations.

Fabry's disease

Fabry's disease is occasionally complicated by ischemic stroke, particularly in the vertebro-basilar territory, but usually not until after other more common features are well established (Meschia *et al.* 2005; Razvi and Bone 2006; Rolfs *et al.* 2005).

Homocystinuria

Homocystinuria is an autosomal recessive inborn error of metabolism that is complicated by cerebral arterial or venous thrombosis (Schimke *et al.* 1965; Visy *et al.* 1991; Rubba *et al.* 1994). Heterozygotes may have an increased risk of vascular disease.

Hypoglycemia

Hypoglycemic drugs, and rarely an insulinoma, are a well-recognized but uncommon cause of transient focal neurological episodes and may be misdiagnosed as TIA (Ch. 8). These episodes tend to occur on waking in the morning or after exercise, and by the time the patient is seen, the blood glucose may well have returned to normal. Persisting focal deficits are unusual (Malouf and Brust 1985; Wallis *et al.* 1985; Service 1995; Shanmugam *et al.* 1997).

Hypercalcemia (Longo and Witherspoon 1980) and **hyponatremia** (Ruby and Burton 1977; Berkovic *et al.* 1984) have been reported to cause TIA-like episodes.

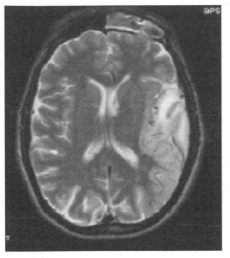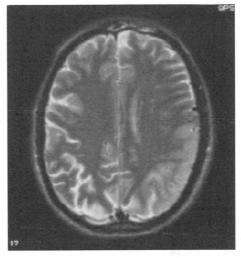

Fig. 6.11. These T_2-weighted MRI images of the brain are from a patient with mitochondrial cytopathy and show primarily cortical hyperintensity in the left temporoparietal region not typical of middle cerebral artery branch infarction.

Fat embolism

Fat embolism, which usually occurs following long bone fracture or surgery, most commonly causes a global encephalopathy, but on occasion there may be focal features, presumably reflecting local ischemia (Jacobson *et al.* 1986; van Oostenbrugge *et al.* 1996).

Fibrocartilaginous embolism

Fibrocartilaginous embolism is a rare and curious disorder where fibrocartilaginous emboli, presumably from degenerative intervertebral disc material, are found in various organs, the spinal cord more often than the brain (Freyaldenhoven *et al.* 2001).

Snake bite

Injection of venom may cause intracranial hemorrhage as a consequence of defibrination and other hemostatic defects, and rarely ischemic stroke (Bashir and Jinkins 1985).

Epidermal naevus syndrome, a sporadic neurocutaneous disorder, can be complicated by stroke (Dobyns and Garg 1991).

Susac's syndrome

Susac's syndrome is a rare triad of branch retinal artery occlusions, hearing loss and microangiopathy of the brain causing a subacute encephalopathy, almost always in women (Gross and Eliashar 2005).

References

Adachi T, Takagi M, Hoshino H *et al.* (1997). Effect of extracranial carotid artery stenosis and other risk factors for stroke on periventricular hyperintensity. *Stroke* 28:2174–2179

Akins PT, Glen S, Nemeth PM *et al.* (1996). Carotid artery thrombus associated with severe iron-deficiency anemia and thrombocytosis. *Stroke* 27:1002–1005

Al-Hakim M, Katirji MB, Osorio I *et al.* (1993). Cerebral venous thrombosis in paroxysmal nocturnal haemoglobinuria: report of two cases. *Neurology* 43:742–746

Amarenco P (2005). Patent foramen ovale and the risk of stroke: smoking gun, guilty by association? *Heart* 91:441–443

Amarenco P, Cohen A, Tzourio C et al. (1994). Atherosclerotic disease of the aortic arch and the risk of ischemic stroke. *New England Journal of Medicine* 331:1474–1479

Aoyagi M, Fukai N, Yamamoto M et al. (1996). Early development of intimal thickening in superficial temporal arteries in patients with Moyamoya disease. *Stroke* 27:1750–1754

Arboix A, Besses C (1997). Cerebrovascular disease as the initial clinical presentation of hematological disorders. *European Neurology* 37:207–211

Arboix A, Besses C, Acin P et al. (1995). Ischemic stroke as first manifestation of essential thrombocythemia. Report of six cases. *Stroke* 26:1463–1466

Arunodaya GR, Vani S, Shankar SK et al. (1997). Fibromuscular dysplasia with dissection of basilar artery presenting as "locked-in-syndrome." *Neurology* 48:1605–1608

Audebert HJ, Planck J, Eisenburg M et al. (2005). Cerebral ischemic infarction in paroxysmal nocturnal haemoglobinuria: report of 2 cases and updated review of 7 previously published patients. *Journal of Neurology* 252:1379–1386

Auer A, Felber S, Schmidauer C et al. (1998). Magnetic resonance angiographic and clinical features of extracranial vertebral artery dissection. *Journal of Neurology, Neurosurgery and Psychiatry* 64:474–481

Ayas N, Wijdicks EFM (1995). Cardiac catheterization complicated by stroke: 14 patients. *Cerebrovascular Diseases* 5:304–307

Bamford J, Sandercock PAG, Jones L et al. (1987). The natural history of lacunar infarction: the Oxfordshire Community Stroke Project. *Stroke* 18:545–551

Bashir R, Jinkins J (1985). Cerebral infarction in a young female following snake bite. *Stroke* 16:328–330

Bathen J, Sparr S, Rokseth R (1978). Embolism in sinoatrial disease. *Acta Medica Scandinavica* 203:7–11

Berkovic SF, Bladin PF, Darby DG (1984). Metabolic disorders presenting as stroke. *Medical Journal of Australia* 140:421–424

Bitzer M, Topka H (1995). Progressive cerebral occlusive disease after radiation therapy. *Stroke* 26:131–136

Boesch SM, Plorer AL, Auer AJ et al. (2003). The natural course of Sneddon syndrome: clinical and magnetic resonance imaging findings in a prospective six year observation study. *Journal of Neurology, Neurosurgery and Psychiatry* 74:542–544

Boiten J, Rothwell PM, Slattery J et al. (1996). Ischemic lacunar stroke in the European Carotid Surgery Trial. Risk factors, distribution of carotid stenosis, effect of surgery and type of recurrent stroke. *Cerebrovascular Diseases* 6:281–287

Boon A, Lodder J, Cheriex E et al. (1996). Risk of stroke in a cohort of 815 patients with calcification of the aortic valve with or without stenosis. *Stroke* 27:847–851

Borhani Haghighi A, Pourmand R, Nikseresht AR (2005). Neuro–Behçet disease. A review. *Neurologist* 11:80–89

Bots ML, van Swieten JC, Breteler MMB et al. (1993). Cerebral white matter lesions and atherosclerosis in the Rotterdam study. *Lancet* 341:1232–1237

Bousser MG (2004). Estrogens, migraine and stroke. *Stroke* 35:2652–2656

Bousser MG, Welch KM (2005). Relation between migraine and stroke. *Lancet Neurology* 4:533–534

Bousser MG, Baron JC, Chiras J (1985). Ischemic strokes and migraine. *Neuroradiology* 27:583–587

Bowen J, Boudoulas H, Wooley CF (1987). Cardiovascular disease of connective tissue origin. *American Journal of Medicine* 82:481–488

Bragoni M, Di Piero V, Priori R et al. (1994). Sjögren's syndrome presenting as ischemic stroke. *Stroke* 25:2276–2279

Brey RL (2005). Antiphospholipid antibodies in young adults with stroke. *Journal of Thrombosis and Thombolysis* 20:105–112

Bruno A, Adams HP, Biller J et al. (1988). Cerebral infarction due to moyamoya disease in young adults. *Stroke* 19:826–833

Cabanes L, Mas JL, Cohen A et al. (1993). Atrial septal aneurysm and patent foramen ovale as risk factors for cryptogenic stroke in patients less than 55 years of age. A study using transoesophageal echocardiography. *Stroke* 24:1865–1873

Calguneri M, Ozturk MA, Ay H et al. (2004). Buerger's disease with multisystem involvement. A case report and a review of the literature. *Angiology* 55:325–328

Caplan LR (1995). Binswanger's disease: revisited. *Neurology* 45:626–633

Catala M, Rancurel G, Koskas F et al. (1993). Ischemic stroke due to spontaneous extracranial vertebral giant aneurysm. *Cerebrovascular Diseases* 3:322–326

Chang CL, Donaghy M, Poulter N et al. (1999). Migraine and stroke in young women: case–control study. *British Medical Journal* 318:13–18

Chapin JE, Davis LE, Kornfeld M et al. (1995). Neurologic manifestations of intravascular lymphomatosis. *Acta Neurology Scandinavica* 91:494–499

Chaves C, Estol C, Esnaola MM et al. (2002). Spontaneous intracranial internal carotid artery dissection: report of 10 patients. *Archives of Neurology* 59:977–981

Chiu D, Shedden P, Bratina P et al. (1998). Clinical features of moyamoya disease in the United States. *Stroke* 29:1347–1351

CODICE Study Group (2006). Recurrent stroke is not associated with massive right-to-left shunt: preliminary results from the 3-year prospective Spanish Multicentre Centre (CODICE study). *Cerebrovascular Diseases* 21:1

Comu S, Verstraeten T, Rinkoff JS et al. (1996). Neurological manifestations of acute posterior multifocal placoid pigment epitheliopathy. *Stroke* 27:996–1001

Coull AJ, Lovett JK, Rothwell PM et al. (2004). Population based study of early risk of stroke after transient ischemic attack or minor stroke: implications for public education and organisation of services. *British Medical Journal* 328:326

Cramer SC, Robertson RL, Dooling EC et al. (1996). Moyamoya and Down syndrome. Clinical and radiological features. *Stroke* 27:2131–2135

Cross SS (1991). How common is cholesterol embolism? *Journal of Clinical Pathology* 44:859–861

D'Cruz DP, Khamashta MA, Hughes GR (2007). Systemic lupus erythematosus. *Lancet* 369:587–596

Davies-Jones GAB (1995). Neurological manifestations of hematological disorders. In *Neurology and General Medicine*, 2nd edn,

Aminoff MJ (ed.), pp. 219–245. New York: Churchill Livingstone.

Davis JM, Zimmerman RA (1983). Injury of the carotid and vertebral arteries. *Neuroradiology* 25:55–69

de Bray JM, Penisson-Besnier I, Dubas F et al. (1997). Extracranial and intracranial vertebrobasilar dissections: diagnosis and prognosis. *Journal of Neurology, Neurosurgery and Psychiatry* 63:46–51

Delalande S, de Seze J, Fauchais AL et al. (2004). Neurologic manifestations in primary Sjögren syndrome: a study of 82 patients. *Medicine (Baltimore)* 83:280–291

Desai B, Toole JF (1975). Kinks, coils and carotids: a review. *Stroke* 6:649–653

De Vries JJ, den Dunnen WF, Timmerman EA et al. (2006). Acute posterior multifocal placoid pigment epitheliopathy with cerebral vasculitis: a multisystem granulomatous disease. *Archives of Ophthalmology* 124:910–913

Diener HC, Weimar C, Katsarava Z (2005). Patent foramen ovale: paradoxical connection to migraine and stroke. *Current Opinion in Neurology* 18:299–304

Dittrich R, Ritter MA, Kaps M et al. (2006). The use of embolic signal detection in multicenter trials to evaluate antiplatelet efficacy: signal analysis and quality control mechanisms in the CARESS (Clopidogrel and Aspirin for Reduction of Emboli in Symptomatic carotid Stenosis) trial. *Stroke* 37:1065–1069

Dobyns WB, Garg BP (1991). Vascular abnormalities in epidermal nevus syndrome. *Neurology* 41:276–278

Donaghy M, Chang CL, Poulter N et al. (2002). European Collaborators of the World Health Organization Collaborative Study of Cardiovascular Disease and Steroid Hormone Contraception. Duration, frequency, recency, and type of migraine and the risk of ischemic stroke in women of childbearing age. *Journal of Neurology, Neurosurgery and Psychiatry* 73:747–750

Dutta M, Hanna E, Das P et al. (2006a). Incidence and prevention of ischemic stroke following myocardial infarction: review of current literature. *Cerebrovascular Diseases* 22:331–339

Dutta M, Karas MG, Segal AZ et al. (2006b). Yield of transoesophageal echocardiography for nonbacterial thrombotic endocarditis and other cardiac sources of embolism in cancer patients with cerebral ischemia. *American Journal of Cardiology* **97**:894–898

Eberhardt RT, Dhadly M (2007). Giant cell arteritis: diagnosis management and cardiovascular implications. *Cardiology Reviews* **15**:55–61

Ekinci EI, Donnan GA (2004). Neurological manifestations of cardiac myxoma: a review of the literature and report of cases. *Internal Medicine Journal* **34**:243–249

Farah S, Al-Shubaili A, Montaser A *et al.* (1998). Behçets syndrome: a report of 41 patients with emphasis on neurological manifestations. *Journal of Neurology, Neurosurgery and Psychiatry* **64**:382–384

Farrell MA, Gilbert JJ, Kaufman JCE (1985). Fatal intracranial arterial dissection: clinical pathological correlation. *Journal of Neurology, Neurosurgery and Psychiatry* **48**:111–121

Feldmann E, Daneault N, Kwan E *et al.* (1990). Chinese–white differences in the distribution of occlusive cerebrovascular disease. *Neurology* **40**:1541–1545

Ferro JM (1998). Vasculitis of the central nervous system. *Journal of Neurology* **245**:766–776

Fisher CM (1979). Capsular infarcts: the underlying vascular lesions. *Archives of Neurology and Psychiatry* **36**:65–73

Fisher CM, Caplan LR (1971). Basilar artery branch occlusion: a cause of pontine infarction. *Neurology* **21**:900–905

Flis CM, Jager HR, Sidhu PS (2007). Carotid and vertebral artery dissections: clinical aspects imaging features and endovascular treatment. *European Radiology* **17**:820–834

Freyaldenhoven TE, Mrak RE, Rock L (2001). Fibrocartilaginous embolization. *Neurology* **56**:1354

Futrell N (1995). Inflammatory vascular disorders: diagnosis and treatment in ischemic stroke. *Current Opinions in Neurology* **8**:55–61

Gan R, Sacco RL, Kargman DE *et al.* (1997). Testing the validity of the lacunar hypothesis: the Northern Manhattan Stroke Study experience. *Neurology* **48**:1204–1211

Gautier JC, Durr A, Koussa S *et al.* (1991). Paradoxical cerebral embolism with a patent foramen ovale. A report of 29 patients. *Cerebrovascular Diseases* **1**:193–202

Genta MS, Genta RM, Gabay C (2006). Systemic rheumatoid vasculitis: a review. *Seminars in Arthritis and Rheumatism* **36**:88–98

Glass J (2006). Neurologic complications of lymphoma and leukemia. *Seminars in Oncology* **33**:342–347

Goldschmidt-Clermont PJ, Creager MA, Lorsordo DW *et al.* (2005). Atherosclerosis 2005: recent discoveries and novel hypotheses *Circulation* **112**:3348–3353

Gorter JW for the Stroke Prevention in Reversible Ischemia Trial (SPIRIT) and the European Atrial Fibrillation Trial (EAFT) Study Groups (1999). Major bleeding during anticoagulation after cerebral ischemia: patterns and risk factors. *Neurology* **53**:1319–1327

Gotto AM Jr., (2005). Evolving concepts of dyslipidaemia, atherosclerosis and cardiovascular disease: the Louis F Bishop Lecture. *Journal of American College of Cardiology* **46**:1219–1224

Griewing B, Guo Y, Doherty C *et al.* (1995). Radiation-induced injury to the carotid artery: a longitudinal study. *European Journal of Neurology* **2**:379–383

Gross M, Eliashar R (2005). Update on Susac's syndrome. *Current Opinions in Neurology* **18**:311–314

Gullapalli D, Phillips LH, II (2004). Neurosarcoidosis. *Current Neurology and Neuroscience Reports* **4**:441–447

Hankey GJ (1991). Isolated angiitis/angiopathy of the central nervous system. *Cerebrovascular Diseases* **1**:2–15

Harrison CN, Linch DC, Machin SJ (1998). Desirability and problems of early diagnosis of essential thrombocythemia. *Lancet* **351**:846–847

Hart RG, Foster JW, Lutner MF *et al.* (1990). Stroke in infective endocarditis. *Stroke* **21**:695–700

Heinzlef O, Cohen A, Amarenco P (1997). An update on aortic causes of ischemic stroke. *Current Opinions in Neurology* **10**:64–72

Helms AK, Kittner SJ (2005). Pregnancy and stroke. *CNS Spectroscopy* **10**:580–587

Hender J, Harris DG, Bu H *et al.* (2006). Stroke in pregnancy. *British Journal of Hospital Medicine* **67**:129–131

Heron E, Fornes P, Rance A *et al.* (1998). Brain involvement in scleroderma. Two autopsy cases. *Stroke* **29**:719–721

Heye N, Hankey GJ (1996). Amphetamine-associated stroke. *Cerebrovascular Diseases* 6:149–155

Hietaharju A, Jantti V, Korpela M *et al.* (1993). Nervous system involvement in systemic lupus erythematus, Sjögren syndrome and scleroderma. *Acta Neurology Scandinavica* 88:299–308

Hilton DA, Footitt D (2003). Neuropathological findings in Sneddon's syndrome. *Neurology* 60:1181–1182

Hoekstra-van Dalen RAH, Cillessen JPM, Kappelle LJ *et al.* (1996). Cerebral infarcts associated with migraine: clinical features, risk factors and follow up. *Journal of Neurology* 243:511–515

Hoffmann M, Corr P, Robbs J (2000). Cerebrovascular findings in Takayasu disease. *Journal of Neuroimaging* 10:84–90

Holmes DR Jr., (2004). Strokes and holes and headaches: are they a package deal? *Lancet* 364:1840–1842

Homma S, Sacco RL (2005). Patent foramen ovale and stroke. *Circulation* 112:1063–1072

Howell SJL, Molyneux AJ (1988). Vertebrobasilar insufficiency in rheumatoid atlanto-axial subluxation: a case report with angiographic demonstration of left vertebral artery occlusion. *Journal of Neurology* 235:189–190

Hsu KC, Wu YR, Lyu RK *et al.* (2006). Aseptic meningitis and ischemic stroke in relapsing polychondritis. *Clinical Rheumatology* 25:265–267

Inzitari D (2003). Leukoariaosis: an independent risk factor for stroke? *Stroke* 34:2067–2071

Iwama T, Hashimoto N, Murai BN *et al.* (1997). Intracranial rebleeding in moyamoya disease. *Journal of Clinical Neuroscience* 4:169–172

Jacobson DM, Terrence CF, Reinmuth OM (1986). The neurological manifestations of fat embolism. *Neurology* 36:847–851

Jeanrenaud X, Kappenberger L (1991). Patent foramen ovale and stroke of unknown origin. *Cerebrovascular Diseases* 1:184–192

Jennekens FG, Kater L (2002a). The central nervous system in systemic lupus erythematous. Part 1. Clinical syndromes: a literature investigation. *Rheumatology (Oxford)* 41:605–618

Jennekens FG, Kater L (2002b). The central nervous system in systemic lups erythematosus.

Part 2. Pathogenic mechanisms of clinical syndromes: a literature investigation. *Rheumatology (Oxford)* 41:619–630

Jones EF, Kalman JM, Calafiore P *et al.* (1995). Proximal aortic atheroma. An independent risk factor for cerebral ischemia. *Stroke* 26:218–224

Jones HR, Siekert RG (1989). Neurological manifestations of infective endocarditis: review of clinical and therapeutic challenges. *Brain* 112:1295–1315

Kalashnikova LA, Nasonov EL, Stoyanovich LZ *et al.* (1994). Sneddon's syndrome and the primary antiphospholipid syndrome. *Cerebrovascular Diseases* 4:76–82

Kanter MC, Hart RG (1991). Neurologic complications of infective endocarditis. *Neurology* 41:1015–1020

Kaposzta Z, Young E, Bath PMW *et al.* (1999). Clinical application of asymptomatic embolic signal detection in acute stroke: a prospective study. *Stroke* 30:1814–1818

Katzav A, Chapman J, Shoenfeld Y (2003). CNS dysfunction in the antiphospholipid syndrome. *Lupus* 12:903–907

Keung YK, Owen J (2004). Iron deficiency and thrombosis: literature review. *Clinical and Applied Thrombolysis and Hemostasis* 10:387–391

Kitahara T, Ariga N, Yamaura A *et al.* (1979). Familial occurrence of moya-moya disease: report of three Japanese families. *Journal of Neurology, Neurosurgery and Psychiatry* 42:208–214

Kizer JR, Devereux RB (2005). Clinical practice. Patent foramen ovale in young adults with unexplained stroke. *New England Journal of Medicine* 353:2361–2372

Koennecke H, Mast H, Trocio SH *et al.* (1998). Frequency and determinants of microembolic signals on transcranial Doppler in unselected patients with acute carotid territory ischemia. A prospective study. *Cerebrovascular Diseases* 8:107–112

Krapf H, Skalej M, Voigt K (1999). Subarachnoid hemorrhage due to septic embolic infarction in infective endocarditis. *Cerebrovascular Diseases* 9:182–184

Krespi Y, Akman-Demir G, Poyraz M *et al.* (2001). Cerebral vasculitis and ischemic stroke in Behçet's disease: report of one case and review of the literature. *European Journal of Neurology* 8:719–722

Kwa VIH, Franke CL, Verbeeten B *et al.* (1998). Silent intracerebral microhemorrhages in patients with ischemic stroke for the Amsterdam Vascular Medicine Group. *Annals of Neurology* **44**:372–377

Labovitz DL, Boden-Albala B, Hauser WA *et al.* (2007). Lacunar infarct or deep intracerebral hemorrhage: who gets which? The Northern Manhattan Study. *Neurology* **68**:606–608

Lammie GA, Brannan F, Slattery J *et al.* (1997). Nonhypertensive cerebral small-vessel disease. An autopsy study. *Stroke* **28**:2222–2229

Lamy C, Giannesini C, Zuber M *et al.* (2002). Clinical and imaging findings in cryptogenic stroke patients with and without patent foramen ovale: the PFO–ASA Study (Atrial Septal Aneurysm). *Stroke* **33**:706–711

Leung SY, Ng THK, Yuen ST *et al.* (1993). Pattern of cerebral atherosclerosis in Hong Kong Chinese: severity in intracranial and extracranial vessels. *Stroke* **24**:779–786

Leys D, Moulin Th, Stojkovic T *et al.* (1995). Follow-up of patients with history of cervical artery dissection. *Cerebrovascular Diseases* **5**:43–49

Lhermitte F, Gautier JC, Derouesne C (1970). Nature of occlusions of the middle cerebral artery. *Neurology* **20**:82–88

Liang P and Hoffmann GS (2005). Advances in the medical and surgical treatment of Takayasu arteritis. *Current Opinions in Rheumatology* **17**:16–24

Lim W, Crowther MA, Eikelboom JW (2006). Management of antiphospholipid antibody syndrome: a systematic review. *Journal of the American Medical Association* **295**:1050–1057

Limburg M, Wijdicks EF, Li H (1998). Ischemic stroke after surgical procedures: clinical features, neuroimaging and risk factors. *Neurology* **50**:895–901

Loh E, St John Sutton MS, Wun CC *et al.* (1997). Ventricular dysfunction and the risk of stroke after myocardial infarction. *New England Journal of Medicine* **336**:251–257

Longo DL, Witherspoon JM (1980). Focal neurologic symptoms in hypercalcemia. *Neurology* **30**:200–201

Lossos A, River Y, Eliakim A, Steiner I (1995). Neurologic aspects of inflammatory bowel disease. *Neurology* **45**:416–421

Lovett JK, Gallagher PJ, Hands LJ *et al.* (2004). Histological correlates of carotid plaque surface morphology on lumen contrast imaging. *Circulation* **110**:2190–2197

Lucivero V, Mezzapesa DM, Petruzzellis M *et al.* (2004). Ischemic stroke in progressive system sclerosis. *Neurology Science* **25**:230–233

MacLaren K, Gillespie J, Shrestha S *et al.* (2005). Primary angitis of the central nervous system: emerging variants. *Quarterly Journal of Medicine* **98**:643–654

Macleod MR, Amarenco P, Davis SM *et al.* (2004). Atheroma of the aortic arch: an important and poorly recognized factor in the aetiology of stroke. *Lancet Neurology* **3**:408–414

Malouf R, Brust JCM (1985). Hypoglycemia: causes, neurological manifestations and outcome. *Annals of Neurology* **17**:421–430

Markus HS (2006). Can microemboli on transcranial Doppler identify patients at increased stroke risk? *Nature Clinical Practice in Cardiovascular Medicine* **3**:246–247

Markus HS, Hambley H (1998). Neurology and the blood: hematological abnormalities in ischemic stroke. *Journal of Neurology, Neurosurgery and Psychiatry* **64**:150–159

Martin R, Bogousslavsky J for the Lausanne Stroke Registry Group (1993). Mechanisms of late stroke after myocardial infarct: the Lausanne Stroke Registry. *Journal of Neurology, Neurosurgery and Psychiatry* **56**:760–764

Mas JL (2003). Specifics of patent foramen ovale. *Advances in Neurology* **92**:197–202

Mas JL, Arquizan C, Lamy C *et al.* (2001). Patent Foramen Ovale and Atrial Septal Aneurysm Study Group. Recurrent cerebrovascular events associated with patent foramen ovale atrial septal aneurysm or both. *New England Journal of Medicine* **345**:1740–1746

Masuda J, Yutani C, Waki R *et al.* (1992). Histopathological analysis of the mechanisms of intracranial haemorrhage complicating infective endocarditis. *Stroke* **23**:843–850

Matijevic N, Wu K (2006). Hypercoagulable states and strokes. *Current Atherosclerosis Reports* **8**:324–329

Mayer SA, Tatemichi TK, Spitz JL *et al.* (1994). Recurrent ischemic events and diffuse white matter disease in patients with pseudoxanthoma elasticum. *Cerebrovascular Diseases* **4**:294–297

Merrill JT (2007). Antiphospholipid syndrome: what's new in understanding antiphospholipid antibydo-related stroke? *Current Rheumatology Reports* **8**:159–161

Meschia JF, Brott TG, Brown RD Jr., (2005). Genetics of cerebrovascular disorders. *Mayo Clinic Proceedings* **80**:122–132

Messe SR, Cucchiara B, Luciano J *et al.* (2005). PFO management: neurologists vs cardiologists. *Neurology* **65**:172–173

Metz H, Murray-Leslie RM, Bannister RG *et al.* (1961). Kinking of the internal carotid artery. *Lancet* **i**:424–426

Millikan C, Futrell N (1990). The fallacy of the lacune hypothesis. *Stroke* **21**:1251–1257

Mills JA (1994). Systemic lupus erythematosus. *New England Journal of Medicine* **330**:1871–1879

Mitchell JRA, Schwartz CJ (1962). Relationship between arterial disease in different sites. A study of the aorta and coronary carotid and iliac arteries. *British Medical Journal* **i**:1293–1301

Mitsias P, Levine SR (1994). Large cerebral vessel occlusive disease in systemic lupus erythematosus. *Neurology* **44**:385–393

Molloy J, Markus HS (1999). Asymptomatic embolization predicts stroke and TIA risk in patients with carotid artery stenosis. *Stroke* **30**:1440–1443

Moore PM (1997). Neuropsychiatric systemic lupus erythematosus. Stress, stroke and seizures. *Annals of the New York Academy of Sciences* **823**:1–17

Mosso M, Georgiadis D, Baumgartner RW (2004). Progressive occlusive disease of large cerebral arteries and ischemic events in a patient with essential thrombocythemia. *Neurology Research* **26**:702–703

Mumford CJ, Fletcher NA, Ironside JW *et al.* (1996). Progressive ataxia, focal seizures and malabsorption syndrome in a 41 year old woman. *Journal of Neurology, Neurosurgery and Psychiatry* **60**:225–230

Munoz DG (2006). Leukoaraiosis and ischemia: beyond the myth. *Stroke* **37**:1348–1349

Naylor AR, Cuffe RL, Rothwell PM *et al.* (2003a). A systematic review of outcomes following staged and synchronous carotid endarterectomy and coronary artery bypass. *European Journal of Vascular Endovascular Surgery* **25**:380–389

Naylor R, Cuffe RL, Rothwell PM *et al.* (2003b). A systematic review of outcome following synchronous carotid endarterectomy and coronary artery bypass: influence of surgical and patient variables. *European Journal of Vascular Endovascular Surgery* **26**:230–241

Neimann J, Haapaniemi HM, Hillbom M (2000). Neurological complications of drug abuse: pathophysiological mechanisms. *European Journal of Neurology* **7**:595–606

Nesher G (2000). Neurologic manifestations of giant cell arteritis. *Clinical Experimental Rheumatology* **18**:S24–S26

Newman MF, Matthew JP, Grocott HP *et al.* (2006). Central nervous system injury associated with cardiac surgery. *Lancet* **368**:694–703

North KN, Whiteman DAH, Pepin MG *et al.* (1995). Cerebrovascular complications in Ehlers–Danlos syndrome type IV. *Annals of Neurology* **38**:960–964

O'Connell BK, Towfighi J, Brennan RW *et al.* (1985). Dissecting aneurysms of head and neck. *Neurology* **35**:993–997

O'Connor AD, Rusyniak DE, Bruno A (2005). Cerebrovascular and cardiovascular complications of alcohol and sympathomimetic drug abuse. *Medical Clinics of North America* **89**:1343–1358

O'Connor MM, Mayberg MR (2000). Effects of radiation on cerebral vasculature: a review. *Neurosurgery* **46**:138–149

Ogata J, Masuda J, Yutani C *et al.* (1994). Mechanisms of cerebral artery thrombosis: a histopathological analysis on eight necropsy cases. *Journal of Neurology, Neurosurgery and Psychiatry* **57**:17–21

Ogata J, Yonemura K, Kimura K *et al.* (2005). Cerebral infarction associated with essential thrombocythemia: an autopsy case study. *Cerebrovascular Diseases* **19**:201–205

Olin JW, Shih A (2006). Thromboangiitis obliterans (Buerger's disease). *Current Opinions in Rheumatology* **18**:18–24

Orencia AJ, Petty GW, Khandheria BK *et al.* (1995a). Risk of stroke with mitral valve prolapse in population-based cohort study. *Stroke* **26**:7–13

Orencia AJ, Petty GW, Khandheria BK, Fallon WM, Whishant JP (1995b). Mitral valve prolapse and the risk of stroke after initial cerebral ischemia. *Neurology* **45**:1083–1086

Pantoni L, Garcia JH (1997). Pathogenesis of leukoariaosis. A review. *Stroke* 28:652–659

Pearson TC, Wetherley-Mein G (1978). Vascular occlusive episodes and venous hematocrit in primary proliferative polycythemia. *Lancet* ii:1219–1222

Powers WJ (1986). Should lumbar puncture be part of the routine evaluation of patients with cerebral ischemia? *Stroke* 17:332–333

Prior AL, Wilson LA, Gosling RG et al. (1979). Retrograde cerebral embolism. *Lancet* ii:1044–1047

Razvi SS, Bone I (2006). Single gene disorders causing ischemic stroke. *Journal of Neurology* 253:685–700

Redgrave JN, Lovett JK, Gallagher PJ et al. (2006). Histological assessment of 526 symptomatic carotid plaques in relation to the nature and timing of ischemic symptoms: the Oxford Plaque Study. *Circulation* 113:2320–2328

Reichart MD, Bogousslavsky J, Janzer RC (2000). Early lacunar strokes complicating polyarteritis nodosa: thrombotic microangiopathy. *Neurology* 54:883–889

Rhodes (1996). Cholesterol crystal embolism: an important "new" diagnosis for the general physician. *Lancet* 347:1641

Rogers LR (2003). Cerebrovascular complications in cancer patients. *Neurology Clinic* 21:167–192

Roldan CA, Shively BK, Crawford MH (1996). An echocardiographic study of valvular heart disease associated with systematic lupus erythematosus. *New England Journal of Medicine* 335:1424–1430

Rolfs A, Bottcher T, Zschiesche M et al. (2005). Prevalence of Fabry disease in patients with cryptogenic stroke: a prospective study. *Lancet* 366:1794–1796

Ronthal M, Gonzalez RG, Smith RN et al. (2003). Case records of the Massachusetts General Hospital. Weekly clinicopathological exercises. Case 21–2003. A 72 year old man with repetitive strokes in the posterior circulation. *New England Journal of Medicine* 349:170–180

Ross R (1999). Atherosclerosis: an inflammatory disease. *New England Journal of Medicine* 340:115–126

Rothwell PM (2001). The inter-relation between carotid, femoral and coronary artery disease. *European Heart Journal* 22:11–14

Rothwell PM, Warlow CP (2005). Timing of TIAs preceding stroke: time window for prevention is very short. *Neurology* 64:817–820

Rothwell PM, Gibson R, Warlow CP (2000a). The inter-relation between plaque surface morphology, degree of stenosis and the risk of ischemic stroke in patients with symptomatic carotid stenosis. *Stroke* 31:615–621

Rothwell PM, Villagra R, Gibson R et al. (2000b). Evidence of a chronic systemic cause of instability of atherosclerotic plaques. *Lancet* 355:19–24

Rubba P, Mercuri M, Faccenda F et al. (1994). Premature carotid atherosclerosis: does it occur in both familial hypercholesterolemia and homocystinuria? Ultrasound assessment of arterial intima-media thickness and blood flow velocity. *Stroke* 25:943–950

Rubinstein SM, Peerdeman SM, van Tulder MW et al. (2005). A systematic review of the risk factors for cervical artery dissection. *Stroke* 36:1575–1580

Ruby RJ, Burton JR (1977). Acute reversible hemiparesis and hyponatremia. *Lancet* i:1212

Sabolek M, Bachus-Banaschak K, Bachus R et al. (2005). Multiple cerebral aneurysms as delayed complication of left cardiac myxoma: a case report and review. *Acta Neurology Scandinavica* 111:345–350

Sacco RL, Kargman DE, Gu Q et al. (1995). Race-ethnicity and determinants of intracranial atherosclerotic cerebral infarction. The Northern Manhattan Stroke Study. *Stroke* 26:14–20

Salgado AV (1991). Central nervous system complications of infective endocarditis. *Stroke* 22:1461–1463

Samuelsson M, Lindell D, Norrving B (1996). Presumed pathogenetic mechanisms of recurrent stroke after lacunar infarction. *Cerebrovascular Diseases* 6:128–136

Sanna G, Bertolaccini ML, Hughes GR (2005). Hughes syndrome the antiphospholipid syndrome: a new chapter in neurology. *Annals of the New York Academy of Sciences* 1051:465–486

Sarkari NBS, Holmes JM, Bickerstaff ER (1970). Neurological manifestations associated with internal carotid loops and kinks in children. *Journal of Neurology, Neurosurgery and Psychiatry* 33:194–200

Savage COS, Harper L, Adu D (1997). Primary systemic vasculitis. *Lancet* 349:553–558

Schievink WI (2001). Spontaneous dissection of the carotid and vertebral arteries. *New England Journal of Medicine* **344**:898–906

Schievink WI, Michels VV, Piepgras DG (1994). Neurovascular manifestations of heritable connective tissue disorders. A review. *Stroke* **25**:889–903

Schimke RN, McKusick VA, Huang T *et al.* (1965). Homocystinuria Studies of 20 families with 38 affected members. *Journal of the American Medical Association* **193**:711–719

Schulz UGR, Rothwell PM (2003). Differences in vascular risk factors between aetiological subtypes of ischemic stroke in population-based incidence studies. *Stroke* **34**:2050–2059

Seko Y (2007). Giant cell and Takayasu arteritis. *Current Opinions in Rheumatology* **19**:39–43

Sempere AP, Duarte J, Cabezas C *et al.* (1998). Aetiopathogenesis of transient ischemic attacks and minor ischemic strokes: a community-based study in Segovia, Spain. *Stroke* **29**:40–45

Service FJ (1995). Hypoglycemic disorders. *New England Journal of Medicine* **332**:1144–1152

Shanmugam V, Zimnowodzki S, Curtin J *et al.* (1997). Hypoglycemic hemiplegia: insulinoma masquerading as stroke. *Journal of Stroke and Cerebrovascular Diseases* **6**:368–369

Silverstein A, Gilbert H, Wasserman LR (1962). Neurologic complications of polycythemia. *Annals of Internal Medicine* **57**:909–916

Siva A, Altintas A, Saip S (2004). Behçet's syndrome and the nervous system. *Current Opinions in Neurology* **17**:347–357

Slovut DP, Olin JW (2004). Fibromuscular dysplasia. *New England Journal of Medicine* **350**:1862–1871

Sotrel A, Lacson AG, Huff KR (1983). Childhood Kohlmeier–Degos disease with atypical skin lesions. *Neurology* **33**:1146–1151

Spencer TS, Campellone JV, Maldonado I *et al.* (2005). Clinical and magnetic resonance imaging manifestations of neurosarcoidosis. *Seminars in Arthritis and Rheumatism* **34**:649–661

Stewart SS, Ashizawa T, Dudley AW *et al.* (1988). Cerebral vasculitis in relapsing polychondritis. *Neurology* **38**:150–152

Stockhammer G, Felber SR, Zelger B *et al.* (1993). Sneddon's syndrome: diagnosis by skin biopsy and MRI in 17 patients. *Stroke* **24**:685–690

Sturzenegger M, Mattle HP, Rivoir A *et al.* (1993). Ultrasound findings in spontaneous extracranial vertebral artery dissection. *Stroke* **24**:1910–1921

Sturzenegger M, Mattle HP, Rivoir A *et al.* (1995). Ultrasound findings in carotid artery dissection: analysis of 43 patients. *Neurology* **45**:691–698

Subbiah P, Wijdicks E, Muenter M *et al.* (1996). Skin lesion with a fatal neurologic outcome (Degos' disease). *Neurology* **46**:636–640

Switzer JA, Hess DC, Nichols FT *et al.* (2006). Pathophysiology and treatment of stroke in sickle-cell disease: present and future. *Lancet Neurology* **5**:501–512

Tatlisumak T, Fisher M (1996). Hematologic disorders associated with ischemic stroke. *Journal of the Neurological Sciences* **140**:1–11

Tegeler CH, Shi F, Morgan T (1991). Carotid stenosis in lacunar stroke. *Stroke* **22**:1124–1128

Tietjen GE (2005). The risk of stroke in patients with migraine and implications for migraine management. *CNS Drugs* **19**:683–692

Turan TN, Stern BJ (2004). Stroke in pregnancy. *Neurology Clinic* **22**:821–840

van der Meulen JH, Weststrate W, van Gijn J *et al.* (1992). Is cerebral angiography indicated in infective endocarditis? *Stroke* **23**:1662–1667

van Oostenbrugge RJ, Freling G, Lodder J *et al.* (1996). Fatal stroke due to paradoxical fat embolism. *Cerebrovascular Diseases* **6**:313–314

Vidailhet M, Piette JC, Wechsler B *et al.* (1990). Cerebral venous thrombosis in systemic lupus erythematosus. *Stroke* **21**:1226–1231

Viles-Gonzalez JF, Fuster V, Badimon JJ (2004). Atherothrombosis: a widespread disease with unpredictable and life-threatening consequences. *European Heart Journal* **25**:1197–1207

Visy JM, Le Coz P, Chadefaux B *et al.* (1991). Homocystinuria due to 5,10-methylenetetrahydrofolate reductase deficiency revealed by stroke in adult siblings. *Neurology* **41**:1313–1315

Vollmer TL, Guarnaccia J, Harrington W *et al.* (1993). Idiopathic granulomatous angiitis of the central nervous system. Diagnostic challenges. *Archives of Neurology* **50**:925–930

Vongpatanasin W, Hillis LD, Lange RA (1996). Prosthetic heart valves. *New England Journal of Medicine* **335**:407–416

Wahl A, Meier B, Haxel B *et al.* (2001). Prognosis after percutaneous closure of patent foramen ovale for paradoxical embolism. *Neurology* **57**:1330–1332

Wallis WE, Donaldson I, Scott RS *et al.* (1985). Hypoglycemia masquerading as cerebrovascular disease (hypoglycemic hemiplegia). *Annals of Neurology* **18**:510–512

Wen PY, Feske SK, Teoh SK *et al.* (1997). Cerebral haemorrhage in a patient taking fenfluramine and phentermine for obesity. *Neurology* **49**:632–633

White H, Boden-Albala B, Wang C *et al.* (2005). Ischemic stroke subtype incidence among whites, blacks and Hispanics: the Northern Manhattan Study. *Circulation* **111**:1327–1331

Wityk RJ, Lehman D, Klag M *et al.* (1996). Race and sex differences in the distribution of cerebral atherosclerosis. *Stroke* **27**:1974–1980

Yonekawa Y, Khan N (2003). Moyamoya disease. *Advances in Neurology* **92**:113–118

Zajicek JP (2000). Neurosarcoidosis. *Current Opinions in Neurology* **13**:323–325

Zuber M, Khoubesserian P, Meder JF *et al.* (1993). A 34-year delayed and focal postirradiation intracranial vasculopathy. *Cerebrovascular Diseases* **3**:181–182

Zuckerman D, Selim R, Hochberg E (2006). Intravascular lymphoma: the oncologist's "great imitator." *Oncologist* **11**:496–502

Causes of spontaneous intracranial hemorrhage

The causes of spontaneous intracerebral hemorrhage are sometimes, but not always, different from those of TIA and ischemic stroke. Spontaneous intracranial hemorrhage may be classified as:

- primary intracerebral hemorrhage: bleeding within the brain substance
- cerebral microbleeds
- intraventricular hemorrhage
- subdural hemorrhage
- subarachnoid hemorrhage (Ch. 30)

It is often difficult to establish the underlying cause of a spontaneous intracranial hemorrhage. The exact site of origin of bleeding may be unclear: a saccular aneurysm may rupture into the brain as well as into the subarachnoid space, or disruption of a small perforating artery may cause intraventricular hemorrhage as well as a basal ganglia hematoma. Even at autopsy there may be uncertainty because the source of the hemorrhage may have been destroyed. The site of bleeding may give some information as to the likely underlying cause (see below) since the relative frequency of the various pathologies causing intracranial hemorrhage varies by site. However, most parts of the brain may be affected by any of the causes listed in Box 7.1.

Primary intracerebral hemorrhage

Primary intracerebral hemorrhage is more common than subarachnoid hemorrhage, and its incidence increases with age (see Fig. 1.1). It is more frequent in Southeast Asian, Japanese and Chinese populations than in whites. The most common causes are intracranial small vessel disease, which is associated with hypertension, cerebral amyloid angiopathy and intracranial vascular malformations (Sutherland and Auer 2006). Rarer causes include saccular aneurysms, hemostatic defects, particularly those induced by anticoagulation or therapeutic thrombolysis, antiplatelet drugs, infective endocarditis, cerebral vasculitis and recreational drug use (Neiman *et al.* 2000; O'Connor *et al.* 2005).

The site of primary intracerebral hemorrhage provides information as to the cause: "hypertensive" hemorrhages (Fig. 7.1a) tend to occur in the basal ganglia, thalamus, and pons, while lobar hemorrhages are more often caused by cerebral amyloid angiopathy, vascular malformations and hemostatic failure (Dickinson 2001; Smith and Eichler 2006; Sutherland and Auer 2006) (Table 7.1) (Fig. 7.1b). Multiple hemorrhages suggest certain specific causes:

- cerebral amyloid angiopathy
- metastasic tumor
- hemostatic defect
- thrombolytic drugs

Box 7.1. Causes of spontaneous intracranial hemorrhage

Hypertension
Cerebral amyloid angiopathy
Intracranial vascular malformations: arteriovenous, venous, cavernous, telangiectasis
Tumors: melanoma, choriocarcinoma, malignant astrocytoma, oligodendroglioma,
  medulloblastoma, hemangioblastoma, choroid plexus papilloma, hypernephroma,
  endometrial carcinoma, bronchogenic carcinoma
Hemostatic failure: hemophilia and other coagulation disorders, anticoagulation therapy,
  thrombolysis, antiplatelet drugs, disseminated intravascular coagulation, thrombocytopenia,
  thrombotic thrombocytopenic purpura, polycythemia rubra vera, essential thrombocythemia,
  paraproteinemias, renal failure, liver failure, snake bite
Aneurysms: saccular, atheromatous, mycotic, myxomatous, dissecting
  Inflammatory vascular disease
Hemorrhagic transformation of cerebral infarction, venous more often than arterial
Intracranial venous thrombosis (Ch. 29)
Recreational drugs (Ch. 6)
Infections: infective endocarditis, herpes simplex, leptospirosis, anthrax
  Sickle cell disease
Moyamoya syndrome (Ch. 6)
Carotid endarterectomy (Ch. 25)
Intracranial surgery
Alcohol
Wernicke's encephalopathy
Chronic meningitis

- multiple hemorrhagic infarcts (usually embolic from the heart)
- intracranial venous thrombosis
- inflammatory vascular disease
- intracranial vascular malformations
- malignant hypertension
- eclampsia
- recreational drug use.

Rarely, primary intracerebral hemorrhage is familial.

The hematoma continues to expand after stroke onset, frequently causing further deterioration (Brott *et al.* 1997; Leira *et al.* 2004). Some brainstem hemorrhages evolve subacutely, particularly those caused by a vascular malformation (O'Laoire *et al.* 1982; Howard 1986). Any large hematoma may cause brain shift, transtentorial herniation, brainstem compression and raised intracranial pressure. Hematomas in the posterior fossa are particularly likely to cause obstructive hydrocephalus. Rupture into the ventricles or on to the surface of the brain is common, causing blood to appear in the subarachnoid space.

Cerebral microbleeds

The increasing use in research and clinical practice of gradient echo MRI (GRE-MRI), which is highly sensitive to hemoglobin degradation products, has led to the frequent detection of small, homogeneous, round foci of low signal intensity (Kidwell and Wintermark 2008) (Fig. 7.2; see also Fig. 7.4, below). The few existing studies of the pathological correlates of these areas of low signal intensity suggest that they correspond to hemosiderin-laden

Table 7.1. Structural causes of primary intracerebral hemorrhage according to location and patient age, listed according to relative frequency (hematological causes excluded)

Patient age	Anterior hemorrhage		Posterior hemorrhage
	Deep	Lobar	
Younger (< 50 years)	AVM	AVM	AVM
	Cavernous malformations	Cavernous malformations	Hypertension
	Hypertension	Tumor	Tumor
	Tumor		
Older (≥ 50 years)	Hypertension	CAA	Hypertension
	CAA	Hypertension	CAA
	Tumor		Tumor

Notes:
CAA, cerebral amyloid angiopathy; AVM, arteriovenous malformation.

(a)

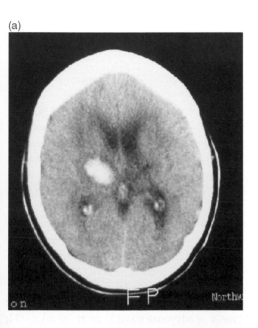

(b)

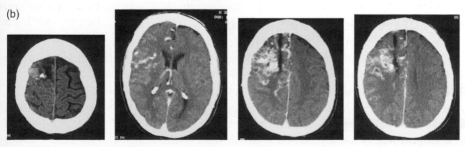

Fig. 7.1. Intracerebral hemorrhage. (a) A CT brain scan showing a typical deep "hypertensive" primary intracerebral hemorrhage. (b) These CT brain scans showing a right frontal arteriovenous malformation causing hemorrhage.

(a) 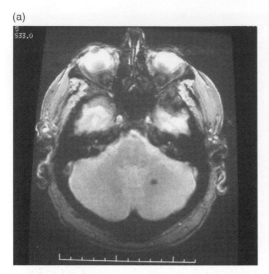 (b)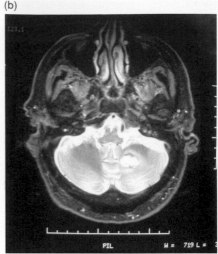

Fig. 7.2. A patient presenting with atrial fibrillation and a transient ischemic attack was found to have a cerebellar microbleed on gradient echo MRI (a) and was started on stroke prevention with aspirin rather than warfarin. Six months later, this patient had a symptomatic hemorrhage at the same site (b).

macrophages adjacent to small vessels and are indicative of previous extravasation of blood (Fazekas *et al.* 1999), so-called "cerebral microbleeds."

Cerebral microbleeds are seen frequently in patients with primary intracerebral hemorrhage, less commonly in patients with ischemic stroke and rarely in "healthy controls" (Cordonnier *et al.* 2007). Risk factors for cerebral microbleeds include hypertension, increasing age, diabetes, cerebral amyloid angiopathy and, less commonly, cerebral autosomal dominant arteriopathy with silent infarcts and leukoaraiosis (CADASIL) (Cordonnier *et al.* 2007). It is unclear whether previous use of antiplatelet agents or anticoagulants is a risk factor for cerebral microbleeds.

The clinical significance of cerebral microbleeds is uncertain. The few data available suggest that their presence and number predict recurrent intracerebral hemorrhage following lobar intracerebral hemorrhage (Greenberg *et al.* 2004) and, possibly, the future occurrence of hemorrhagic stroke (Fan *et al.* 2003) and cerebral infarction (Imaizumi *et al.* 2004) in those with ischemic stroke. Conflicting data exist on the risk of subsequent cerebral hemorrhage in patients with microbleeds treated with antiplatelet agents, anticoagulation and thrombolysis (Kidwell *et al.* 2002; Nighoghossian *et al.* 2002, Derex *et al.* 2004; Kakuda *et al.* 2005).

Primary intraventricular hemorrhage

Primary intraventricular hemorrhage is very unusual, except in premature babies. In adults, a cause is not always found. Some may be secondary to a vascular malformation in the ventricular wall (Gates *et al.* 1986; Darby *et al.* 1988). The clinical features may be indistinguishable from subarachnoid hemorrhage and it may only be differentiated at autopsy.

Subdural hemorrhage

Subdural hemorrhage is usually traumatic rather than spontaneous, although the trauma can be very mild or forgotten in elderly patients and alcoholics. Spontaneous causes of subdural hemorrhage include:

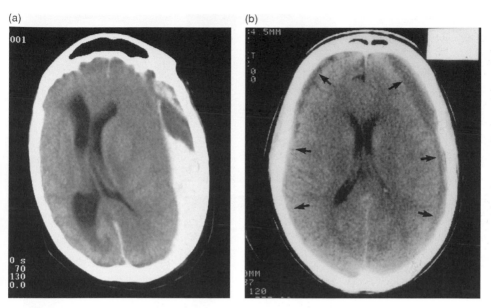

Fig. 7.3. Brain CT scans showing an acute hyperintense left subdural hematoma with mass effect (a) and chronic bilateral hypodense subdural hematoma (b).

- rupture of a vascular malformation in the dura
- rupture of a peripheral aneurysm, mycotic more likely than saccular
- a hemostatic defect, particularly therapeutic anticoagulation
- a superficial cerebral tumor
- rarely lumbar puncture or spontaneous intracranial hypotension.

Often no cause is found. Acute subdural hemorrhage appears hyperintense on CT brain scan whereas chronic subdural hematomas appear hypodense (Fig. 7.3). Hematomas of intermediate age, approximately four to six weeks, are often isodense to gray matter on CT and may be overlooked.

Hypertension

Hypertension causes thickening and disruption of the walls of the small arteries that perforate the base of the brain, particularly the lenticulostriate arteries in the region of the basal ganglia (Ch. 6). Rupture of these abnormal vessels is thought to cause hypertensive primary intracerebral hemorrhage, although it is almost impossible to prove a cause and effect relationship in individuals because the hemorrhage destroys the exact site of the bleeding (Takebayashi and Kaneko 1983). In practice, the clinical diagnosis of "hypertensive" primary intracerebral hemorrhage is based on the lack of any alternative explanation in a patient known to have had hypertension, or who clearly has evidence of hypertensive organ damage. However, it seems very likely that other factors, such as cerebral amyloid angiopathy, may interact with hypertension to cause primary intracerebral hemorrhage in a particular individual.

Cerebral amyloid angiopathy

Cerebral amyloid angiopathy is an organ-specific form of amyloid deposition in small and medium-sized arteries, and less commonly veins, of the cerebral cortex and meninges,

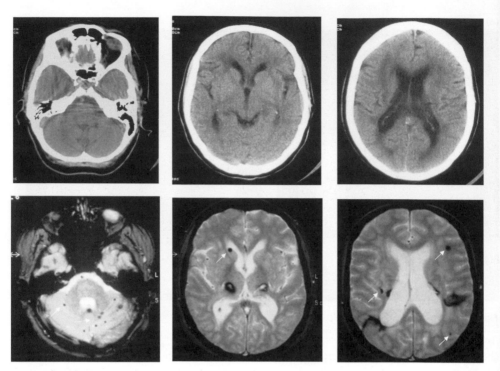

Fig. 7.4. Brain CT scans (top) from a patient with cerebral amyloid angiopathy showing only leukoaraiosis, whereas gradient echo MRI performed on the same day (bottom) shows evidence of several previous intracerebral hemorrhages and multiple microbleeds (arrows).

particularly in the elderly. Frequently, there is associated subcortical small vessel disease and demyelination, and leukoaraiosis and microbleeds on brain imaging (Zhang-Nunes *et al.* 2006; Maia *et al.* 2007) (Figs. 7.2 and 7.4). It is thought to be the cause of lobar hemorrhages in the elderly, which are often multiple and recurrent, and possibly of subarachnoid hemorrhage (Smith and Eichler 2006; Thanvi and Robinson 2006). Patients, with or without lobar hemorrhage, may have progressive dementia and a history of minor stroke-like episodes and TIAs, and even focal epileptic seizures. Cerebral amyloid angiopathy may be associated with Alzheimer's disease, Down's syndrome, cerebral vasculitis, cerebral irradiation and dementia pugilistica. Dominantly inherited forms of cerebral amyloid angiopathy cause primary intracerebral hemorrhage in young adults in Iceland (Jensson *et al.* 1987) and in middle-aged adults in Holland (Bornebroek *et al.* 1997), and a syndrome of progressive dementia, ataxia, and spasticity associated sometimes with stroke in the UK (Plant *et al.* 1990).

Intracranial vascular malformations

Intracranial vascular malformations are uncommon, probably congenital, and sometimes familial (Byrne 2005). Those in the dura, draining into the sinuses rather than cerebral veins, can also be caused by skull fracture, craniotomy or dural sinus thrombosis. The overall intracranial vascular malformations detection rate is approximately 3 per 100 000 population per annum and the prevalence is about 20 per 100 000 (Brown *et al.* 1996).

(a)

(b)

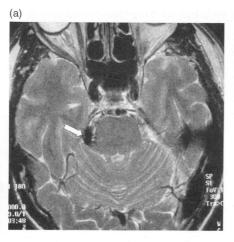
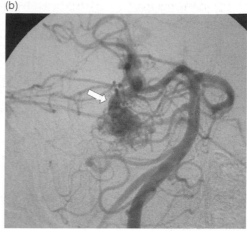

Fig. 7.5. Arteriovenous malformation. A T$_2$-weighted MRI (a) and cerebral angiogram (b) showing a dural arteriovenous malformation (arrows) at the right cerebellopontine angle, causing tinnitus.

Arteriovenous malformations

Arteriovenous malformations present most commonly with signs consistent with a space-occupying lesion or seizures and consist of an abnormal fistulous connection(s) between one or more hypertrophied feeding arteries and dilated draining veins (Clatterbuck *et al.* 2005) (Fig. 7.5). The blood supply is derived from one cerebral artery or, more often, several, sometimes with a contribution from branches of the external carotid artery. Arteriovenous malformations vary from a few millimeters to several centimeters in diameter. Approximately 15% are associated with aneurysms on their feeding arteries. Some grow during life but a few shrink or even disappear, and some are multiple. These fistulae occur in or on the brain, or in the dura of the intracranial sinuses.

Arteriovenous malformations can present at any age with:

- partial or secondarily generalized epileptic seizures
- hemorrhage, which is more often intracerebral than subarachnoid or subdural
- as a mass lesion
- with TIA-like episodes (Ch. 8)
- with a caroticocavernous fistula owing to a dural arteriovenous malformation
- with a self-audible bruit
- with the syndrome of benign intracranial hypertension resulting from increased pressure in cerebral draining veins or sinuses, particularly if a dural arteriovenous malformation is near the transverse/sigmoid sinus and petrous bone
- with high output cardiac failure in neonates and infants.

Headache, although common, is not by itself diagnostically helpful and may well be a coincidence. Rarely, a bruit can be heard over the skull or orbits. A brainstem arteriovenous malformation can present similarly to multiple sclerosis, with fluctuating symptoms and signs of brainstem dysfunction, perhaps caused by recurrent hemorrhage.

A CT scan may show calcification and non-specific hypo- or hyperdensity, while an enhanced scan is likely to show the dilated vessels of large malformations. Magnetic resonance imaging is more sensitive, showing evidence of old hemorrhage and vascular flow voids. Angiography is the definitive investigation but even this may not detect small malformations.

Venous malformations

Venous malformations consist of collections of venous channels and a large draining vein. Most are asymptomatic but they may present with hemorrhage into the ventricles, or seizures. On contrast CT, the draining vein may appear as a linear enhancing streak, but a flow void on MRI is more sensitive. The definitive diagnosis is made on the venous phase of a cerebral angiogram.

Cavernous malformations

Cavernous malformations, or cavernomas, are sharply circumscribed collections of thin-walled sinusoidal vessels lined with a single layer of endothelium without intervening brain parenchyma or identifiable mature vessel wall elements. They are sometimes multiple and occasionally familial (Labauge et al. 2007). Most are asymptomatic and picked up incidentally on MRI. They can present with seizures, recurrent subacute brainstem syndromes, a mass lesion and, less commonly, hemorrhage. The angiogram is usually normal but CT can show a hypo- or hyperdense area that may enhance, perhaps with calcification, usually without surrounding edema or mass effect. A brain MRI reveals sharply circumscribed lesions, typically with evidence of hemosiderin as a result of old but asymptomatic hemorrhage. However, they cannot always be distinguished from small arteriovenous malformations (Kattapong et al. 1995).

Telangiectasias

Telangiectasias are collections of dilated capillaries that are usually of no clinical significance (Milandre et al. 1987). They may be associated with hereditary hemorrhagic telangiectasia (the Osler–Weber–Rendu syndrome), but this is more likely to be associated with neurological complications from a pulmonary arteriovenous malformation with right-to-left shunting, such as cerebral hypoxia, brain abscess, paradoxical and septic embolism, or from an associated intracranial arteriovenous malformation or aneurysm (McDonald et al. 1998).

Caroticocavernous fistula

A caroticocavernous fistula is an abnormal connection between the carotid arterial system and the cavernous sinus. It may occur spontaneously, especially in the elderly, or as a result of a ruptured dural arteriovenous malformation, intracavernous internal carotid artery aneurysm, Ehlers–Danlos syndrome, pseudoxanthoma elasticum or head injury. With a high-flow direct fistulae from the internal carotid artery itself, the onset is dramatic, with unilateral pulsating exophthalmos and an orbital bruit, often audible to the patient. In addition, there may be orbital pain, papilloedema, dilated conjunctival veins and chemosis, glaucoma, monocular visual loss, and involvement of cranial nerves III, IV, VI and I, and sometimes the second sensory division of the trigeminal nerve. The ophthalmoplegia may also be caused by hypoxia and swelling within the extraocular muscles. Dural fistulae present more insidiously because the blood flow is lower from small meningeal branches of the internal or external carotid arteries in the cavernous sinus. If there is no spontaneous resolution, it may be possible to obliterate the fistula with balloon catheterization.

References

Bornebroek M, Westemdorp RGJ, Haan J et al. (1997). Mortality from hereditary cerebral haemorrhage with amyloidosis: Dutch type. The impact of sex parental transmission and year of birth. Brain 120:2243–2249

Brott T, Broderick J, Kothari R et al. (1997). Early haemorrhage growth in patients with intracerebral haemorrhage. Stroke 28:1–5

Brown RD, Wiebers DO, Torner JC et al. (1996). Incidence and prevalence of intracranial vascular malformations in Olmsted, County Minnesota 1965 to 1992. Neurology 46:949–952

Byrne JV (2005). Cerebrovascular malformations. European Radiology 15:448–452

Clatterbuck RE, Hsu FP, Spetzler RF (2005). Supratentorial arteriovenous malformations. Neurosurgery 57:164–167

Cordonnier C, Al-Shahi Salman R, Wardlaw J (2007). Spontaneous brain microbleeds: systematic review, subgroup analyses and standards for study design and reporting. Brain 130:1988–2003

Darby DG, Donnan GA, Saling MA et al. (1988). Primary intraventricular haemorrhage: clinical and neuropsychological findings in a prospective stroke series. Neurology 38:68–75.

Derex L, Nighoghossian N, Hermier M et al. (2004). Thrombolysis for ischemic stroke in patients with old microbleeds on pretreatment MRI. Cerebrovascular Diseases 17:238–241

Dickinson CJ (2001). Why are strokes related to hypertension? Classic studies and hypotheses revisited. Journal of Hypertension 19:1515–1521

Fan YH, Zhang L, Lam WWM et al. (2003). Cerebral microbleeds as a risk factor for subsequent intracerebral haemorrhages among patients with acute ischemic stroke. Stroke 34:2459–2462.

Fazekas F, Kleinert R, Roob G et al. (1999). Histo-pathologic analysis of foci of signal loss on gradient-echo T_2^*-weighted MR images in patients with spontaneous intracerebral haemorrhage: evidence of microangiopathy-related microbleeds. American Journal of Neuroradiology 1999; 20:637–642.

Gates GC, Barnett HJM, Vinters HV et al. (1986). Primary intraventricular haemorrhage in adults. Stroke 17:872–877

Greenberg SM, Eng JA, Ning M et al. (2004). Hemorrhage burden predicts recurrent intracerebral hemorrhage after lobar hemorrhage. Stroke 35:1415–1420.

Howard RS (1986). Brainstem hematoma due to presumed cryptic telangiectasia. Journal of Neurology, Neurosurgery and Psychiatry 49:1241–1245.

Imaizumi T, Horita Y, Hashimoto et al. (2004). Dotlike haemosiderin spots on T_2^*-weighted magnetic resonance imaging as a predictor of stroke recurrence: a prospective study. Journal of Neurosurgery 101:915–920.

Jensson O, Gudmundsson G, Arnason A et al. (1987). Hereditary cystatin C (y-trace) amyloid angiopathy of the CNS causing cerebral haemorrhage. Acta Neurologica Scandinavica 76:102–114.

Kakuda W, Thijs VN, Lansberg MG et al. (2005). Clinical importance of microbleeds in patients receiving IV thrombolysis. Neurology 65:1175–1178

Kattapong VJ, Hart BL, Davis LE (1995). Familial cerebral cavernous angiomas: clinical and radiologic studies. Neurology 45:492–497

Kidwell CS, Wintermark M (2008). Imaging of intracranial haemorrhage. Lancet Neurology 7:256–267

Kidwell CS, Saver JL, Villablanca JP et al. (2002). Magnetic resonance imaging detection of microbleeds before thrombolysis: an emerging application. Stroke 33:95–98

Labauge P, Denier C, Bergametti F et al. (2007). Genetics of cavernous angiomas. Lancet Neurology 6:237–244

Leira R, Davalos A, Silva Y et al. (2004). Early neurologic deterioration in intracerebral hemorrhage: predictors and associated factors. Neurology 63:461–467

Maia LF, MacKenzie IR, Feldman HH (2007). Clinical phenotypes of cerebral amyloid angiopathy. Journal of the Neurological Sciences 257:23–30

McDonald MJ, Brophy BP, Kneebone C (1998). Rendu–Osler–Weber syndrome: a current perspective on cerebral manifestations. Journal of Clinical Neuroscience 5:345–350

Milandre L, Pellissier JF, Boudouresques G et al. (1987). Non-hereditary multiple telangiectasias of the central nervous system. Journal of the Neurological Sciences 82:291–304

Neimann J, Haapaniemi HM, Hillbom M (2000). Neurological complications of drug abuse: pathophysiological mechanisms. *European Journal of Neurology* **7**:595–606

Nighoghossian N, Hermier M, Adeleine P *et al.* (2002). Old microbleeds are a potential risk factor for cerebral bleeding after ischemic stroke: a gradient-echo T_2-weighted brain MRI study. *Stroke* **33**:735–742.

O'Connor AD, Rusyniak DE, Bruno A (2005). Cerebrovascular and cardiovascular complications of alcohol and sympathomimetic drug abuse. *Medical Clinics of North America* **89**:1343–1358

O'Laoire SA, Crockard A, Thomas DGT *et al.* (1982). Brain-stem hematoma. A report of six surgically treated cases. *Journal of Neurosurgery* **56**:222–227

Plant GT, Revesz T, Barnard RO *et al.* (1990). Familial cerebral amyloid angiopathy with non neuritic amyloid plaque formation. *Brain* **113**:721–747

Smith EE, Eichler F (2006). Cerebral amyloid angiopathy and lobar intracerebral hemorrhage. *Archives of Neurology* **63**:148–151

Sutherland GR, Auer RN (2006). Primary intracerebral hemorrhage. *Journal of Clinical Neuroscience* **13**:511–517

Takebayashi S, Kaneko M (1983). Electron microscopic studies of ruptured arteries in hypertensive intracerebral haemorrhage. *Stroke* **14**:28–36

Thanvi B, Robinson T (2006). Sporadic cerebral amyloid angiopathy: an important cause of cerebral haemorrhage in older people. *Age Ageing* **35**:565–571

Zhang-Nunes SX, Maat-Schieman ML, van Duinen SG *et al.* (2006). The cerebral beta-amyloid angiopathies: hereditary and sporadic. *Brain Pathology* **16**:30–39

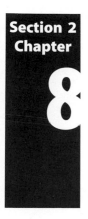
Clinical features, diagnosis and investigation

8 Clinical features and differential diagnosis of a transient ischemic attack

The causes of TIAs are the same as the causes of stroke, with the caveat that the vast majority of TIAs appear to be caused by ischemia rather than hemorrhage (Ch. 9). The differential diagnosis of TIA differs from that of stroke owing to the transient nature of the symptoms (Box 8.1). A careful history and examination is important since this may provide clues to the underlying cause of the TIA (Ch. 9) or may indicate a non-vascular cause for the focal symptoms. Identification of the underlying affected vascular territory from the clinical features of the TIA is important for targeting further investigation and secondary preventive treatments. Localization of the site of ischemia may be aided by brain imaging, which is also used to exclude structural lesions causing "transient focal neurological attacks," and to differentiate between hemorrhage and ischemia (Ch. 10).

Symptoms and ischemic territory

Symptoms are of sudden onset and are "focal," indicating a disturbance in a particular area of brain or in one eye (Flemming *et al.* 2004; Sherman 2004). Motor symptoms are the most common: weakness, clumsiness or heaviness usually on just one side of the body (Table 8.1). Unilateral sensory symptoms are described as numbness, tingling or deadness. Speech may be dysphasic, dysarthric or both. Transient monocular blindness (amaurosis fugax) affects the upper or lower half of vision, or all the vision of one eye, and is often described like a "blind or shutter" coming down from above, or up from below. However, transient monocular ischemia can also cause partial visual loss, such as blurring or dimming. Transient monocular blindness must be distinguished from transient homonymous hemianopia, although this can be difficult even when the patient is a very good historian.

Box 8.1. Causes of transient focal neurological attacks

Transient ischemic attack
Migraine with aura
Partial epileptic seizures
Structural intracranial lesions: tumor, chronic subdural hematoma, vascular malformation, giant aneurysm
Multiple sclerosis
Labyrinthine disorders: Meniere's disease or benign positional vertigo
Peripheral nerve or root lesion
Metabolic: hypo or hyperglycemia, hypercalcemia, hyponatremia
Psychological

Table 8.1. Clinical features and vascular distribution of transient ischemic attacks

Symptoms	Vascular distribution		Frequency (%)
	Carotid	Vertebrobasilar	
Unilateral weakness, heaviness, or clumsiness	+	+	50
Unilateral sensory symptoms	+	+	35
Dysarthria[a]	+	+	23
Transient monocular blindness	+	–	18
Dysphasia	+	(+)	18
Unsteadiness/ataxia[a]	(+)	+	12
Bilateral simultaneous blindness	–	+	7
Vertigo[a]	–	+	5
Homonymous hemianopia	(+)	+	5
Diplopia	–	+	5
Bilateral motor loss	–	+	4
Dysphagia[a]	(+)	+	1
Crossed sensory and motor loss	–	+	1

Note:
[a]In general, if these symptoms are isolated it is best not to diagnose definite transient ischemic attack.

Simultaneous bilateral transient motor or sensory loss is almost always caused by brainstem ischemia. Sudden simultaneous bilateral blindness in elderly patients usually indicates bilateral occipital ischemia. Vertigo, diplopia, dysphagia, unsteadiness, tinnitus, amnesia, drop attacks and dysarthria may be caused by posterior circulation or more global cerebral ischemia, or by non-vascular causes such as motor neuron disease or myesthenia in the case of dysarthria. If these symptoms occur in isolation, the diagnosis of TIA should only be considered after exclusion of other possibilities (Gomez *et al.* 1996; Bos *et al.* 2007). Global symptoms such as a reduced level of consciousness are almost never caused by a TIA. They can only be accepted as resulting from a TIA if there are additional focal symptoms that are unlikely to be epileptic or syncopal.

If more than one body part is involved, the symptoms usually start simultaneously in all parts, persist for a while and then gradually wear off over a few minutes, particularly in the case of transient monocular blindness, or an hour or so. If a patient still has symptoms more than an hour after the onset, the chances are that complete recovery will take more than 24-hours. A mild headache accompanying the neurological symptoms is quite common, usually ipsilateral to the affected carotid territory, but most common in posterior circulation TIAs. If cerebral symptoms last less than a minute, particularly if they are "sensory," the diagnosis of TIA is difficult to sustain. In contrast, symptoms of retinal ischemia may be very short lived.

The symptoms of a TIA enable categorization of attacks by arterial territory affected: carotid in approximately 80% or vertebrobasilar in 20%. This has important implications for further investigation and secondary prevention. Such categorization may be straight-forward where there are definite cortical symptoms such as dysphasia or brainstem symptoms such as diplopia. However, because the motor and sensory pathways are supplied by both vascular systems at different points in their course, it is not always possible to distinguish which territory is involved (Table 8.1). One study found that the agreement between the clinical diagnosis of vascular territory in patients with TIA or minor stroke made by three neurologists compared with the near "gold standard" of lesion location on diffusion-weighted MRI was only moderate, with the kappa statistics varying from 0.48 to 0.54 for each neurologist (Flossmann *et al.* 2006). Interobserver agreement on territory ranged from 0.46 to 0.60, and only the presence of visual symptoms improved the accuracy of vascular territory diagnosis (Flossmann *et al.* 2006). Ischemia in the territory of supply of the deep perforating arteries may be suspected if the patient has a transient lacunar syndrome and no positive evidence of cortical involvement such as dysphasia.

Mechanisms of ischemia

Most TIAs are probably caused by arterial occlusion (Bogousslavsky *et al.* 1986) (Ch. 6). Less commonly, they may be secondary to low flow distal to a severely stenosed or occluded artery in the neck following a fall in blood pressure, as after antihypertensive medication or vasodilators, after standing or sitting up quickly, after a heavy meal or a hot bath, on exercise or during cardiac arrhythmia (Caplan and Sergay 1976; Ruff *et al.* 1981; Ross Russell and Page 1983; Kamata *et al.* 1994). Such low-flow TIAs may be atypical: symptoms may take some minutes to develop; there may be irregular shaking or dystonic posturing of the arm or leg contralateral to the cerebral ischemia; or there is monocular or binocular visual blurring, dimming, fragmentation, or bleaching, often just in bright light (Hess *et al.* 1991; Schulz and Rothwell 2002). Symptoms of focal brainstem ischemia caused by inter-mittent obstruction of a vertebral artery by cervical osteophytes are rare, presumably because collateral blood flow to the brainstem is usually sufficient.

"Subclavian steal" is caused by retrograde flow in the vertebral artery. It is a common angiographic or ultrasound finding when there is stenosis or occlusion of the subclavian artery proximal to the vertebral artery origin, particularly on the left, or of the innominate artery. When the ipsilateral arm is exercised, the increased blood flow to meet the metabolic demand may be enough to "steal" more blood down the vertebral artery, away from the brainstem into the axillary artery. If there is poor collateral blood flow to the brainstem, then symptoms may occur, but this is very rare. The subclavian disease is almost always severe enough to be detectable by unequal radial pulses and blood pressures, and often there is a supraclavicular bruit (Cho *et al.* 2007).

Signs

Owing to their brief duration, patients are rarely examined during a TIA at a time when focal neurological signs might indicate the site of the lesion, although this now occurs more frequently with the advent of acute stroke services and thrombolysis. However, non-neurological signs, including carotid bruits, retinal emboli, cardiac dysrhythmia and signs of peripheral vascular disease, may help to elucidate the cause of the attacks (Ch. 9).

Differential diagnosis and mimics of transient ischemic attacks

Transient ischemic attacks are but one cause of "transient focal neurological attacks" (Box 8.1) and "transient monocular blindness" (Box 8.2). There is no test to confirm a TIA, and the gold standard method of diagnosis remains a thorough clinical assessment as soon as possible after the event by an experienced stroke physician, although the advent of

Box 8.2. Causes of transient monocular blindness (amaurosis fugax)

Transient ischemic attack	Intraorbital tumor
Glaucoma	Caroticocavernous fistula
Uhthoff's phenomenon in retrobulbar neuritis	Retinal migraine
Raised intracranial pressure with papilloedema	Intracranial dural malformation
Retinal hemorrhage	Paraneoplastic retinopathy
Retinal venous thrombosis	Reversible diabetic cataract
Retinal detachment	Uveitis–glaucoma–hyphema syndrome
Macular degeneration	

Table 8.2. Numbers of patients referred to dedicated "TIA clinics" in whom a non-neurovascular diagnosis was eventually made in Oxford Vascular Study (OXVASC; 2002–2004) and the Oxford Community Stroke Project (OCSP; 1981–1986)

Diagnosis	OXVASC ($n=112$)	Diagnosis	OCSP ($n=317$)
Migraine	25	Migraine	52
Anxiety	14	Syncope	48
Seizure	9	"Possible TIA"	46
Peripheral neuropathy	8	"Funny turn"	45
Arrhythmia	6	Isolated vertigo	33
Labyrinthine	6	Epilepsy	29
Postural hypotension	6	Transient global amnesia	17
Transient global amnesia	6	Lone bilateral blindness	14
Syncope	5	Isolated diplopia	4
Tumor or metastases	4	Drop attack	3
Cervical spine disease	3	Meningioma	2
Dementia	2	Miscellaneous	24
Myasthenia gravis	1		
Multiple sclerosis	1		
Parkinson's disease	1		
Miscellaneous	15		

Note:
TIA, transient ischemic attack.
Source: From Martin et al. (1989).

new imaging techniques, particularly diffusion-weighted MRI (Ch. 10), has allowed the diagnosis to be made or excluded with more certainty in some patients. A diagnosis of TIA is supported by a sudden onset and definite focal symptoms in the history and evidence of vascular disease on examination (Hand et al. 2006).

Some conditions and syndromes are particularly frequently misdiagnosed as TIA (Table 8.2), but features in the history are often helpful in distinguishing TIA and minor stroke from mimics (Table 8.3).

Table 8.3. Features of a patient's history that are less typical of a transient ischemic attack and alternative (non-neurovascular) diagnosis suggested

Symptom	Description	Non-neurovascular diagnosis suggested	Notes
Timing	Recurrent/stereotypical episodes	Anxiety related	Especially hemisensory loss
Onset	Stuttering	Tumor	Over hours/days
	Progressive	Migraine	Over minutes
	Ill defined	Delirium	
Symptoms	Prodrome	Aura	Migraine, seizure
	Non-focal	Syncope	Loss of consciousness
		Delirium	Reduced attention
		Labyrinthine dysfunction	Balance disturbance
	Positive	Seizure	Motor symptom
		Migraine	Visual spectra
	Additional symptoms	Migraine	Headache
		Labyrinthine dysfunction	Hearing loss/tinnitus
Course	Fluctuating	Tumor	
		Delirium	
Recall	Absent	Transient global amnesia	
		Seizure	Generalized seizure
	Patchy	Delirium	

Migraine with aura

Migraine is not a major diagnostic problem if the aura is associated with a headache with or without nausea and vomiting or if a known migraineur develops a typical aura without headache. However, occasionally migraine auras start in middle or old age and if there is no headache, they can be confused with TIAs. The time course of the symptoms is the key to distinguishing between TIA and migraine aura: migrainous auras start slowly, spread and intensify over several minutes and usually fade in 20–30 minutes (Dennis and Warlow 1992). The symptoms tend to begin in one domain, particularly vision, fade and move on to another, such as language, and tend to be positive involving flashing lights or tingling rather than the negative symptoms typical of a TIA such as weakness, visual loss, or numbness. However, it is important to note that a progressive or stuttering pattern of symptom onset, positive visual phenomena and headache are also compatible with vertebrobasilar TIA.

Epilepsy

Epilepsy is not a diagnostic problem unless the seizures are partial. Partial sensory seizures tend to cause positive symptoms such as tingling, and symptoms "march" across a hand or foot, and up the limb in around a minute and may eventually be accompanied by focal motor seizures or secondary generalization. Sudden speech arrest seems to be more often epileptic, and not necessarily arising in the dominant hemisphere, than caused by ischemia, which is more likely to cause dysphasic speech (Cascino et al. 1991). Transient inhibitory

(a) 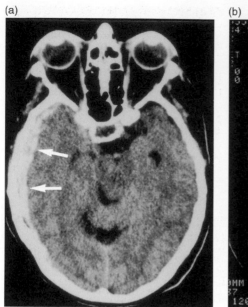 (b)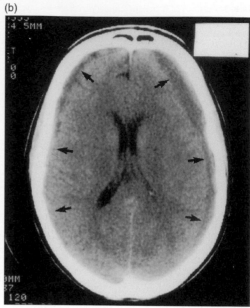

Fig. 8.1. Brain CT scans showing acute (a) and chronic (b) subdural hemorrhage and illustrating that the changes seen in chronic subdural hemorrhage may be subtle.

seizures may mimic the focal motor weakness of TIA but are most unusual (Kaplan 1993). Todd's paresis is a focal neurological deficit that can follow up to 10% of seizures, most commonly grand mal seizures, and typically causes a unilateral motor weakness but can also cause diplopia or speech disturbance. The cause of Todd's paresis is unknown, but "exhaustion" of the primary motor cortex or inactivation of motor fibers by NMDA receptors have been postulated. Like a TIA, Todd's paresis can last for several hours and differentiation can be difficult, but depends mainly on establishing the presence of seizure activity at onset (Gallmetzer *et al.* 2004).

Intracranial structural lesions

Occasionally, but importantly, intracranial structural lesions such as subdural hematoma (Fig. 8.1), or tumor (Fig. 8.2) may cause TIA-like symptoms, although such lesions may sometimes be incidental. Compression of an intracranial artery is perhaps an explanation for those patients with a space-occupying lesion, while focal seizures misdiagnosed as TIAs are another possibility. Intracerebral tumors can suddenly expand in size as a result of in-situ hemorrhage (Fig. 8.2b), edema or both, and these are further causes of symptoms coming on suddenly in an otherwise "chronic" condition. Intracranial vascular malformations might cause local steal of blood, thereby causing a TIA, or perhaps cause focal epileptic attacks that mimic TIAs. Although intracranial structural lesions can cause focal neurological deficits, these are almost never the sole clinical feature. Cerebral imaging with MRI is, therefore, important to exclude space-occupying lesions in patients with stuttering, deficits of gradual onset, more prolonged histories or additional features such as headache or nausea. Imaging with non-contrast CT lacks sensitivity for space-occupying lesions and is not recommended (Ch. 10).

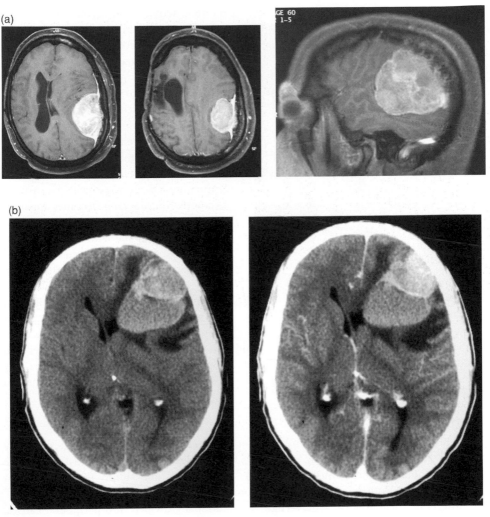

Fig. 8.2. Examples of tumors that may cause symptoms mimicking TIA: (a) meningioma; (b) hemorrhagic melanoma metastasis; and (c) multiple cerebral metastases in a patient with lung adenocarcinoma.

Transient global amnesia

Transient global amnesia is a characteristic but uncommon clinical syndrome, usually occurring in the middle aged or elderly (Hodges and Warlow 1990a, b; Quinette *et al.* 2006). The onset is sudden, with severe anterograde amnesia usually accompanied by retrograde amnesia. The attack lasts several hours, after which the patient recovers the ability to lay down new memories and recall old ones, but never has recall of the period of the attack itself. During the attack, the patient is fully conscious, has no loss of personal identity, looks normal if a little subdued and bewildered, and has no other symptoms apart perhaps from some headache and nausea. The patient can perform normal everyday activities, even driving, but typically asks the same question repetitively because of the anterograde amnesia. A witness account is required to differentiate such attacks from hysterical fugues, alcoholic amnesic states or complex partial seizures. Emotional upset, Valsalva maneuvers, defecation, sexual intercourse and other physical exertions, often

(c)

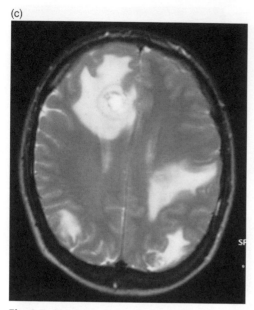

Fig. 8.2. *(cont.)*

outdoor activities on a cold day, may be precipitants (Quinette *et al.* 2006). In most cases, the prognosis is excellent and attacks do not usually recur.

The etiology of transient global amnesia is unclear. Various mechanisms have been proposed, including temporary metabolic abnormality in the medial temporal lobes, venous hypertension and ischemia (Bettermann 2006; Menendez Gonzalez and Rivera 2006; Roach 2006). Sometimes a diagnosis of epilepsy, usually of complex partial type, becomes apparent subsequently. This is particularly likely if the transient global amnesia had been short lived, for less than an hour, had occurred on wakening, and had recurred early (Zeman *et al.* 1998). Recent developments in neuroimaging have confirmed that medial temporal lobe changes accompany transient global amnesia (Sander and Sander 2005). The presence of abnormality on diffusion-weighted MRI (Sander and Sander 2005; Sedlaczek *et al.* 2004) has led to the proposal that transient global amnesia may be an ischemic phenomenon. However such changes are not diagnostic of ischemia and can occur following seizures.

Vestibular dysfunction

The acute onset of vertigo is a common complaint and presents a diagnostic challenge, especially in elderly patients with pre-existing risk factors for vascular disease. An essential part of the evaluation should be the distinction between "true vertigo," put simply the false illusion of movement, and other less-specific symptoms of "unsteadiness" or "light-headedness." The differential diagnosis of "true vertigo" is traditionally divided into peripheral causes, including benign positional vertigo, vestibular neuritis and Meniere's disease, and central causes, one of which is TIA or stroke affecting the brainstem. Generally, peripheral causes of vertigo are more common than central causes and one study found stroke or TIA to be the cause of only 3.2% of presentations with "dizziness symptoms" to an emergency department (Kerber *et al.* 2006).

Important features in the history which help in the differential diagnosis and indicate an alternative cause to TIA or stroke include the recurrent stereotypical episodes, presence of provoking factors (head movement), presence of features of middle ear disease (tinnitus, hearing loss) and absence of other focal neurological symptoms of sudden onset that might be attributable to the brainstem (visual or speech disturbance, weakness or numbness). Features on examination that are thought to identify a central cause of vertigo include nystagmus that is not suppressed by visual fixation, a normal head thrust test and other features of posterior circulation ischemia, including dysphagia, dysarthria, limb or facial weakness, gaze palsies or upgoing plantar responses. Despite these clinical indicators, the differential diagnosis is challenging and is sometimes only made when imaging is suggestive of focal ischemia (Schwartz *et al.* 2007).

Delirium or toxic confusional state

Delirium, toxic confusional state, metabolic encephalopathy or acute confusional state are terms that are used interchangeably and often loosely to describe a syndrome of acutely disordered cognition, sometimes associated with reduced level of consciousness and abnormal attention (see Table 32.1). The syndrome is very common, especially in the elderly and in patients with dementia, and presentations vary widely both in the speed of onset and severity (Siddiqi *et al.* 2006). The differential diagnosis is broad and includes almost any medical condition, but the commonest causes are sepsis, adverse drug reaction and metabolic derangement (Francis *et al.* 1990).

Delirium can be mistaken for a TIA if mild, when the predominant feature is interpreted as language disorder as opposed to confusion and when important clinical details are unclear such as when a witness account is unavailable, the patient has cognitive impairment or there is a long delay between the event and assessment. Reliable differentiation between TIA and delirium is important because each carries a potentially poor prognosis, though for very different reasons and the treatments are dissimilar (Siddiqi *et al.* 2006). Features suggestive of delirium as opposed to TIA include the presence of a causative factor such as urinary tract sepsis, an inability of the patient to remember the event clearly, fluctuating disturbance in attention and consciousness and the absence of a clearly sudden onset.

Syncope and presyncope

Syncope is the abrupt loss of consciousness associated with the loss of postural tone, usually followed by a rapid and complete recovery; presyncope is a premonitory sensation of syncope. The differential diagnosis of syncope is very broad and is divided into cardiovascular causes (most commonly tachy- or bradyarrhythmias) and non-cardiovascular causes (most commonly vasovagal syncope, orthostatic hypotension and carotid sinus hypersensitivity). Although the time course of syncope is consistent with TIA, the lack of focal neurological disturbance is definitely not, and the diagnosis should, therefore, only be made with considerable caution. Diagnostic confusion can sometimes be caused by TIA of the brainstem, causing transient quadriparesis presenting with a sudden loss of postural tone, but loss of consciousness is not a feature. Less infrequently, embolus to the tip of the basilar artery can present with sudden-onset coma, but this is virtually never a transient, self-limiting condition and other signs of brainstem dysfunction are always present and obvious, so this should not cause difficulties in diagnosis (Voetsch *et al.* 2004).

Other neurological disorders

Occasionally, non-structural neurological disorders such as motor neuron disease, multiple sclerosis (Rolak and Fleming 2007) or myasthenia gravis may present with transient symptoms of sudden onset. Although these conditions usually follow progressive courses, at times rapid initial progression can resemble TIA or minor stroke. Both motor neuron disease and myasthenia gravis occur more commonly in the elderly and can present with isolated dysarthria or dysphagia and, unless the diagnosis is made initially, subsequent deterioration can often be put down to 'recurrent stroke' (Libman *et al.* 2002, Kleiner-Fisman and Kott 1998).

Cryptogenic drop attacks

Drop attacks affect middle-aged and elderly women, almost only when walking rather than just standing or sitting (Stevens and Matthews 1973). Without warning, the patient falls to the ground. There is no loss of consciousness or leg weakness. The attacks may recur but then disappear as mysteriously as they came. There is usually no known cause, although carotid sinus syncope and orthostatic hypotension are possibilities (Dey *et al.* 1996). There appear to be no serious prognostic implications. Sudden weakness of both legs can occur in brainstem ischemia and, rarely, if both anterior cerebral arteries are supplied from the same stenosed internal carotid artery. Bilateral motor, sensory or visual impairments can also be caused by bihemispheric boundary zone ischemia distal to severe carotid disease (Sloan and Haley 1990). Finally, spinal cord "TIAs" do occur but are even rarer than spinal cord infarction (Cheshire *et al.* 1996). Cataplexy is almost invariably precipitated by excitement or emotion, seldom causes the patient to fall over and usually presents fairly early in life.

Psychogenic attacks

Psychogenic attacks are usually situational, for instance occurring in open spaces. Suggestive features include age less than 50 years, lack of vascular risk factors, symptoms affecting the non-dominant side (Rothwell 1994), hyperventilation, other medically unexplained symptoms or non-organic motor or sensory signs.

Isolated transient focal neurological disturbance of uncertain significance

In a significant proportion of patients referred to a neurovascular service with suspected TIA or minor stroke, no clear diagnosis of either a cerebrovascular event or a mimic can be reached, even after thorough clinical assessment and investigation. In our experience, these are often presentations with isolated focal neurological disturbance with sudden onset and gradual recovery, over seconds to minutes. Several distinct syndromes can be recognized, for instance isolated and transient vertigo with no other features to suggest a central or peripheral cause, isolated slurred speech, or isolated hemisensory loss.

Currently, little is known about the cause or significance of these syndromes, and rigorous prospective data are required about the risk factors for these presentations, imaging findings and the prognosis. However, our experience is that the outcome is good and, unlike TIA or minor stroke, these are not associated with a high early risk of recurrent stroke.

References

Bettermann K (2006). Transient global amnesia: the continuing quest for a source. *Archives of Neurology* 63:1336–1338

Bogousslavsky J, Hachinski VC, Boughner DR et al. (1986). Clinical predictors of cardiac and arterial lesions in carotid ischaemic attacks. *Archives of Neurology* 43:229–233

Bos MJ, van Rijn MJ, Witteman JC et al. (2007). Incidence and prognosis of transient neurological attacks. *Journal of the American Medical Association.* 298:2877–2885

Caplan LR, Sergay S (1976). Positional cerebral ischaemia. *Journal of Neurology, Neurosurgery and Psychiatry* 39:385–391

Cascino GD, Westmoreland BF, Swanson TH et al. (1991). Seizure-associated speech arrest in elderly patients. *Mayo Clinic Proceedings* 66:254–258

Cheshire WP, Santos CC, Massey EW et al. (1996). Spinal cord infarction: aetiology and outcome. *Neurology* 47:321–330

Cho HJ, Song SK, Lee DW et al. (2007). Carotid-subclavian steal phenomenon. *Neurology* 68:702

Dennis M, Warlow CP (1992). Migraine aura without headache: transient ischaemic attack or not? *Journal of Neurology, Neurosurgery and Psychiatry* 55:437–440

Dennis MS, Bamford JM, Sandercock PA et al. (1989). Incidence of transient ischemic attacks in Oxfordshire, England. *Stroke* 20:333–339.

Dey AB, Stout NR, Kenny RA (1996). Cardiovascular syncope is the commonest cause of drop attacks in the older patient. *European Journal of Cardiac Pacing and Electrophysiology* 6:84–88

Flemming KD, Brown RD Jr., Petty GW *et al.* (2004). Evaluation and management of transient ischaemic attack and minor cerebral infarction. *Mayo Clinic Proceedings* 79:1071–1086

Flossmann E, Redgrave JN, Schulz UG *et al.* (2006). Reliability of clinical diagnosis of the symptomatic vascular territory in patients with recent TIA or minor stroke. *Cerebrovascular Diseases* 21(Suppl 4):18.

Francis J, Martin D, Kapoor WN (1990). A prospective study of delirium in hospitalized elderly. *Journal of the American Medical Association* 263:1097.

Gallmetzer P, Leutmezer F, Serles W *et al.* (2004). Postictal paresis in focal epilepsies – incidence, duration, and causes: a video-EEG monitoring study. *Neurology* 62:2160–2164.

Gomez CR, Cruz-Flores S, Malkoff MD *et al.* (1996). Isolated vertigo as a manifestation of vertebrobasilar ischaemia. *Neurology* 47:94–97

Hand PJ, Kwan J, Lindley RI *et al.* (2006). Distinguishing between stroke and mimic at the bedside: the brain attack study. *Stroke* 37:769–775

Hankey GJ, Warlow CP (1990). Symptomatic carotid ischaemic events: safest and most cost effective way of selecting patients for angiography before carotid endarterectomy. *British Medical Journal* 300:1485–1491

Hess DC, Nichols FT, Sethi KD *et al.* (1991). Transient cerebral ischaemia masquerading as paroxysmal dyskinesia. *Cerebrovascular Diseases* 1:54–57

Hodges JR, Warlow CP (1990a). Syndromes of transient amnesia: towards a classification. A study of 153 cases. *Journal of Neurology, Neurosurgery and Psychiatry* 53:834–843

Hodges JR, Warlow CP (1990b). The aetiology of transient global amnesia. A case–control study of 114 cases with prospective follow-up. *Brain* 113:639–657

Kamata T, Yokata T, Furukawa T *et al.* (1994). Cerebral ischaemic attack caused by postprandial hypotension. *Stroke* 25:511–513

Kaplan PW (1993). Focal seizures resembling transient ischaemic attacks due to subclinical ischaemia. *Cerebrovascular Diseases* 3:241–243

Kerber KA, Brown DL, Lisabeth LD *et al.* (2006). Stroke among patients with dizziness, vertigo, and imbalance in the emergency department: a population-based study. *Stroke* 37:2484–2487

Kleiner-Fisman G, Kott HS (1998). Myasthenia gravis mimicking stroke in elderly patients. *Mayo Clinic Proceedings.* 73:1077–1078

Kroenke K, Hoffman RM, Einstadter D (2000). How common are various causes of dizziness? A critical review. *South Medical Journal* 93:160

Libman R, Benson R, Einberg K (2002). Myasthenia mimicking vertebrobasilar stroke. *Journal of Neurology* 249:1512–1514

Martin MS, Bamford JM, Sandercock PA (1989). Incidence of transient ischemic attacks in Oxfordshire. *Stroke* 20: 333–339.

Menendez Gonzalez M, Rivera MM (2006). Transient global amnesia: increasing evidence of a venous etiology. *Archives of Neurology* 63:1334–1336

Quinette P, Guillery-Girard B, Dayan J *et al.* (2006). What does transient global amnesia really mean? Review of the literature and thorough study of 142 cases. *Brain* 129:1640–1658

Roach ES (2006). Transient global amnesia: look at mechanisms not causes. *Archives of Neurology* 63:1338–1339

Rolak LA, Fleming JO (2007). The differential diagnosis of multiple sclerosis. *Neurologist* 13:57–72

Ross Russell RW, Page NGR (1983). Critical perfusion of brain and retina. *Brain* 106:419–434

Rothwell PM (1994). Investigation of unilateral sensory or motor symptoms: frequency of neurological pathology depends on side of symptoms. *Journal of Neurology, Neurosurgery and Psychiatry* 57:1401–1402

Ruff RL, Talman WT, Petito F (1981). Transient ischaemic attacks associated with hypotension in hypertensive patients with carotid artery stenosis. *Stroke* 12:353–355

Sander K, Sander D (2005). New insights into transient global amnesia: recent imaging and clinical findings. *Lancet Neurology* 4:437–444

Schulz UG, Rothwell PM (2002). Transient ischaemic attacks mimicking focal motor seizures. *Postgraduate Medicine Journal* **78**:246–247

Schwartz NE, Venkat C, Albers GW (2007). Transient isolated vertigo secondary to an acute stroke of the cerebellar nodulus. *Archives of Neurology* **64**:897

Sedlaczek O, Hirsch JG, Grips E *et al.* (2004). Detection of delayed focal MR changes in the lateral hippocampus in transient global amnesia. *Neurology* **62**:2165–2170

Sherman DG (2004). Reconsideration of TIA diagnostic criteria. *Neurology* **62**:S20–S21

Siddiqi N, House AO, Holmes JD (2006). Occurrence and outcome of delirium in medical in-patients: a systematic literature review. *Age Ageing* **35**:350–364

Sloan MA, Haley EC (1990). The syndrome of bilateral hemispheric border zone ischaemia. *Stroke* **21**:1668–1673

Stevens DL, Matthews WB (1973). Cryptogenic drop attacks: an affliction of women. *British Medical Journal* **i**: 439–442

Voetsch B, DeWitt LD, Pessin MS *et al.* (2004). Basilar artery occlusive disease in the New England Medical Center Posterior Circulation Registry. *Archives of Neurology* **61**:496–504

Zeman AZJ, Boniface SJ, Hodges JR (1998). Transient epileptic amnesia: a description of the clinical and neuropsychological features in 10 cases and a review of the literature. *Journal of Neurology, Neurosurgery and Psychiatry* **64**:435–443

9 The clinical features and differential diagnosis of acute stroke

The diagnosis of stroke is often fairly straightforward. However, clinicians should be aware of the conditions that can mimic stroke since diagnostic errors will have important consequences. In common with TIA, determining the site of the cerebrovascular lesion is important since this narrows down the likely underlying etiology and enables appropriate targeting of investigations (Chs. 10–13). There may be important clues from the history and examination suggesting the underlying cause of the stroke, or that there may be a non-vascular cause for the patients's symptoms and signs. Establishing the underlying cause of the stroke enables specific treatment and secondary prevention (see below).

Diagnosis of stroke

The diagnosis of stroke is relatively straightforward if there is focal brain dysfunction of sudden onset or which was first present on waking. There may be some progression over the first few minutes or hours, particularly in posterior circulation stroke (Brandt *et al.* 2000). Usually the deficit stabilizes by 12–24-hours and, if the patient survives, recovery starts within a few days in most cases. Various scoring systems or similar strategies have been developed as aids in diagnosing stroke (Nor *et al.* 2005; Hand *et al.* 2006), but these are not infallible and clinicians should always consider the potential differential diagnoses (Box 9.1).

If the history is consistent with stroke, there is only a 5% chance of a CT or MR brain scan showing an intracranial mass lesion rather than the expected changes consistent with stroke (Sandercock *et al.* 1985). If the history is consistent with TIA, the likelihood of findings on neuroimaging suggestive of an alternative diagnosis is even lower (Ch. 10). This risk is higher when the speed of onset is uncertain. Features indicative of an **intracranial tumor** (see Fig. 8.2) include recent headaches, seizures, papilloedema, a worsening deficit over days or weeks, and the presence of a primary tumor elsewhere. Chronic **subdural hematoma** (see Figs. 7.3 and 8.1) is suggested by prior head injury, more drowsiness, confusion and headache out of proportion to the severity of the neurological deficit, a fluctuating course, use of anticoagulants or chronic alcohol abuse. Other diagnoses are usually obvious: **multiple sclerosis** occurs at a younger age, **peripheral nerve or root lesion** are accompanied by clinical signs and or pain, **postseizure hemiparesis** is suggested by the history, **metabolic encephalopathy** by global rather than focal neurological features, **somatization and hysteria** by young age and inconsistent signs, **encephalitis** by fever, clinical symptoms and signs and a diffusely abnormal EEG, and **intracranial abscess** by fever and a predisposing cause such as sinusitis or a congenital heart lesion (Norris and Hachinski 1982). Very occasionally, more unusual conditions such as Wilson's disease (Pendlebury *et al.* 2004) and Creutzfelt–Jacob disease may present with stroke-like symptoms (Fig. 9.1).

Occasionally, head injury causing intracerebral hemorrhage can be missed, while hemorrhagic stroke may cause a fall and subsequent head injury; consequently the sequence of

> **Box 9.1.** Differential diagnosis of acute stroke
>
> Intracranial tumor, e.g. glioma, meningioma
> Subdural hematoma
> Epileptic seizure
> Metabolic/toxic encephalopathy: hypoglycemia, hepatic failure, alcohol intoxication
> Cerebral abscess
> Viral encephalitis
> Hypertensive encephalopathy
> Multiple sclerosis
> Head injury
> Peripheral nerve lesion
> Psychogenic (somatization, hysteria)
> Creutzfeldt–Jakob disease

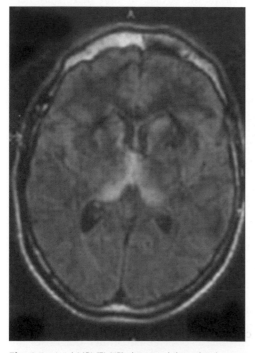

Fig. 9.1. Axial MRI (FLAIR) showing bilateral pulvinar hyperintensity in a patient with new variant Creutzfelt–Jacob disease.

events may be unclear (Berlit *et al.* 1991). Ischemic stroke following head injury may be caused by neck artery dissection (Ch. 6). Residual signs from an old stroke may become more pronounced with intercurrent illness or after a seizure.

Determining the site of the lesion

Determining the location of the stroke provides useful prognostic information and helps to establish the underlying cause for the stroke, since the various clinical syndromes (described below) have differing probabilities of being caused by large or small vessel disease or cardioembolism.

Strokes can be divided into four main clinical syndromes on the basis of symptoms and clinical signs (Bamford *et al.* 1991; Mead *et al.* 1999):

- total anterior circulation syndrome
- partial anterior circulation syndrome
- lacunar syndrome
- posterior circulation syndrome.

These categories provide information on early prognosis, residual disability and risk of recurrence.

Stroke localization using clinical data is not infallible: in about one-quarter of cases where a recent lesion is visible on brain imaging, it is not in the expected place (Mead *et al.* 1999). For example, although most pure motor strokes are caused by a lacunar infarct as a result of small vessel disease, in a few cases the CT or MR scan shows striatocapsular infarction caused by middle cerebral artery occlusion with good cortical collaterals

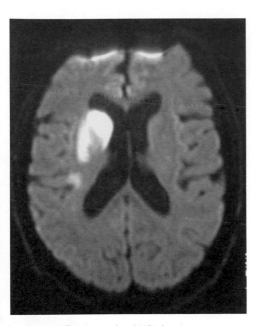

Fig. 9.2. Diffusion-weighted MRI showing a striatocapsular infarct.

(Fig. 9.2). Therefore, patients may need to be reclassified on the basis of the brain imaging results.

Total anterior circulation syndrome

A large hematoma in one cerebral hemisphere, or an infarct affecting a large proportion of the middle cerebral artery territory, causes a characteristic clinical syndrome:

- contralateral hemiparesis, with or without a sensory deficit and involving the whole of at least two of the three body areas: the face, upper limb or lower limb
- a homonymous visual field defect
- a cortical deficit consisting of dysphasia, neglect or visuospatial problems.

Cognitive or visual field defects may have to be assumed in drowsy patients. Deviation of the eyes towards the affected hemisphere is common but recovers in a few days. A large hematoma may cause midline shift, transtentorial herniation and coma within 24-hours (Fig. 9.3). By contrast, these changes take two or three days to evolve with large infarcts as cerebral edema develops.

Total anterior circulation infarcts are usually the result of acute occlusion of the internal carotid artery or embolic occlusion of the proximal middle cerebral artery from a cardiac or proximal arterial source (Caplan 1993; Lindgren *et al.* 1994; Wardlaw *et al.* 1996, Georgiadis *et al.* 2004) (see Fig. 5.1). Sometimes the cortex is relatively spared owing to good pial collaterals or rapid recanalization of the occluded artery, and infarction is largely subcortical in the distribution of several lenticulostriate arteries. This may be seen as a characteristic area of "striatocapsular infarction" on brain imaging (Fig. 9.2). This clinical syndrome is not as severe as a total anterior circulation syndrome, having less cognitive deficit and often being without homonymous hemianopia (Nicolai *et al.* 1996).

Partial anterior circulation syndrome

A lobar hemorrhage, or a cortical infarct, causes a more restricted clinical syndrome (Bassetti *et al.* 1993; Aerden *et al.* 2004):

- any two of the following three components of a total anterior circulation syndrome: hemiparesis or hemiplegia contralateral to hemispheric lesion, homonymous visual field defect, and cortical deficit (dysphasia, neglect or visuospatial problems)

  or
- motor/sensory deficit restricted to one body area or part of one body area
- isolated cortical deficit such as dysphasia.

It may be difficult to distinguish between some partial anterior circulation syndromes and a 'lacunar' stroke.

Partial anterior circulation infarcts (Fig. 9.4) are caused by occlusion of a branch of the middle cerebral artery, or rarely the trunk of the anterior cerebral artery. They are usually

(a)   (b)

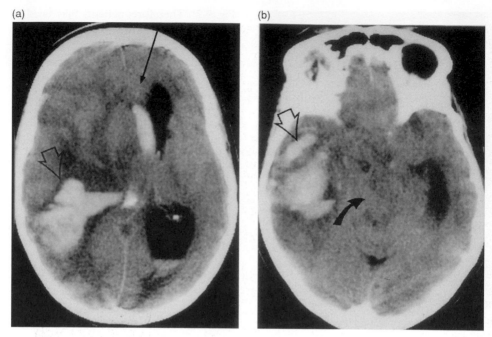

Fig. 9.3. Large intracerebral hematoma with mass effect.

a consequence of embolism from the heart or proximal atherothrombosis as in total anterior circulation infarcts. Investigation should be prompt because of the high risk of recurrence. Anterior cerebral artery infarcts cause contralateral weakness predominantly of the lower limb, sometimes with cortical sensory loss, and aphasia if in the dominant hemisphere. Left, and rarely right, anterior cerebral infarcts can cause a curious dyspraxia of the left upper limb owing to infarction of the corpus callosum disconnecting the right motor centers from the left language centers (Kazui *et al.* 1992). Bilateral leg and even additional bilateral arm weakness has been described when both anterior cerebral arteries are supplied from one stenosed internal carotid artery, or if both anterior cerebral arteries are occluded by embolism, so mimicking a brainstem or spinal cord syndrome (Borggreve *et al.* 1994).

Some anterior circulation syndromes, usually classified as partial anterior circulation syndromes, are caused by boundary zone infarcts. The rare anterior choroidal artery distribution infarcts, which can be defined only by the CT or MRI pattern, are probably caused by microvascular disease as well as embolism, and they can lead to a partial anterior circulation syndrome or lacunar syndrome (Hupperts *et al.* 1994).

Lacunar syndrome

Lacunar syndromes are defined clinically. They are highly predictive of small, deep lesions affecting the motor and/or sensory pathways in the corona radiata, internal capsule, thalamus, cerebral peduncle or pons. Although a few patients have a partial anterior circulation infarct (Bamford *et al.* 1987; Anzalone and Landi 1989; Arboix *et al.* 2007), the great majority have small infarcts, which are sometimes visible on CT, more often on MRI. These are caused by presumed occlusion of a small perforating artery affected by intracranial small vessel disease (see Fig. 10.2). There is no visual field defect, no new cortical

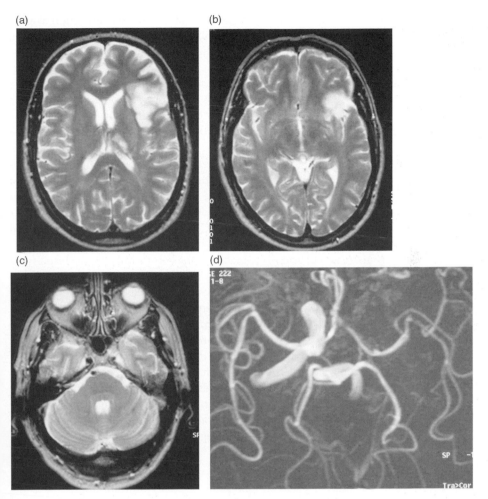

Fig. 9.4. Axial T$_2$-weighted MRI scans (a–c) and a magnetic resonance angiogram (d) showing a right partial anterior circulation infarct secondary to right carotid occlusion.

defect, no impairment of consciousness and nothing to suggest a brainstem syndrome, for instance diplopia or crossed motor and sensory deficits.

The four main lacunar syndromes are:

- pure motor deficit
- pure sensory deficit: involving two or three of the areas face, arm and leg
- sensorimotor deficit
- ataxic hemiparesis.

Pure motor stroke constitutes about 50% of lacunar cases. It consists of a unilateral motor deficit involving two or three areas, the face, upper arm and/or leg, including the whole of each area that is affected. There are often sensory symptoms but no sensory signs. The lesion occurs at locations where the motor pathways are closely packed together and separate from other pathways: usually in the internal capsule or pons, sometimes the corona radiata or cerebral peduncle, and rarely in the medullary pyramid. There may be a flurry of immediately preceding TIAs, the so-called capsular warning syndrome (Donnan *et al.* 1996).

Pure sensory stroke constitutes about 5% of cases. It has the same distribution as pure motor stroke but the symptoms are of sensory loss, with or without sensory signs affecting all modalities equally, or sparing proprioception. The lesion is usually in the thalamus (see Fig. 10.3) but can be in the brainstem.

Sensorimotor stroke constitutes about 35% of cases. It is the combination of a pure motor stroke with sensory signs in the affected body parts. The lesion is usually in the thalamus or internal capsule, but it can be in the corona radiata or pons. A similar clinical picture can be caused by cortical infarcts, leading to misclassification (Blecic et al. 1993).

Ataxic hemiparesis constitutes about 10% of cases. It is the combination of cortico-spinal and ipsilateral cerebellar-like dysfunction affecting the arm and/or leg. It includes a syndrome in which there is little more than dysarthria and one clumsy hand. The lesion is usually in the pons, internal capsule or cerebral peduncle. Dysarthria, with or without upper motor neuron facial weakness, may also be a lacunar syndrome with similar lesion localization as ataxic hemiparesis, but there are other localizing possibilities as well.

Small deep infarcts in the subcortical white matter of the corona radiata may result from small vessel disease affecting the long medullary perforating arteries extending down from cortical branches of the middle cerebral artery or from embolism. Such centrum semiovale infarcts present as either a lacunar syndrome or, occasionally, as a partial anterior cirulation syndrome with "cortical" features (Read et al. 1998; Lammie and Wardlaw 1999). They are not, however, easy to classify or to distinguish from border zone infarcts deeper in the white matter lying between the arterial territories of the deep perforators from the first part of the middle cerebral artery and the superficial medullary perforators.

Various other lacunar syndromes have been described with rather poor clinical–pathological–anatomical correlation; for example, chorea or hemiballismus usually appears to be caused by a lesion in the contralateral subthalamic nucleus or elsewhere in the basal ganglia and tends to get better (Ghika and Bogousslavsky 2001).

Posterior circulation syndrome

Brainstem, cerebellar, thalamic or occipital lobe signs normally indicate infarction in the distribution of the vertebrobasilar circulation or a localized hemorrhage.

The posterior circulation syndrome consists of any one of the following:

- motor and/or sensory deficit and cranial nerve palsy
- bilateral motor and/or sensory deficit
- deficit of conjugate eye movement
- cerebellar deficit
- isolated hemianopia or cortical blindness.

A combination of brainstem and occipital lobe signs is highly suggestive of infarction caused by thromboembolism within the basilar and posterior cerebral artery territories. Occasionally, proximal posterior cerebral artery occlusion causes extensive temporal, thalamic and perhaps midbrain infarction. This results in contralateral hemiparesis and sensory loss, and a marked cognitive deficit such as aphasia, as well as the expected homonymous hemianopia. This syndrome may be confused with occlusion of the middle cerebral artery or one of its branches (Argentino et al. 1996). This is the so-called "walking total anterior circulation syndrome" because although it fulfils the definition of a total anterior circulation syndrome, the motor loss is mild. Cerebellar hematomas have fairly characteristic clinical features except in the case of massive hemorrhage, which is clinically indistinguishable from brainstem stroke, and very small hemorrhages, which may simulate a peripheral disorder of the vestibular system (Jensen and St. Louis 2005).

The causes of infarction in the vertebrobasilar territory are heterogeneous. Often they are difficult to establish since vertebral angiography is seldom carried out, although non-invasive arterial imaging is increasingly helpful. Some lacunar syndromes result from small brainstem or thalamic infarcts following small vessel occlusion: intracranial small vessel disease or atheroma at the mouth of small perforating arteries. However, both small and large infarcts can be caused by embolism from the heart by atherothrombosis, affecting the vertebral and basilar arteries; thrombotic occlusion complicating atheroma of the basilar artery or its major branches; or by low flow distal to vertebral and other arterial occlusions.

Although a large number of posterior circulation syndromes have been described, there is no clear association with a unique pattern of arterial occlusion or with prognosis. Syndromes include the "top of the basilar" syndrome (Caplan 1980), various other mid-brain syndromes (Bogousslavsky *et al.* 1994), the locked-in syndrome (Patterson and Grabois 1986), pontine syndromes (Bassetti *et al.* 1996), lateral medullary syndromes (Kim *et al.* 1998) and medial medullary syndromes (Bassetti *et al.* 1997). Recognition of these is more an exercise in clinical–anatomical correlation rather than being very useful for clinical management. Because thalamic and cerebellar strokes can cause diagnostic confusion, and the latter may require surgical treatment, they are given separate consideration below.

Thalamic stroke

Small thalamic lesions may cause a pure sensory stroke or sensorimotor stroke, sometimes with ataxia in the same limbs (Schmahmann 2003). However, other deficits may occur in isolation, or in combination depending on which thalamic nuclei are involved. These include paralysis of upward gaze, small pupils, apathy, depressed consciousness, hypersomnolence, disorientation, visual hallucinations, aphasia and impairment of verbal memory attributable to the left thalamus, and visuospatial dysfunction attributable to the right thalamus. Occlusion of a single small branch of the proximal posterior cerebral artery can cause bilateral paramedian thalamic infarction with severe retrograde and anterograde amnesia.

Thalamic stroke should be considered when there is a sudden onset of behavioral disturbance. The diagnosis is often missed since patients are thought to have primary psychiatric disorders, especially when neurological dysfunction is lacking. Distinct behavioral patterns can be delineated on the basis of the four main arterial thalamic territories (Schmahmann 2003; Carrera and Bogousslavsky 2006):

- the anterior pattern consists mainly of perseverations, apathy and amnesia; paramedian infarction causes disinhibition and personality change, amnesia and, in the case of extensive lesions, thalamic "dementia"
- after inferolateral lesion, executive dysfunction may develop but is often overlooked, although it may occasionally lead to severe long-term disability
- posterior lesions are known to cause cognitive dysfunction, including neglect and aphasia, but no specific behavioral syndrome has been reported.

Cerebellar strokes

Cerebellar strokes can be mild, with sudden vertigo, nausea, imbalance, and horizontal nystagmus, which soon recovers. They are frequently misdiagnosed as labyrinthitis. More extensive infarction, or hemorrhage, causes additional ipsilateral limb and truncal ataxia, as well as dysarthria. Very severe strokes cause occipital headache, vomiting and depressed consciousness, so making it impossible to detect limb or truncal ataxia. There are often additional brainstem signs such as ipsilateral facial weakness and sensory loss, a gaze palsy to the side of the lesion, ipsilateral deafness and tinnitus, and bilateral extensor plantar responses. These occur because of pressure from a large edematous infarct or hematoma, or because an occluded artery supplying the cerebellum may also supply parts of the brainstem. Mass effect can obstruct flow of cerebrospinal fluid from the fourth ventricle, causing acute or subacute hydrocephalus. The consequent coma and meningism may be mistaken for subarachnoid hemorrhage. A CT scan will reveal a hematoma, but the signs of an infarct are more subtle, with disappearance or shift of the fourth ventricle owing to mass effect before the low density of the lesion itself appears. Magnetic resonance is more sensitive in infarction and provides detail of any additional brainstem involvement. It should be noted that initial mild symptoms may be misleading and patients may deteriorate rapidly. Accordingly, urgent brain imaging is mandatory in suspected cerebellar stroke, irrespective of apparent clinical severity.

Patients who become acutely or subacutely comatose have a very poor prognosis. However, if there is little evidence of primary brainstem infarction, drainage of any hydrocephalus and/or decompression of the posterior fossa may sometimes be followed by relatively good-quality survival.

Boundary zone infarcts

Boundary zone infarcts occur in the border zones *between* arterial territories:

- anterior boundary zone: between the superficial territories of the middle cerebral artery and anterior cerebral artery in the frontoparasagittal region
- posterior boundary zone: between the superficial territories of the middle cerebral artery and posterior cerebral artery in the parieto-occipital region
- subcortical boundary zone: between the superficial medullary penetrators and deep lenticulostriate territories of the middle cerebral artery in the paraventricular white matter of the corona radiation.

There is evidence that both low-flow and microembolism may be important in causing boundary zone infarction (Momjian-Mayor and Baron 2005). The evidence strongly favors a hemodynamic mechanism for internal boundary zone infarction, especially in the centrum semiovale. However, the relationship between cortical boundary zone infarction and hemodynamic compromise appears more complicated, and artery-to-artery embolism may play an important role. Based on the high prevalence of microembolic signals documented by ultrasound in symptomatic carotid disease, embolism and hypoperfusion may play a synergistic role, with small emboli lodging in distal field arterioles being more likely to result in cortical microinfarcts when chronic hypoperfusion prevails. Future studies combining imaging of brain perfusion, diffusion-weighted imaging and ultrasound detection of microembolic signals should help to resolve these issues.

Low flow may occur secondary to systemic hypotension, as during cardiac arrest. This results in bilateral infarcts, usually in the posterior boundary zones, and causes cortical blindness, visual disorientation and agnosia, and amnesia. Alternatively, a relatively small fall in systemic blood pressure in the presence of internal carotid occlusion or stenosis may cause unilateral boundary zone infarction, usually in the anterior and subcortical regions. This causes contralateral weakness of the leg more than the arm, with sparing of the face, some impaired sensation in the same areas, and aphasia if the dominant hemisphere is affected. Unilateral posterior boundary zone infarcts are less common and cause contralateral hemianopia and cortical sensory loss, along with aphasia if the dominant hemisphere is affected.

Miscellaneous clinical features

Cranial nerves

Unilateral supratentorial stroke lesions can cause contralateral weakness of the bulbar muscles, with unilateral weakness of the palate, tongue and forehead musculature, resembling a lower motor-neuron rather than upper motor-neuron facial palsy. Because all these muscles have a strong *bilateral* upper motor-neuron innervation, this weakness tends to disappear quite quickly in most cases. The bulbar muscle weakness may be enough to cause significant dysphagia; therefore, dysphagia is not a symptom exclusively confined to brainstem strokes. Dysarthria is common in supratentorial strokes, usually in proportion to any facial weakness, and is a defining feature of the clumsy hand–dysarthria syndrome, but it can be isolated with no localizing value (Ichikawa and Kageyama 1991). Any weakness of the sternomastoid muscle is ipsilateral to a supratentorial lesion so there is difficulty turning the head away from the side of the lesion. Lower cranial nerve lesions ipsilateral to a supratentorial infarct suggest dissection of the internal carotid artery. Lesions of cranial nerves III, IV and VI have rarely been described ipsilateral to internal carotid artery occlusion or dissection, presumably caused by ischemia of the nerve trunks.

Headache

Headache is not uncommon around the time of stroke onset. It is more often severe in primary intracerebral hemorrhage than ischemic stroke, and more often severe with posterior than anterior circulation strokes. If the headache is localized at all, it tends to be over the site of the lesion. Headache is more common in cortical and posterior circulation than lacunar infarcts (Kumral *et al.* 1995). Severe unilateral neck, orbital or scalp pain suggests internal carotid artery dissection, particularly if there is an ipsilateral Horner's syndrome. Severe occipital headache can occur with vertebral artery dissection. Headache is also a particular feature of venous infarcts. Unusual headache in the days before stroke would suggest giant cell arteritis or perhaps a mass lesion rather than a stroke.

Movement disorders

Acute hemiparkinsonism contralateral to a basal ganglia stroke is rare. Contralateral chorea, hemiballismus and sometimes tremor or dystonia are more common (D'Olhaberriague *et al.* 1995; Scott and Jankovic 1996; Giroud *et al.* 1997). Dystonia often develops gradually in a hemiplegic limb some weeks after the stroke, particularly in children and young adults. Rather nondescript "limb-shaking" has been described in patients with "low flow" TIA and can occur in stroke, particularly in brainstem infarction.

Determining the cause of the stroke: pathophysiological mechanism

The four main classifications described above (Bamford *et al.* 1991; Mead *et al.* 1999) are clinical and can be determined at the bedside and following the results of brain imaging. Further classification is possible in ischemic stroke by etiology, and this is most commonly done according to the TOAST criteria.

TOAST classification

The TOAST system attempts to classify ischemic strokes according to the major causative pathophysiological mechanisms. It assigns ischemic strokes to five subtypes based upon clinical features and the results of investigation including brain and vascular imaging, cardiac tests and laboratory tests for a prothrombotic state (Adams *et al.* 1993). It was originally developed in a clinical trial of heparin (Trial of ORG 10172) but has been used extensively in both research and clinical practice and has been modified only slightly since its first description in 1993 (Adams *et al.* 1993; Ay *et al.* 2005).

The five TOAST subtypes of ischemic stroke are:

- large artery atherosclerosis
- cardioembolism
- small vessel occlusion
- stroke of other determined etiology
- stroke of undetermined etiology.

Large artery atherosclerosis is confirmed by the presence of brain or vascular imaging findings of either significant stenosis ($>50\%$) or occlusion of a major brain artery or branch cortical artery, presumably through atherosclerosis. Cortical, cerebellar, brainstem or large subcortical lesions on CT or MRI are supportive of the diagnosis, as are symptoms or signs of large artery disease elsewhere. The most frequent sources of cardioembolism (Ch. 6) are:

- atrial fibrillation
- a mechanical prosthetic valve
- mitral stenosis
- left atrial or left ventricular thrombus
- recent myocardial infarction
- dilated cardiomyopathy
- infective endocarditis.

The small vessel occlusion category corresponds to the lacunar syndrome described by Bamford *et al.* (1991) and is supported by normal brain imaging or a relevant subcortical or brainstem infarct measuring <1.5 cm. "Other determined etiologies" include non-atherosclerotic vasculopathies, hypercoagulable states and hematological disorders. Stroke of undetermined etiology includes those in which evaluation has been inadequate, adequate evaluation has not revealed a cause ("cryptogenic stroke") and those in which two or more potential causes have been identified (for instance a patient who has atrial fibrillation and an ipsilateral carotid stenosis of 60%, or a patient with a traditional lacunar syndrome and an ipsilateral carotid stenosis of 60%).

Some overlap exists between the clinical classification (Bamford *et al.* 1991) and the etiological TOAST classification. In a large hospital-based series of patients with ischemic stroke, total and partial anterior circulation infarcts were most likely to be caused by large artery atherosclerosis, cardioembolism or both (Wardlaw *et al.* 1999).

Determining the cause of the stroke: clues from the history

In the vast majority of strokes, there is the sudden onset of focal symptoms without any other features. However, it is important to take a detailed history since occasionally there may be a more gradual onset of symptoms, thus widening the differential diagnosis, or there may be points in the history suggesting an underlying cause for the stroke or an indication that the presentation is of a condition mimicking stroke (Table 9.1).

Gradual onset

Gradual onset of stroke over hours or days, rather than seconds or minutes, is unusual and is much more likely to occur in ischemic than in hemorrhagic stroke. If the onset is gradual, and not likely to be caused by low flow or migraine (Ch. 8), then a structural intracranial lesion must be excluded. In younger patients, multiple sclerosis should also be considered. However, focal neurological deficits that develop over hours, or up to two days, in elderly patients are still most likely to have a vascular cause since vascular disease is so common in older patients.

Precipitating factors

The activity being undertaken at stroke onset and the time of onset may both be important. Anything to suggest a fall in cerebral perfusion or blood pressure may be relevant, as is pregnancy and any operative procedure. Activity affecting head position, or head and neck trauma (see Ch. 6), may indicate dissection. Recurrent attacks first thing in the morning or during exercise suggest hypoglycemia (may be the presenting feature of insulinoma or related to drugs such as pentamidine as well as diabetes). Onset during a Valsalva maneuver such as lifting, suggests a low-flow ischemic stroke or paradoxical embolism (Ch. 6).

Headache

Headache at around the onset of ischemic stroke or TIA occurs in about 25% of patients, is usually mild and, if localized at all, tends to be related to the position of the brain/eye lesion. It is more common with ischemia in the vertebrobasilar than carotid distribution and is less common with lacunar ischemia. Severe pain unilaterally in the head, face, neck or eye at around or before the time of stroke onset is highly suggestive of carotid dissection, while vertebral dissection tends to cause unilateral or sometimes bilateral occipital pain (Ch. 6). Migrainous stroke may be accompanied by headache (Chs. 6 and 8) and patients with cerebral autosomal dominant arteriopathy with subcortical infarcts and leukoencephalopathy (CADASIL) usually have a history of migraine. In the context of the differential diagnosis of TIAs, migraine should be fairly obvious, unless there is no headache (Ch. 8). It is important to note that vertebrobasilar ischemia may cause similar symptoms to migraine with headache, gradual onset of focal neurological symptoms and visual disturbance.

Although intracranial venous thrombosis usually causes either a benign intracranial hypertension syndrome or a subacute encephalopathy, sometimes the onset is focal. The diagnosis may be suggested by headache, which occurs in the majority of patients (around 75%) (Ch. 30). Stroke (or TIA) in the context of a headache occurring for days or weeks previously must raise the possibility of giant cell arteritis and other inflammatory vascular disorders (Ch. 6). Pain in the jaw muscles with chewing, which resolves with rest, strongly suggests claudication, caused more frequently by giant cell arteritis than atherothrombosis of the external carotid artery.

Epileptic seizures

Epileptic seizures, partial or generalized, within hours of stroke onset are unusual in adults (5%) and should lead to a reconsideration of non-stroke brain pathologies, particularly since contrast enhancement of a tumor on CT can be misinterpreted as an infarct. The risk of seizure is higher with hemorrhagic than ischemic strokes and if the lesion is large and involves the cerebral cortex (Arboix et al. 2003). Seizures are common in venous infarction (up to 40%) and mitochondrial cytopathy. Partial motor seizures can be confused with limb-shaking TIAs (Ch. 8), but the former are more clonic and the jerking spreads in

Table 9.1. Important clues from the history that may suggest the cause of an ischemic stroke, or that the diagnosis of cerebrovascular disease should be reconsidered

Type	Features
Gradual onset	Low cerebral blood flow without acute occlusion (Ch. 6)
	Migraine (Ch. 8)
	Structural intracranial lesion (Chs. 8 and 9)
	Multiple sclerosis
Precipitating factors	Suspected systemic hypotension or low cerebral perfusion pressure (standing up or sitting up quickly, heavy meal, hot weather, hot bath, warming the face, exercise, coughing, hyperventilation, chest pain or palpitations, starting or changing blood pressure-lowering drugs)
	Pregnancy/puerperium
	Surgery
	Head turning
	Hypoglycemia
	Valsalva maneuver (paradoxical embolism, or low flow)
Recent headache	Carotid/vertebral dissection (Ch. 6)
	Migrainous stroke/transient ischemic attack (Ch. 8)
	Intracranial venous thrombosis (Ch. 29)
	Giant cell arteritis (or other inflammatory vascular disorders) (Ch. 6)
	Structural intracranial lesion (Chs. 8 and 9)
Epileptic seizures	Intracranial venous thrombosis (Ch. 29)
	Mitochondrial diseases (Ch. 6)
	Non-vascular intracranial lesion (Chs. 8 and 9)
Malaise	Inflammatory arterial disorders (Ch. 6)
	Infective endocarditis (Ch. 6)
	Cardiac myxoma (Ch. 6)
	Cancer (Ch. 6)
	Thrombotic thrombocytopenic purpura (Ch. 6)
	Sarcoidosis (Ch. 6)
Chest pain	Myocardial infarction
	Aortic dissection
	Paradoxical embolism (Ch. 6)
Non-stroke vascular disease or vascular risk factors	Ischemic heart disease (Ch. 2)
	Claudication (Ch. 2)
	Hypertension (Ch. 2)
	Smoking (Ch. 2)
Drugs	Oral contraceptives (Ch. 2)
	Estrogens in men (Ch. 2)
	Blood pressure-lowering/vasodilators (Ch. 6)
	Hypoglycemic drugs (Ch. 6)

Table 9.1. (*cont.*)

Type	Features
	Cocaine, ecstasy (Ch. 6)
	Amphetamines (Ch. 6)
	Ephedrine (Ch. 6)
	Phenylpropanolamine (Ch. 6)
	Atypical antipsychotic drugs
Injury	Chronic subdural hematoma (Ch. 7)
	Vertebral/carotid artery dissection (Ch. 6)
	Fat embolism (Ch. 6)
Self-audible bruits	Internal carotid artery stenosis (distal)
	Dural arteriovenous fistula (Ch. 7)
	Glomus tumor
	Caroticocavernous fistula (Ch. 7)
	Raised intracranial pressure
	Intracranial venous thrombosis (Ch. 29)
Past medical history	Inflammatory bowel disease (Ch. 6)
	Coeliac disease (Ch. 6)
	Homocystinuria (Ch. 6)
	Cancer (Ch. 6)
	Irradiation of the head or neck (Ch. 6)
	Recurrent deep venous thrombosis
	Recurrent miscarriages
	Recent surgery/long-distance travel
Family history (Table 3.2)	

a typical jacksonian way from one body part to another and the latter are supposed never to involve the face. Rarely, transient focal ischemia seems to cause partial epileptic seizures, but proving a causal relationship is seldom possible (Kaplan 1993). Interestingly, onset of idiopathic seizures late in life is a powerful independent predictor of subsequent stroke (Cleary *et al.* 2004) and of dementia after stroke (Cordonnier *et al.* 2007). Seizures preceded by malaise, headache and fever suggest encephalitis.

Malaise

Stroke in the context of preceeding malaise for up to some months suggests an inflammatory arterial disorder, particularly giant cell arteritis, infective endocarditis, cardiac myxoma, cancer, thrombotic thrombocytopenic purpura or even sarcoidosis (Ch. 6).

Chest pain

Chest pain may be indicative of a recent myocardial infarction with complicating stroke, aortic dissection (particularly if the pain is also interscapular) or pulmonary embolism and raises the possibility of paradoxical embolism.

Vascular risk factors

Vascular risk factors (Ch. 2) and diseases should be sought. It is unusual for an ischemic stroke or TIA to occur in someone with no vascular risk factors, unless they are very old, or are young with some unusual cause of stroke (Ch. 6). A history of heart disease may be relevant and cardiac symptoms should be specifically inquired about.

Drugs

Drugs may be relevant: oral contraceptives in women, estrogens in men, hypotensive agents, hypoglycemic agents and recreational drugs.

Injury

Any injury in the days and weeks before ischemic stroke or TIA onset is important and may not be spontaneously volunteered by the patient particularly where this occurred some time previously. A head or neck injury might have caused a chronic subdural hematoma (highly unlikely if more than three months previously) or carotid or vertebral dissection (Ch. 6).

Self-audible bruits

Pulsatile self-audible bruits are rare. They can be differentiated from tinnitus because they are in time with the pulse. They may be audible to the examiner on auscultation of the neck, eye or cranium and may indicate:

- distal internal carotid artery stenosis (dissection or, rarely, atherothrombosis)
- dural arteriovenous fistula near the petrous temporal bone
- glomus tumor
- caroticocavernous fistula
- intracranial venous thrombosis
- symptomatic and idiopathic intracranial hypertension
- loop in the internal carotid artery.

Past medical history

Recurrent deep venous thrombosis suggests thrombophilia, particularly if there is a family history, or the antiphospholipid syndrome, the latter being suggested by the accompanying feature of recurrent miscarriage. Any reason for a recent deep vein thrombosis (e.g. a long-haul flight or surgery) should raise the question of paradoxical embolism. Past medical history of a condition predisposing to stroke (Chs. 2, 3 and 6) may be present.

Previous strokes and/or transient ischemic attacks

Previous strokes and/or TIAs in different vascular territories are more likely with a proximal embolic source in the heart, or arch of the aorta, than with a single arterial lesion. Attacks going back months or more make certain causes such as infective endocarditis and arterial dissection unlikely.

Family history

There are several rare familial conditions that may be complicated by ischemic stroke and TIAs (Table 3.2). However, family history of stroke is only a modest risk factor for sporadic ischemic stroke (Flossmann and Rothwell, 2004) and a family history of stroke is associated with little or no increase the risk of future stroke (Flossmann and Rothwell 2005, 2006) (Ch. 3).

Determining the cause of stroke: clues from the examination

Similarly to a detailed history, careful clinical examination of the patient with suspected stroke may provide clues to the underlying cause of the stroke (Table 9.1).

Neurological examination

Neurological examination is primarily to localize the brain lesion but there may also be clues as to the cause of the stroke: a Horner's syndrome ipsilateral to a carotid distribution infarct suggests dissection of the internal carotid artery or sometimes acute atherothrombotic carotid occlusion. Lower cranial nerve lesions ipsilateral to a hemispheric cerebral infarct can also occur in carotid dissection.

Total anterior circulation syndromes or brainstem strokes often cause some drowsiness, but in smaller lesions, consciousness is normal. Therefore if consciousness is impaired and yet the focal deficit is mild, it is important to:

- reconsider the differential diagnosis (particularly chronic subdural hematoma)
- consider the diffuse encephalopathic disorders that have focal features and that may masquerade as stroke, for example cerebral vasculitis, non-bacterial thrombotic endocarditis, intracranial venous thrombosis, mitochondrial cytopathy, thrombotic thrombocytopenic purpura, familial hemiplegic migraine and Hashimoto's encephalitis
- be aware that comorbidity, such as pneumonia, sedative drugs, infection and hypoglycemia, may excacerbate the neurological deficit

Eyes

The eyes may provide general clues to the cause of a stroke (e.g. diabetic or hypertensive retinopathy) or may reveal papilloedema, which would make the diagnosis of ischemic stroke, or even intracerebral hemorrhage, most unlikely. There may be evidence of retinal emboli, which are often asymptomatic. Roth spots in the retina are very suggestive of infective endocarditis. Dislocated lenses should suggest Marfan's syndrome or homocystinuria. Angioid streaks in the retina suggest pseudoxanthoma elasticum, and in hyperviscosity syndromes there is a characteristic retinopathy.

Dilated episcleral vessels are a clue to abnormal anastamoses between branches of the external carotid artery and orbital branches of the internal carotid artery, distal to severe internal carotid artery disease. With extreme ischemia, ischemic oculopathy may develop, with impaired visual acuity, eye pain, rubeosis of the iris (dilated blood vessels), fixed dilated pupil, 'low-pressure' glaucoma, cataract and corneal edema.

Arterial pulses

Both radial pulses should be examined simultaneously since inequality in timing or volume suggests subclavian or innominate stenosis or occlusion and, importantly, aortic dissection.

Tenderness of the branches of the external carotid artery (occipital, facial, superficial temporal) points towards giant cell arteritis. Tenderness of the common carotid artery in the neck can occur in acute carotid occlusion but is more likely to be a sign of dissection, or arteritis. Absence of several neck and arm pulses in a young person occurs in Takayasu's arteritis (Ch. 6). Delayed or absent leg pulses suggest coarctation of the aorta or, much more commonly, peripheral vascular disease. Other causes of widespread disease of the aortic arch are atheroma, giant cell arteritis, syphilis, subintimal fibrosis, arterial dissection and trauma.

Table 9.2. Clues to the cause of ischemic stroke/transient ischemic attack from examination of the skin and nails

Feature	Possible cause
Finger clubbing	Right-to-left intracardiac shunt
	Cancer (Ch. 6)
	Pulmonary arteriovenous malformation (Ch. 6)
	Infective endocarditis (Ch. 6)
	Inflammatory bowel disease (Ch. 6)
Splinter hemorrhages	Infective endocarditis (Ch. 6)
	Cholesterol embolization syndrome (Ch. 6)
	Vasculitis (Ch. 6)
Scleroderma	Systemic sclerosis (Ch. 6)
Livedo reticularis	Sneddon's syndrome (Ch. 6)
	Systemic lupus erythematosus (Ch. 6)
	Polyarteritis nodosa (Ch. 6)
	Cholesterol embolization syndrome (Ch. 6)
Lax skin	Ehlers–Danlos syndrome (Ch. 3)
	Pseudoxanthoma elasticum (Ch. 3)
Skin color	Anemia (Ch. 6)
	Polycythemia (Ch. 6)
	Cyanosis (right-to-left intracardiac shunt, pulmonary arteriovenous malformation) (Ch. 6)
Porcelain-white papules/scars	Kohlmeier–Degos disease (Ch. 6)
Skin scars	Ehlers–Danlos syndrome (Ch. 3)
Petechiae/purpura/bruising	Thrombotic thrombocytopenic purpura (Ch. 6)
	Fat embolism (Ch. 6)
	Cholesterol embolization syndrome (Ch. 6)
	Ehlers–Danlos syndrome (Ch. 3)
Orogenital ulceration	Behçet's disease (Ch. 6)
Rash	Fabry's disease (Ch. 6)
	Systemic lupus erythematosus (Ch. 6)
	Tuberous sclerosis (Ch. 6)
Epidermal naevi	Epidermal naevus syndrome
Café-au-lait patches	Neurofibromatosis
Thrombosed superficial veins, needle marks	Intravenous drug use (Ch. 6)

The prevalence of aortic aneurysm in patients with stroke and TIA is unknown but is likely to be high, particularly if the patient has carotid stenosis (Ch. 6).

Cervical bruits

A localized bruit over the carotid bifurcation (under the jaw) is predictive of some degree of carotid stenosis, but very tight stenosis or occlusion may not cause a bruit at all. Bruits may be asymptomatic, particularly in women, probably owing to sex differences in carotid bifurcation anatomy (Schulz and Rothwell 2001) and less likely to be associated with carotid stenosis.

Cardiac examination

Thorough cardiac examination should look for possible cardiac source of embolism, including atrial fibrillation, mitral stenosis and prosthetic heart valves. Left ventricular hypertrophy suggests hypertension or aortic stenosis, and a displaced apex from a dilated left ventricle indicates underlying cardiac or valvular pathology.

Fever

Fever is unusual in the first few hours after stroke onset, and endocarditis or other infections, inflammatory vascular disorders or cardiac myxoma should be considered. Later fever is quite common and usually reflects a complication of the stroke (Ch. 16).

Other indications

Clues as to the cause of a stroke may be obtained from examination of the skin and nails (Table 9.2).

References

Adams HP Jr., Bendixen BH, Kappelle LJ et al. (1993). Classification of subtype of acute ischemic stroke. Definitions for use in a multicenter clinical trial. TOAST. Trial of Org 10172 in Acute Stroke Treatment. Stroke 24:35–41

Aerden L, Luijckx GJ, Ricci S et al. (2004). Validation of the Oxfordshire Community Stroke Project syndrome diagnosis derived from a standard symptom list in acute stroke. Journal of Neurology Science 220:55–58

Anzalone N, Landi G (1989). Non ischaemic causes of lacunar syndromes: prevalence and clinical findings. Journal of Neurology, Neurosurgery and Psychiatry 52:1188–1190

Arboix, A, Comes, E, Garcia-Eroles et al. (2003). Prognostic value of very early seizures for in-hospital mortality in atherothrombotic infarction. European Neurology 50:78–84

Arboix A, Garcia-Eroles L, Massons J et al. (2007). Haemorrhagic pure motor stroke. European Journal of Neurology 14:219–223

Argentino C, De Michele M, Fiorelli M et al. (1996). Posterior circulation infarcts simulating anterior circulation stroke: perspective of the acute phase. Stroke 27:1306–1309

Ay H, Furie KL, Singhal A et al. (2005). An evidence-based causative classification system for acute ischemic stroke. Annals of Neurology 58:688–697

Bamford J, Sandercock PAG, Jones L et al. (1987). The natural history of lacunar infarction: the Oxfordshire Community Stroke Project. Stroke 18:545–551

Bamford J, Sandercock P, Dennis M et al. (1991). Classification and natural history of clinically identifiable subtypes of cerebral infarction. Lancet 337:1521–1526

Bassetti C, Bogousslavsky J, Regli F (1993). Sensory syndromes in parietal stroke. Neurology 43:1942–1949

Bassetti C, Bogousslavsky J, Barth A, Regli F (1996). Isolated infarcts of the pons. Neurology 46:165–175

Bassetti C, Bogousslavsky J, Mattle H et al. (1997). Medial medullary stroke: report of seven patients and review of the literature. Neurology 48:882–890

Berlit P, Rakicky J, Tornow K (1991). Differential diagnosis of spontaneous and traumatic intracranial haemorrhage. Journal of Neurology, Neurosurgery and Psychiatry 54:1118

Blecic SA, Bogousslavsky J, van Melle et al. (1993). Isolated sensorimotor stroke: a re-evaluation of clinical topographic and aetiological patterns. Cerebrovascular Diseases 3:357–363

Bogousslavsky J, Maeder P, Regli F et al. (1994). Pure midbrain infarction: clinical syndromes MRI and aetiologic patterns. Neurology 44:2032–2040

Borggreve F, de Deyn PP, Marien P et al. (1994). Bilateral infarction in the anterior cerebral artery vascular territory due to an unusual anomaly of the circle of Willis. *Stroke* 25:1279–1281

Brandt T, Steinke W, Thie A et al. (2000). Posterior cerebral artery territory infarcts: clinical features, infarct topography, causes and outcome. Multicenter results and a review of the literature. *Cerebrovascular Diseases* 10:170–182

Caplan LR (1980). "Top of the basilar" syndrome. *Neurology* 30:72–79

Caplan LR (1993). Brain embolism revisited. *Neurology* 43:1281–1287

Carrera E, Bogousslavsky J (2006). The thalamus and behaviour: effects of anatomically distinct strokes. *Neurology* 66:1817–1823

Cleary P, Shorvon S, Tallis R. (2004). Late-onset seizures as a predictor of subsequent stroke. *Lancet* 363:1184–1186

Cordonnier C, Hénon H, Derambure P et al. (2007). Early epileptic seizures after stroke are associated with increased risk of new-onset dementia. *Journal of Neurology, Neurosurgery and Psychiatry* 78:514–516

D'Olhaberriague L, Arboix A, Marti-Vilalta JL et al. (1995). Movement disorders in ischaemic stroke: clinical study of 22 patients. *European Journal of Neurology* 2:553–557

Donnan GA, O'Malley HM, Quang L et al. (1996). The capsular warning syndrome: the high risk of early stroke. *Cerebrovascular Diseases* 6:202–207

Flossman E, Rothwell PM (2004). Systematic review of methods and results of studies of the genetic epidemiology of ischaemic stroke. *Stroke* 35:212–227

Flossmann E, Rothwell, PM (2005). Family history of stroke in patients with TIA in relation to hypertension and other intermediate phenotypes. *Stroke* 36:830–835

Flossmann E, Rothwell PM (2006). Family history of stroke does not predict risk of stroke after transient ischemic attack. *Stroke* 37:544–546

Georgiadis D, Oehler J, Schwarz S et al. (2004). Does acute occlusion of the carotid T invariably have a poor outcome? *Neurology* 63:22–26

Ghika J, Bogousslavsky J (2001). Abnormal movements. In *Stroke Syndromes* Bogousslavsky J, Caplan L (eds.), pp. 162–181. Cambridge, UK: Cambridge University Press

Giroud M, Lemesle M, Madinier G et al. (1997). Unilateral lenticular infarcts: radiological and clinical syndromes, aetiology and prognosis. *Journal of Neurology, Neurosurgery and Psychiatry* 63:611–615

Hand PJ, Kwan J, Lindley RI et al. (2006). Distinguishing between stroke and mimic at the bedside: the brain attack study. *Stroke* 37:769–775

Hennerici M, Aulich A, Sandmann W et al. (1981). Incidence of asymptomatic extracranial arterial disease. *Stroke* 12:750–758

Hupperts RMM, Lodder J, Heuts-van Raak EPM et al. (1994). Infarcts in the anterior choroidal artery territory. Anatomical distribution, clinical syndromes, presumed pathogenesis and early outcome. *Brain* 117:825–834

Ichikawa K, Kageyama Y (1991). Clinical anatomic study of pure dysarthria. *Stroke* 22:809–812

Jensen MB, St. Louis EK (2005). Management of acute cerebellar stroke. *Archives of Neurology* 62:537–544

Kaplan PW (1993). Focal seizures resembling transient ischaemic attacks due to subclinical ischaemia. *Cerebrovascular Diseases* 3:241–243

Kazui S, Sawada T, Naritomi H et al. (1992). Left unilateral ideomotor apraxia in ischaemic stroke within the territory of the anterior cerebral artery. *Cerebrovascular Diseases* 2:35–39

Kim JS, Lee JH, Choi CG (1998). Patterns of lateral medullary infarction. Vascular lesion: magnetic resonance imaging correlation of 34 cases. *Stroke* 29:645–652

Kumral E, Bogousslavsky J, van Melle G et al. (1995). Headache at stroke onset: the Lausanne Stroke Registry. *Journal of Neurology, Neurosurgery and Psychiatry* 58:490–492

Lammie GA, Wardlaw JM (1999). Small centrum ovale infarcts: a pathological study. *Cerebrovascular Diseases* 9:82–90

Lindgren A, Roijer A, Norrving B et al. (1994). Carotid artery and heart disease in subtypes of cerebral infarction. *Stroke* 25:2356–2362

Mead GE, Lewis SC, Wardlaw JM *et al.* (1999). Should CT appearance of lacunar stroke influence patient management? *Journal of Neurology, Neurosurgery and Psychiatry* **67**:682–684

Momjian-Mayor I, Baron JC (2005). The pathophysiology of watershed infarction in internal carotid artery disease: review of cerebral perfusion studies. *Stroke* **36**:567–577

Nicolai A, Lazzarino LG, Biasutti E (1996). Large striatocapsular infarcts: clinical features and risk factors. *Journal of Neurology* **243**:44–50

Nor AM, Davis J, Sen B *et al.* (2005). The Recognition of Stroke in the Emergency Room (ROSIER) scale: development and validation of a stroke recognition instrument. *Lancet Neurology* **4**:727–734

Norris JW, Hachinski VC (1982). Misdiagnosis of stroke. *Lancet* **i**:328–331

Patterson JR, Grabois M (1986). Locked-in syndrome: a review of 139 cases. *Stroke* **17**:758–764

Pendlebury ST, Rothwell PM, Dalton A, Burton EA (2004). Strokelike presentation of Wilson's disease with homozygosity for a novel T766R mutation. *Neurology* **63**:1982–1983

Read SJ, Pettigrew L, Schimmel L *et al.* (1998). White matter medullary infarcts: acute subcortical infarction in the centrum ovale. *Cerebrovascular Diseases* **8**:289–295

Sandercock PAG, Molyneux A, Warlow C (1985). Value of computed tomography in patients with stroke: Oxfordshire Community Stroke Project. *British Medical Journal* **290**:193–197

Schmahmann JD (2003). Vascular syndromes of the thalamus. *Stroke* **34**:2264–2278

Schulz UG, Rothwell PM (2001). Major variation in carotid bifurcation anatomy: a possible risk factor for plaque development? *Stroke* **32**: 2522–2529

Scott BL, Jankovic J (1996). Delayed-onset progressive movement disorders after static brain lesions. *Neurology* **46**:68–74

Wardlaw JM, Merrick MV, Ferrington CM *et al.* (1996). Comparison of a simple isotope method of predicting likely middle cerebral artery occlusion with transcranial Doppler ultrasound in acute ischaemic stroke. *Cerebrovascular Diseases* **6**:32–39

Wardlaw JM, Lewsi SC, Dennis MS *et al.* (1999). Is it reasonable to assume a particular embolic source from the type of stroke? *Cerebrovascular Diseases* **9**(Suppl 1):14

Chapter 10

Brain imaging in transient ischemic attack and minor stroke

The main modalities for imaging the brain parenchyma are CT and MRI, and these are increasingly used to assess the cerebral vasculature in TIA and stroke. They differ in a number of technical aspects (Table 10.1). At present there is little consensus on optimal imaging strategies after TIA or minor stroke, or indeed if imaging is required at all in some cases. The role of imaging differs from that in major stroke for a number of reasons. First, in patients with TIA or minor stroke, the likelihood of alternative, non-neurovascular diagnoses is higher than in patients with major stroke and so imaging is important in identifying mimics. Second, minor stroke is less likely to be caused by hemorrhage than major stroke and the risk is lower still in TIA, although it is not negligible (Gunatilake 1998; Werring *et al.* 2005). Third, although there is little or no neurological deficit, the risk of recurrent and possibly severe ischemic events is high and imaging has a role in identifying high-risk patients. In TIA and minor stroke, brain imaging is required to:

- exclude stroke mimics
- differentiate between ischemic and hemorrhagic events
- determine etiology, for example, carotid stenosis or cardioembolic source with lesions in multiple vascular territories
- identify patients at high risk of early recurrent stroke, in order to target suitable treatment.

The sensitivity and specificity of different imaging modalities varies with the pre-test probability, the nature of the lesion in question and the delay from event to imaging, while the availability of and expertise in imaging techniques will vary from center to center. When making decisions about imaging after TIA and minor stroke, the choice of imaging will depend on all these factors, as well as patient safety, tolerability and contraindications (Table 10.2).

The identification of non-neurovascular diagnoses

The most important mimics to identify with brain imaging after suspected TIA or minor stroke are subdural hematomas and brain tumors (see Figs. 8.1 and 8.2). The likelihood of these diagnoses will depend on the clinical setting. For example, high rates of non-vascular pathology have been reported in early studies conducted in specialist units before CT was widely available, where patients referred for imaging were highly selected (Weisberg and Nice 1977; Weisberg 1986). In cohorts of patients with suspected TIA who were referred directly for scanning by primary care physicians, prior to expert review by a stroke physician, rates of alternative diagnoses were also high, probably reflecting a high rate of pre-imaging misdiagnosis (Lemesle *et al.* 1998). Low rates have been reported in retrospective case series but these studies are likely not to have included patients in whom the initial diagnosis was changed in light of brain imaging results (Rolak *et al.* 1990;

Table 10.1. Technical aspects of imaging using computed tomography (CT) and magnetic resonance imaging (MRI)

Modality	Usage
CT	An X-ray tube rotates helically around the subject while an array of detectors opposite the tube measures the residual radiation that has passed through the body according to the density of local tissues to X-rays. Cross-sectional images are constructed using mathematical algorithms
MRI	The subject is exposed to a strong external magnetic field, causing nuclei containing an odd number of neutrons or protons to align themselves within the field. When a pulse of radiofrequency energy of a particular frequency is applied, the protons are perturbed initially and then realign, producing a radiofrequency signal that is proportional to the surrounding "magnetic micro-environment." Radiofrequency signals are detected and processed to form an image; it provides better contrast between soft tissues than CT
T_1-weighted	Show brain structure
T_2-weighted	Show brain water content (cerebrospinal fluid) and proton density
Gradient echo	Most sensitive to hemoglobin degradation products and detects hemorrhage
Diffusion weighted	Detects abnormalities caused by ischemia in the hyper-acute phase
Perfusion	Quantifies the amount of contrast agent reaching the brain tissue after a fast intravenous bolus

Table 10.2. Advantages and disadvantages of computed tomography (CT) and magnetic resonance imaging (MRI) in minor stroke and transient ischemic attack

Modality	Advantages	Disadvantages
CT	Low cost and wide availability	Low sensitivity for small acute ischemic lesions
	Superior detection of hemorrhage in the early phase[a]	Low sensitivity for mimics, especially early tumor
		Radiation exposure
		Intravenous contrast nephrotoxic and potentially allergenic
MRI	Superior sensitivity for stroke mimics	Patient tolerability and contraindications
	Provides prognostic information	
	Superior detection of hemorrhage in the subacute and chronic phase[a]	

Note:
[a]Although pre-test probability of hemorrhage is low in patients with a high clinical suspicion of transient ischemic attack or minor stroke.

Douglas *et al.* 2003). Secondary prevention trials of aspirin in TIA and minor stroke have also reported very low numbers of patients subsequently shown to have non-vascular pathologies after randomization into the trials but these studies did not report the number of patients with suspected TIAs who were scanned and excluded before randomization because a non-vascular cause was identified (Dutch TIA Study Group 1993; UK TIA Study Group 1993). Finally, many studies have described relatively young cohorts, but the prevalence of non-vascular pathologies is likely to increase with age. Therefore, it is difficult to be either reassured by low rates of non-vascular pathology in cohorts diagnosed with TIA or convinced of the need for routine neuroimaging by high rates.

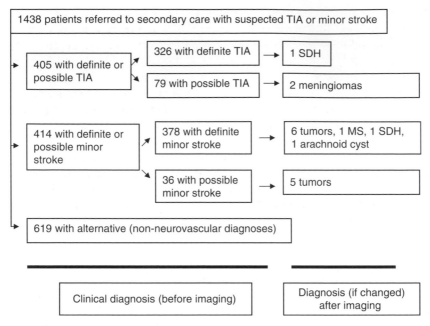

Fig. 10.1. Numbers of patients referred to the Oxford Vascular Study (OXVASC) between 2002 and 2007 with suspected transient ischemic attack (TIA) or minor stroke showing clinical diagnosis (before imaging) and revised diagnosis following brain imaging. SDH, subdural hematoma; MS, multiple sclerosis.

Brain imaging after transient ischemic attack and minor stroke: The Oxford Vascular Study (OXVASC)

The Oxford Vascular Study (OXVASC) is a population-based study in which all patients with suspected TIA or stroke are ascertained prospectively and reviewed by an experienced stroke physician who determines the probability of a vascular diagnosis before brain imaging. Events are described as definite, when the diagnosis is clearly neurovascular in origin, or possible, when an alternative explanation for the event could be found but a minor stroke or TIA could not be completely excluded on clinical grounds. This study has the advantages that all patients are studied irrespective of whether they are referred to the clinic or hospital, pre-imaging diagnoses are reliably recorded and imaging is near complete.

Over a five year period, 1438 patients were referred either to the hospital or to the study clinic with a suspected TIA or minor stroke (defined on assessment as a score of ≤ 3 on the National Institutes of Health Stroke Scale [NIHSS]) (Wityk *et al.* 1994) (Fig. 10.1). Of these, a pre-scan diagnosis of definite or possible TIA was made in 405 patients (46% male, mean age 74 years), and definite or possible minor stroke in 414 patients (54% male, mean age 76 years). Overall, 97% underwent brain imaging for definite or possible events (699 CT, 93 MRI).

Of 326 patients with a clinical diagnosis of definite TIA, only one patient (0.3%; confidence interval [CI], 95% 0.1–1.7) was subsequently found to have symptomatic non-vascular pathology, a small subdural hematoma. Of 79 patients with a clinical diagnosis of possible TIA, two patients (2.5%; 95% CI, 0.7–8.8) were subsequently diagnosed with symptomatic non-vascular pathology, a meningioma in both cases.

Of 378 patients with a clinical diagnosis of definite minor stroke, there were nine (2.4%; 95% CI, 1.3–4.5) with non-vascular pathology (six intracranial tumors, one demyelination, one arachnoid cyst, one subdural hematoma). Possible minor stroke was diagnosed in 36, and non-vascular pathology was identified in five (13.9%; 95% CI, 6.1–28.7), all of whom had intracranial tumors.

Importantly, of the 11 patients in total with intracranial tumors, five were not identified on initial non-contrast CT and the correct diagnosis was only made after the patient deteriorated and repeat neuroimaging was performed. The yield of CT imaging for non-vascular pathology in patients with definite TIA or minor stroke is, therefore, low and it is only slightly higher in possible events where additional clinical features such as seizure at the time of ictus or prominent confusion cast doubt on the pre-imaging diagnosis. Imaging with CT, therefore, does not add significantly to bedside assessment by an expert clinician, and MRI is recommended as first-line brain imaging in recent guidelines (European Stroke Organization Executive Committee and Writing Committee 2008; National Institute for Health and Clinical Excellence 2008).

The identification of infarction and hemorrhage

The rapid and accurate identification of intracerebral hemorrhage with brain imaging in patients with TIA or minor stroke is essential to direct timely, safe and effective secondary prevention. For example, the misdiagnosis of a cerebral hemorrhage as an infarct may lead to a patient erroneously receiving antithrombotic or anticoagulant medication, with consequent increased risk of further hemorrhage, while a delay to rapid initiation of secondary preventive medication while imaging is awaited may expose a patient with an infarct to an unacceptably high risk of further ischemia. These scenarios are particularly relevant as the initiation of aspirin before brain imaging is recommended in some guidelines (National Institute for Health and Clinical Excellence 2008).

As mentioned above, the sensitivity and specificity of different imaging modalities for infarction versus hemorrhage varies with pre-test probability and delay from event to imaging. Acute primary intracerebral hemorrhage is seen on CT scanning as an area of well-defined hyperintensity. Soon, a surrounding area of low density appears that is attributable to edema, clot retraction and infarction of the surrounding brain. The hemoglobin in the hematoma itself is broken down to oxyhemoglobin through deoxyhemoglobin and methemoglobin prior to red cell lysis and breakdown into ferritin and haemosiderin, causing the initial area of hyperintensity to become isodense and then hypointense, at which stage it becomes indistinguishable from an infarct (see Fig. 11.1). When the volume of hemorrhage is small, as in minor stroke, the rate of change of imaging abnormalities is faster and so the sensitivity of CT for hemorrhage diminishes more quickly with time (Fig. 10.2) (Dennis et al. 1987). In cases when there is a delay from event to imaging, MRI becomes more sensitive for the detection of hemorrhage than CT, although the exact timing of this process is not clear and will vary with size of hemorrhage. Decisions about choice of imaging modality should be made according to these factors and local availability and expertise.

Rates of hemorrhage in transient ischemic attack and minor stroke

The risk associated with a policy of "blind" treatment prior to imaging depends on the frequency of intracranial hemorrhage among patients with TIA or minor stroke. However, few published studies have reported this frequency.

Table 10.3. Rates of infarction, primary hemorrhage or hemorrhagic infarction on CT scan among subjects with probable or definite transient ischemic attack or minor stroke in the Oxford Vascular Study (OXVASC)

Event	Appropriate infarction (%; 95% CI)	Primary hemorrhage or hemorrhagic infarction (%; 95% CI)
Transient ischemic attack		
Definite	10.1 (7.0–14.3)	0
Possible	3.0 (0.8–10.40)	0
Minor stroke		
Definite	40.4 (35.3–45.7)	5.9 (3.9–8.9)
Possible	19.2 (8.5–379)	3.9 (0.7–18.9)

Note:
CI, confidence interval.

Day 1   Day 3

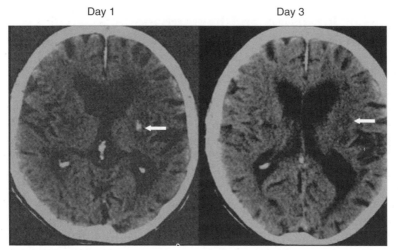

Fig. 10.2. These CT brain scans show a small hemorrhage in the left basal ganglia/ internal capsule (arrow) visible as a hyperintense area on day 1 that has become hypodense by day 3.

One prospective study of consecutive patients (both inpatients and outpatients) presenting to a single center with mild stroke after a delay of over four days reported imaging findings after both CT and MRI scanning were performed (Wardlaw *et al.* 2003). Among 228 patients scanned after a median delay of 20 days, primary intracerebral hemorrhage was identified by CT in two patients (0.9%; 95% CI, 0.1–3.1) and MRI in eight (3.5%; 95% CI, 1.5–6.8). Both hemorrhages identified by CT were identified on MRI. The study concluded with the recommendation that MRI was the modality of choice in patients with minor stroke where there is a delay to imaging, owing to the unacceptable rate of misdiagnosis with CT.

In the OXVASC cohort of patients with probable or definite TIA or minor stroke, 699 were imaged with CT. Rates of infarction and hemorrhage detected with CT are listed in Table 10.3.

Among 334 patients with definite or possible minor stroke in OXVASC in whom hemorrhage could be detected reliably by either CT performed within 10 days or MRI (regardless of delay), primary hemorrhage was detected in 17 (5.1%; 95% CI, 3.2–8.0), and hemorrhagic transformation of an infarct in four (1.2%; 95% CI, 0.5–3.0).

Similar rates of primary intracerebral hemorrhage were reported in an unpublished study of consecutive patients with minor stroke attending a neurovascular clinic in Buckinghamshire, UK, who were all imaged with MRI on the day of attendance. Of 280 patients (59% male, mean age 72 years), primary intracerebral hemorrhage was detected in 15 (5.4%; 95% CI, 3.3–8.7) and hemorrhagic transformation in six (2.1%; 95% CI, 1.0–4.6). The median delay to assessment and scanning was 15 days (interquartile range, 10–23).

In the OXVASC and Buckinghamshire neurovascular clinic cohorts of minor stroke patients, the clinical factors identified as being predictive of hemorrhage were blood pressure on initial assessment $\geq 180/110$ mmHg, vomiting and confusion at onset, and premorbid anticoagulation. Headache was only very weakly predictive and age was not predictive at all. In settings where access to MRI is limited and delays from event to presentation and imaging do occur, these factors might be used to identify patients with a high pre-test probability of hemorrhage and in whom MRI imaging will have a higher positive yield.

Microbleeds and transient ischemic attack and minor stroke

Echoplanar gradient-echo T_2-weighted imaging (GRE) MRI, which exploits the paramagnetic effects of deoxyhemoglobin, has a high sensitivity for detecting primary intracerebral hemorrhage. Studies comparing CT and GRE MRI for detection of hemorrhage in acute stroke show that GRE MRI is as good or better than CT, particularly for small or chronic bleeds (Schellinger *et al.* 1999, 2007; Fiebach *et al.* 2004; Kidwell *et al.* 2004; Chalela *et al.* 2007). Use of GRE MRI has led to the increasing detection of apparently spontaneous cerebral microbleeds, which are small, round, homogeneous foci of low signal intensity (see Figs. 7.2 and 7.4). They were first described in the mid 1990s (Chan *et al.* 1996; Greenberg *et al.* 1996; Offenbacher *et al.* 1996) and have led to considerable research interest, although their pathological and clinical significance is still unclear (Ch. 7).

The few pathological data available indicate that cerebral microbleeds are small areas of old hemorrhage, often associated with lipohyalinosis in the deep perforating arteries feeding the affected area of the brain (Fazekas *et al.* 1999). It is unclear whether the presence of microbleeds increases the risk of intracerebral hemorrhage in patients treated with antiplatelet or anticoagulant therapy (Cordonnier *et al.* 2007) although they seem not to be associated with increased risk in thrombolysis (Ch. 11).

In a rigorous systematic review, microbleeds were found to be infrequent in "healthy adults," with a prevalence of 5.0% (95% CI, 3.9–6.2) pooled across four studies of 1411 individuals, and more common in patients with ischemic stroke, with a prevalence of 33.5%; (95% CI, 30.7–36.4) pooled across 16 studies of 1075 individuals. It should be noted that individual studies of ischemic stroke reported prevalences ranging from 12% to 71% (Cordonnier *et al.* 2007). To date, only one study has described the presence of cerebral microbleeds specifically in patients with TIAs. In a cohort of 129 consecutive patients attending a neurovascular clinic, microbleeds were detected in 1/43 (2%) with TIA and 20/86 (23%) with stroke, although patients with TIA but who had suffered a previous stroke were excluded (Werring *et al.* 2005). Given that the cohort was recruited from an outpatient setting, it is likely that the stroke patients included had suffered non-disabling strokes, although specific data on severity were not described.

At present, further research is required with better designed studies to assess the clinical determinants of microbleeds and their influence on prognosis

Imaging: diagnosis and prognostication

Recent studies have demonstrated the usefulness of MRI in patients with suspected TIA, particularly diffusion-weighted imaging (DWI) (Figs. 10.3–10.9) (Schulz *et al.* 2003; Schulz *et al.* 2004). This modality relies on changes in the Brownian motion of water molecules to generate contrast. During early ischemia, there is decreased water proton movement caused by cytotoxic edema as water moves from the less-restricted extracellular environment into the more-restricted intracellular environment. Reduced proton diffusion leads to

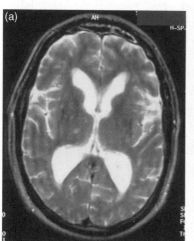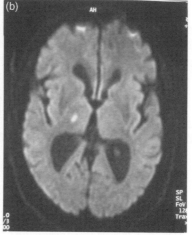

Fig. 10.3. Images with T$_2$-weighted (a) and diffusion-weighted (b) MRI in a 70-year-old man who presented with a history of sudden-onset numbness and tingling in the left face arm and leg. On examination there was sensory loss over the left hand but nothing else. The diffusion-weighted images confirm a thalamic infarct consistent with the clinical diagnosis of pure sensory stroke.

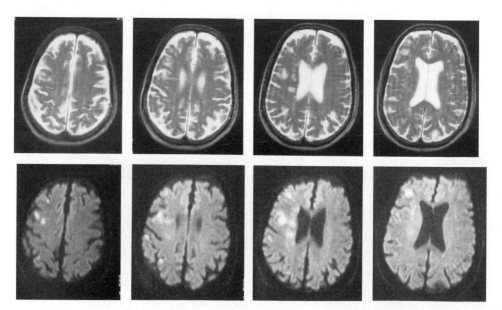

Fig. 10.4. These T$_2$-weighted (top) and diffusion-weighted (bottom) scans were taken of an 81-year-old man with a fall 10 days previously that was followed by difficulty using his left leg, confusion and slurred speech. The diffusion-weighted image confirms multiple acute lesions in the right hemisphere and carotid imaging confirmed severe right carotid stenosis.

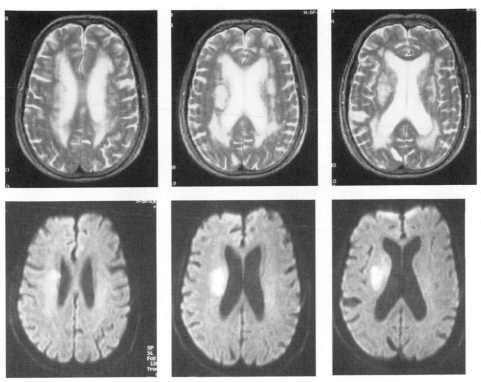

Fig. 10.5. These T$_2$-weighted (top) and diffusion-weighted (bottom) MRI scans were taken of an 80-year-old woman who had developed dysarthria and left-sided weakness two weeks previously. The T$_2$-weighted images show extensive leukoaraiosis, making it impossible to be certain which is the acute lesion this, however, is clearly shown in the diffusion-weighted images.

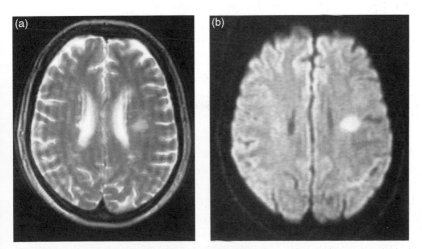

Fig. 10.6. A T$_2$-weighted (a) and diffusion-weighted (b) MRI in a 60-year-old woman who had awoken three weeks before with slurred speech. On examination, there was very mild dysarthria. Several white matter hyperintensities are seen on the T$_2$-weighted image but the acute causative lesion in seen clearly in the diffusion-weighted image.

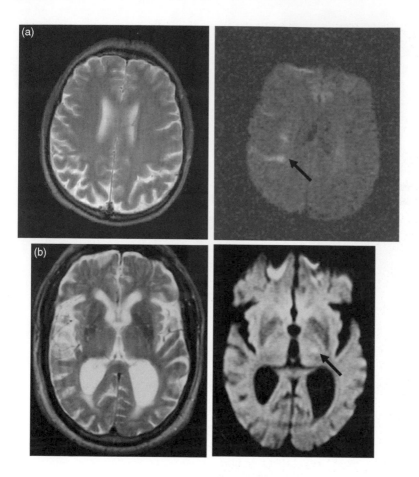

Fig. 10.7. Use of T_2-weighted and diffusion-weighted (DWI) MRI. (a) A patient without vascular risk factors presented with a history of transient left arm and facial weakness 10 days earlier. The T_2-weighted image (left) is normal but DWI (right) shows an acute right parietal infarction (arrow). (b) A patient presented with a history of transient right arm and facial weakness and sensory loss nine days before presentation. The T_2-weighted image (left) is normal but the DWI (right) shows an acute left thalamic infarction (arrow).

a bright, high-signal DWI lesion. The degree of water proton restriction can be quantitatively measured using maps of the apparent diffusion coefficient (ADC). In contrast to DWI, ADC maps depict reduced diffusion as a dark, low signal. The value of the ADC changes with time after stroke onset, being reduced for the first few days after which it rises (pseudonormalization) to become hyperintense in the chronic phase when there is vasogenic edema and cellular necrosis. This allows DWI to distinguish between acute and chronic infarction, unlike conventional MRI (Schaefer *et al.* 2005), although it should be noted that the DWI-detectable lesion persists for at least a week since it detects prolonged T_2 signal "T_2 shine-through" so correct interpretation of DWI including identifying acute recurrence of ischemia requires consideration of the ADC map.

Approximately 50% of patients with TIA have a focal abnormality on DWI if scanned within 24-hours; of these 25% do not have a lesion correlate on T_2-weighted MRI (Kidwell *et al.* 1999; Ay *et al.* 2002). Presence of DWI abnormalities is associated with some clinical characteristics of the presenting event. For example, in a systematic review of all studies

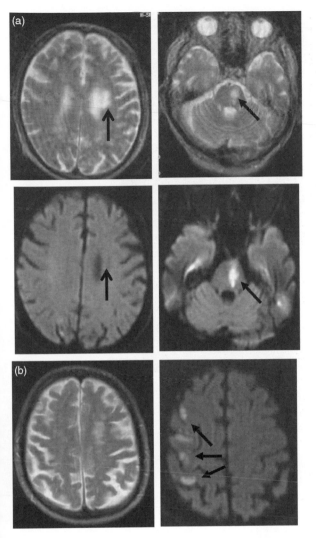

Fig. 10.8. Distinguishing the region of circulation affected (a) Anterior circulation or posterior circulation event? A patient presented with right-arm weakness that developed eight days previous and a history of a previous stroke with a right hemiparesis. The T_2-weighted MRI (upper images) shows two possibly relevant lesions (left corona radiata and left pons, arrows). The diffusion-weighted images (lower images) show that the pontine lesion is recent (arrow). (b) Lacunar or cortical event? A patient presented with a 12 day history of left hemiparesis involving face, arm and leg. The T_2-weighted MRI (left) shows widespread "small vessel disease" throughout both hemispheres, but diffusion-weighted MRI (right) shows acute right hemispheric cortical infarcts (arrows).

reporting DWI findings and clinical characteristics of presenting TIA, symptom duration over one hour, dysarthria, dysphasia and weakness were all significantly associated with abnormalities on DWI, as were atrial fibrillation and carotid stenosis > 50%, while hypertension, diabetes and patient age were not (Redgrave *et al.* 2007). Use of DWI alters the attending physician's opinion regarding vascular localization, anatomical localization and probable TIA/minor stroke mechanism in a significant number of patients (Figs. 10.3–9) (Albers *et al.* 2000; Schulz *et al.* 2004; Gass *et al.* 2004).

Approximately 25% of patients with TIA have cerebral infarction with transient signs in which DWI positivity corresponds to cytotoxic edema; this progresses to permanent parenchymal injury and increased tissue water content visible as a lesion on T_2-weighted MRI. Approximately 20% of patients have early DWI abnormality but no evidence of later T_2-weighted abnormality. This suggests reversibility of the initial DWI abnormality if blood flow is restored early enough to prevent permanent parenchymal injury, as seen in patients with stroke in whom the DWI-detected lesion may regress with reperfusion.

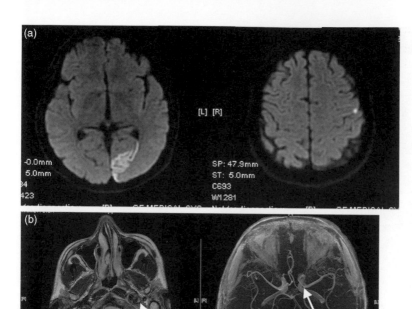

Fig. 10.9. (a) Diffusion-weighted MRI showing two areas of acute infarction in the left parietal and occipital regions. (b) Magnetic resonance angiography shows aberrant arterial anatomy with the posterior cerebral artery arising directly from the internal carotid artery (arrow) (c) This was confirmed on catheter angiography.

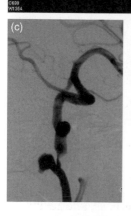
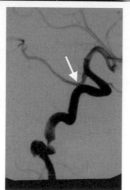

In patients with negative DWI, a very brief period of ischemia may have been sufficient to disrupt neuronal activity but insufficient to cause cytotoxic edema.

Many patients with TIA or minor stroke delay seeking medical attention. Often there is a further delay before they are seen by specialist stroke services. In these patients, a clear history may be more difficult to obtain; clinical signs may have resolved, and it may be difficult to make a definite diagnosis of a cerebral ischemic event or to be certain of the vascular territory or territories involved. Recent studies suggest that DWI is also of use in diagnosis and management of patients presenting later with TIA or minor stroke symptoms (Schulz *et al.* 2003, 2004) (Fig. 10.3). Clinically appropriate ischemic lesions are detected by DWI in a high proportion of patients with minor stroke when they are scanned two weeks or more after their event (Schulz *et al.* 2004). Interobserver agreement for identifying recent ischemic lesions in this patient group is much higher for DWI than for T$_2$-weighted scans, and DWI provides useful information over and above T_2-weighted imaging in approximately a third of patients, most commonly by increasing diagnostic certainty and by indicating the vascular territory involved (Figs. 10.3–9). The presence of lesions seen with DWI decreases with time since symptom onset and increases with NIHSS and age and is positively associated with stroke rather than TIA, motor deficit and dysarthria (Schulz *et al.* 2004).

Preliminary studies using DWI suggest that the presence, absence and pattern of DWI-detectable lesions in patients with TIA and minor stroke provide prognostic information (Ch. 14) (Wen *et al.* 2004; Purroy *et al.* 2004; Bang *et al.* 2005; Coutts *et al.* 2005; Sylaja *et al.* 2007).

References

Albers GW, Lansberg MG, Norbash AM *et al.* (2000). Yield of diffusion-weighted MRI for detection of potentially relevant findings in stroke patients. *Neurology* **54**:1562–1567

Ay H, Oliveira-Filho J, Buonanno FS *et al.* (2002). "Footprints" of transient ischemic attacks: a diffusion-weighted MRI study. *Cerebrovascular Digest* **14**:177–186

Bang OY, Lee PH, Heo KG *et al.* (2005). Specific DWI lesion patterns predict prognosis after acute ischaemic stroke within the MCA territory. *Journal of Neurology, Neurosurgery and Psychiatry* **76**:1222–1228

Chalela JA, Kidwell CS, Nentwich L *et al.* (2007). Magnetic resonance imaging and computed tomography in emergency assessment of patients with suspected acute stroke: a prospective study. *Lancet* **369**:293–298

Chan S, Kartha K, Yoon SS *et al.* (1996). Multifocal hypointense cerebral lesions on gradient-echo MR are associated with chronic hypertension. *American Journal of Neuroradiology* **17**:1821–1827

Cordonnier C, Al-Shahi Salman R, Wardlaw J (2007). Spontaneous brain microbleeds: systematic review, subgroup analyses and standards for study design and reporting. *Brain* **130**:1988–2003

Coutts SB, Simon JE, Eliasziw M *et al.* (2005). Triaging transient ischemic attack and minor stroke patients using acute magnetic resonance imaging. *Annals of Neurology* **57**:848–854

Dennis MS, Bamford JM, Molyneux AJ *et al.* (1987). Rapid resolution of signs of primary intracerebral hemorrhage in computed tomograms of the brain. *British Medical Journal* **295**:379–381

Douglas VC, Johnston CM, Elkins J *et al.* (2003). Head computed tomography findings predict short-term stroke risk after transient ischemic attack. *Stroke* **34**:2894–2898

Dutch TIA Trial Study Group (1993). Predictors of major vascular events in patients with a transient ischemic attack or nondisabling stroke. *Stroke* **24**:527–531

European Stroke Organization Executive Committee and Writing Committee (2008). Guidelines for Management of Ischaemic Stroke 2008. *Cerebrovascular Diseases* **25**:457–507

Fazekas F, Kleinert R, Roob G *et al.* (1999). Histopathologic analysis of foci of signal loss on gradient-echo T_2-weighted MR images in patients with spontaneous intracerebral hemorrhage: evidence of microangiopathy-related microbleeds. *American Journal of Neuroradiology* **20**:637–642

Fiebach JB, Schellinger PD, Gass A *et al.* (2004). Stroke magnetic resonance imaging is accurate in hyperacute intracerebral hemorrhage: a multicenter study on the validity of stroke imaging. *Stroke* **35**:502–506

Gass A, Ay H, Szabo K *et al.* (2004). Diffusion-weighted MRI for the "small stuff": the details of acute cerebral ischaemia. *Lancet Neurology* **3**:39–45

Greenberg SM, Finklestein SP, Schaefer PW (1996). Petechial hemorrhages accompanying lobar hemorrhage: detection by gradient-echo MRI. *Neurology* **46**:1751–1754

Gunatilake SB (1998). Rapid resolution of symptoms and signs of intracerebral hemorrhage: case reports. *British Medical Journal* **316**:1495–1496

Kidwell CS, Alger JR, Di Salle F *et al.* (1999). Diffusion MRI in patients with transient ischemic attacks. *Stroke* **30**:1174–1180

Kidwell CS, Chalela JA, Saver JL *et al.* (2004). Comparison of MRI and CT for detection of acute intracerebral hemorrhage. *JAMA* **292**:1823–1830

Lemesle M, Madinier G, Menassa M et al. (1998). Incidence of transient ischemic attacks in Dijon, France. A 5-year community-based study. *Neuroepidemiology* **17**:74–79

National Institute for Health and Clinical Excellence (2008). *Stroke: Diagnosis and Initial Management of Acute Stroke and Transient Ischaemic Attack (TIA): Draft Guidance for Consultation.* London: NICE

Offenbacher H, Fazekas F, Schmidt R et al. (1996). MR of cerebral abnormalities concomitant with primary intracerebral hematomas. *American Journal of Neuroradiology* **17**:573–578

Purroy F, Montaner J, Rovira A et al. (2004). Higher risk of further vascular events among transient ischaemic attack patients with diffusion-weighted imaging acute lesions. *Stroke* **35**:2313–2319

Redgrave JN, Coutts SB, Schulz UG et al. (2007). Systematic review of associations between the presence of acute ischemic lesions on diffusion-weighted imaging and clinical predictors of early stroke risk after transient ischemic attack. *Stroke* **38**:1482–1488

Rolak LA, Gilmer W, Strittmatter WJ (1990). Low yield in the diagnostic evaluation of transient ischemic attacks. *Neurology* **40**:747–748

Schaefer PW, Copen WA, Lev MH et al. (2005). Diffusion-weighted imaging in acute stroke. *Neuroimaging Clinics of North American* **15**:503–530

Schellinger PD, Jansen O, Fiebach JB et al. (1999). A standardized MRI stroke protocol: comparison with CT in hyperacute intracerebral hemorrhage. *Stroke* **30**:765–768

Schellinger PD, Thomalla G, Fiehler J et al. (2007). MRI-based and CT-based thrombolytic therapy in acute stroke within and beyond established time windows: an analysis of 1210 patients. *Stroke* **38**:2640–2645

Schulz UGR, Briley D, Meagher T et al. (2003). Abnormalities on diffusion weighted magnetic resonance imaging performed several weeks after a minor stroke or transient ischaemic attack. *Journal of Neurology, Neurosurgery and Psychiatry* **74**:734–738

Schulz UG, Flossman E, Rothwell PM (2004). Heritability of ischemic stroke in relation to age, vascular risk factors and subtypes of incident stroke in population-based studies. *Stroke* **35**:819–824

Sylaja PN, Coutts SB, Subramaniam S et al. (2007). Acute ischemic lesions of varying ages predict risk of ischemic events in stroke/TIA patients. *Neurology* **68**:415–419

UK TIA Study Group (1993). Intracranial tumours that mimic transient cerebral ischaemia: lessons from a large multicentre trial. *Journal of Neurology, Neurosurgery and Psychiatry* **56**:563–566

Wardlaw JM, Keir SL, Dennis MS (2003). The impact of delays in computed tomography of the brain on the accuracy of diagnosis and subsequent management in patients with minor stroke. *Journal of Neurology, Neurosurgery and Psychiatry* **74**:77–81

Weisberg LA (1986). Computerized tomographic abnormalities in patients with hemispheric transient ischemic attacks. *South Medical Journal* **79**:804–807

Weisberg LA, Nice CN (1977). Intracranial tumors simulating the presentation of cerebrovascular syndromes. Early detection with cerebral computed tomography (CCT). *American Journal of Medicine* **63**:517–524

Wen HM, Lam WW, Rainer T et al. (2004). Multiple acute cerebral infarcts on diffusion-weighted imaging and risk of recurrent stroke. *Neurology* **63**:1317–1319

Werring DJ, Coward LJ, Losseff NA et al. (2005). Cerebral microbleeds are common in ischemic stroke but rare in TIA. *Neurology* **65**:1914–1918

Wityk RJ, Pessin MS, Kaplan RF et al. (1994). Serial assessment of acute stroke using the NIH Stroke Scale. *Stroke* **25**:362–365

11

Brain imaging in major acute stroke

In patients with major stroke, investigations are required to:

- differentiate between infarction and hemorrhage
- exclude stroke mimics
- inform treatment decisions: identify vascular occlusion or stenosis; identify areas of completed and threatened infarction
- provide prognostic information.

Brain imaging is required to distinguish between primary intracerebral hemorrhage and cerebral infarction since this distinction cannot be made reliably on clinical criteria alone (Hawkins *et al.* 1995). Recent developments in brain imaging, in particular new MRI sequences, and to a lesser extent CT techniques, have enabled visualization of the pathophysiological processes involved in brain infarction. These new techniques are being developed to select patients suitable for thrombolytic treatment beyond the three-hour time window (Ch. 21) and may in the future enable targeting of treatments such as neuroprotection.

At present in most centers in most countries, CT remains the imaging modality used routinely to distinguish between hemorrhage and infarction in acute stroke: it is better tolerated, easier to perform in sick patients and is more widely available than MRI. Further, the various randomized trials of thrombolysis in ischemic stroke used CT criteria to guide treatment decisions and showed thrombolysis to be effective if given within three hours of stroke (Ch. 21). Consequently, CT is felt to be sufficient to select patients for thrombolysis within three hours of stroke onset by most centers. Although conventional T_1- and T_2-weighted MR sequences have a low sensitivity acutely for intracranial hemorrhage, newer MR sequences have greater sensitivity for hemorrhage than CT. Consequently, some centers advocate the use of multi-modal MRI as the imaging modality of choice in acute stroke (Chalela *et al.* 2007) particularly beyond the three-hour time window, although the use of perfusion CT to image cerebral blood flow is also becoming more common (Table 11.1).

Computed tomography and conventional magnetic resonance imaging

Hemorrhage

Hemorrhage is seen as a hyperdense region by CT, often in the form of a space-occupying mass (Fig. 9.3). The sensitivity of CT for parenchymal hemorrhage is almost 100% but small parenchymal hemorrhage or subarachnoid hemorrhage may be missed (Schriger *et al.* 1998). With increasing passage of time after the onset of the hemorrhage, CT becomes progressively less good at distinguishing between hemorrhage and infarction as the initial hyperdensity becomes iso- and then hypodense (Fig. 11.1). Consequently, MRI is better

Table 11.1. Advantages and disadvantages of computed tomography (CT) and magnetic resonance imaging (MRI) in major stroke

Modality	Advantages	Disadvantages
CT	Low cost and wide availability	Radiation exposure
	Safe for medically unstable patients	Poor image resolution for posterior structures
	Rapid acquisition of images	
	High sensitivity for hemorrhage in the acute phase	
MRI	High sensitivity for stroke mimics	Patient tolerability and contraindications
	High sensitivity for ischemia (with DWI) and cerebral perfusion	Low sensitivity for cerebral hemorrhage, but now much improved with GRE
	High resolution for imaging of vasculature	Slower image acquisition

Notes:
DWI, diffusion-weighted imaging; GRE, gradient-echo.

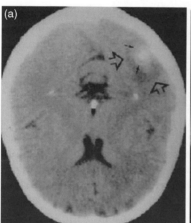
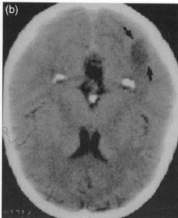

Fig. 11.1. These CT brain scans show an acute right cortical hemorrhage on the day of the stroke (a; open arrow), which has become hypodense on repeat scanning seven days later (b; black arrow).

than CT for diagnosing hemorrhage more than a week after onset, particularly in defining possible underlying pathology.

There is usually not a large amount of edema early after intracerebral hemorrhage, and the finding of edema should prompt a search for an underlying tumor or venous obstruction. Hemorrhages related to coagulopathies, anticoagulants or to cerebral amyloid angiopathy are often inhomogeneous with fluid levels. The location and number of hemorrhages may provide clues as to the underlying cause and hence guide further investigation and treatment (see Ch. 7).

As stated above, conventional MRI is not the modality of choice for distinguishing between hemorrhage and infarction in acute stroke. The appearance of primary intracerebral hemorrhage on conventional MRI sequences at different time periods following stroke onset is complex since the T_1 and T_2 relaxation rates vary with the concentration of breakdown products of hemoglobin. As the hematoma ages, it is converted from oxyhemoglobin to deoxyhemoglobin and then to methemoglobin prior to red cell lysis and breakdown into ferritin and hemosiderin. Acute hematoma is characterized by central hypointensity on T_2-weighted and isointensity on T_1-weighted MRI. Methemoglobin formation leads to

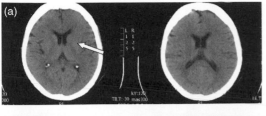

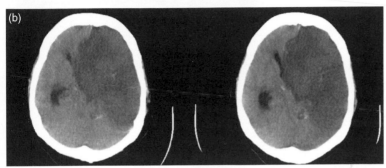

Fig. 11.2. Early ischemic change on CT (a) showing very subtle loss of white/gray matter differentiation in the internal capsule/basal ganglia (arrow) in a patient with a massive infarction in the right territory middle cerebral artery. This is seen clearly on CT scan three days after stroke onset (b).

shortening of T_1 relaxation and to central hyperintensity on T_1-weighted images, with hyperintensity on T_2-weighted images. Days and weeks after onset of bleeding, a hypo-intense border zone caused by the paramagnetic rim of methemoglobin demarcates the border zone of the hematoma. The complexity and subtlety of these changes has resulted in a strong preference by clinicians and radiologists for CT over conventional MRI in the acute evaluation of intracerebral hemorrhage.

Ischemic changes

Knowledge of the nature and time course of ischemic changes on CT and conventional MRI is necessary as an aid to diagnosis, infarct localization and selection of patients for acute stroke therapy. While hemorrhage is visible almost immediately on CT, ischemia takes longer to manifest, although changes have been reported as early as 22 minutes in one study (von Kummer *et al.* 2001). Consistent with its end-artery vascular system, the striatocapsular area exhibits irreversible damage very early in patients with middle cerebral artery stem occlusion whereas the cortical areas usually fall within the penumbra. The earliest signs of ischemia are of brain tissue swelling, as shown by effacement of cortical sulci, asymmetry of the sylvian fissures and ventricular distortion (Fig. 11.2) (Kucinski *et al.* 2002). Occasionally the segment of the artery occluded by the thrombus, particularly in the case of the main trunk of the middle cerebral artery, may appear hyperdense, although inter-observer agreement on such signs is only moderate (von Kummer *et al.* 1996; Grotta *et al.* 1999). Early brain swelling is followed by the development of parenchymal hypodensity, corresponding to cytotoxic edema, and is seen on CT as loss of the normal gray/white matter differentiation in the cortex, insular ribbon or basal ganglia.

The early ischemic changes on CT are subtle and the CT may appear normal if performed in the first few hours. The sensitivity of CT within five hours of ischemic stroke was reported as 58% in one early study (Horowitz *et al.* 1991) although a higher rate of 68% has been reported within two hours (von Kummer *et al.* 1994) and even higher of 75% within three hours with middle cerebral artery infarction (Barber *et al.* 2000). The inter-observer reliability and reproducibility of CT in the estimation of the degree of ischemic

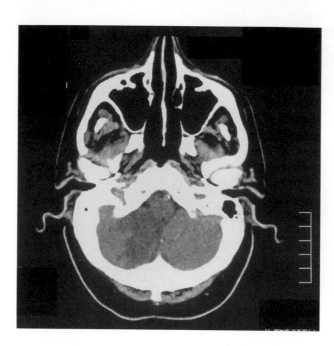

Fig. 11.3. Later ischemic change with hypodensity indicating a cerebellar stroke.

change is modest (von Kummer *et al.* 1996; von Kummer *et al.* 1997; Grotta *et al.* 1999; Schriger *et al.* 1998) although use of a systematic CT review system, the Alberta Stroke Program Early CT Score (ASPECTS) by trained observers has better inter-rater reliability (Coutts *et al.* 2004). Sensitivity is less for small infarcts and infarcts in the posterior fossa, and a significant minority of clinically definite strokes are not associated with an appropriate lesion on CT even after two or three days.

One to two days after stroke onset, the infarcted area appears as an ill-defined hypodense area as vasogenic edema becomes predominant. Within two or three days, the attenuation values become lower, the ischemic area is better demarcated and there may be evidence of mass effect (Figs. 5.1 and 11.3). Later, there may be ipsilateral ventricular dilatation owing to loss of brain substance. Hemorrhagic transformation usually occurs a few days after stroke onset in large infarcts, but it may develop within hours and result in appearances very similar to primary intracerebral hemorrhage (Fig. 16.1) (Bogousslavsky 1991).

The site of any hypodensity relates to the underlying arterial distribution, allowing for differences between individuals in arterial anatomy. A small proportion of patients with first-ever strokes have focal hypodensities on CT in areas inconsistent with the presenting symptoms. Others have widespread diffuse periventricular hypodensity, making any new infarcts difficult to delineate (Chodosh *et al.* 1988). Further, despite the temporal sequence of ischemic changes on CT, it is often difficult to determine the age of an infarct from the CT appearance. Diffusion-weighted MR imaging overcomes these limitations (Figs. 10.3–10.9).

In summary, the main role of CT in acute stroke is to exclude hemorrhage. Owing to the limitations in visualization of ischemia, especially in the early stages, CT cannot be used to stratify participants reliably according to infarct location or size in trials of acute stroke therapy, although it is currently used to exclude major completed infarction prior to early thrombolysis.

The earliest ischemic change on conventional MRI, immediately detectable, is loss of the normal flow void in the affected artery, the MRI equivalent of the hyperdense artery sign on

CT, and arterial enhancement if contrast has been used (Mohr *et al.* 1995). Subsequent changes are swelling on T_1-weighted images caused by cytotoxic edema, which is present in up to half of patients within six hours, hyperintensity on T_2-weighted images from vasogenic edema, present within eight hours, and T_1-weighted signal change, within 16 hours (Yuh *et al.* 1991). Consequently, the sensitivity of conventional MRI is low in the first few hours following the onset of stroke symptoms, with values similar to CT (Mohr *et al.* 1995; Mullins *et al.* 2002). In subacute ischemic stroke, conventional MRI has higher sensitivity than CT owing to its better spatial resolution and lack of posterior fossa artefact (Simmons *et al.* 1986; Bryan *et al.* 1991) but conventional MRI may still be normal in clinically definite stroke.

Conventional MRI is poor at distinguishing acute from chronic infarction. This is a particular problem in patients with multiple infarcts and in the elderly, in whom multiple T_2-weighted abnormalities in the corona radiata, basal ganglia and brainstem are common and in whom neurological symptoms may develop with intercurrent illness on a background of previous stroke. This, together with the poor sensitivity in the acute stroke period, means that, as for CT, conventional MRI is often unable to stratify patients according to infarct presence, ischemic stroke subtype, size or location prior to therapy or randomization in acute stroke trials. Both MRI and MR venography will help where there is a possibility of venous rather than arterial infarction.

Gradient-echo and primary intracerebral imaging hemorrhage

There are limitations to the information on cerebrovascular pathophysiology in vivo that can be provided by CT and conventional MRI. Specifically, these include lack of sensitivity for acute ischemic stroke, difficulty in determining infarct age, lack of demonstration of the ischemic penumbra and low sensitivity and specificity for primary intracerebral hemorrhage in the case of MRI. New imaging techniques address some of these deficiencies and thereby impact on the management of patients with acute stroke.

Recent advances in new MRI sequences that allow further characterization of ischemia have led to increased interest in using gradient-echo (GRE) MRI to detect hemorrhage (Ch. 10). This would avoid having to perform two imaging modalities in acute stroke, CT followed by MRI, in patients in whom further characterization of pathophysiology is necessary, for instance to determine selection for thrombolysis.

Diffusion-weighted imaging

Diffusion-weighted imaging (DWI) has a high sensitivity for acute ischemic stroke, at approximately 90% (Baird and Warach 1998), although other conditions such as seizure, encephalitis and multiple sclerosis can all cause lesions detected by DWI lesions. Diffusion-weighted imaging is abnormal within minutes of stroke onset (Hjort *et al.* 2005a). Inter-observer agreement is better for DWI than with conventional MRI, with sensitivity and specificity of 95% and nearly 100%, respectively (Lutsep *et al.* 1997; Lansberg *et al.* 2000). However, there appears to be a lower sensitivity for DWI in posterior circulation acute stroke, with a 19–31% false-negative rate, particularly where lesions are small and within the first 24-hours after stroke onset (Oppenheim *et al.* 2000).

The fact that DWI distinguishes between acute and chronic infarction and has high sensitivity in acute stroke makes it a valuable tool in the diagnosis and management of patients with acute stroke. It has been reported to show localization in a different vascular

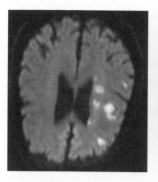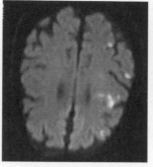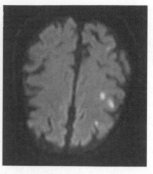

Fig. 11.4. Diffusion-weighted MRI showing multiple areas of acute infarction in a patient with a right carotid dissection.

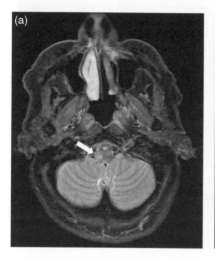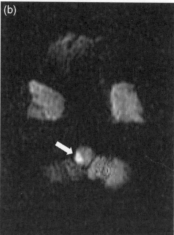

Fig. 11.5. A patient with lateral medullary infarction (arrows) as seen in T_2-weighted (a) and diffusion-weighted (b) MRI.

territory from that initially suspected on the basis of clinical features and conventional MRI in 18% of patients (Albers *et al.* 2000; Schulz *et al.* 2004). It can confirm that a new ischemic cerebrovascular event has occurred in a confused elderly patient with previous strokes or in patients with non-specific symptoms such as confusion or dizziness. The presence of bilateral multiple acute infarcts as shown on DWI may suggest cardioembolism, prompting further cardiac investigation, whereas one acute infarct with several old infarcts might be more suggestive of a thromboembolic event. Multiple recent infarcts in the anterior circulation of the same hemisphere (Fig. 10.4) suggest critical carotid stenosis (Gass *et al.* 2004), dissection (Fig. 11.4) or proximal middle cerebral artery stenosis (Lee *et al.* 2005) and warrant urgent imaging of the anterior circulation vessels with referral for surgery where appropriate. Demonstration of posterior circulation infarction may prompt further assessment of the vertebrobasilar vessels (Fig. 11.5). Symptomatic vertebrobasilar stenosis may warrant specific secondary preventive therapy (Ch. 24).

Diffusion and perfusion imaging and the ischemic penumbra

There is a need to identify those patients with a small infarct but a large ischemic penumbra, in whom the risk – benefit ratio of thrombolysis is likely to be favorable, and to exclude

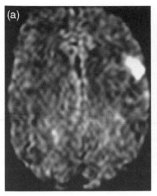 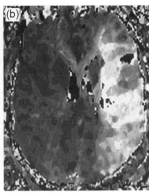

Fig. 11.6. A patient with acute ischemic stroke where MRI shows a perfusion–diffusion mismatch with a relatively small area of high signal on diffusion-weighted imaging (a) but a large area of reduced perfusion on perfusion weighted imaging (b).

from treatment patients at high risk of hemorrhagic transformation or with small lacunar infarcts. Qualitative information on the ischemic penumbra can be obtained using DWI in combination with perfusion-weighted imaging (Kidwell and Hsia 2006; Muir *et al.* 2006).

Perfusion-weighted imaging measures the relative blood flow rate through the brain and can be achieved using an injected contrast agent such as gadolinium or endogenous techniques. The latter have the advantage that they can be used for multiple repeat investigations, but at present the level of contrast produced is less than that obtained with exogenous agents. Nearly all published studies of perfusion-weighted imaging in acute stroke have used exogenous contrast agents. In contrast to lesion volumes seen with DWI, those with perfusion-weighted imaging are typically largest acutely and resolve over time. Consistent with earlier positron emission tomography studies, perfusion changes precede the development of DWI-detected lesions. In the absence of reperfusion, lesions detected by DWI progressively extend over 24-hours into the area of reduced perfusion-weighted imaging (see below).

Two patterns of DWI and perfusion-weighted imaging abnormalities have been observed in acute ischemic stroke:

- perfusion-weighted imaging shows less damage than DWI: the volume of abnormal perfusion is less than that of the hyperintense DWI signal
- perfusion-weighted imaging shows more damage than DWI: the volume of abnormal perfusion is greater than the volume of hyperintense DWI change.

When perfusion-weighted imaging shows a larger abnormality than DWI, at least half of patients show an increase in DWI-detectable lesion volume over the 3–11 days after stroke onset (Sorensen *et al.* 1996; Baird *et al.* 1997; Barber *et al.* 1998; van Everdingen *et al.* 1998; Beaulieu *et al.* 1999; Karonen *et al.* 1999). Lesion growth is amplified by hyperglycemia, high hematocrit, old age and hypoxia (Baird *et al.* 2003; Allport *et al.* 2005; Ay *et al.* 2005; Singhal *et al.* 2005). When perfusion-weighted imaging shows less abnormality than does DWI initially, no significant lesion growth occurs (Barber *et al.* 1998). Consequently, it has been proposed that when there is "perfusion–diffusion mismatch," that is, where there is reduced perfusion but not yet DWI signal change, this tissue area represents the ischemic penumbra and thus tissue that may be salvaged if perfusion can be restored quickly enough (Fig. 11.6).

However, it has recently become apparent that simple perfusion–diffusion mismatch does not delineate the ischemic penumbra accurately. The DWI signal change does not correspond exactly to irreversibly infarcted tissue, tending to overestimate it; consequently, part of the lesion detected by DWI appears to lie within the ischemic penumbra (Kidwell *et al.* 2003). Hence, patients with matched diffusion and perfusion deficits may actually have a significant penumbra. Deficits detectable by DWI have been shown to be reversible both spontaneously (Lecouvet *et al.* 1999; Krueger *et al.* 2000) and following reperfusion with thrombolysis (Kidwell *et al.* 2000; Parsons *et al.* 2001). In some cases, this initial resolution was temporary, with development of recurrent lesions within a week (Kidwell *et al.* 2002).

Regarding perfusion-weighted imaging, the size of the hypoperfused area will vary according to the method of measurement used: prolonged mean transit time, reduced cerebral blood volume or reduced cerebral blood flow, of which only the last reflects true hypoperfusion. This hampers comparisons between studies. Hypoperfused areas will include oligemic areas as well as areas at risk of infarction and thus perfusion-weighted imaging will tend to overestimate the boundary of the penumbra. Given the fact that DWI change does not correspond exactly to irreversibly damaged tissue, severity of perfusion deficit has been proposed as a surrogate for subsequent infarction (Thijs *et al.* 2001; Fiehler *et al.* 2002; Shih *et al.* 2003) and as a potential tool for use in clinical selection of patients for thrombolysis.

Perfusion computed tomography

Recently, there has been increasing interest in the use of new CT methods (Wintermark and Bogousslavsky 2003) to examine cerebral blood flow. Cerebral blood flow measurement using CT can be achieved using existing CT-based technology; it is easier to perform in sick patients than MRI and is not contraindicated in those with pacemakers, ferromagnetic implants, mechanical heart valves and those with claustrophobia. The CT perfusion technique uses exogenous contrast and enables calculation of cerebral blood flow, cerebral blood volume and mean transit time. However, quantification of cerebral blood flow is problematic, as it is in perfusion-weighted imaging, and most studies use ratios comparing values with homologous areas of the contralateral hemisphere, which itself may show a reduced cerebral blood flow in the acute stroke period owing to diaschisis. In addition, current technology allows only limited brain coverage of two to four slices, which means that large areas of ischemia are imaged inadequately and small ones may be missed altogether.

Despite the limitations described above, there is evidence that perfusion CT values correlate with angiographic findings and DWI/perfusion-weighted imaging changes, can predict infarction and clinical outcome (Nabavi *et al.* 2002; Meuli 2004; Parsons *et al.* 2005; Wintermark *et al.* 2007) and may be able to identify patients likely to benefit from thrombolysis.

Radiological selection of patients for thrombolysis

Radiological investigation to exclude hemorrhage is essential in selecting patients for thrombolysis. It may also help to identify patients with large completed infarcts, a small ischemic penumbra or TIA, in whom thrombolysis would not be beneficial. The majority of centers currently rely on CT rather than MRI as the first-line investigation in stroke.

Retrospective analysis of CT scans has suggested that early signs of extensive infarction on CT, corresponding to a very poor ASPECTS score of ≤ 2 (Weir *et al.* 2006) are associated with 85% mortality without thrombolysis and poor outcome, including hemorrhagic transformation, after thrombolysis (von Kummer *et al.* 1994, 1997; Hacke *et al.* 1998; Dzialowski *et al.* 2006). These observations have led to the introduction of the "one-third rule," that is, patients with signs of infarction of greater than one-third of the middle cerebral artery territory on CT should not receive thrombolytic therapy. However, overestimation of the degree of ischemic change on CT may lead to thrombolytic treatment being inappropriately withheld (Barber *et al.* 1999). Initial small studies investigating cerebral microbleeds and the risk of hemorrhagic transformation after thrombolysis showed an uncertain relationship (Derex *et al.* 2005; Koennecke 2006; Cordonnier *et al.* 2007), but more recent data do not show an increased thrombolysis risk (Fiehler *et al.* 2007). In contrast, the presence of a large lesion on DWI (Singer *et al.* 2007) or high permeability (Bang *et al.* 2007) is associated with hemorrhage.

The theory that the ischemic penumbra represents salvageable tissue has led to the proposal that thrombolysis is likely to be most effective in those patients with diffusion–perfusion mismatch. Despite the fact that the area of diffusion–perfusion mismatch does not precisely delineate the penumbra, it appears reasonably robust in representing tissue at risk of infarction. Use of recombinant tissue plasminogen activator is associated with early resolution of perfusion-weighted imaging lesions in less than 36 hours, reduced DWI lesion growth, smaller final stroke volumes and better clinical outcome on follow-up (Hjort *et al.* 2005b). It has been suggested that diffusion–perfusion mismatch might be mirrored by a clinical–diffusion mismatch, but current data suggest that this is not the case (Lansberg *et al.* 2007; Messe *et al.* 2007).

In patients with matched images by DWI and perfusion-weighted imaging, it is unclear whether reperfusion will be of benefit since it is uncertain whether the area detected by DWI still contains a significant penumbra. In these cases, MR angiographic findings and the clinical picture should be taken into account. A severe neurological deficit and middle cerebral artery occlusion predicts a malignant middle cerebral artery infarction. A DWI lesion with normal or increased perfusion indicates spontaneous recanalization and is inappropriate for thrombolysis.

Both MR and CT angiography have been used to assess patients in the acute phase after stroke and have been proposed as possible means of selecting patients for thrombolysis. It has been observed that patients with a patent middle cerebral artery typically have smaller perfusion-weighted imaging volumes than patients with evidence of large vessel occlusion: absent middle cerebral artery flow on MR angiogram is significantly associated with a greater perfusion–diffusion mismatch, larger acute DWI lesions, secondary lesion growth, larger final infarct size and worse final outcome (Barber *et al.* 1999). However, a significant minority of the 30–35% of patients with middle cerebral artery occlusion do not show progressive lesion enlargement and patients without middle cerebral artery occlusion may show significant mismatch.

At present, there is no consensus on the exact criteria to use in patient selection for thrombolysis using multimodal MRI (Hand *et al.* 2006). Many centers offer thrombolytic therapy to selected patients within three hours of stroke onset according to local criteria, including brain imaging findings, often CT based. Beyond the three to six hour time window, there are few data to guide treatment decisions, although thrombolysis has been shown to be potentially effective when given three to nine hours after stroke onset (Furlan *et al.* 2006). In the phase II Desmoteplase In Acute Ischemic Stroke trial (DIAS), patients with MRI evidence of perfusion–diffusion mismatch were randomized to escalating doses of desmoteplase administered three to nine hours after acute ischemic stroke (Hacke *et al.* 2005). High doses of desmoteplase were associated with unacceptably high intracerebral hemorrhage rates, but lower doses produced a higher rate of reperfusion and suggested better clinical outcome compared with placebo.

In the observational DEFUSE (Diffusion and Perfusion Imaging Evaluation for Understanding Stroke Evolution) study, an MRI scan was obtained immediately before and three to six hours after treatment with intravenous tissue plasminogen activator, which was given three to six hours after symptom onset (Albers *et al.* 2006). Baseline MRI profiles were used to categorize patients into subgroups, and clinical responses were compared based on whether early reperfusion was achieved. Early reperfusion was associated with significantly increased odds of achieving a favorable clinical response in patients with a perfusion–diffusion mismatch (odds ratio, 5.4; $p = 0.039$) and an even more favorable response in patients with the "target mismatch" profile (odds ratio, 8.7; $p = 0.011$). Patients with the "no mismatch" profile did not appear to benefit from early reperfusion. Early reperfusion was associated with fatal intracranial hemorrhage in patients with the "malignant" profile.

The recent Echoplanar Imaging Thrombolytic Evaluation Trial (EPITHET; Davis *et al.* 2008) randomly assigned 101 patients to receive alteplase or placebo three to six hours after onset of ischemic stroke. Perfusion and diffusion imaging were done before and three to five days after therapy, with T_2-weighted MRI. The primary endpoint was infarct growth between baseline diffusion imaging and the day 90 T_2-weighted lesion in mismatch patients. Major secondary endpoints were reperfusion, good neurological outcome and good functional outcome. Alteplase was non-significantly associated with lower infarct growth and significantly associated with increased reperfusion in patients who had mismatch.

The DIAS, DEFUSE and EPITHET studies were small and used different thrombolytic agents (and different doses in DIAS), and further studies are needed before it is certain that diffusion–perfusion mismatch on MRI is a reliable surrogate for the presence of a penumbra that might benefit from thrombolysis beyond the three-hour time window.

Transcranial Doppler ultrasonography aimed at the occluded part of a vessel may help to expose thrombi to the effect of thrombolytic agents and thus augment the effect of thrombolysis. The CLOTBUST II (ultrasound-enhanced systemic thrombolysis for acute ischemic stroke) trial tested this hypothesis (Alexandrov *et al.* 2004). Patients with acute ischemic stroke and middle cerebral artery occlusion presenting within three hours after stroke onset received intravenous tissue plasminogen activator and were randomized to receive additional transcranial Doppler ultrasonography or placebo. The treatment group showed a significantly higher rate of recanalization and a non-significant trend towards more favorable outcome, suggesting that transcranial Doppler ultrasonography may indeed enhance the effectiveness of intravenous thrombolysis. There are two ongoing trials assessing this technique further: MUST (Microbubbles and Ultrasound in Stroke Trial), and PULSE (Pilot UltraSound Lysis Early Treatment Study).

References

Albers GW, Lansberg MG, Norbash AM *et al.* (2000). Yield of diffusion-weighted MRI for detection of potentially relevant findings in stroke patients. *Neurology* **54**:1562–1567

Albers GW, Thijs VN, Wechsler L for the DEFUSE Investigators (2006). Magnetic resonance imaging profiles predict clinical response to early reperfusion: the diffusion and perfusion imaging evaluation for understanding stroke evolution (DEFUSE) study. *Annals of Neurology* **60**:508–517

Alexandrov AV, Molina CA, Grotta JC *et al.* (2004). Ultrasound-enhanced systemic thrombolysis for acute ischemic stroke. *New England Journal of Medicine* **351**:2170–2178

Allport LE, Parsons MW, Butcher KS *et al.* (2005). Elevated hematocrit is associated with reduced reperfusion and tissue survival in acute stroke. *Neurology* **65**:1382–1387

Ay H, Koroshetz WJ, Vangel M *et al.* (2005). Conversion of ischemic brain tissue into infarction increases with age. *Stroke* **36**:2632–2636

Baird AE, Warach S (1998). Magnetic resonance imaging of acute stroke. *Journal of Cerebral Blood Flow and Metabolism* **18**:583–609

Baird AE, Benfield A, Schlaug G et al. (1997). Enlargement of human cerebral ischemic lesion volumes measured by diffusion-weighted magnetic resonance imaging. *Annals of Neurology* **41**:581–589

Baird TA, Parsons MW, Phanh T et al. (2003). Persistent poststroke hyperglycemia is independently associated with infarct expansion and worse clinical outcome. *Stroke* **34**:2208–2214

Bang OY, Buck BH, Saver JL et al. (2007). Prediction of hemorrhagic transformation after recanalization therapy using T_2^*-permeability magnetic resonance imaging. *Annals of Neurology* **62**:170–176

Barber PA, Darby DG, Desmond PM et al. (1998). Prediction of stroke outcome with echoplanar perfusion-and diffusion-weighted MRI. *Neurology* **51**:418–426

Barber PA, Davis SM, Darby DG et al. (1999). Absent middle cerebral artery flow predicts the presence and evolution of the ischemic penumbra. *Neurology* **52**:1125–1132

Barber PA, Demchuk AM, Zhang J et al. (2000). Validity and reliability of a quantitative computed tomography score in predicting outcome of hyperacute stroke before thrombolytic therapy. ASPECTS Study Group. Alberta Stroke Programme Early CT Score. *Lancet* **355**:1670–1674

Beaulieu C, de Crespigny A, Tong DC et al. (1999). Longitudinal magnetic resonance imaging study of perfusion and diffusion in stroke: evolution of lesion volume and correlation with clinical outcome. *Annals in Neurology* **46**:568–578

Bogousslavsky J (1991). Topographic patterns of cerebral infarcts: correlation with aetiology. *Cerebrovascular Diseases* **1**:61–68

Bryan RN, Levy LM, Whitlow WD et al. (1991). Diagnosis of acute cerebral infarction: comparison of CT and MR imaging. *American Journal of Neuroradiology* **12**:611–620

Chalela JA, Kidwell CS, Nentwich LM et al. (2007). Magnetic resonance imaging and computed tomography in emergency assessment of patients with suspected acute stroke: a prospective comparison. *Lancet* **369**:293–298

Chodosh EH, Foulkes MA, Kase CS et al. (1988). Silent stroke in the NINCDS stroke data bank. *Neurology* **38**:1674–1679

Cordonnier C, Al-Shahi Salman R, Wardlaw J (2007). Spontaneous brain microbleeds: systematic review subgroup analyses and standards for study design and reporting. *Brain* **130**:1988–2003

Coutts SB, Demchuk AM, Barber PA et al. (2004). Interobserver variation of ASPECTS in real time. *Stroke* **35**:103–105

Davis SM, Donnan GA, Parsons MW for the EPITHET Investigators (2008). Effects of alteplase beyond 3 h after stroke in the Echoplanar Imaging Thrombolytic Evaluation Trial (EPITHET): a placebo-controlled randomised trial. *Lancet Neurology* **7**:299–309

Derex L, Hermier M, Adeleine P et al. (2005). Clinical and imaging predictors of intracerebral hemorrhage in stroke patients treated with intravenous tissue lasminogen activator. *Journal of Neurology, Neurosurgery and Psychiatry* **76**:70–75

Dzialowski I, Hill MD, Coutts SB et al. (2006). Extent of early ischemic changes on computed tomography (CT) before thrombolysis: prognostic value of the Alberta Stroke Program Early CT Score in ECASS II. *Stroke* **37**:973–978

Fiehler J, Foth M, Kucinski T et al. (2002). Severe ADC decreases do not predict irreversible tissue damage in humans. *Stroke* **33**:79–86

Fiehler J, Albers GW, Boulanger JM for the MR Stroke Group (2007). Bleeding Risk Analysis in Stroke Imaging before thromboLysis (BRASIL): pooled analysis of T_2^* weighted magnetic resonance imaging data from 570 patients. *Stroke* **38**:2738–2744

Furlan AJ, Eyding D, Albers GW et al. (2006). Dose Escalation of Desmoteplase for Acute Ischemic Stroke (DEDAS): evidence of safety and efficacy 3 to 9 hours after stroke onset. *Stroke* **37**:1227–1231

Gass A, Ay H, Szabo K et al. (2004). Diffusion-weighted MRI for the "small stuff": the details of acute cerebral ischemia. *Lancet Neurology* **3**:39–45

Grotta JC, Chiu D, Lu M et al. (1999). Agreement and variability in the interpretation of early CT changes in stroke patients qualifying for intravenous rtPA therapy. *Stroke* **30**:1528–1533

Gunatilake SB (1998). Rapid resolution of symptoms and signs of intracerebral hemorrhage: case reports. *British Medical Journal* **316**:1495–1496

Hacke W, Kaste M, Fieschi C *et al.* (1998). Randomised double-blind placebo-controlled trial of thrombolytic therapy with intravenous alteplase in acute ischemic stroke (ECASS II) Second European–Australasian Acute Stroke Study Investigators. *Lancet* **352**:1245–1251

Hacke W, Albers G, Al-Rawi Y for the DIAS Study Group (2005). The Desmoteplase in Acute Ischemic Stroke Trial (DIAS): a phase II MRI-based 9-hour window acute stroke thrombolysis trial with intravenous desmoteplase. *Stroke* **36**:66–73

Hand PJ, Wardlaw JM, Rivers CS *et al.* (2006). MR diffusion-weighted imaging and outcome prediction after ischemic stroke. *Neurology* **66**:1159–1163

Hawkins GC, Bonita R, Broad JB *et al.* (1995). Inadequacy of clinical scoring systems to differentiate stroke subtypes in population-based studies. *Stroke* **26**:1338–1342

Hjort N, Christensen S, Solling C *et al.* (2005a). Ischemic injury detected by diffusion imaging 11 minutes after stroke. *Annals of Neurology* **58**:462–465

Hjort N, Butcher K, Davis SM *et al.* (2005b). Magnetic resonance imaging criteria for thrombolysis in acute cerebral infarct. *Stroke* **36**:388–397

Horowitz SH, Zito JL, Donnarumma R *et al.* (1991). Computed tomographic–angiographic findings within the first five hours of cerebral infarction. *Stroke* **22**:1245–1253

Karonen JO, Vanninen RL, Liu Y *et al.* (1999). Combined diffusion and perfusion MRI with correlation to single-photon emission CT in acute ischemic stroke. Ischemic penumbra predicts infarct growth. *Stroke* **30**:1583–1590

Kidwell CS, Hsia AW (2006). Imaging of the brain and cerebral vasculature in patients with suspected stroke: advantages and disadvantages of CT and MRI. *Current Neurology and Neuroscience Reports* **6**:9–16

Kidwell CS, Saver JL, Mattiello J *et al.* (2000). Thrombolytic reversal of acute human cerebral ischemic injury shown by diffusion/perfusion magnetic resonance imaging. *Annals of Neurology* **47**:462–469

Kidwell CS, Saver JL, Starkman S *et al.* (2002). Late secondary ischemic injury in patients receiving intraarterial thrombolysis. *Annals of Neurology* **52**:698–703

Kidwell CS, Alger JR, Saver JL (2003). Beyond mismatch: evolving paradigms in imaging the ischemic penumbra with multimodal magnetic resonance imaging. *Stroke* **34**:2729–2735

Koennecke HC (2006). Cerebral microbleeds on MRI: prevalence associations and potential clinical implications. *Neurology* **66**:165–171

Krueger K, Kugel H, Grond M *et al.* (2000). Late resolution of diffusion-weighted MRI changes in a patient with prolonged reversible ischemic neurological deficit after thrombolytic therapy. *Stroke* **31**:2715–2718

Kucinski T, Vaterlein O, Glauche V *et al.* (2002). Correlation of apparent diffusion coefficient and computed tomography density in acute ischemic stroke. *Stroke* **33**:1786–1791

Lansberg MG, Norbash AM, Marks MP *et al.* (2000). Advantages of adding diffusion-weighted magnetic resonance imaging to conventional magnetic resonance imaging for evaluating acute stroke. *Archives of Neurology* **57**:1311–1316

Lansberg MG, Thijs VN, Hamilton S for the DEFUSE Investigators (2007). Evaluation of the clinical–diffusion and perfusion–diffusion mismatch models in DEFUSE. *Stroke* **38**:1826–1830

Lecouvet FE, Duprez TP, Raymackers JM *et al.* (1999). Resolution of early diffusion-weighted and FLAIR MRI abnormalities in a patient with TIA. *Neurology* **52**:1085–1087

Lee DK, Kim JS, Kwon SU *et al.* (2005). Lesion patterns and stroke mechanism in atherosclerotic middle cerebral artery disease: early diffusion-weighted imaging study. *Stroke* **36**:2583–2588

Lee SH, Bae HJ, Kwon SJ *et al.* (2004). Cerebral microbleeds are regionally associated with intracerebral hemorrhage. *Neurology* **62**:72–76

Lutsep HL, Albers GW, DeCrespigny A *et al.* (1997). Clinical utility of diffusion-weighted magnetic resonance imaging in the assessment of ischemic stroke. *Annals of Neurology* **41**:574–580

Messe SR, Kasner SE, Chalela JA *et al.* (2007). CT–NIHSS mismatch does not correlate with MRI diffusion–perfusion mismatch. *Stroke* **38**:2079–2084

Meuli RA (2004). Imaging viable brain tissue with CT scan during acute stroke. *Cerebrovascular Disease* 17:28–34

Mohr JP, Biller J, Hilal SK *et al.* (1995). Magnetic resonance versus computed tomographic imaging in acute stroke. *Stroke* 26:807–812

Muir KW, Buchan A, von Kummer R *et al.* (2006). Imaging of acute stroke. *Lancet Neurology* 5:755–768

Mullins ME, Schaefer PW, Sorensen AG *et al.* (2002). CT and conventional and diffusion-weighted MR imaging in acute stroke: study in 691 patients at presentation to the emergency department. *Radiology* 224:353–360

Nabavi DG, Kloska SP, Nam EM *et al.* (2002). MOSAIC: multimodal stroke assessment using computed tomography: novel diagnostic approach for the prediction of infarction size and clinical outcome. *Stroke* 33:2819–2826

Nighoghossian N, Hermier M, Adeleine P *et al.* (2002). Old microbleeds are a potential risk factor for cerebral bleeding after ischemic stroke: a gradient-echo T_2^* weighted brain MRI study. *Stroke* 33:735–742

Oppenheim C, Stanescu R, Dormont D *et al.* (2000). False-negative diffusion-weighted MR findings in acute ischemic stroke. *American Journal of Neuroradiology* 21:1434–1440

Parsons MW, Yang Q, Barber PA *et al.* (2001). Perfusion magnetic resonance imaging maps in hyperacute stroke: relative cerebral blood flow most accurately identifies tissue destined to infarct. *Stroke* 32:1581–1587

Parsons MW, Pepper EM, Chan V *et al.* (2005). Perfusion computed tomography: prediction of final infarct extent and stroke outcome. *Annals of Neurology* 58:672–679

Schriger DL, Kalafut M, Starkman S *et al.* (1998). Cranial computed tomography interpretation in acute stroke: physician accuracy in determining eligibility for thrombolytic therapy. *JAMA* 279:1293–1297

Schulz UG, Flossman E, Rothwell PM (2004). Heritability of ischemic stroke in relation to age, vascular risk factors and subtypes of incident stroke in population-based studies. *Stroke* 35:819–824

Shih LC, Saver JL, Alger JR *et al.* (2003). Perfusion-weighted magnetic resonance imaging thresholds identifying core, irreversibly infarcted tissue. *Stroke* 34:1425–1430

Simmons Z, Biller J, Adams HP, Jr., *et al.* (1986). Cerebellar infarction: comparison of computed tomography and magnetic resonance imaging. *Annals of Neurology* 19:291–293

Singer OC, Humpich MC, Fiehler J for the MR Stroke Study Group Investigators (2007). Risk for symptomatic intracerebral hemorrhage after thrombolysis assessed by diffusion-weighted magnetic resonance imaging. *Annals of Neurology* 63:52–60

Singhal AB, Benner T, Roccatagliata L *et al.* (2005). A pilot study of normobaric oxygen therapy in acute ischemic stroke. *Stroke* 36:797–802

Sorensen AG, Buonanno FS, Gonzalez RG *et al.* (1996). Hyperacute stroke: evaluation with combined multisection diffusion-weighted and haemodynamically weighted echo-planar MR imaging. *Radiology* 199:391–401

Thijs VN, Adami A, Neumann-Haefelin T *et al.* (2001). Relationship between severity of MR perfusion deficit and DWI lesion evolution. *Neurology* 57:1205–1211

van Everdingen KJ, van der Grond J, Kappelle LJ *et al.* (1998). Diffusion-weighted magnetic resonance imaging in acute stroke. *Stroke* 29:1783–1790

von Kummer R, Meyding-Lamade U, Forsting M *et al.* (1994). Sensitivity and prognostic value of early CT in occlusion of the middle cerebral artery trunk. *American Journal of Neuroradiology* 15:9–15

von Kummer R, Holle R, Gizyska U *et al.* (1996). Interobserver agreement in assessing early CT signs of middle cerebral artery infarction. *American Journal of Neuroradiology* 17:1743–1748

von Kummer R, Allen KL, Holle R *et al.* (1997). Acute stroke: usefulness of early CT findings before thrombolytic therapy. *Radiology* 205:327–333

von Kummer R, Bourquain H, Bastianello S *et al.* (2001). Early prediction of irreversible brain damage after ischemic stroke at CT. *Radiology* 219:95–100

Weir NU, Pexman JH, Hill MD *et al.* (2006). How well does ASPECTS predict the outcome of acute stroke treated with IV tPA? *Neurology* 67:516–518

Wintermark M, Bogousslavsky J (2003).
Imaging of acute ischemic brain injury:
the return of computed tomography. *Current
Opinions in Neurology* **16**:59–63

Wintermark M, Meuli R, Browaeys P *et al.* (2007).
Comparison of CT perfusion and angiography
and MRI in selecting stroke patients for
acute treatment. *Neurology* **68**:694–697

Yuh WT, Crain MR, Loes DJ *et al.* (1991). MR
imaging of cerebral ischemia: findings in the
first 24 hours. *American Journal of
Neuroradiology* **12**:621–629

Chapter 12

Vascular imaging in transient ischemic attack and stroke

The main clinical indications for imaging the cerebral circulation are TIA (e.g. to identify arterial stenosis), acute ischemic stroke (e.g. to identify vessel occlusion), intracerebral hemorrhage (e.g. to identify an underlying vascular malformation) and possible arterial dissection, fibromuscular dysplasia or other arteriopathies, cerebral aneurysm, intracranial venous thrombosis or cerebral vasculitis.

In contrast to pharmaceutical products, diagnostic and imaging technologies are not subject to stringent regulatory control, and no standards are set for validation; as a result, the evidence base on important issues such as diagnostic sensitivity and specificity is often poor. For example, although several hundred studies of carotid imaging have been published over the last few decades, most are undermined by poor design, inadequate sample size and inappropriate analysis and presentation of data (Rothwell *et al.* 2000a).

Catheter angiography

Cerebral angiography, introduced by Moniz in Portugal in the 1930s, was the first method to display the cerebral circulation during life (Ch. 25). Originally it required the intra-carotid injection of material that was opaque to X-rays. Over the years, the technology has improved, with less-toxic contrast material, femoral artery catheterization, digital imaging and catheters that can be controlled and introduced into vessels as small as the cortical branches of the middle cerebral artery.

Before the introduction of axial imaging of the brain in the early 1970s, first by CT and then by MRI, catheter angiography was used to identify intracranial mass lesions, hydro-cephalus and other structural abnormalities. Nowadays, with the increased use of CT angiography, MR angiography and ultrasound imaging, catheter angiography is more or less confined to displaying arterial stenosis and occlusions caused by vascular disease (atheroma, vasculitis, dissection, etc.), intracranial venous thrombosis, small intracranial aneurysms and intracranial vascular malformations. The reasons for this diminishing role are that although catheter angiography remains the "gold standard" technique in many situations, it is inconvenient, invasive, uncomfortable and costly and it requires hospital admission and carries a risk (Table 12.1). For example, a systematic review of prospective studies of the risks of catheter angiography in patients with cerebrovascular disease reported a 0.1% risk of death and a 1.0% risk of permanent neurological sequelae (Hankey and Warlow 1990), although more recent studies have reported lower risks (Johnston *et al.* 2001).

Compared with cut-film selective intra-arterial catheter angiography recorded directly on to X-ray film, intra-arterial digital subtraction angiography (DSA) (Fig. 12.1) is quicker; the images are easier to manipulate and store and contrast resolution is better although spatial resolution is less. However, there is no evidence that less contrast is used or that it is much safer (Warnock *et al.* 1993). Even for imaging only as far as the carotid bifurcation,

Table 12.1. Complications of catheter angiography

	Complication
Related to the catheter placement	TIA, stroke or death as a result of dislodgement of atheromatous plaque by the catheter tip; dissection of the arterial wall; thrombus formation on the catheter tip; air embolism
Related to arterial puncture and cannulation	Hematoma
	Aneurysm
	Nerve injury
	Exacerbation of peripheral vascular disease distal to puncture site
Related to intravenous contrast	Allergic reaction
	Cardiac failure owing to the volume of injected contrast
	Renal toxicity

Note:
TIA, transient ischemic attack.
Source: From Gerraty *et al.* (1996).

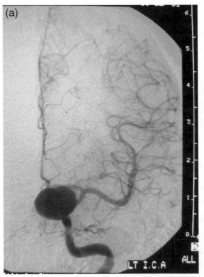 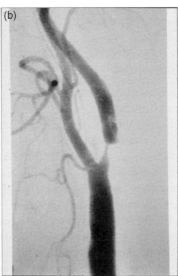

Fig. 12.1. Digitally subtracted arterial angiograms showing a large distal internal carotid artery aneurysm (a) and a severe stenosis of the proximal internal carotid artery (b).

neither intravenous DSA nor arch aortography is a satisfactory alternative to selective intra-arterial angiography (Pelz *et al.* 1985; Rothwell *et al.* 1998; Cuffe and Rothwell 2006).

Even with selective catheter angiography, there can be difficulty in distinguishing occlusion from extreme internal carotid artery stenosis, and then late views are needed to see contrast eventually passing up into the head. Moreover, because of the localized and non-concentric nature of atherosclerotic plaques, biplanar, and preferably triplanar (Jeans *et al.* 1986; Cuffe and Rothwell 2006), views of the carotid bifurcation are required to measure the degree of carotid stenosis accurately: that is, to visualize the residual lumen without overlap of other vessels, to measure at the narrowest point and to compare with a suitable denominator to derive the percentage diameter stenosis.

Catheter angiography can also provide information about ulceration of carotid plaque and complicating luminal thrombosis, albeit with only moderate interobserver agreement (Streifler *et al.* 1994; Rothwell *et al.* 1998). However, angiographic irregularity and ulceration predict a higher risk of stroke than if the plaque is smooth, given the same degree of stenosis (Eliasziw *et al.* 1994; Rothwell *et al.* 2000b), and there is good correlation between catheter angiographic plaque morphology and histology when the latter is rigorously evaluated (Lovett *et al.* 2004). Luminal thrombus is relatively unusual but is thought to be associated with a high risk of stroke (Martin *et al.* 1992).

Catheter angiography is still widely used to reveal a vascular malformation or aneurysm in young patients with intracerebral hemorrhage. In older patients, bleeds from either hypertension or amyloid angiopathy are predominant. Vascular malformations and aneurysms are most likely if the cerebral hemorrhage is lobar or intraventricular and there is no hypertension (Zhu *et al.* 1997). However, MRI can be more sensitive than catheter angiography in detecting vascular malformations (particularly cavernomas), and MR and CT angiography are increasingly able to detect aneurysms of a size likely to rebleed.

Until recently, catheter angiography was the standard imaging modality to confirm or exclude carotid or vertebral artery dissection (Fig. 12.2) because ultrasound was neither specific nor sensitive enough. However, there is now a widespread consensus that cross-sectional MRI, to show thrombus within the widened arterial wall, combined with MR angiography is the safest and best option.

Catheter angiography versus non-invasive imaging

Although non-invasive methods of imaging continue to improve, catheter angiography remains the gold standard against which other vessel imaging methods must be compared, and it is also the underpinning method for the interventional neuroradiological treatment of arterial stenoses, aneurysms and vascular malformations. However, the clinician is often faced with the question as to whether to base decision making on non-invasive imaging alone or whether to proceed to catheter angiography. For example, multislice CT angiography is widely used in the screening for cerebral aneurysms because of its speed, tolerability, safety and potential for three-dimensional reconstructions. The sensitivity of CT angiography for aneurysms >3 mm diameter is approximately 96% but it is much less for smaller aneurysms. The sensitivity for detecting ruptured aneurysms with CT angiography, with conventional angiography as the gold standard, is approximately 95% (Villablanca *et al.* 2002; Chappell *et al.* 2003; Wintermark *et al.* 2003). Magnetic resonance angiography has similar resolution to CT angiography but is less easy to use in sick patients. Four-vessel catheter angiography may still, therefore, be required when non-invasive imaging is negative.

A similar trade-off between diagnostic accuracy and risk is necessary when imaging the carotid bifurcation in patients with TIA or ischemic stroke. Performing intra-arterial catheter angiography in everyone is clearly unacceptable because of the risks and cost. Fewer than 20% of patients will have an operable carotid stenosis; even if only those with "cortical" rather than "lacunar" events are selected (Hankey and Warlow 1991; Hankey *et al.* 1991; Mead *et al.* 1999). Confining angiography to patients with a carotid bifurcation bruit will miss some patients with severe stenosis and still subject too many with mild or moderate stenosis to the risks. Nor will a combination of a cervical bruit with various clinical features do much better (Mead *et al.* 1999).

Therefore, non-invasive imaging is required at least as an initial screening tool. In many centers, decisions about endarterectomy are now based solely on non-invasive imaging.

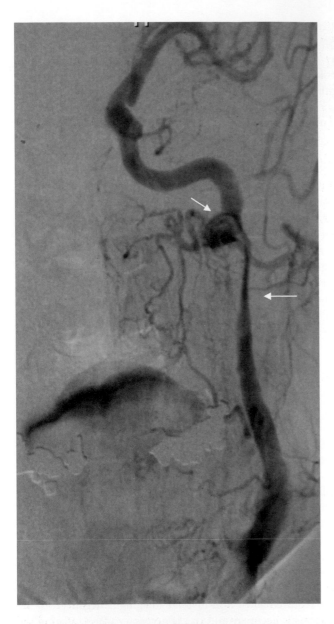

Fig. 12.2. Digitally subtracted arterial angiogram showing a distal internal carotid artery dissection (tapering lumen; lower arrow) and a complicating aneurysm (upper arrow).

However, because benefit from endarterectomy is highly dependent on the degree of symptomatic carotid stenosis as measured on catheter angiography, misclassification of stenosis with non-invasive methods will lead to some patients being operated on unnecessarily, and others being denied appropriate surgery. A meta-analysis of studies of non-invasive carotid imaging published prior to 1995 concluded that non-invasive methods could not substitute for catheter angiography as the sole pre-endarterectomy imaging because of the frequency with which the degree of stenosis was misclassified (Blakeley *et al.* 1995). More recent studies have confirmed this (Johnston and Goldstein 2001; Norris *et al.* 2003; Norris and Halliday 2004; Chappell *et al.* 2006). For example, in a comparison of catheter angiography with Doppler ultrasound in 569 consecutive patients in "accredited"

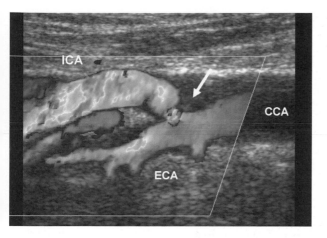

Fig. 12.3. A color-flow Doppler ultrasound of the carotid bifurcation showing a plaque (arrow) at the origin of the internal carotid artery (ICA) and the resulting stenosis. ECA, external carotid artery; CCA, common carotid artery. (See the color plate section.)

laboratories with experienced radiologists, 28% of decisions about endarterectomy based on Doppler ultrasound alone were inappropriate (Johnston and Goldstein 2001). However, the combination of Doppler ultrasound with another non-invasive method of imaging, such as MR angiography, reduced inappropriate decisions in comparison with catheter angiography to less than 10% in patients for whom the results of Doppler ultrasound and MR angiography were concordant (Johnston and Goldstein, 2001). Similar approaches based on two different methods of non-invasive imaging have been shown by other groups to be effective in routine clinical practice (Johnston *et al.* 2002; Barth *et al.* 2006). Catheter angiography is still required in the patients in whom Doppler ultrasound and MR angiography do not produce concordant results.

Duplex sonography

Duplex sonography combines real-time ultrasound imaging to display the arterial anatomy with pulsed Doppler flow analysis at any point of interest in the vessel lumen. Its accuracy is enhanced and it is technically easier to carry out if the Doppler signals are color coded to show the direction of blood flow and its velocity (Fig. 12.3). Power Doppler and intravenous echocontrast may also help (Droste *et al.* 1999; Gaitini and Soudack 2005; Wardlaw and Lewis 2005). The degree of carotid luminal stenosis is calculated not only from the real-time ultrasound image, which can be inaccurate when the lesion is echolucent or calcification scatters the ultrasound beam, but also from the blood flow velocities derived from the Doppler signal. If color Doppler is not available, only gray-scale duplex, it is usually helpful to insonate the supraorbital artery first with a simple continuous-wave Doppler probe, because *inward* flow of blood strongly suggests severe internal carotid artery stenosis or occlusion, although not necessarily at the origin.

Although duplex sonography is non-invasive and widely available, there are some difficulties that any ultrasound service must deal with (Box 12.1). Nonetheless, with stringent quality control and ideally with confirmation of stenosis by an independent observer, duplex sonography is now the most common way that carotid stenosis severe enough to warrant surgery is diagnosed (Chappell *et al.* 2006).

There are no standard and commonly used definitions for the ultrasound appearance of plaques (soft, hard, calcified, etc.) and there is also considerable variation in reporting

Box 12.1. Difficulties encountered with carotid duplex sonography

Operator dependent so requires training, skill and experience to ensure accuracy of and
  consistency in measurement of stenosis
Plaque or peri-arterial calcification causes difficulty in interpretation
Lack of reliability in distinguishing very severe stenosis (>90%) from occlusion, and resultant
  uncertainty in decision making about surgery
Only moderate-to-good sensitivity and specificity for severe internal carotid artery stenosis
  (70–99%)
Variability between machines in accuracy of measurement of carotid stenosis
Little information provided about proximal or distal arterial anatomy (although this is
  sometimes not relevant to the surgeon nor affected by disease)

between and even within the same observers at different times (Arnold *et al.* 1999).
Therefore, although unstable and ulcerated plaques are more likely to be symptomatic than
stable plaques with fibrous caps, the ultrasound inaccuracy compromises any study of the
relationship between plaque characteristics on duplex sonography and the risk of later
stroke, and so the selection for carotid surgery (Gronholdt 1999). In asymptomatic stenosis,
there is some evidence that a hypoechoic plaque predicts an increased risk of stroke
(Polak *et al.* 1998), but this was not confirmed in the Asymptomatic Carotid Surgery Trial
(Halliday *et al.* 2004). Until it becomes possible to translate carotid plaque irregularity as
seen on catheter angiography, which does add to the risk of stroke over and above the
degree of stenosis, into what is seen on duplex sonography, it will remain difficult to use
anything other than stenosis to predict stroke risk if only duplex is being used.

Despite these limitations, duplex sonography is a remarkably quick and simple investigation in experienced hands, and it is neither unpleasant nor risky. Very rarely, the pressure
of the Doppler probe on the carotid bifurcation can dislodge thrombus, or cause enough
carotid sinus stimulation to lead to bradycardia or hypotension (Rosario *et al.* 1987; Friedman
1990). The same conceivably applies to the various arterial compression maneuvers that
may be carried out during transcranial Doppler, and any such compression should be
avoided in patients who may have carotid bifurcation disease.

Computed tomography angiography and perfusion imaging

Computed tomography is now a widely used method for imaging the carotid arteries and
cerebral circulation (Brink *et al.* 1997, Bartlett *et al.* 2006). It is easier to perform in sick
patients than MRI and is not contraindicated in those with pacemakers, ferromagnetic
implants, mechanical heart valves and those with claustrophobia. However, it does require
a large dose of intravenous contrast to outline the arterial lumen; there is X-ray exposure;
the images obtained depend on the proficiency of the operator in their selection, and it
tends to underestimate vessel stenosis. Nevertheless, it does provide multiple viewing angles,
three-dimensional reconstruction (Fig. 12.4), and imaging of calcium deposits separately
from the vessel lumen outlined by the contrast (Heiken *et al.* 1993; Leclerc *et al.* 1995;
Nandalur *et al.* 2006).

Computed tomography perfusion studies can also be used to examine cerebral blood
flow (Wintermark and Bogousslavsky 2003) using existing CT technology. This technique
uses exogenous contrast and allows calculation of cerebral blood flow, cerebral blood
volume and mean transit time. However, quantification of cerebral blood flow is problematic,
and most studies use ratios comparing values with homologous areas of the contralateral

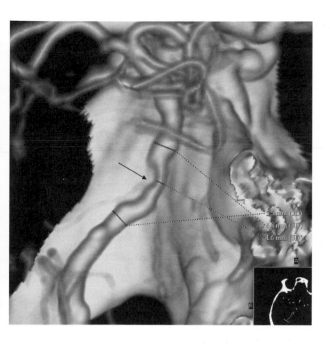

Fig. 12.4. A CT angiogram three-dimensional reconstruction showing a stenosis (arrow) of the distal vertebral artery. (See the color plate section.)

hemisphere, which itself may show a reduced cerebral blood flow in acute stroke, for example in diaschisis. In addition, current technology allows only limited brain coverage of two to four slices, which means that large areas of ischemia are imaged inadequately and small ones may be missed altogether. Nevertheless, there is evidence in acute stroke that perfusion CT values correlate with angiographic findings and can predict infarction and clinical outcome (Nabavi *et al.* 2002; Meuli 2004; Parsons *et al.* 2005; Wintermark *et al.* 2007). It is likely, therefore, that CT measurements of cerebral blood flow will become increasingly important in selecting patients for acute stroke therapy owing to the speed and relative ease of performing CT compared with MRI.

Magnetic resonance angiography and perfusion imaging

Magnetic resonance angiography is non-invasive and safe if done without contrast ("time of flight" imaging) (Fig. 12.5). Contrast-enhanced imaging provides improved resolution and reduces problems with flow voids at points of stenosis, and it is necessary for detecting cerebral aneurysms or determining the severity of carotid stenosis. However, even with contrast, MR angiography is unlikely to be accurate enough in estimating carotid stenosis, at least at the present stage of development (Graves 1997; Chappell *et al.* 2006; DeMarco *et al.* 2006). The pictures are not always adequate to allow measurement of the carotid stenosis (movement and swallowing artefacts are particular problems); the severity of the stenosis tends to be overestimated; there may be a flow gap distal to a stenosis of as little as 60%, making precise stenosis measurement impossible even in the posterior part of the carotid bulb, in both cases probably because of loss of laminar flow and increased residence times of the blood; irregularity/ulceration are not well seen; and severe stenosis can be confused with occlusion (Siewert *et al.* 1995; Levi *et al.* 1996; Fox *et al.* 2005). However, image quality and reproducibility of measurement of stenosis are significantly improved with contrast-enhanced MR angiography (DeMarco *et al.* 2006; Mitra *et al.* 2006). So far, there have not been enough methodologically sound comparisons of MR angiography with

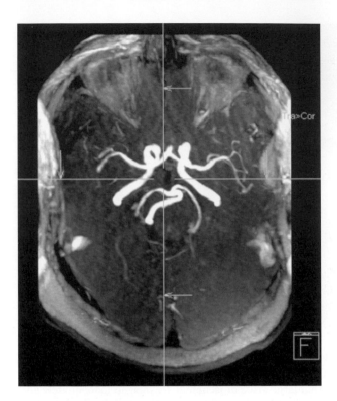

Fig. 12.5. A "time of flight" MR angiogram of the circle of Willis in a patient with no posterior communicating arteries.

catheter angiography (U-King-Im *et al.* 2005; Chappell *et al.* 2006). The comparative studies that have been carried out have frequently been overtaken by changes in MR technology.

Perfusion imaging can also be achieved with MRI using an injected contrast agent such as gadolinium or endogenous techniques. The latter have the advantage that they can be used for multiple repeat investigations, but at present the level of contrast produced is less that that obtained with exogenous agents. The MRI techniques can measure mean transit time, cerebral blood volume and cerebral blood flow. It has been proposed as a potential tool for use in clinical selection of patients for thrombolysis in acute stroke (Thijs *et al.* 2001; Fiehler *et al.* 2002; Shih *et al.* 2003), particularly in combination with diffusion weighted imaging (Kidwell and Hsia 2006; Muir *et al.* 2006), but there is still no consensus on the criteria for patient selection (Hand *et al.* 2006).

Imaging the posterior circulation

Vertebrobasilar TIAs were thought for many years to be associated with a lower risk of stroke than carotid territory TIAs, but recent work has shown that the risk of stroke is at least as high (Flossmann and Rothwell 2003; Flossmann *et al.* 2006). There is, therefore, an increasing interest in angioplasty and stenting of atherothrombotic stenoses of the vertebral or proximal basilar arteries. Angiography with MR or CT is the most useful non-invasive method of imaging the posterior circulation, although catheter angiography is often still necessary to confirm or exclude significant stenosis.

Although asymptomatic **subclavian steal** is quite common (reversed vertebral artery flow detected by ultrasound or vertebral angiography), *symptomatic* subclavian steal is rare, presumably because collateral blood flow to the brainstem is enough to compensate for the reversed vertebral artery blood flow distal to ipsilateral subclavian stenosis or occlusion. The clinical syndrome is quite easily recognized by unequal blood pressures between the two arms, a supraclavicular bruit and vertebrobasilar TIAs, which may or may not be brought on by exercise of the arm ipsilateral to the subclavian stenosis or occlusion, so increasing blood flow down the vertebral artery from the brainstem to the arm muscles (Bornstein and Norris 1986; Hennerici et al. 1988). It is only this type of symptomatic patient who may require surgery and, therefore, who has to accept the risk of any preceding angiography. **Innominate artery steal** is even rarer, with retrograde vertebral artery flow distal to innominate rather than subclavian artery occlusion (Kempczinski and Hermann 1979; Grosveld et al. 1988).

Transcranial Doppler sonography

Transcranial Doppler sonography provides information on the velocity of blood flow, and its direction in relation to the ultrasound probe, in the major intracranial arteries at the base of the brain, and so whether they are occluded or stenosed. It is non-invasive, safe, repeatable, not too difficult to perform accurately, can be performed at the bedside and is not expensive. However, the patient has to keep reasonably still; the examination can take as long as an hour; the skull is impervious to ultrasound in 5–10% of individuals, more with increasing age and in females, but less if intravenous echocontrast is used; exact vessel identification may be difficult, but color-flow real-time imaging makes this easier; spatial resolution is poor; diagnostic criteria vary; and the technique is not always accurate in comparison with cerebral catheter angiography (Baumgartner et al. 1997; Baumgartner 1999; Gerriets et al. 1999; Markus 1999).

Despite the fact that transcranial Doppler sonography, like positron emission tomography, has increased our knowledge of the cerebral circulation in health and disease, and even though it is inexpensive and quite widely available and repeatable on demand (unlike positron emission tomography), it still has rather a minor role in *routine* clinical management.

Possible indications for transcranial Doppler ultrasound in routine clinical practice (Babikian et al. 1997; Molloy and Markus 1999; Alexandrov et al. 2004; Kim et al. 2005; Dittrich et al. 2006; Markus 2006) include:

- operative monitoring during carotid endarterectomy
- diagnosis of patent foramen ovale and other right-to-left shunts
- identification of patients with carotid stenosis at high risk of stroke
- display of intracranial arterial occlusion and stenosis
- assessment of cerebrovascular reactivity
- acceleration of clot lysis during or after thrombolysis for acute ischemic stroke.

Detection of emboli as high-intensity transient signals on the sonogram, so-called microembolic signals, might be of clinical relevance in certain situations. The vast majority of such signals appear to be from asymptomatic emboli but their detection may help in distinguishing cardiac and aortic arch emboli from carotid emboli, because with the first two, emboli should be detected in several arterial distributions, whereas with the last in only the one arterial distribution distal to the supposed embolic source (Markus et al. 1994; Sliwka et al. 1997; Markus 2006). However, the frequency of microembolic signals can be so frustratingly low and variable and so their detection requires prolonged monitoring and automation (Markus 1999, 2006; Dittrich et al. 2006). Consequently, their detection is currently used mainly as a research tool, most usefully perhaps as a surrogate outcome in trials of secondary prevention of stroke (Dittrich *et al.* 2006; Markus 2006).

Transcranial Doppler sonography can also be used to assess cerebrovascular reactivity as indicated by the capacity for intracranial vasodilatation in response to acetazolamide, carbon dioxide inhalation or breath holding, although these three methods do not always produce concordant results (Bishop *et al.* 1986; Markus and Harrison 1992; Dahl *et al.* 1995; Derdeyn *et al.* 2005). However, there is still debate about exactly how to standardize this test and it is not widely used in routine clinical practice. Impaired reactivity may have some prognostic significance for identifying individual patients at particularly high risk of stroke from amongst those with carotid stenosis and internal carotid artery occlusion, although the numbers studied have been small and the situation is not yet clear-cut (Derdeyn *et al.* 1999, 2005; Vernieri *et al.* 2001). With time, and presumably increasing collateralization, any impairment of reactivity can return to normal (Kleiser and Widder 1992; Widder *et al.* 1994; Gur *et al.* 1996; Vernieri *et al.* 1999).

References

Alexandrov AV, Molina CA, Grotta JC *et al.* (2004). Ultrasound-enhanced systemic thrombolysis for acute ischemic stroke. *New England Journal of Medicine* **351**:2170–2178

Arnold JA, Modaresi KB, Thomas N *et al.* (1999). Carotid plaque characterization by duplex scanning: observer error may undermine current clinical trials. *Stroke* **30**:61–65

Babikian VL, Wijman CAC, Hyde C *et al.* (1997). Cerebral microembolism and early recurrent cerebral or retinal ischemic events. *Stroke* **28**:1314–1318

Bartlett ES, Symons SP, Fox AJ (2006). Correlation of carotid stenosis diameter and cross-sectional areas with CT angiography. *American Journal of Neuroradiology* **27**:638–642

Barth A, Arnold M, Mattle HPC *et al.* (2006). Contrast-enhanced 3-D MRA in decision making for carotid endarterectomy: a 6-year experience. *Cerebrovascular Diseases* **21**:393–400

Baumgartner RW (1999). Transcranial color-coded duplex sonography. *Journal of Neurology* **246**:637–647

Baumgartner RW, Mattle HP, Aaslid RC *et al.* (1997). Transcranial colour-coded duplex sonography in arterial cerebrovascular disease. *Cerebrovascular Diseases* **7**:57–63

Bishop CCR, Powell S, Insall MC *et al.* (1986). Effect of internal carotid artery occlusion on middle cerebral artery blood flow at rest and in response to hypercapnia. *Lancet* **i**:710–712

Blakeley DD, Oddone EZ, Hasselblad VC *et al.* (1995). Non-invasive carotid artery testing: a meta-analytic review. *Annals of Internal Medicine* **122**:360–367

Bornstein NM, Norris JW (1986). Subclavian steal: a harmless haemodynamic phenomenon? *Lancet* **ii**:303–305

Brink JA, McFarland EG, Heiken JP (1997). Helical/spiral computed body tomography. *Clinical Radiology* **52**:489–503

Chappell ET, Moure FC, Good MC (2003). Comparison of computed tomographic angiography with digital subtraction angiography in the diagnosis of cerebral aneurysms: a meta-analysis. *Neurosurgery* **52**:624–631

Chappell F, Wardlaw J, Best JKK *et al.* (2006). Non-invasive imaging compared with intra-arterial angiography in the diagnosis of symptomatic carotid stenosis: a meta-analysis. *Lancet* **376**:1503–1512

Cuffe R, Rothwell PM (2006). Effect of non-optimal imaging on the relationship between the measured degree of symptomatic carotid stenosis and risk of ischemic stroke. *Stroke* **37**:1785–1791

Dahl A, Russell D, Rootwelt KC *et al.* (1995). Cerebral vasoreactivity assessed with transcranial Doppler and regional cerebral blood flow measurements: dose serum concentration and time course of the response to acetazolamide. *Stroke* **26**:2302–2306

DeMarco JK, Huston J III, Nash AK (2006). Extracranial carotid MR imaging at 3T.

Magnetic Resonance Imaging Clinics of North America **14**:109–1021

Derdeyn CP, Grubb RL, Powers WJ (1999). Cerebral haemodynamic impairment: methods of measurements and association with stroke risk. *Neurology* **53**:251–259

Derdeyn CP, Grubb RL Jr., Powers WJ (2005). Indications for cerebral revascularization for patients with atherosclerotic carotid occlusion. *Skull Base* **15**:7–14

Dittrich R, Ritter MA, Kaps MC *et al.* (2006). The use of embolic signal detection in multicenter trials to evaluate antiplatelet efficacy: signal analysis and quality control mechanisms in the CARESS (Clopidogrel and Aspirin for Reduction of Emboli in Symptomatic carotid Stenosis) trial. *Stroke* **37**:1065–1069

Droste DW, Jurgens R, Nabavi DGC *et al.* (1999). Echocontrast-enhanced ultrasound of extracranial internal carotid artery high-grade stenosis and occlusion. *Stroke* **30**:2302–2306

Eliasziw M, Streifler JY, Fox AJC for the North American Symptomatic Carotid Endarterectomy Trial (1994). Significance of plaque ulceration in symptomatic patients with high-grade carotid stenosis. *Stroke* **25**:304–308

Fiehler J, von Bezold M, Kucinski T *et al.* (2002). Cerebral blood flow predicts lesion growth in acute stroke patients. *Stroke* **33**:2421–2425

Flossmann E, Rothwell PM (2003). Prognosis of verterobrobasilar transient ischemic attack and minor ischemic stroke. *Brain* **126**:1940–1954

Flossmann E, Redgrave JN, Schulz UGC *et al.* (2006). Reliability of clinical diagnosis of the symptomatic vascular territory in patients with recent TIA or minor stroke. *Cerebrovascular Diseases* **21**(Suppl 4):18

Fox AJ, Eliasziw M, Rothwell PMC *et al.* (2005). Identification prognosis and management of patients with carotid artery near occlusion. *American Journal of Neuroradiology* **26**:2086–2094

Friedman SG (1990). Transient ischemic attacks resulting from carotid duplex imaging. *Surgery* **107**:153–155

Gaitini D, Soudack M (2005). Diagnosing carotid stenosis by Doppler sonography: state of the art. *Journal of Ultrasound Medicine* **24**:1127–1136

Gerraty RP, Bowser DN, Infeld BC *et al.* (1996). Microemboli during carotid angiography: association with stroke risk factors or subsequent magnetic resonance imaging changes? *Stroke* **27**:1543–1547

Gerriets T, Seidel G, Fiss IC *et al.* (1999). Contrast-enhanced transcranial colour-coded duplex sonography: efficiency and validity. *Neurology* **52**:1133–1137

Graves MJ (1997). Magnetic resonance angiography *British Journal of Radiology* **70**:6–28

Gronholdt MLM (1999). Ultrasound and lipoproteins as predictors of lipid-rich rupture-prone plaques in the carotid artery. *Arteriosclerosis Thrombosis and Vascular Biology* **19**:2–13

Grosveld WJ, Lawson JA, Eikelboom BCC *et al.* (1988). Clinical and haemodynamic significance of innominate artery lesions evaluated by ultrasonography and digital angiography. *Stroke* **19**:958–962

Gur AY, Bova I, Bornstein NM (1996). Is impaired cerebral vasomotor reactivity a predictive factor of stroke in asymptomatic patients? *Stroke* **27**:2188–2190

Halliday A, Mansfield A, Marro JC for the MRC Asymptomatic Carotid Surgery Trial (ACST) Collaborative Group (2004). Prevention of disabling and fatal strokes by successful carotid endarterectomy in patients without recent neurological symptoms: randomised controlled trial *Lancet* **363**:1491–1502

Hand PJ, Wardlaw JM, Rivers CS *et al.* (2006). MR diffusion-weighted imaging and outcome prediction after ischemic stroke. *Neurology* **66**:1159–1163

Hankey GJ, Warlow CP (1990). Symptomatic carotid ischemic events: safest and most cost effective way of selecting patients for angiography before carotid endarterectomy. *British Medical Journal* **300**:1485–1491

Hankey GJ, Warlow CP (1991). Lacunar transient ischemic attacks: a clinically useful concept? *Lancet* **337**:335–338

Hankey GJ, Slattery JM, Warlow CP (1991). The prognosis of hospital-referred transient ischemic attacks. *Journal of Neurology, Neurosurgery and Psychiatry* **54**:793–802

Heiken JP, Brink JA, Vannier MW (1993). Spiral (helical) CT. *Radiology* **189**:647–656

Hennerici M, Klemm C, Rautenberg W (1988). The subclavian steal phenomenon: a common vascular disorder with rare neurologic deficits. *Neurology* **38**:669–673

Jeans WD, Mackenzie S, Baird RN (1986). Angiography in transient cerebral ischemia using three views of the carotid bifurcation. *British Journal of Radiology* **59**:135–142

Johnston DC, Goldstein LB (2001). Clinical carotid endarterectomy decision making: noninvasive vascular imaging versus angiography. *Neurology* **56**:1009–1015

Johnston DC, Chapman KM, Goldstein LB (2001). Low rate of complications of cerebral angiography in routine clinical practice. *Neurology* **57**:2012–2014

Johnston DC, Eastwood JD, Nguyen TC *et al.* (2002). Contrast-enhanced magnetic resonance angiography of carotid arteries: utility in routine clinical practice. *Stroke* **33**:2834–2838

Kempczinski R, Hermann G (1979). The innominate steal syndrome. *Journal of Cardiovascular Surgery* **20**:481–486

Kidwell CS, Hsia AW (2006). Imaging of the brain and cerebral vasculature in patients with suspected stroke: advantages and disadvantages of CT and MRI. *Current Neurology and Neuroscience Reports* **6**:9–16

Kim YS, Garami Z, Mikulik RC for the CLOTBUST Collaborators (2005). Early recanalization rates and clinical outcomes in patients with tandem internal carotid artery/middle cerebral artery occlusion and isolated middle cerebral artery occlusion. *Stroke* **36**:869–871

Kleiser B, Widder B (1992). Course of carotid artery occlusions with impaired cerebrovascular reactivity. *Stroke* **23**:171–174

Leclerc X, Godefroy O, Pruvo JPC *et al.* (1995). Computed tomographic angiography for the evaluation of carotid artery stenosis. *Stroke* **26**:1577–1581

Levi CR, Mitchell A, Fitt GC *et al.* (1996). The accuracy of magnetic resonance angiography in the assessment of extracranial carotid artery occlusive disease. *Cerebrovascular Diseases* **6**:231–236

Lovett JK, Gallagher PJ, Hands LJC *et al.* (2004). Histological correlates of carotid plaque surface morphology on lumen contrast imaging. *Circulation* **110**:2190–2197

Markus HS (1999). Transcranial Doppler ultrasound. *Journal of Neurology, Neurosurgery and Psychiatry* **67**:135–137

Markus HS (2006). Can microemboli on transcranial Doppler identify patients at increased stroke risk? *Nature Clinical Practice in Cardiovascular Medicine* **3**:246–247

Markus HS, Harrison MJG (1992). Estimation of cerebrovascular reactivity using transcranial Doppler, including the use of breath-holding as the vasodilatory stimulus. *Stroke* **23**:668–673

Markus HS, Droste DW, Brown MM (1994). Detection of asymptomatic cerebral embolic signals with Doppler ultrasound. *Lancet* **343**:1011–1012

Martin R, Bogousslavsky J, Miklossy J *et al.* (1992). Floating thrombus in the innominate artery as a cause of cerebral infarction in young adults. *Cerebrovascular Diseases* **2**:177–181

Mead GE, Wardlaw JM, Lewis SCC *et al.* (1999). Can simple clinical features be used to identify patients with severe carotid stenosis on Doppler ultrasound? *Journal of Neurology, Neurosurgery and Psychiatry* **66**:16–19

Meuli RA (2004). Imaging viable brain tissue with CT scan during acute stroke. *Cerebrovascular Diseases* **17**:28–34

Mitra D, Connolly D, Jenkins SC *et al.* (2006). Comparison of image quality, diagnostic confidence and interobserver variability in contrast enhanced MR angiography and 2D time of flight angiography, in evaluation of carotid stenosis. *British Journal of Radiology* **79**:201–207

Molloy J, Markus HS (1999). Asymptomatic embolization predicts stroke and TIA risk in patients with carotid artery stenosis. *Stroke* **30**:1440–1443

Muir KW, Buchan A, von Kummer R *et al.* (2006). Imaging of acute stroke. *Lancet Neurology* **5**:755–768

Nabavi DG, Kloska SP, Nam EM *et al.* (2002). MOSAIC: multimodal stroke assessment using computed tomography: novel diagnostic approach for the prediction of infarction size and clinical outcome. *Stroke* **33**:2819–2826

Nandalur KR, Baskurt E, Hagspiel KDC *et al.* (2006). Carotid artery calcification on CT may independently predict stroke risk. *American Journal of Radiology* **186**:547–552

Norris JW, Halliday A (2004). Is ultrasound sufficient for vascular imaging prior to carotid endarterectomy? *Stroke* **35**:370–371

Norris JW, Morriello F, Rowed DW *et al.* (2003). Vascular imaging before carotid endarterectomy. *Stroke* **34**:e16

Parsons MW, Pepper EM, Chan V *et al.* (2005). Perfusion computed tomography: prediction of final infarct extent and stroke outcome. *Annals of Neurology* **58**:672–679

Pelz DM, Fox AJ, Vinuela F (1985). Digital subtraction angiography: current clinical applications. *Stroke* **16**:528–536

Polak JF, Shemanski L, O'Leary DH for the Cardiovascular Health Study (1998). Hypoechoic plaque at US of the carotid artery: an independent risk factor for incident stroke in adults aged 65 years or older. *Radiology* **208**:649–654

Rosario JA, Hachinski VA, Lee DH *et al.* (1987). Adverse reactions to duplex scanning. *Lancet* **ii**:1023

Rothwell PM, Gibson RJ, Villagra RC *et al.* (1998). The effect of angiographic technique and image quality on the reproducibility of measurement of carotid stenosis and assessment of plaque surface morphology. *Clinical Radiology* **53**:439–443

Rothwell PM, Pendlebury ST, Wardlaw J *et al.* (2000a). Critical appraisal of the design and reporting of studies of the imaging and measurement of carotid stenosis. *Stroke* **31**:1444–1450

Rothwell PM, Gibson R, Warlow CP on behalf of the European Carotid Surgery Trialists' Collaborative Group (2000b). Interrelation between plaque surface morphology and degree of stenosis on carotid angiograms and the risk of ischemic stroke in patients with symptomatic carotid stenosis. *Stroke* **31**:615–621

Shih LC, Saver JL, Alger JR *et al.* (2003). Perfusion-weighted magnetic resonance imaging thresholds identifying core, irreversibly infarcted tissue. *Stroke* **34**:1425–1430

Siewert B, Patel MR, Warach S (1995). Magnetic resonance angiography. *Neurologist* **1**:167–184

Sliwka U, Lingnau A, Stohlmann WD *et al.* (1997). Prevalence and time course of microembolic signals in patients with acute stroke: a prospective study. *Stroke* **28**:358–363

Streifler JY, Eliaziw M, Fox AJ, for the North American Symptomatic Carotid Endarterectomy Trial (1994). Angiographic detection of carotid plaque ulceration: comparison with surgical observations in a multicentre study. *Stroke* **25**:1130–1132

Thijs VN, Adami A, Neumann-Haefelin T *et al.* (2001). Relationship between severity of MR perfusion deficit and DWI lesion evolution. *Neurology* **57**:1205–1211

U-King-Im JM, Hollingworth W, Trivedi RAC *et al.* (2005). Cost-effectiveness of diagnostic strategies prior to carotid endarterectomy. *Annals of Neurology* **58**:506–515

Vernieri F, Pasqualetti P, Passarelli FC *et al.* (1999). Outcome of carotid artery occlusion is predicted by cerebrovascular reactivity. *Stroke* **30**:593–598

Vernieri F, Pasqualetti P, Matteis MC *et al.* (2001). Effect of collateral blood flow and cerebral vasomotor reactivity on the outcome of carotid artery occlusion. *Stroke* **32**:1552–1558

Villablanca JP, Hooshi P, Martin N *et al.* (2002). Three-dimensional helical computerized tomography angiography in the diagnosis characterization and management of middle cerebral artery aneurysms: comparison with conventional angiography and intraoperative findings. *Journal of Neurosurgery* **97**:1322–1332

Wardlaw JM, Lewis S (2005). Carotid stenosis measurement on colour Doppler ultrasound: agreement of ECST NASCET and CCA methods applied to ultrasound with intra-arterial angiographic stenosis measurement. *European Journal of Radiology* **56**:205–211

Warnock NG, Gandhi MR, Bergvall UC *et al.* (1993). Complications of intra-arterial digital subtraction angiography in patients investigated for cerebral vascular disease. *British Journal of Radiology* **66**:855–858

Widder B, Kleiser B, Krapf H (1994). Course of cerebrovascular reactivity in patients with carotid artery occlusions. *Stroke* **25**:1963–1967

Wintermark M, Uske A, Chalaron M *et al.* (2003). Multislice computerized tomography angiography in the evaluation of intracranial aneurysms: a comparison with intraarterial digital subtraction angiography. *Journal of Neurosurgery* **98**:828–836

Wintermark M, Bogousslavsky J (2003). Imaging of acute ischemic brain injury: the return of computed tomography. *Current Opinions in Neurology* **16**:59–63

Wintermark M, Meuli R, Browaeys P *et al.* (2007). Comparison of CT perfusion and angiography and MRI in selecting stroke patients for acute treatment. *Neurology* **68**:694–697

Zhu XL, Chan MSY, Poon WS (1997). Spontaneous intracranial hemorrhage: which patients need diagnostic cerebral angiography? A prospective study of 206 cases and review of the literature. *Stroke* **28**:1406–1409

13

Non-radiological investigations for transient ischemic attack and stroke

The clinical syndrome – total anterior circulation stroke, partial anterior circulation stroke, lacunar infarction or posterior circulation stroke – gives an indication as to the site and size of the lesion, which, together with brain imaging findings, often gives clues as to the likely underlying cause, for example large vessel disease versus small vessel disease (Chs. 6 and 9). Although brain imaging is of paramount importance in TIA and stroke (Chs. 10–12), non-radiological investigations may help to identify the cause of the cerebrovascular event, eliminate stroke and TIA mimics and enable appropriate secondary preventive therapy. Investigations are likely to be more extensive in patients without evidence of vascular disease or embolism from the heart, in whom there may be a rare underlying cause for the stroke.

First-line investigations

In general, all patients with a TIA or stroke should have basic blood and urine tests at presentation (Table 13.1). Patients with hemorrhagic stroke should have a clotting screen, particularly if they are already taking anticoagulation medication. The likelihood of finding a relevant abnormality may be low for some tests, such as full blood count and erythrocyte sedimentation rate, but such straightforward tests may reveal a serious treatable disorder, such as giant cell arteritis. Many patients are hypercholesterolemic, although immediately after stroke, but probably not TIA, there is a transient fall in plasma cholesterol, which will lead to underestimation of the usual level (Mendez et al. 1987; Woo et al. 1990).

Second-line investigations

Second-line investigations (Table 13.2) must be targeted appropriately since the likelihood of a relevant result depends on the selection of patients and further investigation will incur more cost. There are numerous rare causes of stroke (Ch. 6) for which highly specialized tests may be required.

Routine lumbar puncture is not indicated after stroke and may be dangerous in the presence of a large intracerebral hematoma, or edematous infarct causing brain shift. Examination of the cerebrospinal fluid may be necessary in diagnostic uncertainty where there is a possibility of encephalitis or multiple sclerosis or if the stroke is thought to have been caused by infective endocarditis or by chronic meningitis in syphilis or tuberculosis. The cerebrospinal fluid after stroke is usually acellular, but there may be up to 100×10^6 cells/l. Levels above this suggest septic emboli to the brain (Powers 1986). Lumbar puncture is mandatory in sudden-onset headache with negative CT brain scan, to exclude subarachnoid hemorrhage (Ch. 30).

Routine electroencephalography is not indicated in stroke but may be helpful where there is a possibility of encephalitis or generalized encephalopathy, or focal seizure activity.

Table 13.1. Baseline non-imaging tests for transient ischemic attack and stroke

Investigation	Disorders detected
Full blood count	Anemia
	Polycythemia
	Leukemia
	Thrombocythemia/thrombocytopenia
Erythrocyte sedimentation rate/C-reactive protein	Vasculitis
	Infective endocarditis
	Hyperviscosity
	Myxoma
Electrolytes	Hyponatremia
	Hypokalemia
Urea	Renal impairment
Plasma glucose	Diabetes
	Hypoglycemia
Plasma lipids	Hyperlipidemia
Urine analysis	Diabetes
	Renal disease
	Vasculitis

It should be noted that there may be transient focal weakness after a seizure "Todd's paresis" (Ch. 8).

Temporal artery biopsy may be required in suspected temporal arteritis (Ch. 6).

Cardiac investigations

Given the high prevalence of cardiovascular disease in patients with cerebrovascular disease (about one-third have angina or have had a myocardial infarction) (Ch. 6), there is a strong likelihood of electrocardiography (ECG) abnormalities in patients presenting with TIA and stroke. The ECG may show evidence of coronary vascular disease, previous or current myocardial infarction, or disorders of rhythm, including atrial fibrillation. It should be noted that stroke can itself cause ECG changes, in approximately 15–20% of patients, ranging from left-axis deviation to a variety of repolarization abnormalities including QT prolongation, septal U waves and ST segment changes. The ECG changes are thought to be neurally mediated and not a result of coexisting coronary artery disease. The insular cortex may be a possible cortical site of generation of some of these changes. Patients with left insular stroke may be prone to ECG changes and an increase in cardiac sympathetic nervous activity (assessed by spectral analysis) (Oppenheimer *et al.* 1996). Such changes may contribute to the excess cardiac mortality in stroke patients.

Many patients will require cardiac investigation beyond ECG (Table 13.3) although the likelihood of finding a cardiac abnormality on routine transthoracic echocardiography in patients without prior known cardiac abnormality is low (Table 13.4) (Beattie *et al.* 1998). Patients with a suspected cardiac source of embolism should certainly have transthoracic

Table 13.2. Second-line investigations for selected with transient ischemic attack (TIA) or stroke patients

Investigation	Comments
Blood	
Liver function	Fever, malaise, raised ESR, suspected malignancy, temporal arteritis
Calcium	Recurrent focal neurological symptoms are occasionally caused by hypercalcemia
Thyroid function tests	Atrial fibrillation
Body red cell mass	Raised hematocrit
Activated partial thromboplastin time, anticardiolipin antibody,[a] antinuclear and other autoantibodies	Young (<50 years) and no other cause found; past history or family history of venous thrombosis, especially if unusual site (cerebral, mesenteric, hepatic veins); recurrent miscarriage; thrombocytopenia; cardiac valve vegetations; livedo reticularis; raised ESR; malaise; positive syphilis serology
Serum proteins, serum protein electrophoresis, plasma viscosity	Myeloma
Hemoglobin electrophoresis	Hemoglobinopathies, e.g. sickle cell anemia
Protein C and S, antithrombin III, activated protein C resistance, thrombin time[b]	Thrombophilia: personal or family history of thrombosis (usually venous, particularly in unusual sites such as hepatic vein) at unusually young age
Blood cultures	Infective endocarditis: fever, cardiac murmur, hematuria, deranged liver function, raised ESR, malaise
HIV serology	Unexplained stroke in the young, drug addiction, homosexuality, blood product transfusion, lymphadenopathy, pneumonia, cytomegalovirus retinitis
Lipoprotein fractionation	Elevated cholesterol or strong family history, hyperlipoproteinemia
Serum homocysteine	Marfanoid habitus, high myopia, dislocated lenses, osteoporosis, mental retardation
Leukocyte α-galactosidase A	Corneal opacities, cutaneous angiokeratomas, paresthesias and pain, renal failure
Blood/cerebrospinal fluid lactate	MELAS/mitochondiral cytopathy: young patient, basal ganglia calcification, epilepsy, parieto-occipital ischemia
Syphilis serology	Young patient, high risk of sexually transmitted disease
Cardiac enzymes	History or ECG evidence of recent electrocardiographic myocardial infarction
Drug screen	Cocaine/amphetamine/Ecstasy: young patient, no other obvious cause
Urine	
Amino acids	Marfanoid habitus, high myopia, dislocated lenses, osteoporosis, mental retardation
Drug screen	Young patient, no other obvious cause, cocaine/amphetamine, etc.

Table 13.2. (*cont.*)

Investigation	Comments
Others	
Electroencephalography	Doubt about diagnosis of TIA or stroke: ?epilepsy
Temporal artery biopsy	Age >60 years, jaw claudication, headache, polymyalgia, malaise, anemia, raised ESR[a]

Notes:
ESR, erythrocyte sedimentation rate.
[a]Repeat to ensure persistently raised.
[b]Transient falls occur after stroke so any low level must be repeated and family members investigated.

Table 13.3. Cardiac investigations in stroke

Investigation	Comments
ECG	Left ventricular hypertrophy
	Arrhythmia
	Conduction block
	Myocardial infarction
Chest X-ray	Hypertension, finger clubbing, cardiac murmur or abnormal ECG, ill patient
Echocardiography (transthoracic)	Possible cardiac source of embolism, or clinical, ECG, transesophageal evidence of embologenic heart ultrasound or radiographic disease, aortic arch dissection
24-hour ECG	Palpitations or blackout during a suspected TIA, suspicious resting ECG

Notes:
ECG, electrocardiography; TIA, transient ischemic attack.

Table 13.4. Pooled prevalence of various cardiac abnormalities on transthoracic echocardiography in patients with ischemic stroke without prior known cardiac disease

Abnormality	Pooled prevalence (%)	
	<45 years	>45 years
Myxoma	0.7	0.1
Vegetations	1	1
Mitral stenosis	2	2
Left atrial thrombus	0.5	0.3
Left ventricular thrombus/cardiomyopathy	3	10

Source: From Beattie *et al.* (1998).

echocardiography and or transesophageal examination (Table 13.5). Specific echocardiographic techniques may be required where there is the possibility of patent foramen ovale (Table 13.5; Ch. 6). Prolonged ECG recording using ambulatory machines is required where there is suspected dysrhythmia such as paroxysmal atrial fibrillation.

Table 13.5. Comparison of transthoracic and transesophageal echocardiography for detecting potential cardiac sources of embolism

Transthoracic preferred	Transesophageal preferred
Left ventricular thrombus	Left atrial thrombus
Left ventricular dyskinesis	Left atrial appendage thrombus
Mitral stenosis	Spontaneous echo contrast
Mitral annulus calcification	Intracardiac tumors
Aortic stenosis	Atrial septal defect[a]
	Atrial septal aneurysm
	Patent foramen ovale[a]
	Mitral and aortic valve vegetations
	Prosthetic heart valve malfunction
	Aortic arch atherothrombosis/dissection
	Mitral valve prolapse

Notes:
[a]A less-invasive alternative is to inject air bubbles or other echocontrast material intravenously; if there is a patent foramen ovale, they can be detected by transcranial Doppler sonography of the middle cerebral artery, particularly with a provocative Valsalva maneuver. There is considerable variation in the methods used to detect patent foramen ovale and this influences the diagnostic sensitivity and specificity. It is also uncertain what size of shunt is "clinically relevant" and some bubbles may pass to the brain through pulmonary rather than cardiac shunts (Droste *et al.* 1999, 2002; Schwarze *et al.* 1999).

References

Beattie JR, Cohen DJ, Manning WJ, Douglas PS (1998). Role of routine transthoracic echocardiography in evaluation and management of stroke. *Journal of Internal Medicine* **243**:281–291

Droste DW, Kriete JU, Stypmann J *et al.* (1999). Contrast transcranial Doppler ultrasound in the detection of right-to-left shunts: comparison of different procedures and different procedures and different contrast agents. *Stroke* **30**:1827–1832

Droste DW, Lakemeier S, Wichter T *et al.* (2002). Optimizing the technique of contrast transcranial Doppler ultrasound in the detection of right-to-left shunts. *Stroke* **33**:2211–2216

Mendez I, Hachinski V, Wolfe B (1987). Serum lipids after stroke. *Neurology* **37**:507–511

Oppenheimer SM (1994). Neurogenic cardiac effects of cerebrovascular disease. *Current Opinions in Neurology* **7**:20–24

Oppenheimer SM, Martin WM, Kedem G (1996). Left insular cortex lesions perturb cardiac autonomic tone. *Clinical Autonomic Research* **6**:131–140

Powers WJ (1986). Should lumbar puncture be part of the routine evaluation of patients with cerebral ischemia? *Stroke* **17**:332–333

Schwarze JJ, Sander D, Kukla C *et al.* (1999). Methodological parameters influence the detection of right-to-left shunts by contrast transcranial Doppler ultrasonography. *Stroke* **30**:1234–1239

Woo J, Lam CWK, Kay R *et al.* (1990). Acute and long term changes in serum lipids after acute stroke. *Stroke* **21**:1407–1411

Prognosis of transient ischemic attack and stroke
Methods of determining prognosis

Why study prognosis?

Once a diagnosis has been made, the issue of prognosis is as important to patients as treatment. There are many examples in neurology of the usefulness of simple prognostic studies of groups of patients, such as the demonstrations of the relatively benign long-term outcome after transient global amnesia (Hodges and Warlow 1990a, b), after cryptogenic drop-attacks in middle-aged women (Stevens and Matthews 1973), and the more recent data on the risks of major congenital malformations when taking various antiepileptic drugs in pregnancy (Morrow *et al.* 2006). Prognostic studies not only provide patients with useful information on the average risk of a poor outcome but also provide data that can be used to inform decisions for individuals about treatment by allowing an estimation of the likely absolute risk reduction (ARR) of a poor outcome with treatment, derived from the relative risk reduction provided by clinical trials. The ARR indicates what the chance of benefit from treatment is (e.g. an ARR of 25% – from 50% to 25% – tells us that one in four patients has to be treated for one to avoid a poor outcome, or put in another way there is a 1 in 4 chance of benefit for the individual treated patient). In contrast, a relative risk reduction gives no information about the likelihood of benefit. For example, the relative reductions in the risk of stroke in the Swedish Trial in Old Patients with Hypertension (STOP-hypertension) (Dahlof *et al.* 1991) and MRC (Medical Research Council Working Party 1985) trials of blood pressure lowering in primary prevention were virtually identical (47% versus 45%). However, there was a 12-fold difference in the ARR and so probability of benefit for individual patients. All other things being equal, 166 of the young hypertensives in the MRC trial would have to be treated for five years to prevent one stroke, compared with 14 of the elderly hypertensives in STOP-hypertension. Therefore, without an understanding of prognosis (i.e. absolute risk of a poor outcome), the likelihood that a treatment is worth having is impossible to judge (unless of course it is to relieve a symptom such as pain).

Why predict an individual's prognosis?

Patients and their doctors are understandably keen to go further than simply defining average or overall prognosis. They want to understand how a combination of particular factors might determine prognosis for the individual concerned: "How do *my* particular characteristics influence the likely outcome, doctor?"

Where possible, treatments should always be targeted at those individuals who are likely to benefit and be avoided in those with little chance of benefit, or in whom the risks of complications are too great compared with the expected benefit. A targeted approach based on risk is most useful for treatments with modest benefits (e.g. lipid lowering in primary prevention of vascular disease), for costly treatments with moderate overall benefits

Table 14.1. Prerequisites for the clinical credibility of a prognostic model

	Prerequisites
Use of relevant data	All clinically relevant patient data should have been tested for inclusion in the model. Many models are developed in retrospective studies using those variables that happen to have been collected already for other reasons. Thus, potentially valuable variables may be omitted if data for them are unavailable
Simplicity of data collection	It should be simple for doctors to obtain all of the patient data required in the model reliably and without expending undue resources in time to generate the prediction and so guide decisions. Data should be obtainable with high reliability, particularly in those patients for which the model's prediction are most likely to be needed
Avoidance of arbitrary thresholds	Model builders should avoid arbitrary thresholds for continuous variables because categorization discards potentially useful information
Derivation	The statistical modeling method must be correctly applied. Black box models, such as artificial neural networks, are less suitable for clinical applications
Simplicity of use	It should be simple and intuitive for doctors to calculate the model's prediction for a patient. The model's structure should be apparent and its predictions should make sense to the doctors who will rely on it. This will increase the likelihood of uptake of a model in routine practice

Sources: From Wyatt and Altman 1995; Altman and Royston 2000.

(e.g. beta-interferon in multiple sclerosis), if the availability of treatment is limited (e.g. organ transplantation), in developing countries with limited healthcare budgets and, most importantly, for treatments that although of overall benefit are associated with a significant risk of harm (such as carotid endarterectomy or anticoagulation).

However, without formal risk models, clinicians are often inaccurate in assessment of risk in their patients (Grover *et al.* 1995). Moreover, the absolute risk of a poor outcome for patients with multiple specific characteristics cannot simply be derived arithmetically from data on the effect of each individual characteristic such as age or severity of illness: that is, one cannot simply multiply risk ratios for these characteristics together as if they were independent. Even if one could, it would still be rather complicated. In a patient with symptomatic carotid stenosis, for example, what would the risk of stroke without endarterectomy be in a 78-year-old (high risk) female (lower risk) with 80% stenosis who presented within two days (high risk) of an ocular ischemic event (low risk) and was found to have an ulcerated carotid plaque (high risk)?

Models that combine prognostic variables to predict risk are, therefore, essential if we want reliable prognostication at the individual level.

What is a prognostic model?

A prognostic model is the mathematical combination of two or more patient or disease characteristics to predict outcome. Confusingly, prognostic models are also termed prognostic indexes, risk scores, probability models, risk stratification schemes or clinical prediction rules (Reilly and Evans 2006). To be useful, they must be shown to predict clinically relevant outcomes reliably. They must, therefore, be derived from a representative cohort in which outcome has been measured accurately. Next, they must be validated, not just in the data from which they were derived (internal validation) but also on data from independent cohorts (external validation) (Wyatt and Altman 1995; Justice *et al.* 1999; Altman and Royston 2000). Lastly, a model must be simple to use and have clinical credibility, otherwise it is unlikely to be taken up in routine clinical practice (Table 14.1).

A model for prediction of stroke on medical treatment in patients with recently symptomatic carotid stenosis is shown in Table 14.2 (Rothwell *et al.* 2005). The numeric weights for each variable are coefficients from a fitted regression model (Lewis 2007) and the model can be simplified to produce a simple risk score. Examples of other models are also given showing prediction of stroke in patients with non-valvular atrial fibrillation (the CHADS2 scheme; Box 14.1; Gage *et al.* 2004; Hart 2007), prediction of recurrence after a single seizure or in early epilepsy (Kim *et al.* 2007; Box 14.2) and the prediction of outcome in the Guillain–Barré syndrome (van Koningsveld *et al.* 2007; Box 14.3). Further examples of prognostic models are given elsewhere in the book, including the ABCD tool (Ch. 15).

The best evidence of the impact of using prognostic models comes from stratification of the results of randomized trials by predicted baseline risk, and the usefulness of this approach in targeting treatment has been demonstrated particularly well in patients with vascular disease. Predictable qualitative heterogeneity of relative treatment effect (i.e. benefit in some patients and harm in others) in relation to baseline risk has been demonstrated for anticoagulation therapy in primary prevention of stroke in patients with non-valvular atrial fibrillation (Laupacis *et al.* 1994), carotid endarterectomy for symptomatic stenosis (Rothwell *et al.* 2005), coronary artery bypass grafting (Yusuf *et al.* 1994), and anti-arrhythmic drugs following myocardial infarction (Boissel *et al.* 1993). Clinically important heterogeneity has also been demonstrated for blood pressure lowering (Li *et al.* 1998), aspirin (Sanmuganathan *et al.* 2001), lipid lowering in primary prevention of vascular disease (West of Scotland Coronary Prevention Group 1996), and in many other areas of medicine and surgery (Pagliaro *et al.* 1992; International Study of Unruptured Intracranial Aneurysms Investigators 1998).

How to measure prognosis

In order to develop a prognostic model, prognosis itself must first be measured reliably, although there is limited consensus on the ideal methodology required to achieve this. As there is little evidence to support the importance of features of study method that might affect the reliability of findings, particularly the avoidance of bias, researchers have tended to devise their own criteria or to ignore the issue altogether. As a result, many prognostic studies have been found to be of poor quality in both TIA and stroke (Kernan *et al.* 1991) and other fields of medicine (Altman 2001; Hayden *et al.* 2006). Despite the lack of accepted criteria, both theoretical considerations and common sense point towards the importance of various aspects of study method that would be required for the reliable measurement of prognosis (Sackett and Whelan 1980; Kernan *et al.* 1991; Altman 2001) (Table 14.3).

In the case of TIA and stroke, the diagnostic criteria used and by whom the diagnosis was made must be adequately described, especially because the definition of TIA has changed over time (Ch. 1) and diagnostic sensitivity may vary between individuals and groups of clinicians, for example between neurologists and emergency department physicians. Methods of ascertainment of cases from the study population should be described as should all demographic and clinical characteristics of the cohort; where relevant, this includes the methods of measurement themselves. Adequate description of the derivation cohort allows an assessment of how representative it is of the population in which the prognostic tool is intended for use. Only patients at a similar point in the course of the condition should be included, a point that has previously been taken to be the time of diagnosis, referral to secondary care or initiation of treatment. However, ideally, this point should be as early as possible into the condition ("inception cohort") and this is the reason

Table 14.2. A Cox model for the five-year risk of ipsilateral ischemic stroke on medical treatment in patients with recently symptomatic carotid stenosis[a]

Model			Scoring system		
Risk factor	Hazard ratio (95% CI)	p value	Risk factor	Score	Example
Stenosis (per 10%)	1.18 (1.10–1.25)	< 0.0001	Stenosis (%)		
			50–59	2.4	2.4
			60–69	2.8	
			70–79	3.3	
			80–89	3.9	
			90–99	4.6	
Near occlusion	0.49 (0.19–1.24)	0.1309	Near occlusion	0.5	No
Male sex	1.19 (0.81–1.75)	0.3687	Male sex	1.2	No
Age (per 10 years)	1.12 (0.89–1.39)	0.3343	Age (years)		
			31–40	1.1	
			41–50	1.2	
			51–60	1.3	
			61–70	1.5	1.5
			71–80	1.6	
			81–90	1.8	
Time since last event (per 7 days)	0.96 (0.93–0.99)	0.0039	Time since last event (days)		
			0–13	8.7	8.7
			14–28	8.0	
			29–89	6.3	
			90–365	2.3	
Presenting event		0.0067	Presenting event		
Ocular	1.000		Ocular	1.0	
Single TIA	1.41 (0.75–2.66)		Single TIA	1.4	
Multiple TIAs	2.05 (1.16–3.60)		Multiple TIAs	2.0	
Minor stroke	1.82 (0.99–3.34)		Minor stroke	1.8	
Major stroke	2.54 (1.48–4.35)		Major stroke	2.5	2.5
Diabetes	1.35 (0.86–2.11)	0.1881	Diabetes	1.4	1.4
Previous MI	1.57 (1.01–2.45)	0.0471	Previous MI	1.6	No
PVD	1.18 (0.78–1.77)	0.4368	PVD	1.2	No
Treated hypertension	1.24 (0.88–1.75)	0.2137	Treated hypertension	1.2	1.2
Irregular/ulcerated plaque	2.03 (1.31–3.14)	0.0015	Irregular/plaque ulcerated	2.0	2.0
Total risk score					263
Predicted 5-year risk of stroke (derived using a nomogram)					37%

Notes:
CI, confidence interval; MI, myocardial infarction; PVD, peripheral vascular disease; TIA, transient ischemic attack.
[a]Hazard ratios derived from the model are used for the scoring system. The score for the five-year risk of stroke is the product the individual scores for each of the risk factors present. The score is converted into a risk with a graph.
Source: Rothwell et al. (2005).

Box 14.1. Prediction of stroke in patients with non-valvular atrial fibrillation

Why predict risk?

The absolute risk of stroke varies 20-fold among patients with non-valvular atrial fibrillation, depending on age and associated vascular diseases. Estimating an individual's stroke risk is, therefore, essential when considering potentially hazardous anticoagulation therapy. More than 10 similar stroke risk models for patients with atrial fibrillation have been published, but the CHADS2 scheme is now the most widely used.

What is the score?

The CHADS2 scheme awards 1 point each for **c**ongestive heart failure, **h**ypertension, **a**ge ≥ 75 years and **d**iabetes mellitus and 2 points for prior **s**troke or TIA.

Does it work?

The CHADS2 score has been validated in many groups of patients, three of which are shown below (Gage *et al.* 2004; Hart 2007). In each of the validation studies, those with CHADS2 scores of 0 or 1 had stroke rates of $\leq 3\%$ per year, whereas those with higher scores had progressively increasing risks. The lower risks in the outpatient cohort very likely reflect the small numbers of patients with previous TIA or stroke compared with the other groups.

	Hospital discharge cohort	Outpatient cohort	Aspirin-treated clinical trial participants
No.	1733	5089	2580
Prior stroke No. [%]	433 (25)	204 (4)	568 (22)
Overall annual stroke rate	4.4	2.0	4.2
CHADS2 score (95% CI)	Stroke + TIA rate (%/year)	Stroke + systemic embolism rate (%/year)	Stroke rate (%/year)
0	1.9 (1.2–3.0)	0.5 (0.3–0.8)	0.8 (0.4–1.7)
1	2.8 (2.0–3.8)	1.5 (1.2–1.9)	2.2 (1.6–3.1)
2	4.0 (3.1–5.1)	2.5 (2.0–3.2)	4.5 (3.5–5.9)
3	5.9 (4.6–7.3)	5.3 (4.2–6.7)	8.6 (6.8–11.0)
4	8.5 (6.3–11)	6.0 (3.9–9.3)	10.9 (7.8–15.2)
5–6	>12	6.9 (3.4–13.8)	>12

Note:
CI, confidence interval.

What are its potential deficiencies?

For patients with prior stroke/TIA who have no other risk factors, a CHADS2 score of 2 yields an estimated stroke risk of 2.5–4.5% per year, which is probably too low. All patients with atrial fibrillation and prior stroke or TIA, recent or remote, should be considered high risk. The stroke risk associated with a CHADS2 score of 2 is very different according to primary versus secondary prevention. The use of a CHAD score (i.e. dropping "S2") for primary prevention or a CHADS3 score for secondary prevention appears to fit available data better. If echocardiographic data are available, the Stroke Prevention in Atrial Fibrillation (SPAF) III risk stratification scheme has also been validated in several, albeit smaller, groups of patients (Stroke Prevention in Atrial Fibrillation Investigators 1995).
Sources: From Gage *et al.* 2004; Hart 2007.

Box 14.2. Prediction of recurrence after a single seizure and in early epilepsy

Why predict risk?

Outcome after a first seizure varies, with approximately 65% of newly diagnosed people rapidly entering remission after starting treatment and approximately 25% developing drug-resistant epilepsy. Treatment for most patients is with antiepileptic drugs, which carry risks of acute idiosyncratic reactions, dose-related and chronic toxic effects and teratogenicity. The benefits of treatment will outweigh the risks for most patients, but for those who have had only a single seizure the risk–benefit ratio is more finely balanced.

What is the score?

A prognostic model was developed based on individual patient data from the Multicentre Trial for Early Epilepsy and Single Seizures (MESS) to enable identification of patients at low, medium or high risk of seizure recurrence (Kim *et al.* 2007). A 60:40 split-sample approach was used in which the model was developed on a subsample (885 patients) of the full dataset and validated on the remainder of the sample (535 patients). The significant predictors of future seizures, on which the score was based, were number of seizures of all types at presentation (one scored 0; two or three scored 1 and four or more scored 2 points), presence of a neurological disorder or learning disability (1 point), and an abnormal electroencephalogram (1 point).

Does it work?

Patients with a single seizure and no other high-risk characteristics (i.e. 0 points) were classified as low risk, those with two or three seizures, a neurological disorder or an abnormal EEG (1 point) were classified as medium risk, and those with ≥ 2 points were classified as high risk. In trial patients randomized to delayed treatment, the probabilities of a recurrent seizure were 19%, 35% and 59%, respectively, at one year, and 30%, 56% and 73%, respectively, at five years. The score was also used to stratify the analysis of the effect of antiepileptic treatment in the trial (patients had been randomized to immediate treatment or delayed treatment if required). There was no benefit to immediate treatment in patients at low risk of seizure recurrence, but there were potentially worthwhile benefits in those at medium and high risk.

What are its potential deficiencies?

The split sample approach is not an independent validation and so further validations are required, preferably in non-trial groups of patients.
Source: From Kim *et al.* 2007.

that some studies of the prognosis of TIA that ascertained patients some weeks or months after the initial event underestimated the immediate risk of stroke (Rothwell 2003). Intensity and setting of treatment should be described as both of these factors will have an impact on prognosis (Giles and Rothwell 2007). Methods of follow-up must be appropriately sensitive to identify outcomes and criteria for such outcomes, and methods of adjudication must be fully described.

Although, in general, prospective cohort studies of well-defined groups of patients are superior, retrospective studies may have the advantage of longer follow-up, which might be necessary for a clinically relevant prognosis or simply in order to have a sufficient number of outcome events to construct a reasonably precise prediction model. However,

Box 14.3. Prediction of outcome in the Guillain–Barré syndrome

Why predict risk?
Guillain–Barré syndrome (GBS) is characterized by rapidly progressive weakness, which is usually followed by slow clinical recovery but outcome is variable, with some patients remaining bedridden or wheelchair bound. Previous studies showed that preceding infection, age, rapid progression, disability at nadir and electrophysiological characteristics were associated with long-term prognosis, but a readily applicable and validated model was required to predict outcome.

What is the score?
The score was derived and validated on patients in the acute phase of GBS who were unable to walk independently (van Koningsveld *et al.* 2007). The derivation set included 388 patients from randomized controlled trials and the outcome was inability to walk independently at six months. A simple score was developed from the coefficients in a regression model: age, preceding diarrhea and GBS disability score at 2 weeks after entry. Scores range from 1 to 7, with three categories for age (≤ 40, 41–60 and >60 years scoring 0, 0.5 and 1, respectively), 1 point for recent diarrhea and 1–5 points for disability score at 2 weeks.

Does it work?
The score was validated in a set of 374 patients from another randomized trial. Predictions of the inability to walk independently at six months ranged from 1% for a score of 1 to 83% for patients with a score of 7. Predictions agreed well with observed outcome frequencies (i.e. good calibration) and showed very good discriminative ability (C statistic $= 0.85$).

Score	Derivation set ($n = 388$)	Validation set ($n = 374$)	Combined set ($n = 762$)
1–3	1/107 (1%)	0/86 (0%)	1/193 (0.5%)
3.5–4.5	7/116 (6%)	9/110 (8%)	16/226 (7%)
5	20/81 (25%)	23/80 (29%)	43/161 (27%)
5.5–7	43/84 (51%)	51/98 (22%)	94/182 (53%)
Total	71/388 (18%)	83/374 (22%)	154/762 (20%)

What are its potential deficiencies?
The score was derived and validated on patients from randomized controlled trials, who may have been unrepresentative. The score was also derived and validated on patients with moderately severe GBS (unable to walk independently) and might work less well in milder cases – but then the prognosis for full recovery is known to be good in mild cases and so a score is not necessary. There are also geographical differences in the type of GBS and its outcome. This score was derived and validated on European populations, and so further validations in other areas would be helpful. It has not yet been validated by independent researchers.
Source: From van Koningsveld *et al.* 2007.

retrospective studies often have vague inclusion criteria, selection biases, incomplete baseline data, variable use of diagnostic tests, non-standard methods of measurement and inconsistent treatment (Laupacis *et al.* 1997).

Table 14.3. Table of quality criteria for study method for reliable measurement of prognosis

Study feature	Qualities sought
Sample of patients	Methods of patient selection from study population described
	Inclusion and exclusion criteria defined
	Diagnostic criteria defined
	Clinical and demographic characteristics fully described
	Representative
	Assembled at common (usually early) point in course of disease
	Complete (all eligible patients included)
Follow-up of patients	Sufficiently long, thorough and sensitive to outcomes of interest
	Loss to follow-up provided
Outcome	Objective, unbiased and fully defined (e.g. assessment blinded to prognostic information)
	Appropriate
	Known for all or high proportion of patients
Prognostic variable	Fully defined
	Details of measurement available (methods if relevant)
	Available for all or high proportion of patients
Analysis	Continuous predictor variable analyzed appropriately
	Statistical adjustment for all important prognostic factors
Treatment subsequent to inclusion in cohort	Fully described
	Treatment standardized or randomized

Source: From Altman and Royston 2000.

Developing a prognostic model

The purpose of a prognostic model is usually to predict the risk of an event. Although the outcome is, therefore, binary (i.e. yes or no), the predictions are almost always intermediate probabilities, rather than 0% (will definitely not happen) or 100% (definitely will happen). A model should, therefore, successfully distinguish between high and low risk *groups*, but the ability to predict an *individual's* outcome is almost always limited (Henderson and Keiding 2005). Nevertheless, even relatively modest risk stratification can be clinically useful. For example, given a 5% operative risk of stroke and death for endarterectomy for patients with asymptomatic carotid stenosis and an average five-year risk of stroke on medical treatment of about 10%, simply separating patients into a group with a mere 5% five-year unoperated risk and a group with a more worrying 20% five-year risk would substantially improve the targeting of treatment (avoid for the former, recommend for the latter perhaps).

The quality of the data is also important. Measurements should ideally have been made with reliable and reasonably standard methods, preferably without categorization (i.e. they should be recorded as continuous variables as opposed to ad hoc categories, which might limit their predictive value). In multicenter trials or cohorts, it is particularly important to have consistent methods of measurements and similar definitions of variables across centers (e.g. are the centers all using the same definitions of hypertension?). As complete a set of data as possible is also essential for the development of reliable prognostic models. Even when each variable is reasonably complete, many patients will have missing data for at least one variable, often the majority of patients (Clark and Altman 2003). Excluding such cases, as standard statistical packages would automatically do, reduces statistical power and may also introduce bias. The alternative to exclusion of patients with missing data is to impute the missing values (Vach 1997; Schafer and Graham 2002). Although imputation requires certain assumptions about why data are missing, it can often be preferable to risking selection bias by using only cases with complete data (Schafer and Graham 2002; Burton and Altman 2004).

Prognostic models are usually derived using logistic regression (for predicting binary outcomes) or Cox regression (for time-to event data). The sample size required depends on the number of outcomes and *not* the number of patients (Feinstein 1996; Schmoor *et al.* 2000). Cohorts with few events per prognostic variable studied are likely to produce unreliable results. It is generally recommended that there should be at least 10–20 outcome events per prognostic variable studied (i.e. *not* 10–20 per variable eventually included in the model), although reliable models have been derived on smaller numbers (Harrell *et al.* 1984; Feinstein 1996). However, with a small derivation cohort there will always be a risk of selecting unimportant variables and missing important ones by chance.

Before performing multivariable analysis, many researchers try to reduce the number of candidate variables by means of univariate analyses, eliminating those variables that are not significant univariate predictors (often with a cut-off of $p < 0.1$). However, this step is not strictly necessary and it may introduce bias (Sun *et al.* 1996; Babyak 2004). It makes more sense to reduce the number of candidate variables using clinical criteria, such as by eliminating variables that are difficult to measure in routine practice (e.g. emboli on transcranial Doppler) or a variable that is likely to be closely correlated with another (e.g. systolic and diastolic blood pressure).

The initial selection of variables can be further reduced automatically using a selection algorithm (often backward elimination or forward selection). Such an automated procedure sounds as though it should produce the optimal choice of predictive variables, but it is often necessary in practice to use clinical knowledge to over-ride the statistical process, either to ensure inclusion of a variable that is known from previous studies to be highly predictive or to eliminate variables that might lead to overfitting (i.e. overestimation of the predictive value of the model by inclusion of variables that appear to be predictive in the derivation cohort, probably by chance, but are unlikely to be predictive in other cohorts).

It is also important to look for potential interactions between the predictive value of particular variables (i.e. the predictive value of one variable may depend on the presence or absence of another), especially if there is some a priori clinical or biological reason to suspect an interaction. For example, the predictive value of cholesterol level is likely to fall with age in a model predicting the risk of vascular events (total cholesterol is highly predictive of myocardial infarction in patients in their 40s and 50s, of less value in 60s and early 70s, and of little value in the 80s). Such interactions can be taken into account in the model by including an interaction term, which will increase the predictive power of the model, assuming that the interaction is generalizable to future patients.

Studies developing models should be reported in adequate detail. Several reviews of papers presenting prognostic models have found common deficiencies in methodology and reporting, including a lack of information on the method for selecting the variables in the model and on the coding of variables, and a tendency to have too few events per variable in the derivation cohort (Concato *et al.* 1993; Coste *et al.* 1995; Laupacis *et al.* 1997; Counsell and Dennis 2001; Hackett and Anderson 2005; Jacob *et al.* 2005). Authors must report the model in enough detail so that someone else can use it in the clinic and can validate it with their own data. The main issues in assessing studies reporting prognostic models are internal validity, external validity, statistical validity, evaluation of the model and practicality of the model (Counsell and Dennis 2001; Jacob *et al.* 2005).

How to derive a simple risk score

Ideally, in order for risk scores to be useful in clinical practice, they should be simple enough to be calculated without the need for a calculator or computer and to be memorized and so should be based only on a small number of variables (Table 14.3). In practice, a few variables with strong predictive effects usually account for most of the prognostic power, with the remaining weaker variables contributing relatively little. However, a large number of candidate variables are often available for initial consideration, and so a balance is required between fitting the current data as well as possible and developing a model that will be generalizable *and* will actually be used in day-to-day practice. On the one hand, models that are "over-fitted" to the derivation cohort often perform badly when independently validated (Harrell *et al.* 1984; Babyak 2004). This is because they generally contain some variables that were only marginally statistically significant predictors in the derivation cohort, often through chance, or they overestimated the predictive value of genuinely predictive variables, both of which will result in a model that "overpredicts."

On the other hand, a potential problem with simple risk scores is that they may not use the full information from the prognostic variables (Christensen 1987; Royston *et al.* 2006). If continuous predictors such as age are dichotomized (e.g. old versus young), power is usually reduced (Altman and Royston 2000). Furthermore, if the dichotomy is data derived at the point where "it looks best," it may also compromise the generalizability of the score. However, although some loss of prognostic power is almost inevitable, simple scores often perform almost as well as more complex models. One reason for this is that a simple score based on a small number of highly predictive variables is much less likely to be overfitted than a complex score with additional weakly predictive variables and interaction terms.

Assuming that there are no complex interaction terms in a multivariable model, it is relatively easy to convert a model to a simple score. The numeric weights allocated to each variable in the model (i.e. the coefficients from the fitted regression model) provide the basis of the score. Simply using the same numeric weights and adding them up to produce a simple score will actually result in the same ranking of patients as the more complex mathematical model. The only thing that is lost is the exact predicted risk. However, the exact predicted risk can be obtained from a simple graph of score versus risk.

Validation of a prognostic model or score

A prognostic model or score must always be independently validated. Simply because a model seems to include appropriately modeled powerful predictors does not mean that it will necessarily validate well, because associations might just occur by chance, and predictors may not be as powerful as they appear.

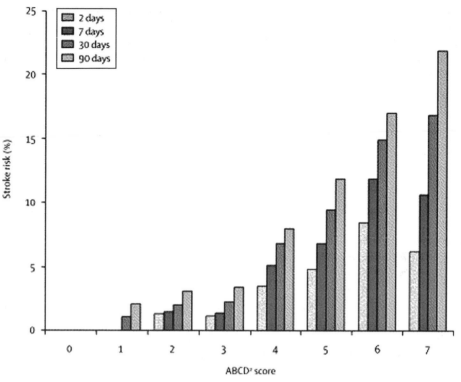

Fig. 14.1. Short-term stroke risk stratified by ABCD^2 score in six cohort studies combined ($n = 4799$ patients). Stroke risks are shown at 2, 7, 30 and 90 days (Johnston *et al.* 2007).

External validation of a model means determining whether it performs well in groups of patients other than those on whom it was derived: that is, how is it likely to do in real clinical practice. These other groups almost certainly will differ in case mix, referral patterns, treatment protocols, methods of measurement of variables and definition of outcomes. Nevertheless, if a prognostic model includes powerful predictive variables, appropriately modeled, it should validate reasonably well in other groups of patients. For example, Fig. 14.1 shows the validation of the ABCD^2 score on pooled individual patient data from six independent groups of patients with TIA (Johnston *et al.* 2007) (Ch. 15).

The two main aims of a validation are to calibrate the model (i.e. to compare observed and predicted event rates for groups of patients) and to assess its discrimination (i.e. how well it distinguishes between patients who do or do not have an outcome event) (Harrell *et al.* 1996; Mackillop and Quirt 1997; Altman and Royston 2000).

Calibration is assessed by comparing the observed with the predicted proportions of events in groups defined by the risk prediction or score.

Discrimination can be summarized by various single statistics, such as the area under the receiver operating characteristic curve (or the equivalent C statistic), R^2 measures, or the d statistic, although all of these measures have limitations (Royston and Sauerbrei 2004; Altman and Royston 2007; Lewis 2007).

In reality, the best measure of the performance of a model is whether the risk stratification that it provides is likely to be useful in routine clinical practice. A relatively poorly predictive model can be useful when, for example, the overall risks of treatment versus no treatment are finely balanced, whereas a very powerfully predictive model may be unhelpful if a very high or low probability of a poor outcome is needed to affect clinical management. For example, use of a model predicting risk of death in a patient with prolonged refractory septic shock would only be helpful in the decision to withdraw active treatment if it could reliably predict probabilities of death of 95% or higher.

Internal validation of a model uses the same dataset as was used for derivation and will, therefore, almost inevitably overestimate its discriminatory power – sadly, this rather lazy approach is all too common and no external validation is ever attempted. Better, in the absence of a new group of patients, is to use new data from the same source as the derivation sample. Several approaches are possible and will give useful information about predictive power (although *not* about generalizability):

- split the dataset into two parts before the modeling begins: the model is derived on the first portion of the data (the "training" set) and its ability to predict outcome is evaluated on the second portion (the "test" set)
- a bootstrapping approach i.e. leave-one-out cross-validation
- split the data in a non-random way, such as by time period or source of referral
- prospective validation on subsequent patients from the same center(s).

These types of partially independent validation are of course tempting, and they do allow refinement of models and scores (Verweij and van Houwelingen 1993; Schumacher *et al.* 1997; Babyak 2004), but they are not a sufficient validation. Clearly, with each of the approaches listed above, there will be many similarities between the derivation and validation sets of patients, and between the clinical and laboratory techniques used in evaluating them. Indeed, this lack of true independence of the validation group of patients probably explains, in part, the fact that researchers tend to confirm the validity of their own models more often than do independent researchers (Altman and Royston 2000; Altman and Royston 2007). The likely generalizability and so usefulness of a model can usually only be shown convincingly in a completely independent group of patients.

Even when a model has been independently validated and performs well, it must still be shown that it is useful in clinical practice. For helping treatment decisions in individual patients, usefulness is generally best tested by stratifying patients in a randomized controlled trial by estimated baseline risk of a poor outcome. Fig. 14.2 shows an external validation in an independent trial of the model detailed in Table 14.2 for the five-year risk of stroke on medical treatment in patients with recently symptomatic carotid stenosis (Rothwell *et al.* 2005). Predicted medical risk is plotted against observed risk of stroke or death in patients randomized to medical or surgical treatment. Given that surgical treatment is associated with an additional 1–2% stroke risk per year over and above the operative risk, it is clear that surgery should probably only be considered in patients in the top two quintiles of predicted risk on medical treatment. Surgery will be harmful, or of no benefit, in the lower-risk individuals. This type of stratification of trial data using an independently derived model is usually essential to convince clinicians that the risk modeling approach is clinically useful. It is important to recognize, however, that even if the model has been validated previously in several non-trial groups of patients, it may perform differently in a trial because of the tendency to recruit relatively low-risk individuals. The distribution of risks in patients who are considered for treatment in routine clinical practice may be closer to that in the non-trial observational groups of patients used for derivation and validation of the model.

Reilly and Evans (2006) have defined five levels of evidence to assess the usefulness of a clinical prediction model (Box 14.4).

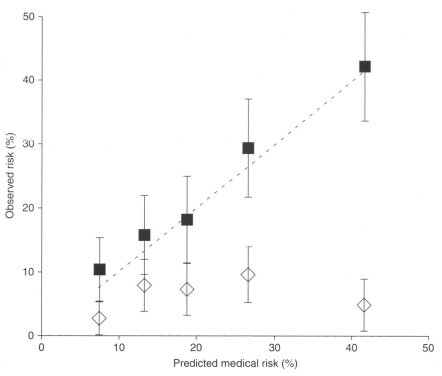

Fig. 14.2. An external validation of the model detailed in Table 14.2 for the five-year risk of stroke on medical treatment in an independent randomized trial of endarterectomy versus medical treatment for symptomatic carotid stenosis (Rothwell *et al.* 2005). Predicted risk of stroke on medical treatment is plotted against the observed risk of stroke in patients randomized to medical treatment in the trial (squares) and against the observed operative risk of stroke and death in patients randomized to surgical treatment (diamonds). Groups are quintiles of predicted risk.

Box 14.4. Five levels of evidence suggested by Reilly and Evans (2006) to assess the usefulness of a clinical prediction rule

1. Derivation of the prediction rule
2. Narrow validation of the prediction rule (i.e. prospective evaluation in one setting)
3. Broad validation of the prediction rule (i.e. prospective evaluation in varied settings with a wide spectrum of patients and physicians)
4. Narrow impact analysis of the prediction rule used as a decision rule (i.e. prospective demonstration in one setting that the use of the prediction rule improves clinical decision making)
5. Broad impact analysis of the prediction rule used as a decision rule (i.e. prospective demonstration in varied settings that use of the prediction rule improves clinical decision making in a wide spectrum of patients).

Another important issue is the need for updating of predictive models and scores if new predictors are discovered, requiring the addition of new variables to the model, or if new treatments reduce the risk of a poor outcome in general, requiring recalibration of the model. In general, minor recalibration of the prognostic index from the original model would be preferable to complete reconstruction (van Houwelingen and Thorogood 1995).

References

Altman DG (2001). Systematic reviews of evaluations of prognostic variables. *British Medical Journal* **323**:224–228

Altman DG, Royston P (2000). What do we mean by validating a prognostic model? *Statistics in Medicine* **19**:453–473

Altman DG, Royston P (2007). Evaluating the performance of prognostic models. In *Treating Individuals: from Randomized Trials to Personalised Medicine*, Rothwell PM (ed.), pp. 213–30. London: Elsevier

Babyak MA (2004). What you see may not be what you get: a brief, nontechnical introduction to overfitting in regression-type models. *Psychosomatic Medicine* **66**:411–421

Boissel JP, Collet JP, Lievre M *et al.* (1993). An effect model for the assessment of drug benefit: example of antiarrhythmic drugs in postmyocardial infarction patients. *Journal of Cardiovascular Pharmacology* **22**:356–363

Burton A, Altman DG (2004). Missing covariate data within cancer prognostic studies: a review of current reporting and proposed guidelines. *British Journal of Cancer* **91**:4–8

Christensen E (1987). Multivariate survival analysis using Cox's regression model. *Hepatology* **7**:1346–1358

Clark TG, Altman DG (2003). Developing a prognostic model in the presence of missing data: an ovarian cancer case study. *Journal of Clinical Epidemiology* **56**:28–37

Concato J, Feinstein AR, Holford TR (1993). The risk of determining risk with multivariable models. *Annals of Internal Medicine* **118**:201–210

Coste J, Fermanian J, Venot A (1995). Methodological and statistical problems in the construction of composite measurement scales: a survey of six medical and epidemiological journals. *Statistics in Medicine* **14**:331–345

Counsell C, Dennis M (2001). Systematic review of prognostic models in patients with acute stroke. *Cerebrovascular Diseases* **12**:159–170

Dahlof B, Lindholm LH, Hansson L *et al.* (1991). Morbidity and mortality in the Swedish trial in old patients with hypertension (STOP-hypertension). *Lancet* **338**:1281–1285

Feinstein AR (1996). *Multivariable Analysis: An Introduction*. New Haven, CT: Yale University Press

Gage BF, van Walraven C, Pearce LA *et al.* (2004). Selecting patients with atrial fibrillation for anticoagulation. Stroke risk stratification in patients taking aspirin. *Circulation* **110**:2287–2292

Giles MF, Rothwell PM (2007). Risk of stroke early after transient ischaemic attack: a systematic review and meta-analysis. *Lancet Neurology* **6**:1063–1072

Grover SA, Lowensteyn I, Esrey KL *et al.* (1995). Do doctors accurately assess coronary risk in their patients? Preliminary results of the coronary health assessment study. *British Medical Journal* **310**:975–978

Hackett ML, Anderson CS (2005). Predictors of depression after stroke: a systematic review of observational studies. *Stroke* **36**:2296–2301

Harrell FE Jr., Lee KL, Califf RM *et al.* (1984). Regression modelling strategies for improved prognostic prediction. *Statistics in Medicine* **3**:143–152

Harrell FE Jr., Lee KL, Mark DB (1996). Multivariable prognostic models: issues in developing models, evaluating assumptions and adequacy, and measuring and reducing errors. *Statistics in Medicine* **15**:361–387

Hart RG (2007). Antithrombotic therapy to prevent stroke in patients with atrial fibrillation. In *Treating Individuals: From Randomized Trials to Personalised Medicine*, Rothwell PM (ed.) pp. 265–278. London: Elsevier

Hayden JA, Côté P, Bombardier C (2006). Evaluation of the quality of prognosis studies in systematic reviews. *Annals of Internal Medicine* **144**:427–437

Henderson R, Keiding N (2005). Individual survival time prediction using statistical models. *Journal of Medical Ethics* **31**:703–706

Hodges JR, Warlow CP (1990a). Syndromes of transient amnesia: towards a classification. A study of 153 cases. *Journal of Neurology, Neurosurgery Psychiatry* **53**:834–843

Hodges JR, Warlow CP (1990b). The aetiology of transient global amnesia. A case–control study of 114 cases with prospective follow-up. *Brain* **113**:639–657

International Study of Unruptured Intracranial Aneurysms Investigators (1998). Unruptured intracranial aneurysms: risks of rupture and risks of surgical intervention. *New England Journal of Medicine* 1998 **339**:1725–1733

Jacob M, Lewsey JD, Sharpin C *et al.* (2005). Systematic review and validation of prognostic models in liver transplantation. *Liver Transplantation* **11**:814–825

Johnston SC, Rothwell PM, Nguyen-Huynh MN *et al.* (2007). Validation and refinement of scores to predict very early stroke risk after transient ischaemic attack. *Lancet* **369**:283–292

Justice AC, Covinsky KE, Berlin JA (1999). Assessing the generalizability of prognostic information. *Annals of Internal Medicine* **130**:515–524

Kernan WN, Feinstein AR, Brass LM (1991). A methodological appraisal of research on prognosis after transient ischemic attacks. *Stroke* **22**:1108–1116

Kim LG, Johnson TL, Marson AG, for the MRC MESS Study group (2007). Prediction of risk of seizure recurrence after a single seizure and early epilepsy: further results from the MESS trial. *Lancet Neurology* **5**:317–322

Laupacis A, Boysen G, Connolly S *et al.* (1994). Risk factors for stroke and efficacy of antithrombotic therapy in atrial fibrillation. Analysis of pooled data from five randomised controlled trials. *Archives of Internal Medicine* **154**:1449–1457

Laupacis A, Sekar N, Stiell IG (1997). Clinical prediction rules. A review and suggested modifications of methodological standards. *Journal of the American Medical Association* **277**:488–494

Lewis S (2007). Regression analysis. *Practical Neurology* **7**:259–264

Li W, Boissel JP, Girard P *et al.* (1998). Identification and prediction of responders to a therapy: a model and its preliminary application to actual data. *Journal of Epidemiology and Biostatistics* **3**:189–197

Mackillop WJ, Quirt CF (1997). Measuring the accuracy of prognostic judgments in oncology. *Journal of Clinical Epidemiology* **50**:21–29

Medical Research Council Working Party (1985). MRC trial of treatment of mild hypertension: principal results. *British Medical Journal* **291**:97–104

Morrow J, Russell A, Guthrie E *et al.* (2006). Malformation risks of antiepileptic drugs in pregnancy: a prospective study from the UK Epilepsy and Pregnancy Register. *Journal of Neurology, Neurosurgery Psychiatry* **77**:193–198

Pagliaro L, D'Amico G, Soronson TIA *et al.* (1992). Prevention of bleeding in cirrhosis. *Annals of Internal Medicine* **117**:59–70

Reilly BM, Evans AT (2006). Translating clinical research into clinical practice: impact of using prediction rules to make decisions. *Annals of Internal Medicine* **144**:201–209

Rothwell PM (2003). Incidence, risk factors and prognosis of stroke and TIA: the need for high-quality, large-scale epidemiological studies and meta-analyses. *Cerebrovascular Diseases* **16**(Suppl 3):2–10

Rothwell PM, Mehta Z, Howard SC *et al.* (2005). From subgroups to individuals: general principles and the example of carotid endarterectomy. *Lancet* **365**:256–265

Royston P, Sauerbrei W (2004). A new measure of prognostic separation in survival data. *Statistics in Medicine* **23**:723–748

Royston P, Altman DG, Sauerbrei W (2006). Dichotomizing continuous predictors in multiple regression: a bad idea. *Statistics in Medicine* **25**:127–141

Sackett DL, Whelan G (1980). Cancer risk in ulcerative colitis: scientific requirements for the study of prognosis. *Gastroenterology* **78**:1632–1635

Sanmuganathan PS, Ghahramani P, Jackson PR *et al.* (2001). Aspirin for primary prevention of coronary heart disease: safety and absolute benefit related to coronary risk derived from meta-analysis of randomised trials. *Heart* **85**:265–271

Schafer JL, Graham JW (2002). Missing data: our view of the state of the art. *Psychological Methods* **7**:147–177

Schmoor C, Sauerbrei W, Schumacher M (2000). Sample size considerations for the evaluation of prognostic factors in survival analysis. *Statistics in Medicine* **19**:441–452

Schumacher M, Hollander N, Sauerbrei W (1997). Resampling and cross-validation techniques: a tool to reduce bias caused by model building? *Statistics in Medicine* **16**:2813–2827

Stevens DL, Matthews WB (1973). Cryptogenic drop attacks: an affliction of women. *British Medical Journal* **1**:439–442

Stroke Prevention in Atrial Fibrillation Investigators (1995). Risk factors for thromboembolism during aspirin therapy in patients with atrial fibrillation: the Stroke Prevention in Atrial Fibrillation study. *Journal of Stroke and Cerebrovascular Diseases* 1995; **5**:147–157

Sun GW, Shook TL, Kay GL (1996). Inappropriate use of bivariable analysis to screen risk factors for use in multivariable analysis. *Journal of Clinical Epidemiology.* **49**:907–916

Vach W (1997). Some issues in estimating the effect of prognostic factors from incomplete covariate data. *Statistics in Medicine* **16**:57–72

van Houwelingen HC, Thorogood J (1995). Construction, validation and updating of a prognostic model for kidney graft survival. *Statistics in Medicine* **14**: 1999–2008

van Koningsveld R, Steyerberg EW, Hughes RA *et al.* (2007). A clinical prognostic scoring system for Guillain–Barré syndrome. *Lancet Neurology* **6**:589–594

Verweij PJ, van Houwelingen HC (1993). Cross-validation in survival analysis. *Statistics in Medicine* **12**:2305–2314

West of Scotland Coronary Prevention Group (1996). West of Scotland Coronary Prevention Study: identification of high-risk groups and comparison with other cardiovascular intervention trials. *Lancet* **348**:1339–1342

Wyatt JC, Altman DG (1995). Commentary. Prognostic models: clinically useful or quickly forgotten? *British Medical Journal* **311**:1539–1541

Yusuf S, Zucker D, Peduzzi P *et al.* (1994). Effect of coronary artery bypass graft surgery on survival: overview of 10-year results from randomised trials by the Coronary Artery Bypass Graft Surgery Trialists' Collaboration. *Lancet* **344**:563–570

Chapter 15

Short-term prognosis after transient ischemic attack and minor stroke

Recent research has shown that the risk of stroke immediately after TIA or minor stroke is considerable (Giles and Rothwell 2007; Wu *et al.* 2007). However, this poses a challenge to clinical services because although the majority of patients will, by definition, have suffered a transient illness with no immediate major sequelae, an important minority are at risk of a major stroke in the short term. Prognostic tools have, therefore, been developed to identify patients at high (and low) risk in order to inform public education, aid effective triage to secondary care and direct secondary preventive treatment.

Early risk of stroke after transient ischemic attack or minor stroke

Patients with major stroke often report earlier short-lived neurological symptoms, and data from population-based studies and trials suggest that approximately 20% of patients with stroke have a preceding TIA (Rothwell and Warlow 2005). A similar proportion of major strokes are probably preceded by a minor stroke. However, the prospective estimation of risk after TIA or minor stroke is challenging, and in the past the risk has been considered to be low (approximately 1–2% at one week and 2–4% at one month) (Hankey *et al.* 1991; Gubitz *et al.* 1999; Gubitz and Sandercock 2000; Warlow *et al.* 2001). However, these risks are now considered underestimates because they were calculated from cohort studies and clinical trials in which patients were recruited some time after their initial event and patients who experienced subsequent stroke before recruitment were excluded (Rothwell 2003).

Accurate estimation of the early risk of stroke after TIA or minor stroke requires particular study methods. First, potential patients must be recruited as rapidly as possible after the event so that strokes following very early after TIA are included. Second, patients should be assessed initially by an expert stroke physician to ensure that the diagnosis is made reliably and mimics are excluded. Third, follow-up should be in person and outcome events should be independently adjudicated to ensure correct identification of subsequent strokes. Lastly, patients should ideally be recruited from a defined population as opposed to a particular clinical setting in order to reduce selection bias.

A number of more recent studies have met most or all of these criteria. The first was published in 2000 (Johnston *et al.* 2000). All patients presenting to emergency departments (ED) with a diagnosis of TIA within a health maintenance organization in California, USA, were studied over a year, starting in February 1997. Of 1707 patients, almost all presenting within 24-hours of the event, 180 (10.5%) returned to the ED within 90 days of the index TIA with a stroke, half of which occurred in the first two days after the TIA. Also, within the first 90 days, 2.6% of patients were hospitalized for cardiovascular events 2.6% of patients died, and 12.7% suffered recurrent TIAs. In this study, patients were included if they had a diagnosis of TIA made by an ED physician, but these estimates of risk did not change substantially when the charts were examined by a neurologist and patients in whom the diagnosis was in doubt were excluded from the analysis.

Comparable risks of stroke after TIA were measured in population-based studies in Oxfordshire, UK (Lovett *et al.* 2003; Coull *et al.* 2004). In a cohort of 249 consecutive patients with a TIA ascertained in the Oxford Vascular Study (OXVASC) over a 30-month period, stroke risks at two and seven days were 6.8% (95% confidence interval [CI], 3.7–10.0) and 12.0% (95% CI, 8.0–16.1), respectively (Rothwell *et al.* 2007). Although this cohort was smaller than the Californian cohort, it had the advantages of being population based and, therefore, included patients who were treated as inpatients, as outpatients and managed solely in primary care; diagnoses were made by an experienced stoke physician; and follow-up was face to face with independent adjudication of outcome events.

A recent systematic review identified 18 independent cohorts, all published since 2000, reporting stroke risk in 10 126 patients with TIA (Giles and Rothwell 2007). The pooled stroke risks were 3.1% (95% CI, 2.0–4.1) at two days and 5.2% (95% CI, 3.9–6.5) at seven days, but there was considerable heterogeneity between studies ($p < 0.0001$), with risks ranging from 0% to 12.8% at seven days. However, the risks observed in individual studies over different intervals of follow-up were highly consistent, and the heterogeneity between studies was almost fully explained by study method, setting and treatment. The lowest stroke risks at seven days were seen in studies in specialist stroke services offering emergency access and treatment (0.9%; 95% CI, 0.0–1.9 [four studies]) and highest risks in population-based without urgent treatment (11.0%; 95% CI, 8.6–13.5 [three studies]). Intermediate risks were measured by studies recruiting from single EDs (5.8%; 95% CI, 3.7–8.0 [three studies]) and low risks in studies recruiting from routine neurovascular clinics (3.3%; 95% CI, 1.6–5.0 [two studies]) (Fig. 15.1). Findings were similar for stroke risks at two days. These differences in measured risk reflect a combination of patient selection by different care settings, with higher-risk patients being managed in emergency care; exclusion of high-risk individuals when there is a delay to recruitment; and modification of risk in patients who are urgently and aggressively treated with secondary preventive medication (Table 15.1).

The risk of stroke following minor stroke has not been studied in such depth. However, in a provisional report from the first year of OXVASC, the risk of stroke among 87 patients with minor stroke (defined as a score of ≤ 3 on the National Institutes of Health Stroke Scale (NIHSS)) was 11.5% (95% CI, 4.8–11.2) at seven days and 18.5% (95% CI, 10.3–26.7) at 90 days (Coull *et al.* 2004). Among patients with minor stroke who were referred to the dedicated neurovascular clinic in the EXPRESS study and did not need immediate admission to hospital, the rates of recurrent stroke at 90 days were 10·8% (17/158) in phase 1, without urgent intervention, and 4.0% (5/125) in phase 2, with urgent intervention (Rothwell *et al.* 2007) (Ch. 20).

Identification of high-risk patients: simple risk scores

Patients with TIA and minor stroke are very heterogeneous in terms of symptoms, risk factors, underlying pathology and early prognosis. Effective management requires the reliable identification of patients at high (and low) risk in order to inform public education, aid effective triage to specialist services and direct secondary preventive treatment. There is evidence that clinical features of a TIA provide substantial prognostic information, as do some other methods.

Five risk factors were found to be independently associated with high risk of recurrent stroke at three months in a large ED cohort of patients with TIA (Johnson *et al.* 2000).

Table 15.1. Advantages and disadvantages of different clinical settings in studies of early prognosis after transient ischemic attack or minor stroke

Setting	Advantages	Disadvantages
ED	Short delay between clinical event and presentation to medical attention	Selection bias: patients managed in alternative settings not studied
	Large cohorts in different departments can be identified and studied	Data collected retrospectively
	Computerized databases can be searched rapidly	Diagnosis and management by ED physician and may not be consistent/fully described
		Patients with a TIA and then a stroke before attending ED not included
		Non-standardized follow-up
Population-based	No selection bias	Costly and labor and time intensive
	Uniform diagnosis, management and follow-up	
	Sensitive follow-up to detect outcome events	
	Complete data available on patient cohort	
	Some data available on study population	
Outpatient clinic	Standardized diagnosis and management	Frequent delay between event and clinic attendance

Notes:
ED, emergency department; TIA, transient ischemic attack.

These included age over 60 years, symptom duration >10 minutes, motor weakness, speech impairment and diabetes mellitus. Recurrent stroke risk at three months varied from 0% for those with none of these factors to 34% for those with all five factors. Isolated sensory or visual symptoms were associated with low risk.

These and other factors identified as being associated with early stroke risk (Gladstone et al. 2004; Hill et al. 2004) were used to derive the ABCD score, a predictive tool of stroke risk within seven days after TIA (Rothwell et al. 2005). Briefly, all clinical features that had previously been found to be independently predictive of stroke after TIA were tested in a derivation cohort of 209 patients recruited from the Oxfordshire Community Stroke Project (OCSP, Lovett et al. 2003). Any variable that was a univariate predictor of the seven-day risk of stroke with a significance of $p \leq 0.1$ assessed with the log rank test was incorporated into the score. The score was then validated in three further independent cohorts.

The score is based on four clinical features and is out of a total of 6 (Table 15.2). The score was found to be highly predictive with areas under the receiver operating characteristic (ROC) curves of 0.85 (95% CI, 0.78–0.91), 0.91 (95% CI, 0.86–0.95) and 0.80 (95% CI, 0.72–0.89) for each of the validation cohorts. In the OXVASC population-based validation cohort of all 377 referrals with suspected, possible or definite TIA, there were 20 strokes at seven days after the initial event: 19 (95%) of these occurred in the 101 patients (27%) with a risk score ≥ 5. The seven-day risks were 0.4% (95% CI, 0–1.1) in 274 patients (73%) with a score of < 5, 12.1% (95% CI, 4.2–20.0) in 66 patients (18%) with a score of 5, and 31.4% (95% CI, 16.0–46.8) in 35 patients (9%) with a score of 6.

2-day stroke risk

Study	Strokes/patients	Risk (%)	95% CI

Population based using face to face follow-up

Lovett *et al.* 2003 (OCSP)	9/209	4.3	1.6–7.1
Rothwell *et al.* 2005 (ABCD)	13/190	6.8	3.3–10.4
Correia *et al.* 2006	14/141	10.2	5.1–15.3
TOTAL	36/540	6.7	3.6–9.7

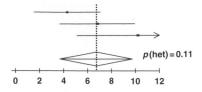

p(het) = 0.11

Population based using administrative follow-up (without exclusions)

Johnston *et al.* 2007	91/1707	5.3	4.3–6.4
Kleindorfer *et al.* 2005	40/1023	3.9	2.7–5.1
Johnston *et al.* 2007 ED	51/1084	4.7	3.4–6.0
TOTAL	182/3814	4.8	4.0–5.6

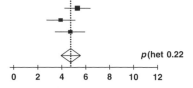

p(het 0.22

Population based using administrative follow-up (with exclusions)

Gladstone *et al.* 2004	7/265	2.6	0.7–4.6
Hill *et al.* 2004	32/2285	1.4	0.9–1.9
Whitehead *et al.* 2005 (BASIC)	7/362	1.9	0.5–3.4
TOTAL	46/2912	1.6	1.1–2.1

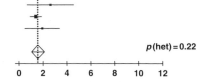

p(het) = 0.22

Single emergency departments

Tsivgoulis *et al.* 2006	Data unavailable		
Bray *et al.* 2007	3/98	3.1	0.0–6.5
Purroy *et al.* 2007	Data unavailable		
TOTAL	3/98	3.1	

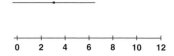

Routine outpatient

Whitehead *et al.* 2005	Data unavailable		
Johnston clinic *et al.* 2007	16/962	1.7	0.9–2.5
TOTAL	16/962	1.7	

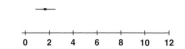

Specialist stroke service

Cucchiara *et al.* 2006	2/117	1.7	0.0–4.1
Calvet *et al.* 2007	4/201	2.0	0.1–3.9
Rothwell *et al.* 2007 (EXPRESS)	1/160	0.6	0.0–1.8
Lavellée *et al.* 2007 (SOS-TIA)	0/629	0.0	0.0–0.3
TOTAL	7/1107	0.6	0.0–1.6

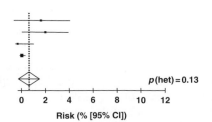

p(het) = 0.13

Risk (% [95% CI])

Fig. 15.1. Stroke risks at two and seven days measured in a systematic review of 18 independent cohorts, stratified according to study method and setting (Giles and Rothwell 2007). CI, confidence interval; *p* (het), *p* value for heterogeneity between studies; *p* (sig), *p* value for overall significance of the meta-analysis of comparisons between studies.

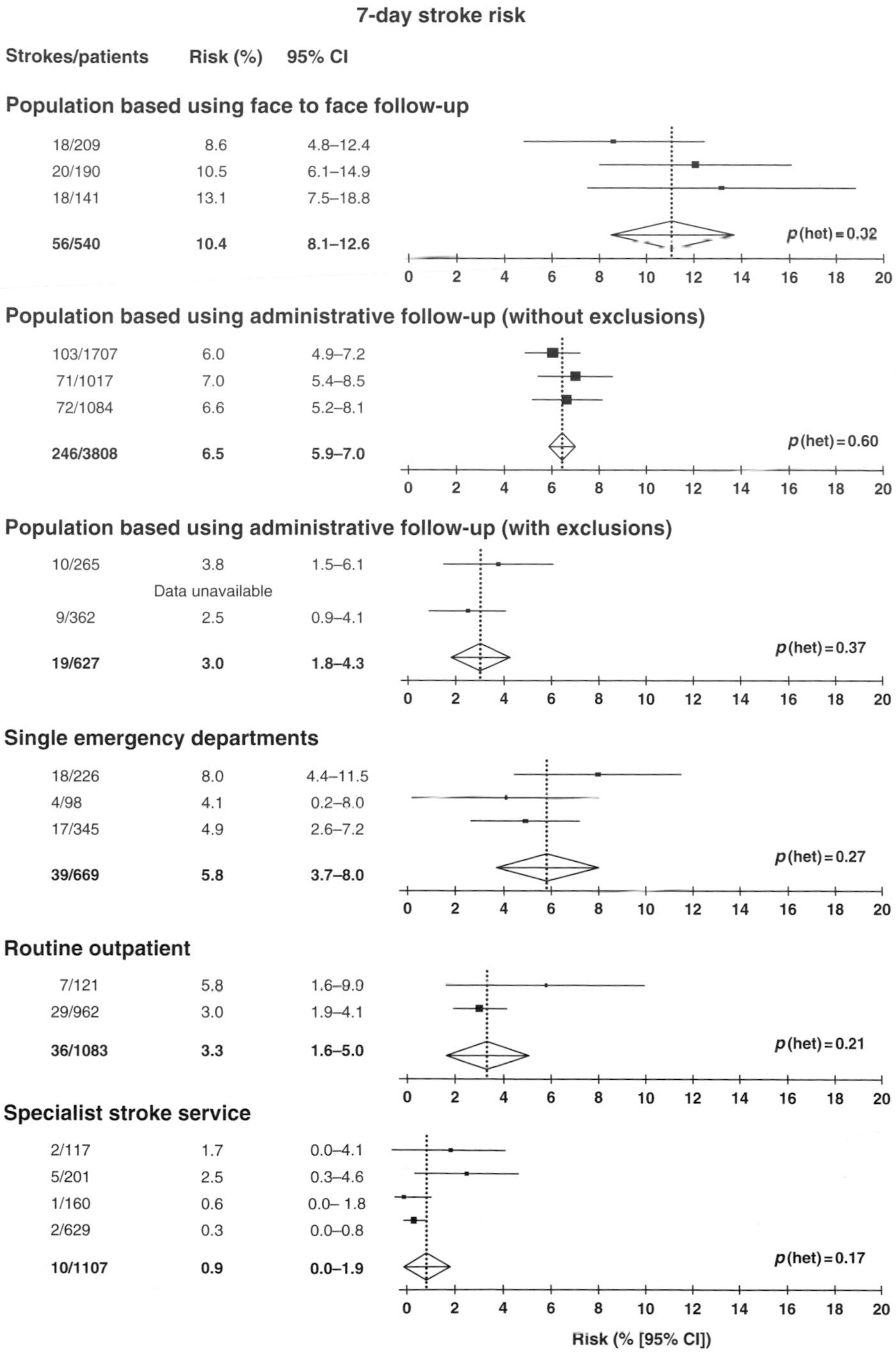

7-day stroke risk

Strokes/patients	Risk (%)	95% CI

Population based using face to face follow-up

18/209	8.6	4.8–12.4
20/190	10.5	6.1–14.9
18/141	13.1	7.5–18.8
56/540	**10.4**	**8.1–12.6**

p(het)=0.32

0 2 4 6 8 10 12 14 16 18 20

Population based using administrative follow-up (without exclusions)

103/1707	6.0	4.9–7.2
71/1017	7.0	5.4–8.5
72/1084	6.6	5.2–8.1
246/3808	**6.5**	**5.9–7.0**

p(het)=0.60

0 2 4 6 8 10 12 14 16 18 20

Population based using administrative follow-up (with exclusions)

10/265	3.8	1.5–6.1
	Data unavailable	
9/362	2.5	0.9–4.1
19/627	**3.0**	**1.8–4.3**

p(het)=0.37

0 2 4 6 8 10 12 14 16 18 20

Single emergency departments

18/226	8.0	4.4–11.5
4/98	4.1	0.2–8.0
17/345	4.9	2.6–7.2
39/669	**5.8**	**3.7–8.0**

p(het)=0.27

0 2 4 6 8 10 12 14 16 18 20

Routine outpatient

7/121	5.8	1.6–9.9
29/962	3.0	1.9–4.1
36/1083	**3.3**	**1.6–5.0**

p(het)=0.21

0 2 4 6 8 10 12 14 16 18 20

Specialist stroke service

2/117	1.7	0.0–4.1
5/201	2.5	0.3–4.6
1/160	0.6	0.0–1.8
2/629	0.3	0.0–0.8
10/1107	**0.9**	**0.0–1.9**

p(het)=0.17

0 2 4 6 8 10 12 14 16 18 20

Risk (% [95% CI])

Fig. 15.1. (cont.)

Table 15.2. The clinical features and scoring for the ABCD system of assessing risk of stroke in the seven days after a transient ischemic attack

	Clinical feature	Category	Score
A	Age	$\geq$ 60 years	1
		< 60 years	0
B	Blood pressure at assessment[a]	SBP > 140 mmHg or DBP $\geq$ 90 mmHg	1
		Other	0
C	Clinical features	Unilateral weakness	2
		Speech disturbance (no weakness)	1
		Other	0
D	Duration	$\geq$ 60 minutes	2
		10–59 minutes	1
		< 10 minutes	0
	Total (maximum)		6

Notes:
SBP, systolic blood pressure; DBP, diastolic blood pressure.
[a]Measured at earliest assessment after the attack.
Source: From Rothwell et al. (2005).

The score was originally designed to facilitate triage between primary and secondary care, and to inform public education of "high risk" scenarios in which medical attention should be sought urgently (Rothwell et al. 2005), although its use has been extended to treatment decisions (National Institute for Health and Clinical Excellence 2008).

Although diabetes was found to be predictive of early stroke in the ABCD score (Rothwell et al. 2005), it lacked statistical significance and was not included. However, the ABCD scoring system has been refined in larger cohorts of patients with the subsequent addition of one point for diabetes to make the ABCD^2 score out of 7 (Rothwell et al. 2005; Johnston et al. 2007) (Table 15.3).

Both the ABCD and the ABCD^2 scores have been further validated in independent cohorts since publication in 2005 and 2007, respectively. In a systematic review, 11 studies were identified that reported the performance of one or both scores in 13 cohorts including 5938 subjects with 332 strokes at seven days (Giles and Rothwell 2008). Pooled estimates of the areas under the ROC curves for the ABCD and ABCD^2 scores, respectively, were 0.70 (95% CI, 0.66–0.73) and 0.70 (95% CI, 0.66–0.74) for stroke risk at seven days and 0.68 (95% CI, 0.65–0.71) and 0.69 (95% CI, 0.66–0.72) for stroke risk at 90 days. Predictive power was independent of clinical setting (ED, specialist neurovascular units and population-based studies) but was greater in two additional cohorts that included patients with both suspected and confirmed TIA than in cohorts of patients with confirmed TIA only. These findings imply that the scores works partly by providing diagnostic information, but this cannot fully explain their prognostic power.

In conclusion, the ABCD and ABCD^2 scores are reliable tools to predict the early risk of stroke after TIA. However, although they are sensitive and easily calculable using clinical information readily available at the time of assessment, they have a high false-positive rate and were deliberately designed to include only clinical data so that they could be used for initial triage. Further information may, therefore, be required to refine risk prediction.

Table 15.3. The clinical features and scoring for the ABCD^2 system

	Clinical feature	Category	Score
A	Age	≥ 60 years	1
		< 60 years	0
B	Blood pressure at assessment[a]	SBP > 140 mmHg or DBP ≥ 90 mmHg	1
		Other	0
C	Clinical Features	Unilateral weakness	2
		Speech disturbance (no weakness)	1
		Other	0
D	Duration	≥ 60 minutes	2
		10–59 minutes	1
		< 10 minutes	0
D	Diabetes	Present	1
		Absent	0
	Total (maximum)		7

Notes:
SBP, systolic blood pressure; DBP, diastolic blood pressure.
[a]Measured at earliest assessment after the attack.
Sources: From Rothwell et al. (2005) and Johnston et al. (2007).

Risk of recurrence by vascular territory

The early risk of stroke after TIA also depends on the vascular territory of the event. Monocular events are associated with a low risk of subsequent cerebral stroke (Hankey et al. 1991, Benavente et al. 2001). Posterior circulation TIAs, which make up approximately 25% of all attacks, were thought for many years to be associated with a lower risk of stroke than carotid territory TIAs (Sivenius et al. 1991; Mohr et al. 1992; Caplan 1996). Correspondingly, they were often managed less aggressively.

However, a recent systematic review of 37 published cohort studies and five unpublished studies reporting the risk of stroke after a TIA or minor stroke by territory of presenting event found no major differences in prognosis between vertebrobasilar events and carotid events. In fact, studies that recruited during the acute phase after the presenting event found a higher risk of subsequent stroke in patients with vertebrobasilar events (odds ratio [OR], 1.47; 95% CI, 1.1–2.0; $p = 0.014$) (Flossman and Rothwell 2003). More recent observations from OXVASC suggest that TIAs attributable to the posterior circulation have higher rates of recurrent stroke than those attributable to the anterior circulation (Flossman et al. 2006). Among 256 consecutive patients with TIA, 212 (82.5%) with an anterior event and 44 (17.1%) with a posterior event, rates of stroke were 15.9% and 9.4%, respectively ($p = 0.22$), at seven days and 31.8% and 17.0%, respectively ($p = 0.03$), at one year (Fig. 15.2). In a further series of patients with TIA and minor stroke in OXVASC, the rate of symptomatic large artery stenosis was higher among patients with posterior circulation events than among those with carotid territory events (Marquardt et al. 2008).

These findings increase interest in imaging the posterior circulation and in angioplasty or stenting any atherothrombotic stenosis detected in the vertebral or proximal basilar arteries.

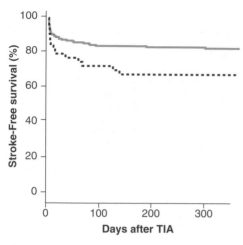

Fig. 15.2. Stroke-free survival curves for consecutive patients with transient ischemic attacks (TIAs) and anterior (—) versus posterior (---) circulation events in the Oxford Vascular Study (OXVASC) (log rank $p = 0.04$) (Flossman *et al.* 2006).

Risk by underlying pathology

Several population-based studies of stroke have shown that recurrent stroke risk is highest in those with large arterial territory stroke and lowest in those with lacunar stroke (Lovett *et al.* 2004a) (Fig. 15.3). Although large artery pathology accounted for only 14% of the initial strokes in a pooled analysis of data from four such studies, 37% of the recurrences at seven days occurred in this group (Lovett *et al.* 2004a). Subtype differences in early recurrent risk are probably smaller in patients with TIA, where some patients with small vessel disease can have a very high risk of early stroke, for instance the "capsular warning syndrome" (Donnan *et al.* 1993; Farrar and Donnan 1993). Nevertheless, several other observations highlight the high early risk of stroke after large artery TIA, including the very high risk of stroke during delays to carotid endarterectomy in patients with recently symptomatic stenosis $\geq 50\%$ of the carotid artery (Fairhead and Rothwell 2005; Rantner *et al.* 2005). Patients with cardioembolic TIA or stroke, predominantly consisting of patients with non-valvular atrial fibrillation, are at intermediate early risk of recurrence (Lovett *et al.* 2004b).

Imaging and prognosis

Some early studies suggested that the presence of infarction on CT in patients with TIA or minor stroke predicts an increased risk of stroke recurrence (Evans *et al.* 1991; van Swieten *et al.* 1992; Dutch TIA Trial Study Group 1993), although others have failed to confirm this finding (Davalos *et al.* 1988; Dennis *et al.* 1990). Interpretation of these studies is difficult as scans were often performed some time after the clinical event and new and old infarction was not differentiated. A more recent study of TIA patients who had CT scans performed within 48 hours of their clinical event showed that appearances consistent with recent infarction on CT predicted recurrent stroke (OR, 4.06; 95% CI, 1.16–14.14; $p = 0.028$) (Douglas *et al.* 2003), and it has been suggested that the presence of infarction detected by CT scanning after TIA may improve the prediction of early stroke (Sciolla and Melis 2008).

As reviewed in Ch. 10, diffusion-weighted MRI (DWI) is a particularly sensitive (although somewhat non-specific) technique for identifying acute cerebral ischemia. It is, therefore, likely that the presence of abnormalities on DWI in a patient with TIA or minor stroke would suggest an active "vascular process" such as a source of emboli or large artery atheromatous disease and would, therefore, signify a high risk of further thromboembolism and so recurrent stroke (Tong and Caplan 2007). Several studies have indeed demonstrated an association between abnormalities on DWI in the acute phase and the development of further abnormalities (Sylaja *et al.* 2007). However, although DWI technology has been available since the mid 1990s, the association between abnormalities on DWI in patients with TIA and minor stroke and those with recurrent stroke has only recently been demonstrated.

1 month risks

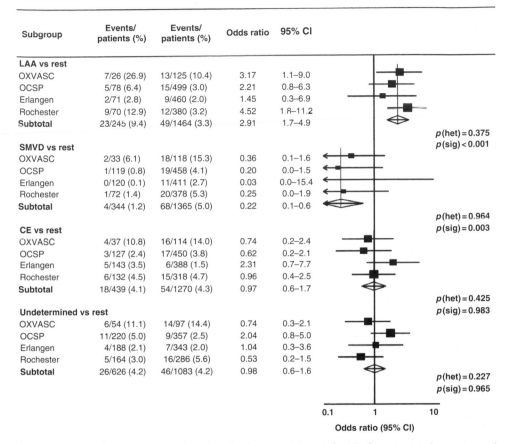

Subgroup	Events/ patients (%)	Events/ patients (%)	Odds ratio	95% CI
LAA vs rest				
OXVASC	7/26 (26.9)	13/125 (10.4)	3.17	1.1–9.0
OCSP	5/78 (6.4)	15/499 (3.0)	2.21	0.8–6.3
Erlangen	2/71 (2.8)	9/460 (2.0)	1.45	0.3–6.9
Rochester	9/70 (12.9)	12/380 (3.2)	4.52	1.8–11.2
Subtotal	23/245 (9.4)	49/1464 (3.3)	2.91	1.7–4.9
				p(het) = 0.375
				p(sig) < 0.001
SMVD vs rest				
OXVASC	2/33 (6.1)	18/118 (15.3)	0.36	0.1–1.6
OCSP	1/119 (0.8)	19/458 (4.1)	0.20	0.0–1.5
Erlangen	0/120 (0.1)	11/411 (2.7)	0.03	0.0–15.4
Rochester	1/72 (1.4)	20/378 (5.3)	0.25	0.0–1.9
Subtotal	4/344 (1.2)	68/1365 (5.0)	0.22	0.1–0.6
				p(het) = 0.964
				p(sig) = 0.003
CE vs rest				
OXVASC	4/37 (10.8)	16/114 (14.0)	0.74	0.2–2.4
OCSP	3/127 (2.4)	17/450 (3.8)	0.62	0.2–2.1
Erlangen	5/143 (3.5)	6/388 (1.5)	2.31	0.7–7.7
Rochester	6/132 (4.5)	15/318 (4.7)	0.96	0.4–2.5
Subtotal	18/439 (4.1)	54/1270 (4.3)	0.97	0.6–1.7
				p(het) = 0.425
				p(sig) = 0.983
Undetermined vs rest				
OXVASC	6/54 (11.1)	14/97 (14.4)	0.74	0.3–2.1
OCSP	11/220 (5.0)	9/357 (2.5)	2.04	0.8–5.0
Erlangen	4/188 (2.1)	7/343 (2.0)	1.04	0.3–3.6
Rochester	5/164 (3.0)	16/286 (5.6)	0.53	0.2–1.5
Subtotal	26/626 (4.2)	46/1083 (4.2)	0.98	0.6–1.6
				p(het) = 0.227
				p(sig) = 0.965

Odds ratio (95% CI)

Fig. 15.3. Meta-analysis of population-based studies showing odds ratios for risk of recurrent stroke at one month according to pathological subtype (Lovett *et al.* 2004a). CI, confidence interval; p (het), p value for heterogeneity between studies; p (sig), p value overall significance of the meta-analysis of comparisons between studies; LAA, large vessel atherosclerotic stroke; SMVD, small vessel disease; CE, cardioembolic stroke. *Sources*: Flossman *et al.* 2006 (OXVASC); Lovett *et al.* 2003 (OCSP); Petty *et al.* 2000 (Rochester study); Kolominsky–Rabas *et al.* 2001 (Erlingen study).

This is partly because of the small size of studies in relation to the patient numbers required to demonstrate such an association, as illustrated by the main studies described below.

In one cohort of 83 consecutive patients with a TIA attending an ED who were scanned with DWI, abnormalities were identified in 27. The combination of DWI abnormalities and symptoms lasting over an hour was found to be predictive of a combined endpoint of stroke or other vascular event (Purroy *et al.* 2004). In another cohort of 120 patients with TIA or minor stroke, all of whom received DWI within 24-hours, the presence of abnormalities on DWI was associated with a higher risk of stroke at 90 days, as was vessel occlusion (Coutts *et al.* 2005). In a further cohort of 87 patients with TIA and 74 with ischemic stroke, the rate of recurrent stroke was highest in the group with TIA and infarction on DWI (Ay *et al.* 2005). Lastly, in a retrospective cohort study of 146 patients with TIA, 37 (25%) had abnormalities on DWI; the presence of these abnormalities was shown to be independently associated with a higher risk of in-hospital recurrent TIA or stroke (OR, 11.2; $p < 0.01$) (Prabhakaran *et al.* 2007).

Although the association between DWI-identified lesions and early risk of stroke is fairly clear, it is uncertain what additional prognostic information over and above the clinical characteristics in the risk scores it provides. Indeed, focal motor weakness, speech disturbance and symptoms lasting longer than one hour are all associated with DWI-detected lesions in patients with TIA (Redgrave *et al.* 2007a, b), while DWI abnormalities are also associated with large vessel disease (Coutts *et al.* 2005). Larger studies are, therefore, needed to address the interplay between the prognostic information available from clinical features and imaging.

Lastly, the presence of solid microembolic signals in the middle cerebral artery detected by transcranial Doppler has been shown to be associated with a high risk of stroke following TIA or minor stroke in patients with recently symptomatic carotid stenosis, although this technique is not readily available in everyday clinical practice. In one study of 73 patients with minor stroke or TIA in whom transcranial Doppler imaging of the symptomatic cerebral artery was performed within seven days, the presence of microembolic signals was a predictor of the early recurrence of ischemia after adjustment for the presence of carotid stenosis, antiplatelet therapy during follow-up and other confounding variables (relative risk, 8.7; 95% CI, 2.0–38.2; $p = 0.0015$) (Valton *et al.* 1998). In another study of 111 subjects with both symptomatic and asymptomatic carotid stenosis > 60%, the presence of microembolic signals was predictive of TIA and stroke risk during follow-up (Molloy and Markus 1999).

The role of perfusion imaging in short-term risk prediction after TIA and minor stroke is uncertain (Latchaw *et al.* 2003).

References

Ay H, Koroshetz WJ, Benner T *et al.* (2005). Transient ischemic attack with infarction: a unique syndrome? *Annals of Neurology* 57:679–686

Benavente O, Eliasziw M, Streifler JY *et al.* (2001). for the NASCET Collaborators: prognosis after transient monocular blindness associated with carotid artery stenosis. *New England Journal of Medicine* 345:1084–1090

Bray JE, Coughlan K, Bladin C (2007). Can the ABCD score be dichotomised to identify high-risk patients with transient ischaemic attack in the emergency department?, *Emergency Medicine Journal* 24:92–95

Calvet D, Lamy C, Touzé E *et al.* (2007). Management and outcome of patients with transient ischemic attack admitted to a stroke unit, *Cerebrovascular Diseases* 24:80–85

Caplan LR (1996). *Posterior Circulation Disease: Clinical Findings, Diagnosis and Management*, pp. 20–1. Boston, MA: Blackwell Science.

Correia M, Silva MR, Magalhaes R, Guimaraes L, Silva MC (2006). Transient ischemic attacks in rural and urban northern Portugal: incidence and short-term prognosis. *Stroke* 37:50–55

Coull AJ, Lovett JK, Rothwell PM for the Oxford Vascular Study (2004). Population based study of early risk of stroke after transient ischaemic attack or minor stroke: implications for public education and organisation of services. *British Medical Journal* 328:326

Coutts SB, Simon JE, Eliasziw M *et al.* (2005). Triaging transient ischemic attack and minor stroke patients using acute magnetic resonance imaging. *Annals of Neurology* 57:848–854

Cucchiara BL, Messe SR, Taylor RA *et al.* (2006). Is the ABCD score useful for risk stratification of patients with acute transient ischemic attack? *Stroke* 37:1710–1714

Davalos A, Matias-Guiu J, Torrent O *et al.* (1988). Computed tomography in reversible ischaemic attacks: clinical and prognostic correlations in a prospective study. *Journal of Neurology* 235:155–158

Dennis M, Bamford J, Sandercock P *et al.* (1990). Computed tomography in patients with transient ischaemic attacks: when is a transient ischaemic attack not a transient ischaemic attack but a stroke? *Journal of Neurology* 237:257–261

Donnan GA, O'Malley HM, Quang L *et al.* (1993). The capsular warning syndrome: pathogenesis and clinical features. *Neurology* 43:957–962

Douglas CD, Johnston CM, Elkins J *et al.* (2003). Head computed tomography findings predict short-term stroke risk after transient ischemic attack. *Stroke* 34:2894–2899

Dutch TIA Trial Study Group (1993). Predictors of major vascular events in patients with a transient ischemic attack or nondisabling stroke: the Dutch TIA Trial Study Group. *Stroke* **24**:527–531

Evans GW, Howard G, Murros KE *et al.* (1991). Cerebral infarction verified by cranial computed tomography and prognosis for survival following transient ischemic attack. *Stroke* **22**:431–436

Fairhead JF, Rothwell PM (2005). The need for urgency in identification and treatment of symptomatic carotid stenosis is already established. *Cerebrovascular Diseases* **19**:355–358

Farrar J, Donnan GA (1993). Capsular warning syndrome preceding pontine infarction. *Stroke* **24**:762

Flossman E, Rothwell PM (2003). Prognosis of vertebrovasilar transient ischaemic attack and minor ischaemic stroke. *Brain* **126**:1940–1954

Flossman E, Touze E, Giles MF *et al.* (2006). The early risk of stroke after vertebrobasilar TIA is higher than after carotid TIA. *Cerebrovascular Diseases* **21**(Suppl 4):6

Giles MF, Rothwell PM (2007). Risk of stroke early after transient ischaemic attack: a systematic review and meta-analysis. *Lancet Neurology* **6**:1063–1072

Giles MF, Rothwell PM (2008). Systematic review and meta-analysis of validations of the ABCD and ABCD^2 scores in prediction of stroke risk after transient ischaemic attack. *Cerebrovascular Diseases*, in press

Gladstone DJ, Kapral MK, Fang J Laupacis A, Tu JV (2004). Management and outcomes of transient ischaemic attacks in Ontario. *Canadian Medical Association Journal CMAJ* **1707**:1099–1104

Gubitz G, Sandercock P (2000). Prevention of ischaemic stroke. *British Medical Journal* **321**:1455–1459

Gubitz G, Phillips S, Dwyer V (1999). What is the cost of admitting patients with transient ischaemic attacks to hospital? *Cerebrovascular Diseases* **9**:210–214

Hankey GJ, Slattery JM, Warlow CP (1991). The prognosis of hospital-referred transient ischaemic attacks. *Journal of Neurology, Neurosurgery Psychiatry* **54**:793–802

Hill MD, Yiannakoulias N, Jeerakathil T *et al.* (2004). The high risk of stroke immediately after transient ischemic attack. A population-based study. *Neurology* **62**:2015–2020

Johnston SC, Gress DR, Browner WS *et al.* (2000). Short-term prognosis after emergency department diagnosis of TIA. *Journal of the American Medical Association* **284**:2901–2906

Johnston SC, Rothwell PM, Nguyen-Huynh MN *et al.* (2007). Validation and refinement of scores to predict very early stroke risk after transient ischaemic attack. *Lancet* **369**:283–292

Kleindorfer D, Panagos P, Pancioli A *et al.* (2005). Incidence and short-term prognosis of transient ischemic attack in a population-based study, *Stroke* **36**:720–723

Kolominsky-Rabas PL, Weber M, Gefeller O, Neundoerfer B, Heuschmann PU (2001). Epidemiology of ischemic stroke subtypes according to TOAST criteria: incidence, recurrence, and long-term survival in ischemic stroke subtypes: a population-based study. *Stroke* **32**:2735–2740

Latchaw RE, Yonas H, Hunter GJ *et al.* (2003). Guidelines and recommendations for perfusion imaging in cerebral ischemia: a scientific statement for healthcare professionals by the Writing Group on Perfusion Imaging, from the Council on Cardiovascular Radiology of the American Heart Association. *Stroke* **34**:1084–1104

Lavallée PC, Mesegaur E, Abboud F *et al.* (2007). A transient ischaemic attack clinic with round-the-clock access (SOS-TIA): Feasibility and effects. *Lancet Neurology* **6**:953–960

Lovett JK, Dennis MS, Sandercock PA *et al.* (2003). Very early risk of stroke after a first transient ischemic attack. *Stroke* **34**:e138–e140

Lovett JK, Coull AJ, Rothwell PM (2004a). Early risk of recurrence by subtype of ischemic stroke in population-based incidence studies. *Neurology* **62**:569–573

Lovett JK, Gallagher PJ, Hands LJ *et al.* (2004b). Histological correlates of carotid plaque surface morphology on lumen contrast imaging. *Circulation* **110**:2190–2197

Marquardt L, Chandratheva A, Geraghty O *et al.* (2008). Population-based study of the frequency of $\geq 50\%$ symptomatic stenosis in vertebrobasilar TIA or minor stroke. *Cerebrovascular Diseases*, in press

Mohr JP, Gautier JC, Pessin MS (1992). Internal carotid artery disease. In *Stroke*, Barnett HJM Mohr JP Stein BM Yatsu FM (eds.), p. 311. New York: Churchill Livingstone

Molloy J, Markus HS (1999). Asymptomatic embolization predicts stroke and TIA risk in patients with carotid artery stenosis. *Stroke* **30**:1440–1443

National Institute for Health and Clinical Excellence (2008). *Stroke: Diagnosis and Initial Management of Acute Stroke and Transient Ischaemic Attack (TIA). Draft Guidance for Consultation.* London: NICE

Petty GW, Brown R-DJ, Whisnant JP et al. (2000). Ischemic stroke subtypes: a population-based study of functional outcome, survival, and recurrence. *Stroke* **31**:1062–1068

Prabhakaran S, Chong JY, Sacco RL (2007). Impact of abnormal diffusion-weighted imaging results on short-term outcome following transient ischemic attack. *Archives of Neurology* **64**:1105–1109

Purroy F, Montaner J, Rovira A et al. (2004). Higher risk of further vascular events among transient ischaemic attack patients with diffusion-weighted imaging acute lesions. *Stroke* **35**:2313–2319

Purroy F, Molina CA, Montaner J, Alvarez-Sabin J (2007). Absence of usefulness of ABCD score in the early risk of stroke of transient ischemic attack patients. *Stroke* **38**:855–856

Rantner B, Pavelka M, Posch L (2005). Carotid endarterectomy after ischemic stroke: is there a justification for delayed surgery? *European Journal of Vascular Endovascular Surgery* **30**:36–40

Redgrave JN, Schulz UG, Briley D et al. (2007a). Presence of acute ischaemic lesions on diffusion-weighted imaging is associated with clinical predictors of early risk of stroke after transient ischaemic attack. *Cerebrovascular Diseases* **24**:86–90

Redgrave JN, Coutts SB, Schulz UG et al. (2007b). Systematic review of associations between the presence of acute ischemic lesions on diffusion-weighted imaging and clinical predictors of early stroke risk after transient ischaemic attack. *Stroke* **38**:1482–1488

Rothwell PM (2003). Incidence, risk factors and prognosis of stroke and transient ischaemic attack: the need for high-quality large-scale epidemiological studies. *Cerebrovascular Diseases* **16**(Suppl 3):2–10

Rothwell PM, Warlow CP (2005). Timing of TIAs preceding stroke: time window for prevention is very short. *Neurology* **64**:817–820

Rothwell PM, Giles MF, Flossmann E et al. (2005). A simple score (ABCD) to identify individuals at high early risk of stroke after transient ischaemic attack. *Lancet* **366**:29–36

Rothwell PM, Giles MF, Chandratheva A on behalf of the Early use of Existing Preventive Strategies for Stroke (EXPRESS) Study (2007). Major reduction in risk of early recurrent stroke by urgent treatment of TIA and minor stroke: EXPRESS Study. *Lancet* **370**:1432–1442

Sciolla R, Melis F for the SINPAC Group (2008). Rapid identification of high-risk transient ischemic attacks: prospective validation of the ABCD score. *Stroke* **39**:297–302

Sivenius J, Riekkinen PJ, Smets P et al. (1991). The European Stroke Prevention Study (ESPS): results by arterial distribution. *Annals of Neurology* **29**:596–600

Sylaja PN, Coutts SB, Subramaniam S for the VISION Study Group (2007). Acute ischemic lesions of varying ages predict risk of ischemic events in stroke/TIA patients. *Neurology* **68**:415–419

Tong DC, Caplan LR (2007). Determining future stroke risk using MRI: new data, new questions. *Neurology* **68**:398–399

Tsivgoulis G, Spengos K, Manta P et al. (2006). Validation of the ABCD score in identifying individuals at high early risk of stroke after a transient ischemic attack: a hospital-based case series study. *Stroke* **37**:2892–2897

Valton L, Larrue V, le Traon AP (1998). Microembolic signals and risk of early recurrence in patients with stroke or transient ischemic attack. *Stroke* **29**:2125–2128

van Swieten JC, Kappelle LJ, Algra A et al. (1992). Hypodensity of cerebral white matter in patients with transient ischaemic attack or minor stroke: influence on the rate of subsequent stroke: Dutch TIA Study Group. *Annals of Neurology* **32**:177–183

Warlow CP, Dennis MS, van Gijn J et al. (2001). *Stroke: A Practical Guide to Management*, Ch. 16: Preventing recurrent stroke and other serious vascular events, pp. 653–722. Oxford: Blackwell

Whitehead MA, McManus J, McAlpine C, Langhorne P (2005). Early recurrence of cerebrovascular events after transient ischaemic attack. *Stroke* **36**:1

Wu CM, McLaughlin K, Lorenzetti DL et al. (2007). Early risk of stroke after transient ischemic attack: a systematic review and meta-analysis. *Archives of Internal Medicine* **167**:2417–2422

Chapter 16

Short-term prognosis after major stroke

The short term prognosis after major stroke depends on stroke subtype (Table 16.1), the occurrence of stroke-associated complications, stroke extension or recurrence. Whilst stroke subtype is fixed, optimal acute stroke treatment can impact on stroke morbidity and mortality through minimizing the likelihood of neurological deterioration and the occurrence of complications such as pulmonary embolus and pneumonia (Ch. 20) as well as through the administration of specific therapies (Ch. 21).

Mortality

The prognosis of hospitalized patients tends to be worse than that of patients in the population at large because mild strokes are more likely to be cared for at home. In the community, about 20% of all patients with first-ever stroke are dead within a month. Deaths in the first few days are almost all caused by the brain lesion itself. Deaths after the first week are more likely to be indirect consequences of the brain lesion, such as bronchopneumonia, pulmonary embolism, coincidental cardiac disease or recurrence.

The prognosis is much better for ischemic stroke overall than for intracranial hemorrhage, with approximately 10% and 50% dying, respectively (Bamford *et al.* 1990; Lovelock *et al.* 2007). Early characteristics predicting death in patients with primary intracerebral hemorrhage are:

- level of consciousness assessed by the Glasgow Coma Scale.
- age.
- volume of hematoma.
- intraventricular extension of hemorrhage.

So far predictive models only apply to a small proportion of patients and are not sufficiently accurate to inform treatment decisions in routine clinical practice. The various subtypes of ischemic stroke have very different outcomes: patients with total anterior circulation infarction (TACI) have just as poor an outcome as those with primary intracerebral hemorrhage (Table 16.1). The best single predictor of early death is impaired consciousness, but many other predictors of survival have been identified (Table 16.2). Many of these variables are inter-related, but prognostic models based on independent variables do not provide much more information than an experienced clinician's estimate (Counsell and Dennis 2001; Counsell *et al.* 2002).

Although stroke onset is usually abrupt, the neurological deficit often worsens over the following minutes, hours and sometimes days. Deterioration may be caused by neurological factors (Table 16.3) or systemic factors (Table 16.4) (Karepov *et al.* 2006) but progressive non-stroke pathologies should also be reconsidered.

Table 16.1. Outcomes at 30 days, six months and one year by ischemic stroke subtype

	Outcome (No. [%])				
	LACI	TACI	PACI	POCI	All
30 Days					
Dead	3 (2)	36 (39)	8 (4)	9 (7)	56 (10)
Dep	49 (36)	52 (56)	73 (39)	40 (31)	214 (39)
Indep	85 (62)	4 (4)	104 (56)	80 (62)	273 (50)
6 Months					
Dead	10 (7)	52 (56)	19 (10)	18 (14)	99 (18)
Dep	36 (26)	36 (39)	64 (34)	23 (18)	159 (29)
Indep	91 (66)	4 (4)	102 (55)	88 (68)	285 (52)
1 Year					
Dead	15 (11)	55 (60)	30 (16)	24 (19)	124 (23)
Dep	39 (28)	33 (36)	52 (29)	26 (19)	150 (28)
Indep	83 (60)	4 (4)	103 (55)	79 (62)	269 (49)

Notes:
LACI, lacunar infarct; TACI, total anterior circulation infarct; PACI, partial anterior circulation infarct; POCI, posterior circulation infarct; Dep, functionally dependent (Rankin 3–5); Indep, functionally independent (Rankin 0–2).
Source: From Bamford et al. (1991).

Table 16.2. Factors predictive of early death after major stroke

	Factors
Demographic factors	Increasing age
	Male sex
Previous medical/social history	Myocardial infarction
	TIA or stroke
	Diabetes
	Atrial fibrillation
	Pre-stroke handicap
Clinical features at presentation	Reduced level of consciousness
	Fever
	High or low blood pressure
	Severe motor deficit
Investigation results	High plasma glucose
	High white blood cell count
	Visible infarction on brain imaging
	Large stroke lesion on brain imaging (hematoma or infarction)
	Intraventricular blood

Table 16.3. Neurological causes of deterioration after stroke

	Ischemic stroke	Primary intracerebral hemorrhage
Hemorrhagic transformation	+	–
Cerebral edema	+	(+)
Brain shift (mass effect)	+	+
"Vasospasm"	–	–
Thrombus propagation	+	–
Recurrent embolism	+	–
Hemorrhage growth/recurrence	–	+
Hydrocephalus	(+)	+
Epileptic seizures	+	+

Table 16.4. Systemic causes of neurological deterioration after stroke

Factor	Sequelae
Hypoxia	Pneumonia
	Pulmonary embolism
	Cardiac failure
	Chronic respiratory disease
Hypotension	Pulmonary embolism
	Cardiac failure
	Cardiac arrhythmia
	Pneumonia
	Dehydration
	Septicemia
	Hypotensive drugs/vasodilators
	Bleeding peptic ulcer
Infection and fever	Pneumonia
	Urinary tract infection
	Septicemia
Others	Water and electrolyte imbalance
	Hypo/hyperglycemia
	Depression
	Sedative/hypnotic drugs
	Anticonvulsant drugs

Disability and dependency

Nearly all patients who do not die as a result of their stroke recover to some extent. The mechanisms of recovery are discussed further in Ch. 23. Table 16.1 shows the numbers of patients with ischemic stroke who are functionally dependent at 30 days, six months and

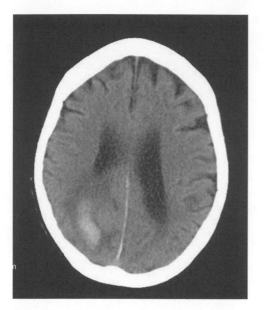

Fig. 16.1. A CT brain scan of a patient with stroke taken on day three after onset, illustrating the difficulty of distinguishing between primary intracerebral hemorrhage and hemorrhagic transformation of an infarct.

one year by subtype of ischemic stroke. The prognosis is poorest for those with TACI, with high rates of dependency and best for those with a posterior circulation infarct. Patients with a lacunar infarct have lower rates of dependency than those with TACI but within this group there is wide variation in outcome, with some patients remaining severely disabled. Rates of dependency are high overall for hemorrhagic stroke, but some of these patients do well. At present, it is difficult to predict outcome in an individual patient and models using clinical criteria appear as good (or bad) as any other methods including brain imaging (Ch. 23).

Early deterioration after ischemic stroke: neurological factors

Very early worsening after stroke is more likely to be caused by neurological factors than systemic ones. The mechanism of worsening may not be clear in an individual patient and is likely to be the result of complex interactions between hemodynamic and other physiological factors. High or low blood pressure, diabetes, coronary heart disease, early CT signs of infarction and middle cerebral artery occlusion have all been associated with increased risk of early deterioration after stroke.

Hemorrhage into cerebral infarcts or hemorrhagic transformation

At autopsy, spontaneous petechial hemorrhages are very common in infarcts. During life they are seen on brain CT in around 15% of patients in the absence of thrombolytic therapy (Fig. 16.1). However incidence rates must be considered in the context of the timing and mode of imaging, the definition of clinically significant hemorrhagic transformation and the fact that there is interobserver variability in identifying hemorrhage (Khatri *et al.* 2007). Hemorrhagic transformation is said to be more common in cardioembolic infarcts, particularly when associated with infective endocarditis (Alexandrov *et al.* 1997), perhaps because the infarcts are often large and patients are frequently receiving anticoagulation therapy (Ch. 6). Hemorrhagic transformation is not often symptomatic unless there is confluent hematoma (Larrue *et al.* 1997; Berger *et al.* 2001).

Hemorrhagic transformation is of particular interest in acute stroke therapy since thrombolysis is associated with increased risk (Khatri *et al.* 2007). Other factors increasing risk of hemorrhagic transformation include heparin use (International Stroke Trial Collaborative Group 1997), edema or mass effect, stroke severity and age (Kent *et al.* 2001; Khatri *et al.* 2007); possibly other risk factors include hyperglycemia, timing of thrombolytic therapy and successful recanalization. Thrombolytic therapy three hours or more after stroke onset and late spontaneous recanalization are associated with high rates of hemorrhage (Molina *et al.* 2001).

Microvascular damage leading to loss of vessel wall integrity is thought to be the cause of hemorrhage into an infarct. The mechanisms for this include plasmin-generated laminin degradation, matrix metalloproteinase activation and transmigration of leukocytes through the vessel wall (Lapchak 2002; Wang *et al.* 2004). It has been suggested that use of tissue plasminogen activator may increase the risk of hemorrhagic transformation not just by reperfusion but also through a direct effect on the molecular processes leading to vessel damage (Wang *et al.* 2004).

Peri-infarct edema
Peri-infarct edema reduces local cerebral blood flow and causes brain shift and herniation, the last being the most common "neurological" cause of death. This complication is a common explanation for worsening over the first few days and can often be detected by CT scan. Intravenous mannitol may reduce the deficit for a while but is unlikely to have a major impact on outcome. Recently, surgical decompression using hemicraniectomy has been shown to improve survival, with satisfactory functional outcome in many patients (Ch. 21).

Propagating thrombosis
Propagating thrombosis proximal or distal to a thrombotic, embolic or any other type of occlusion, or within collateral vessels, is often assumed to explain neurological deterioration if other causes have been excluded. However direct evidence is almost impossible to obtain, except perhaps with transcranial Doppler.

Recurrent embolization
In theory, recurrent embolization may cause deterioration. However, the distinction between propagating thrombosis and embolization is very difficult. There is only anecdotal evidence that full anticoagulation with intravenous heparin slows progression and improves outcome if no other cause of deterioration is evident (Slivka *et al.* 1989).

Epileptic seizures
Partial or generalized epileptic seizures occur for the first time in about 2% of those with acute strokes at around the time of onset, rising to approximately 10% at five years, more with large cortical infarcts or intracranial hemorrhage (Ch. 9) (Ferro and Pinto 2004). Seizures are more common with large strokes, especially if hemorrhagic, and with cortical as opposed to lacunar strokes. Cerebrovascular disease is the most common cause of epilepsy in the elderly, and late-onset epilepsy is a predictor of subsequent stroke (Cleary *et al.* 2004). Seizures may cause neurological deterioration or be mistaken for recurrent stroke. Intractable recurrent seizures are distinctly unusual.

Early deterioration after ischemic stroke: systemic factors
Systemic factors commonly causing deterioration after stroke are shown in Table 16.4 (Ch. 20). Systemic illness usually becomes important from two days or so after stroke onset. A history and careful general examination should reveal features such as confusion, shortness of breath, cough, hypoxia or leg swelling. Simple investigations including full blood count, inflammatory markers, renal function, blood cultures, urine examination and chest X-ray will usually be required to confirm a coexistent medical disorder. Close monitoring of patients with stroke, ideally on a stroke unit, should aim to enable rapid diagnosis of coexistent medical conditions so that treatment can be instituted (Ch. 20) and deterioration prevented.

It is important to note that systemic illness will make a given neurological syndrome worse: a patient with a lacunar infarction may become drowsy and confused such that the clinical features are more consistent with a TACI. This may result in a falsely pessimistic prognosis being given to the patient and family.

References

Alexandrov AV, Black SE, Ehrlich LE *et al.* (1997). Predictors of hemorrhagic transformation occurring spontaneously and on anticoagulants in patients with acute ischemic stroke. *Stroke* **28**:1198–1202

Bamford J, Sandercock PAG, Dennis M *et al.* (1990). A prospective study of acute cerebrovascular disease in the community: the Oxfordshire Community Stroke Project 1981–86. 2. Incidence, case fatality rates and overall outcome at one year of cerebral infarction, primary intracerebral and subarachnoid haemorrhage. *Journal of Neurology, Neurosurgery and Psychiatry* **53**:16–22

Bamford J, Sandercock P, Dennis M *et al.* (1991). Classification and natural history of clinically identifiable subtypes of cerebral infarction. *Lancet* **337**:1521–1526.

Berger C, Fiorelli M, Steiner T *et al.* (2001). Hemorrhagic transformation of ischemic brain tissue: asymptomatic or symptomatic? *Stroke* **32**:1330–1335

Cleary P, Shorvon S, Tallis R (2004). Late-onset seizures as a predictor of subsequent stroke. *Lancet* **363**:1184–1186

Counsell, Dennis M (2001). Systematic review of prognostic models in patients with acute stroke. *Cerebrovascular Diseases* **12**:159–170

Counsell C, Dennis M, McDowall M *et al.* (2002). Predicting outcome after acute and subacute stroke: development and validation of new prognostic models. *Stroke* **33**:1041–1047

Ferro JM, Pinto F (2004). Poststroke epilepsy: epidemiology pathophysiology and management. *Drugs and Aging* **21**:639–653

International Stroke Trial Collaborative Group (1997). The International Stroke Trial (IST): a randomised trial of aspirin subcutaneous heparin both or neither among 19435 patients with acute ischaemic stroke. *Lancet* **349**:1569–1581

Karepov VG, Gur AY, Bova I *et al.* (2006). Stroke-in-evolution: infarct-inherent mechanisms versus systemic causes. *Cerebrovascular Diseases* **21**:42–46

Kent TA, Soukup VM, Fabian RH (2001). Heterogeneity affecting outcome from acute stroke therapy: making reperfusion worse. *Stroke* **32**:2318–2327

Khatri P, Wechsler LR, Broderick JP (2007). Intracranial hemorrhage associated with revascularization therapies. *Stroke* **38**:431–440

Lapchak PA (2002). Hemorrhagic transformation following ischemic stroke: significance causes and relationship to therapy and treatment. *Current Neurology and Neuroscience Reports* **2**:38–43

Larrue V, von Kummer R, del Zoppo G *et al.* (1997). Haemorrhagic transformation in acute ischemic stroke. Potential contributing factors in the European Cooperative Acute Stroke Study. *Stroke* **28**:957–960

Lovelock CE, Molyneux AJ, Rothwell PM *et al.* (2007). Change in incidence and aetiology of intracerebral haemorrhage in Oxfordshire, UK, between 1981 and 2006: a population-based study. *Lancet Neurology* **6**:487–493

Molina CA, Montaner J, Abilleira S *et al.* (2001). Timing of spontaneous recanalization and risk of hemorrhagic transformation in acute cardioembolic stroke. *Stroke* **32**:1079–1084

Slivka A, Levy D, Lapinski RH (1989). Risk associated with heparin withdrawal in ischaemic cerebrovascular disease. *Journal of Neurology, Neurosurgery and Psychiatry* **52**:1332–1336

Wang X, Tsuji K, Lee SR *et al.* (2004). Mechanisms of hemorrhagic transformation after tissue plasminogen activator reperfusion therapy for ischemic stroke. *Stroke* **35**:2726–2730

Wardlaw JM, Lewis SC, Dennis MS *et al.* (1998). Is visible infarction on computed tomography associated with an adverse prognosis in acute ischaemic stroke? *Stroke* **29**:1315–1319

Long-term prognosis after transient ischemic attack and stroke

In the same way that data on the short-term risk of stroke following TIA are essential for informing the early management of patients, data on the medium-term (one to five years) and long-term (five years and beyond) prognosis are required to counsel patients and direct secondary prevention.

Medium- and long-term stroke risks after a transient ischemic attack

Many studies have addressed the question of medium-term prognosis after TIA, but because the condition is heterogeneous and patients have been recruited in a number of different clinical settings, the findings have been difficult to interpret. For example, in 1991, a paper critically reviewed all studies after 1950 of the prognosis after TIA that included over 50 patients and were published in English (Kernan *et al.* 1991). Eligible studies were tested against six key quality methodological principles:

- specified diagnostic criteria and procedures
- "inception cohort" by inclusion of all patients at a specified time after the event (ideally as soon as possible after TIA)
- appropriate endpoints
- adequate description of endpoint surveillance
- adequate reporting and analysis of censored patients
- multivariate analysis of predictive variables.

A total of 60 eligible papers were identified: 22 were observational studies of patients receiving specific treatment; 32 were observational studies, not based on specific treatments; 6 were randomized controlled trials. No studies adhered to all six methodological principles. When the principles were "relaxed" to include only an inception cohort with adequate reporting and analysis of censored patients and appropriate endpoints, only two reports met these criteria, both from the Oxfordshire Community Stroke Project (OCSP: 184 patients, follow-up over 3.7 years) (Dennis *et al.* 1989, 1990).

Since the above review, two further high-quality, prospective, population-based studies of the medium-term prognosis of TIA have been published, one from Söderhamn, Sweden (97 patients, follow-up over three years) (Terent 1990) and the other from Perugia, Italy (94 patients, follow-up over nine years) (Ricci *et al.* 1998). The mean age of patients in all three cohorts was 69 years.

In the Söderhamn cohort, the risk of stroke was approximately 5% per year and the overall mortality was 24.7% over a mean of three years (Terent 1990). No data were reported on cardiovascular morbidity or mortality. In the Perugia cohort, the annual risk of stroke after TIA was 2.4% (95% confidence interval [CI] 0.7–4.7) (Ricci *et al.* 1998). The actuarial risk of death was 28.6% (95% CI, 19.2–37.8) at five years and 49.5% (95% CI,

38.9–60.0) at 10 years, with roughly equal numbers of cerebrovascular, cardiovascular and non-vascular deaths. In OCSP, the annual stroke risk was 4.4% (95% CI, 5.0–7.3) although this was "front-loaded" – being highest in the first year after initial TIA (Dennis *et al.* 1990). The risk of death at five years was 31.3% (95% CI, 23.3–39.3) and the annual risk of death was 6.3% (95% CI, 4.7–7.9). Again, there were roughly equal numbers of cerebrovascular, cardiovascular and non-vascular deaths. The risk of either fatal or non-fatal myocardial infarction was 12.1% (95% CI, 5.8–18.4) at five years and the approximate annual risk was 2.4%.

There are similarly few high-quality prospective hospital-based cohort studies of the medium-term prognosis of TIA (Hankey 2003). Of the four main studies that recruited patients with TIA from hospital as opposed to population-based recruitment, the mean age tended to be younger owing to referral bias, with elderly patients being less likely to be referred to secondary care services (Heyman *et al.* 1984; Hankey *et al.* 1991; Carolei *et al.* 1992; Howard *et al.* 1994). However, in these studies, the annual rate of stroke was 2.2–5.0% over four to five years, which is similar to the risk of myocardial infarction (1.1–4.6%) over the same period. Of note in these studies is the high early risk of stroke measured when patients are recruited very early after the event, which falls after a year or so, in contrast to a steady background risk of acute coronary disease (Hankey *et al.* 1991). It has been argued that the early risk of stroke reflects an active, unstable plaque, which heals with time, while the risk of coronary disease reflects the underlying "athermanous burden" (Hankey 2003).

These studies indicate that, the risk of stroke and other vascular events is appreciable in the medium term, but a question that has recently been addressed is the vascular risk in the longer term and whether there is a need for ongoing aggressive secondary prevention. Only two studies provide reliable data on prognosis up to 15 years after a TIA.

The first study examined the long-term vascular risk starting some time after the initial TIA (Clark *et al.* 2003). The study comprised 290 patients with TIA, diagnosed by a neurologist, who had participated either in OCSP (Dennis *et al.* 1990) or a contemporaneous hospital-referred cohort study (Hankey *et al.* 1991). Patients were followed up over a 10-year period starting in 1988, a median time of 3.8 years (interquartile range, 2.2–5.8) after their most recent TIA. Mean age at baseline was 69 years. At the end of the 10-year follow-up, the risk of stroke was 18.8% (95% CI, 13.6–23.7); the risk of myocardial infarction or death from coronary heart disease was 27.8% (95% CI, 21.8–33.3), and risk of death from any cause was 50.7% (95% CI not given) (Fig. 17.1). The risk of any first stroke, myocardial infarction or vascular death was 42.8% (95% CI, 36.4–48.5). Compared with the rates in the general population standardized for age and sex, only the rate of fatal coronary events was significantly higher than expected (standardized mortality ratio 1.47; 95% CI, 1.10–1.93; $p = 0.009$). The risk of major vascular events was found to be constant throughout the follow-up.

The Life Long After Cerebral Ischemia (LILAC) study reported near complete follow-up on 2473 participants from the Dutch TIA Trial (van Wijk *et al.* 2005). Mean age was 65 years and 759 had a TIA while the remainder suffered a minor stroke (defined as a score on the modified Rankin scale ≤ 3) at enrolment. The trial recruited patients between 1986 and 1989, all of whom were assessed by a neurologist and randomized to two different dosages of aspirin. After a mean follow-up of 10.1 years, 1489 (60%) had died and 1336 (54%) had suffered at least one vascular event. At 10 years, the cumulative risk of recurrent stroke was 18.4% (95% CI, 16.7–20.1), of first major vascular event was 44.1% (95% CI, 42.0–46.1) and of death was 46.6% (95% CI, 44.2–51.3). The corresponding figures for those presenting with TIA at inception (as opposed to minor stroke) were 35.8% (95% CI, 32.3–39.3) for first vascular event and 34.1% (95% CI, 30.7–37.4) for death. The 10-year risk of stroke

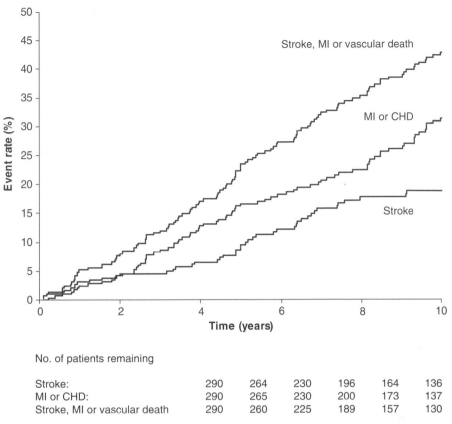

Fig. 17.1. Kaplan–Meier event rates for any stroke, any myocardial infarction (MI) or death from coronary heart disease (CHD), and any stroke, MI or vascular death in a cohort of 290 patients with transient ischemic attack (Clark *et al.* 2003).

for patients with TIA was not reported. Importantly, because of the inclusion criteria of the original trial, only 22% of patients were randomized within a week of the initial vascular event (median time to randomization was 18 days), so much of the very high acute risk described above was missed from these estimates.

These studies both reveal a high vascular risk compared with the "normal population," with this risk continuing up to 10 or 15 years and probably beyond following TIA. They, therefore, support the ongoing use of secondary preventive medication.

Medium- and long-term stroke risks after stroke

The risks of stroke, other acute vascular events and death after stroke have been studied in six population-based cohorts over a follow-up period of five or more years (Scmidt *et al.* 1988; Burn *et al.* 1994; Hankey *et al.* 2000; Petty *et al.* 2000; Brønnum-Hansen *et al.* 2001; Hartmann *et al.* 2001). Two of these studies included ischemic stroke only (Petty *et al.* 2000; Hartmann *et al.* 2001) and the remaining four included both ischemic and hemorrhagic stroke. One study included incident and recurrent events (Brønnum-Hansen *et al.* 2001) and the remaining five included incident stroke only. The risks of death at five years varied between 41% and 72%, while the proportion of deaths caused by acute coronary disease and stroke (either inception event or recurrent stroke) were similar. As in the TIA outcome

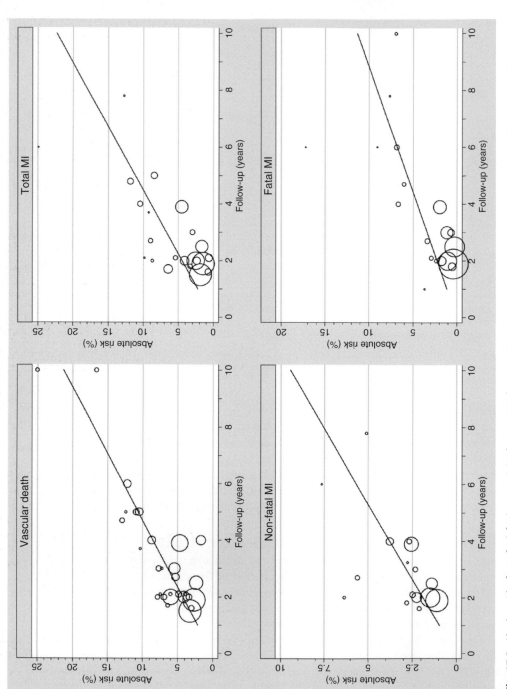

Fig. 17.2. Absolute risk of non-fatal, fatal myocardial infarction (MI), all MI and any vascular death plotted against mean follow-up with fitted regression lines obtained through weighted meta-regressions from a systematic review of 39 studies reporting relevant risks in patients with transient ischemic attack and ischemic stroke. Each circle

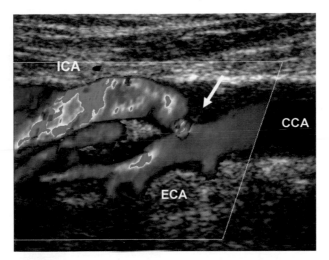

Fig. 12.3. A color-flow Doppler ultrasound of the carotid bifurcation showing a plaque (arrow) at the origin of the internal carotid artery (ICA) and the resulting stenosis. ECA, external carotid artery; CCA, common carotid artery.

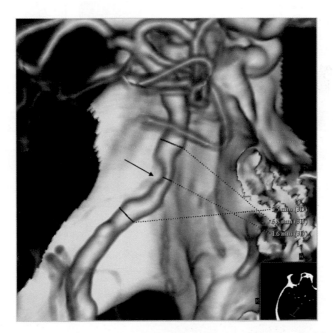

Fig. 12.4. A CT angiogram three-dimensional reconstruction showing a stenosis (arrow) of the distal vertebral artery.

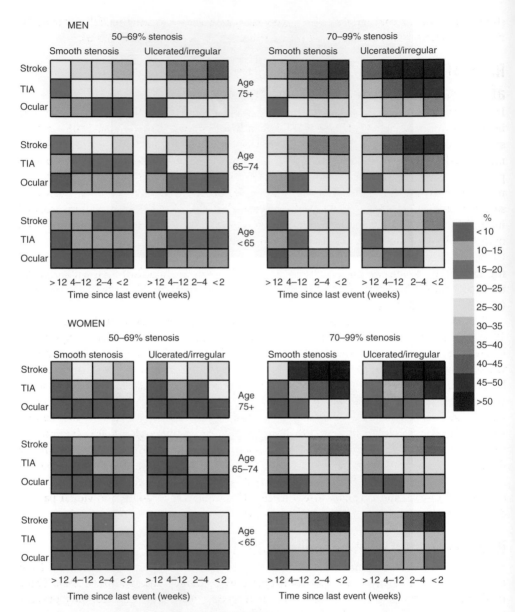

Fig. 27.8. A risk table for the five-year risk of ipsilateral ischemic stroke in patients with recently symptomatic carotid stenosis on medical treatment derived from the ECST model. European Carotid Surgery Trial (ECST) method. TIA, transient ischemic attack.

studies, the risk of stroke tended to be highest early after the event and then fell, whereas the risk of coronary events was constant over the follow-up period (Hankey 2003).

Risks of myocardial infarction and vascular death after transient ischemic attack and stroke

In a recent systematic review and meta-analysis of studies of the risk of myocardial infarction and vascular death after TIA and ischemic stroke (Touzé *et al.* 2005), cohort studies including over 100 patients with TIA or ischemic stroke and reporting risks of myocardial infarction or non-stroke vascular death over at least one year of follow-up published between 1980 and 2005 were identified. The analysis included 39 studies reporting outcomes in 65 996 patients. The ranges of annual risks reported in individual studies were 0.4% to 3.8% for non-stroke vascular death, 0.5% to 4.7% for total myocardial infarction, 0.4% to 3.2% for non-fatal myocardial infarction and 0.2% to 3.7% for fatal myocardial infarction. The annual risks obtained through meta-regression were 2.1% (95% CI, 1.9–2.4) for non-stroke vascular death (29 studies), 2.2% (95% CI, 1.7–2.7) for total myocardial infarction (22 studies), 0.9% (95% CI, 0.7–1.2) for non-fatal myocardial infarction (16 studies), and 1.1% (95% CI, 0.8–1.5) for fatal myocardial infarction (19 studies) (Touzé *et al.* 2005) (Fig. 17.2).

The risk of non-stroke vascular death was lower in studies that enrolled patients after 1990 than in those that enrolled patients before 1990. However, there was no significant heterogeneity in the risk of non-fatal, fatal and total myocardial infarction or non-stroke vascular death according to the other baseline study characteristics, including population-based studies versus randomized controlled trials and mean age of the cohort under 65 years versus more than 65 years. Perhaps surprisingly, the risks of myocardial infarction and non-stroke vascular death were similar in studies of patients with TIA or stroke caused specifically by atherosclerosis as in other studies. However, although several observations would support an association between stroke related to atherosclerosis and coronary artery disease, particularly the positive correlation between carotid, vertebral and coronary vascular disease (Mathur *et al.* 1963; Solberg *et al.* 1968) and the correlation between asymptomatic carotid disease and coronary artery disease (Joakimsen *et al.* 2000), individual patient data were lacking to study this association in full.

Risk prediction in the medium and long term

Several published models have addressed risk prediction in the medium and long term following TIA but many have methodological flaws (Hankey and Warlow 1994). Three models that have been proposed for use in the targeting of longer-term secondary prevention for patients after initial TIA are reviewed below (Table 17.1).

The first was derived from a cohort of 451 patients consecutively admitted to a hospital in North Carolina, USA, between 1977 and 1983 and predicts survival at one and five years (Howard *et al.* 1987). Using regression modeling to identify independent risk factors, age over 60 years, carotid territory TIA, cigarette smoking, previous contralateral stroke, ischemic heart disease and diabetes mellitus were found to predict an increased risk of death. On internal validation, patients under 60 years of age with none of the above risk factors had a five-year survival of over 95%, while patients over 60 years of age with all of these risk factors had a five-year survival of less than 25%.

Hankey and colleagues (1992) studied 469 patients referred to hospital in Oxfordshire, UK, with TIA between 1976 and 1986 and used regression modeling to identify

Table 17.1. Comparison of variables used in different prognostic models for medium- to long-term outcome after transient ischemic attack and stroke in the Hankey, Kernan (SPI-II) and Howard models

Risk factor	Model (outcome of interest)		
	Hankey (stroke)	Kernan (stroke or death)	Howard (death)
Demographic			
Increasing age	+	+	+
Previous medical history			
Cerebrovascular disease	+ (multiple TIAs)	+ (stroke)	+ (stroke)
Ischemic heart disease	–	+	+
Congestive cardiac failure	–	+	–
Left ventricular failure	+	–	–
Peripheral vascular disease	+	–	–
Diabetes	–	+	+
Hypertension	–	+	–
Smoking	–	–	+
Event			
Territory	TIA of brain (versus eye)	–	Anterior versus posterior
		–	

Note:
TIA, transient ischemic attack.
Sources: From Hankey *et al.* (1992), Kernan *et al.* (2000) and Howard *et al.* (1987).

independent risk factors for stroke, coronary events and the combination of stroke, myocardial infarction or vascular death at one and five years. Risk factors for stroke were an increasing number of TIAs in the three months before presentation, increasing age, peripheral vascular disease, left ventricular hypertrophy and TIAs of the brain (compared with the eye). The contribution of each of these factors was weighted and combined in mathematical equations to predict relative and absolute risks for each endpoint at one and five years.

The Stroke Prognosis Instrument II (SPI-II) is a simple score for predicting risk of stroke or death within two years after TIA or non-disabling stroke (Kernan *et al.* 2000). It was derived in 525 patients participating in the Women's Estrogen for Stroke Trial (WEST) and validated in three other cohorts. Multivariate analysis was used to identify independent risk factors for stroke and death and these were then combined into a risk score: congestive heart failure (3 points), diabetes (3 points), prior stroke (3 points), age >70 years (2 points), stroke for the index event (as opposed to TIA) (2 points), hypertension (1 point), and coronary artery disease (1 point). Risk groups I, II and III contained patients with 0 – 3, 4 – 7 and 8 – 15 points, respectively. On testing in pooled data from the validation cohorts, rates of stroke or death at two years were 10%, 19% and 31%, respectively, for each of the different risk groups. In receiver operator characteristic analysis, the area under the curve was 0.63 (95% CI, 0.62–0.65).

From these studies, it appears that the medium- and long-term prognosis after TIA is more dependent on underlying vascular risk factors than characteristics of the event itself,

Table 17.2. Independent predictors of long-term vascular event risk in 2362 individuals with transient ischemic attack[a] or minor stroke

Risk factor	Hazard ratio (95% CI)		
	Model 1	Model 2	Model 3
Demographic characteristics			
Male	1·42 (1·26–1·60)	1·40 (1·25–1·58)	1·38 (1·22–1·56)
Age[b]	1·06 (1·05–1·06)	1·06 (1·05–1·06)	1·05 (1·05–1·06)
History			
Myocardial infarction	1·13 (1·05–1·22)	1·14 (1·06–1·23)	1·11 (1·02–1·21)
Intermittent claudication	1·68 (1·34–2·10)	1·73 (1·38–2·16)	1·77 (1·42–2·19)
Diabetes	2·19 (1·84–2·61)	2·11 (1·77–2·51)	2·05 (1·72–2·44)
Hypertension	1·12 (1·05–1·20)	1·11 (1·04–1·19)	1·09 (1·02–1·17)
Peripheral vascular surgery	1·39 (0·96–2·01)	1·39 (0·96–2·02)	–
Event characteristics			
Minor stroke versus TIA	–	1·22 (1·07–1·40)	1·14 (0·99–1·30)
Vertigo	–	0·75 (0·62–0·90)	0·77 (0·64–0·93)
Amaurosis fugax	–	0·71 (0·49–1·02)	–
Dysarthria	–	1·10 (0·97–1·25)	1·13 (1·00–1·28)
CT brain scan			
White matter lesions	–	–	1·42 (1·22–1·66)
Any infarct	–	–	1·28 (1·14–1·44)
12-lead ECG			
Q wave on ECG	–	–	1·38 (1·20–1·60)
Negative T wave	–	–	1·19 (1·00–1·42)
ST depression	–	–	1·15 (0·96–1·39)
AUC-ROC	0·70 (0·68–0·72)	0·70 (0·68–0·72)	0·72 (0·70–0·74)

Notes:
CI, confidence interval; TIA, transient ischemic attack; CT, computed tomography; ECG, electrocardiography; AUC-ROC, area under the curve of the received operator characteristic.
[a]Model 1 includes baseline risk factor and demographic data; model 2 incorporates event characteristics, and model 3 adds investigation results. Note that the simplest model has very similar discriminatory power, as measured by the AUC-ROC, as the more complex models.
[b]Age was entered as a continuous variable; the increase in hazard is for every incremental year.
Source: From van Wijk *et al.* (2005).

in contrast to the prognosis in the short term. This observation is supported by independent predictors of vascular risk and modeling as reported in the LILAC study, in which models of increasing complexity were devised to predict longer-term risk (van Wijk *et al.* 2005) (Table 17.2). It is noteworthy that the predictive power of each model, as measured by the area and the curve for the receiver operator characteristic, is only minimally improved compared with model 1 (based on established demographics and vascular risk factors) first by the inclusion of clinical characteristics in model 2 and second by the inclusion of CT and electrocardiology findings in model 3.

Although intracerebral hemorrhage is rare, it is a potentially devastating condition. Patients with TIA are unlikely to be at much higher short-term risk of intracranial hemorrhage than age- and sex-matched controls, unlike patients with ischemic stroke, in whom hemorrhagic transformation of an ischemic lesion is more likely. Recent analysis of data from 12 648 individuals with TIA or minor stroke from the Cerebrovascular Cohort Studies Collaboration showed that the incidence of intracranial hemorrhage was 1% over a five-year follow-up after the event (Ariesen *et al.* 2006). Independent risk factors for intracranial hemorrhage were age (> 60 years; hazard ratio [HR], 2.07), blood glucose level (> 7 mmol/l; HR, 1.33), systolic blood pressure (> 140 mmHg; HR, 2.17) and antihypertensive drugs (HR, 1.53). In addition, the Stroke Prevention in Reversible Ischemia Trial (SPIRIT) identified the presence of leukoariosis as a risk factor for intracranial hemorrhage in patients receiving anticoagulation (Stroke Prevention in Reversible Ischemia Trial (SPIRIT) Study Group 1997).

Risk prediction in specific circumstances

Risk prediction in specific conditions following stroke or TIA using modeling is helpful in targeting secondary preventive treatments that might themselves be associated with benefit and harm. Models can provide data on the risk for a specific patient, which can then more reliably inform the risk – benefit ratio for that individual and guide decision making about treatment. Risk models have been developed in symptomatic carotid disease (Ch. 27) and atrial fibrillation (Ch. 14) and these will be discussed below.

Symptomatic carotid stenosis

The risk models described above were derived and validated in populations with a low prevalence of symptomatic carotid disease and, therefore, did not include the degree of carotid stenosis. Given the importance of carotid stenosis in determining the risk of stroke in patients with recently symptomatic carotid disease, models are required for use in this specific clinical situation. This is particularly important because the treatment for carotid stenosis, carotid endarterectomy, itself has important risks associated with it. Risk models have, therefore, been derived to predict the risks associated with medical and surgical treatment in patients with carotid stenosis in order to inform decision making surrounding treatment options.

Risk prediction in carotid stenosis is more fully discussed in Ch. 27.

Atrial fibrillation

Atrial fibrillation is a well-recognized risk factor for TIA and stroke, and many studies have identified independent prognostic factors for stroke in all patients with non-rheumatic atrial fibrillation (NRAF), irrespective of previous cerebrovascular disease (Stroke Prevention in Atrial Fibrillation Investigators 1992a, b; Atrial Fibrillation Investigators 1994). The CHADS2 score has been derived and validated to predict the risk of stroke for patients with atrial fibrillation and includes previous cerebrovascular disease as one of the independent risk factors (Gage *et al.* 2001) (Ch. 2).

However, there is only one report specifically on which patients with a previous TIA or stroke and NRAF are at high (and low) risk, based on 375 patients with NRAF and TIA or non-disabling stroke treated in the placebo arm of the European Atrial Fibrillation Trial (van Latum *et al.* 1995). Independent risk factors for vascular death, stroke and other major vascular events included increasing age, previous thromboembolism, ischemic heart disease, enlarged cardiothoracic ratio on chest radiograph, systolic blood pressure > 160 mmHg at study entry, NRAF for more than one year and presence of an ischemic lesion on CT scan. There are no corresponding studies of predictors of risk in patients with previous TIA or stroke and NRAF who are treated with anticoagulation. However, as mentioned above, the SPIRIT trial identified the presence of leukoariosis as a risk factor for intracranial hemorrhage in patients receiving anticoagulation (Stroke Prevention in Reversible Ischemia Trial [SPIRIT] Study Group 1997), while a recent systematic review of anticoagulation-related bleeding complications in patients with atrial fibrillation irrespective of previous cerebrovascular disease identified advanced age, uncontrolled hypertension, history of ischemic heart disease, cerebrovascular disease, anemia or bleeding and the concomitant use of antiplatelet agents as independently predictive (Hughes and Lip 2007).

References

Ariesen MJ, Algra A, Warlow CP et al. (2006). Predictors of risk of intracerebral haemorrhage in patients with a history of TIA or minor ischaemic stroke. *Journal of Neurology, Neurosurgery and Psychiatry* 77:92–94

Atrial Fibrillation Investigators (1994). Risk factors for stroke and efficacy of antithrombotic therapy in atrial fibrillation: analysis of pooled data from five randomized controlled trials. *Archives of International Medicine* 154:1449–1457

Brønnum-Hansen H, Davidsen M, Thorvaldsen P et al. (2001). Long-term survival and causes of death after stroke. *Stroke* 32:2131–2136

Burn J, Dennis M, Bamford J et al. (1994). Long-term risk of recurrent stroke after a first-ever stroke. The Oxfordshire Community Stroke Project. *Stroke* 25:333–337

Carolei A, Candelise L, Fiorelli M et al. (1992). Long-term prognosis of transient ischemic attacks and reversible ischemic neurologic deficits: A hospital-based study. *Cerebrovascular Diseases* 2:266–272

Clark TG, Murphy MFG, Rothwell PM (2003). Long term risks of stroke, myocardial infarction, and vascular death in "low risk" patients with a non-recent transient ischaemic attack. *Journal of Neurology, Neurosurgery and Psychiatry* 74:577–580

Dennis MS, Bamford JM, Sandercock PAG et al. (1989). Incidence of transient ischemic attacks in Oxfordshire, England. *Stroke* 20:333–339

Dennis MS, Bamford J, Sandercock P et al. (1990). Prognosis of transient ischemic attacks in the Oxfordshire Community Stroke Project. *Stroke* 21:848–853

European Carotid Surgery Trialists' Collaborative Group (1991). MRC European Carotid Surgery Trial. Interim results for symptomatic patients with severe (70–99%) or with mild (0–29%) carotid stenosis. *Lancet* 337:1235–1243

Gage BF, Waterman AD, Shannon W et al. (2001). Validation of clinical classification schemes for predicting stroke: results from the National Registry of Atrial Fibrillation. *Journal of the American Medical Association* 285:2864–2870

Hankey GJ (1991). Isolated angiitis/angiopathy of the central nervous system. *Cerebrovascular Diseases* 1:2–15

Hankey GJ (2003). Long term outcome after ischaemic stroke/transient ischaemic attack. *Cerebrovascular Diseases* 16(Suppl 1):14–19

Hankey GJ, Warlow CP (1994). *Major Problems in Neurology*, Vol. 27: *Transient Ischaemic Attacks of the Brain and Eye.* London: Saunders

Hankey GJ, Slattery JM, Warlow CP (1991). The prognosis of hospital-referred transient ischaemic attacks. *Journal of Neurology, Neurosurgery and Psychiatry* 54:793–802

Hankey GJ, Slattery JM, Warlow CP (1992). Transient ischaemic attacks: which patients are at high (and low) risk of serious vascular events? *Journal of Neurology, Neurosurgery and Psychiatry* 55:640–652

Hankey GJ, Jamrozik K, Broadhurst RJ et al. (2000). Five-year survival after first-ever stroke and related prognostic factors in the Perth Community Stroke Study. *Stroke* 31:2080–2086

Hartmann A, Rundek T, Mast H et al. (2001). Mortality and causes of death after first ischemic stroke. *Neurology* 57:2000–2005

Heyman A, Wilkinson WE, Hurwitz BJ *et al.* (1984). Risk of ischemic heart disease in patients with TIA. *Neurology* 34:626–630

Howard G, Toole JF, Frye-Pierson J *et al.* (1987). Factors influencing the survival of 451 transient ischemic attack patients. *Stroke* 18:552–557

Howard G, Evans GW, Rouse JR III *et al.* (1994). A prospective re-evaluation of transient ischemic attacks as a risk factor for death and fatal or nonfatal cardiovascular events. *Stroke* 25:342–345

Hughes M, Lip GY (2007). Guideline Development Group for the NICE national clinical guideline for management of atrial fibrillation in primary and secondary care. Risk factors for anticoagulation-related bleeding complications in patients with atrial fibrillation: a systematic review. *Quarterly Journal of Medicine* 100:599–607

Joakimsen O, Bonaa KH, Mathiesen EB *et al.* (2000). Prediction of mortality by ultrasound screening of a general population for carotid stenosis: the Tromso Study. *Stroke* 31:1871–1876

Kernan WN, Feinstein AR, Brass LM (1991). A methodological appraisal of research on prognosis after transient ischemic attacks. *Stroke* 22:1108–1116

Kernan WN, Viscoli CM, Brass LM *et al.* (2000). The Stroke Prognosis Instrument II (SPI II): a clinical prediction instrument for patients with transient ischaemia and non-disabling ischaemic stroke. *Stroke* 31:456–462

Mathur KS, Kashyap SK, Kumar V (1963). Correlation of the extent and severity of atherosclerosis in the coronary and cerebral arteries. *Circulation* 27:929–934

Petty GW, Brown RD Jr., Whisnant JP *et al.* (2000). Ischemic stroke subtypes. A population-based study of functional outcome, survival and recurrence. *Stroke* 31:1062–1068

Ricci S, Cantisani AT, Righetti E *et al.* (1998). Long term follow up of TIAs: the SEPIVAC Study. *Neuroepidemiology* 17:54

Rothwell PM, Warlow CP For the ECST Collaborators (1999). Prediction of benefit from carotid endarterectomy in individual patients: a risk-modelling study. *Lancet* 353:2105–2110

Rothwell PM, Mehta Z, Howard SC *et al.* (2005). From subgroups to individuals: general principles and the example of carotid endarterectomy. *Lancet* 365:256–265

Scmidt EV, Smirnov VE, Ryabova VS (1988). Results of the seven-year prospective study of stroke patients. *Stroke* 19:942–949

Solberg LA, McGarry PA, Moossy J *et al.* (1968). Severity of atherosclerosis in cerebral arteries, coronary arteries, and aortas. *Annals of the New York Academy of Sciences* 149:956–973

Stroke Prevention in Atrial Fibrillation Investigators (1992a). Predictors of thromboembolism in atrial fibrillation, I: clinical features of patients at risk. *Annals of Internal Medicine* 116:1–5

Stroke Prevention in Atrial Fibrillation Investigators (1992b). Predictors of thromboembolism in atrial fibrillation, II: echocardiographic features of patients at risk. *Annals of Internal Medicine* 116:6–12

Stroke Prevention in Reversible Ischemia Trial (SPIRIT) Study Group (1997). A randomized trial of anticoagulants versus aspirin after cerebral ischemia of presumed arterial origin. *Annals of Neurology* 42:857–865

Terent A (1990). Survival after stroke and transient ischemic attacks during the 1970s and 1980s. *Stroke* 21:848–853

Touzé E, Varenne O, Chatellier G *et al.* (2005). Risk of myocardial infarction and vascular death after transient ischemic attack and ischemic stroke: a systematic review and meta-analysis. *Stroke* 36:2748–2755

van Latum JC, Koudstaal P, Venables GS *et al.* (1995). Predictors of major vascular events in patients with a transient ischemic attack or minor ischemic stroke and with non-rheumatic atrial fibrillation. *Stroke* 26:801–806

van Wijk I, Kappelle LJ, van Gijn J *et al.* (2005) for the LILAC study group. Long-term survival and vascular event risk after transient ischaemic attack or minor stroke: a cohort study. *Lancet* 365:2098–2104

Treatment of transient ischemic attack and stroke
Methods of assessing treatments

It is clearly important that treatments used in neurological disease are properly assessed before being introduced into routine clinical practice. There are many examples throughout medicine of interventions that were considered beneficial on the basis of theory or uncontrolled observational studies but were subsequently shown to be harmful in randomized controlled trials (Table 18.1).

The justification for randomized trials is not that no worthwhile observations can be made without them, but that important biases can occur in non-randomized comparisons which are particularly problematic if the benefits of treatment are, in reality, small or absent. For example, a non-randomized comparison of the effect of aspirin dosage on the operative risk of carotid endarterectomy (Table 18.2) reported a clinically and statistically significant lower operative risk in patients on high-dose aspirin (1300 mg) than taking low-dose aspirin (325 mg or less) (Barnett *et al.* 1998); however, a subsequent randomized trial (Taylor *et al.* 1999), performed to confirm this observation, showed that high-dose aspirin was, in fact, harmful (Table 18.1). It is likely that the non-randomized comparison had been biased by unmeasured differences between the patients in the low-dose and high-dose aspirin groups.

Randomized trials and systematic reviews of trials, therefore, provide the most reliable data on the effects of treatment. That is not to say, however, that non-randomized studies cannot sometimes provide reliable evidence on the benefits of intervention. Few people would doubt the validity of the observational data on the benefits of antibiotic treatment in bacterial meningitis or the benefits of treatment with levodopa in Parkinson's disease. Similarly, clinical guidelines have been revised worldwide on the basis of the non-randomized evidence of the substantial reduction in the risk of early recurrent stroke (see Fig. 19.2, p. 245) as a result of the urgent initiation of standard secondary prevention (Rothwell *et al.* 2007).

However, such large treatment effects are rare. Most treatments used in medicine have smaller effects that require assessment in randomized controlled trials if they are to be reliably quantified. Specifically, randomization has two main advantages over a non-randomized comparison. First, it ensures that clinicians do not know which treatment the patient will receive, and cannot select certain types of patient for one particular treatment. Second, it tends to result in an equal balance of baseline risk across the treatment groups.

Assessment of the internal validity of a randomized controlled trial

Randomized controlled trials have the potential to produce reliable estimates of the effects of treatments, but they will not inevitably do so. There are many potential sources of bias

Table 18.1. Examples of interventions that were thought initially to be beneficial (or harmful) a view changed by randomized controlled trials

	Examples
Considered beneficial, shown to be harmful	High-dose oxygen therapy in neonates
	Antiarrhythmic drugs after myocardial infarction
	Fluoride treatment for osteoporosis
	Bedrest in twin pregnancy
	Hormone replacement therapy in vascular prevention
	Extracranial to intracranial arterial bypass surgery in stroke prevention
	High-dose aspirin for carotid endarterectomy
Considered harmful, shown to be beneficial	Beta-blockers in heart failure
	Digoxin after myocardial infarction

Source: From Rothwell (2005a).

Table 18.2. The relationship between aspirin dose and the risk of stroke and death within 30 days of carotid endarterectomy in a non-randomized comparison within the North American Symptomatic Carotid Endarterectomy Trial (Barnett *et al.* 1998) and in a subsequent randomized controlled trial (Taylor *et al.* 1999)

	Operative risk of stroke and death with aspirin dosage (%)		Relative risk	*P*-value
	$< 650\,mg$	$> 650\,mg$		
Non-randomized study	7.1	3.9	1.8	< 0.001
Randomized trial	3.7	8.2	0.45	0.002

that must be addressed in the design and performance of a trial in order to ensure that results are reliable. The extent to which bias has been avoided is usually termed *internal validity,* the assessment of which is detailed below. The extent to which the results of a trial can be generalized to other settings, usually meaning routine clinical practice, is termed *external validity*, and is considered later in this chapter.

How was randomization performed?

It is important that the method of randomization is actually *random*. Treatment allocation according to day of the week, date of birth, date of admission or by alternate cases, is not random. The investigator will often know what treatment the patient will get if they enter the trial and so these methods are open to bias. Randomization must be based on tables of random numbers or computer-generated random allocation. It is also important that randomization is secure. Central telephone randomization is preferable to other methods, such as sealed envelopes containing the treatment allocation.

Were the treatment groups balanced?

Randomization will not inevitably result in an adequate balance of clinical characteristics and prognostic factors between the treatment groups in a trial, particularly if the sample size is relatively small. Details of the important clinical characteristics of the patients should,

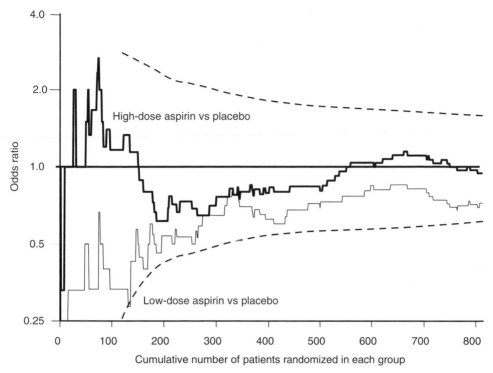

Fig. 18.1. The evolution of the estimates of treatment effect in the UKTIA-Aspirin Trial (Farrell *et al.* 1991) of high-dose aspirin versus low-dose aspirin versus placebo in patients with transient ischemic attack or minor stroke. The treatment effect (odds ratio) calculated at each point was based on the outcomes at final follow-up for patients randomized to that point (PM Rothwell, unpublished data). The dashed lines represent the level at which the apparent treatment effect approached statistical significance at the $p = 0.05$ level.

therefore, be reported by treatment group. If a prognostic variable is particularly important, a relatively minor (and not necessarily statistically significant) imbalance between the treatment groups may have a major effect on the trial result.

Was the trial sufficiently powered?

Sample sizes for randomized controlled trials in neurology may need to be large, either because treatment effects are relatively small or because the progression of disease is slow. Table 18.3 shows the effect of sample size on the reliability of the result of a trial of a hypothetical neurological treatment that is assumed to reduce the risk of a poor outcome by 20%, from 10% to 8%. The risk of getting the wrong result when a trial has an inadequate sample size is illustrated in Fig. 18.1. In this trial, there was considerable variability in the apparent effect of treatment until several hundred patients had been randomized. If the trial had been small, misleading trends in treatment effect could easily have been reported.

Was the trial stopped early?

A trial may need to be stopped early if a treatment has serious adverse effects, or if there is clear benefit. However, as is seen in Fig. 18.1, the chance fluctuations during the early stages of a trial can easily reach statistical significance at the $p = 0.05$ level. If the stopping rule is based on a p value of 0.05, it is quite possible that the trial will be stopped early, and the wrong conclusions drawn. Stopping rules should be based on significance levels of $p < 0.01$

Table 18.3. Effect of sample size on the reliability of the result of a trial of a hypothetical treatment that is expected to reduce the risk of a poor outcome by 20%: from 10% to 8%

Total patients	P^a	Trial power (%)	Comments on trial size
200	0.99	1	Completely hopeless
400	0.98	2	Still hopeless
800	0.96	4	Completely inadequate
1600	0.90	10	Still inadequate
3200	0.75	25	Not really adequate
6400	0.43	57	Barely adequate
12 800	0.09	91	Probably adequate
20 000	0.01	99	Definitely adequate

Note:
^{a}Probability of failing to achieve $p < 0.01$ significance if true relative risk reduction is 20%.

or ideally $p < 0.001$, and the evolving results should be assessed on only a limited number of pre-specified occasions.

Was outcome assessment blind to treatment allocation?

There are two main reasons for blinding the trial clinicians: first, so that the use of non-trial treatments and interventions is not influenced by a knowledge of whether or not the patients received the trial treatment; second, so that clinicians are not biased in their assessment of clinical outcomes. The potential for bias depends on the subjectivity of the trial outcome. Biased assessment of neurological impairment and disability was clearly demonstrated in a multiple sclerosis trial in which blind and non-blind outcome assessment produced very different results (Noseworthy *et al.* 1994). Trials with blind assessment should also report whether or not blinding was effective. It is, of course, sometimes impossible to blind clinical assessment, but non-blind trials should report data on non-trial treatments given to patients during follow-up to ensure that these were not biased.

Were serious complications of treatment included in the main outcome?

Some treatments have serious complications that should be included in the primary outcome, rather than relegated to a table of "side-effects," for example life-threatening gastrointestinal bleeding in trials of antiplatelet agents and anticoagulants.

Was the main analysis an intention-to-treat analysis?

The primary analysis in any randomized trial should be an intention-to-treat analysis: that is, patients remain in the treatment group to which they were originally randomized irrespective of the treatment they eventually received. The alternative, an efficacy analysis (an analysis that is confined to patients who complied with the randomized treatment), is prone to bias. This was illustrated by the Coronary Drug Project (Coronary Drug Project Research Group 1980), a randomized trial comparing several different lipid-lowering regimens with placebo following myocardial infarction. By intention-to-treat analysis, the five-year mortality in the clofibrate group was 20.0% versus 20.9% in the placebo group. However, when patients who complied with treatment in the clofibrate group were compared with non-compliers, the results seemed to suggest that there was a treatment effect:

five-year mortality was 15.0% in the compliers versus 24.6% in the non-compliers. Perhaps clofibrate was beneficial. However, the same analysis in patients in the placebo group showed the same trend: 15.1% mortality in compliers versus 28.2% mortality in non-compliers. The apparent effect of clofibrate in the treatment group was simply a bias generated by the fact that patients who do not comply with treatment tend to have a worse prognosis.

Were any patients excluded from the main analysis?

It is not uncommon in reports of trials to find that a certain number of the patients who were randomized initially were excluded from the final analysis. Common reasons for exclusion are that following randomization it was found that a number of patients did not actually fit the eligibility criteria (so called *protocol violators*) or that some patients never received the randomized treatment because they developed a clear indication for a specific treatment or because they withdrew from the trial for other reasons. However, the interpretation of what is a protocol violation can be rather subjective, and since the decision will often be made towards the end of the trial, and may not be blind to outcome, it is open to abuse. For example, 71 of 1629 patients randomized in a trial of an antiplatelet agent following myocardial infarction were excluded from the final analysis, apparently because they did not meet the eligibility criteria (Anturane Reinfarction Trial Research Group 1980). It subsequently transpired that there was a large excess of deaths in the exclusions from the treatment group compared with the placebo group (Temple and Pledger 1980). Exclusion of these patients led to a bias that had contributed to the statistically significant apparent benefit in the treatment group. A second trial failed to confirm any benefit.

How many patients were lost to follow-up?

Another important potential cause of bias in the analysis of trial results is loss of patients to follow-up. Just as patients who comply with treatment are different from patients who do not, patients who are lost to follow-up are usually different from those who remain in the trial. For example, it may not be possible to contact patients because they are either incapacitated in some way, or even dead. It is, therefore, very difficult to interpret the results of a trial with significant loss to follow-up.

Assessment of the external validity of a randomized controlled trial

Randomized controlled trials must be internally valid (i.e. design and conduct must eliminate the possibility of bias), but to be clinically useful the result must also be relevant to a definable group of patients in a particular clinical setting (i.e. they must be externally valid). Lack of external validity is the most frequent criticism by clinicians of trials, systematic reviews and guidelines, and is one explanation for the widespread underuse in routine practice of many treatments that have been shown to be beneficial in trials and are recommended in guidelines (Rothwell 2005a). Yet medical journals, funding agencies, ethics committees, the pharmaceutical industry and governmental regulators give external validity a low priority. Admittedly, whereas the determinants of internal validity are intuitive and can generally be worked out from first principles, understanding of the determinants of the external validity requires clinical rather than statistical expertise and often depends on a detailed understanding of the particular clinical condition under study and its management in routine clinical practice. However, reliable judgements about the external validity of randomized trials are essential if treatments are to be used correctly in as many patients as possible in routine clinical practice.

Whether the results of a trial can be applied in routine clinical practice depends to some extent on the type of trial. Generally speaking, explanatory (phase II) trials measure the *effectiveness* of treatment, whereas pragmatic (phase III) trials measure the *usefulness* of treatment. A treatment may be *effective* but it may not be *useful* because it is too poorly tolerated, too expensive or too complex to administer. Explanatory trials are often small, include a tightly defined group of patients and frequently have non-clinical (surrogate) measures of outcome. Pragmatic trials seek to measure the usefulness of treatments in situations that, as far as possible, mimic normal clinical practice. However, it would be wrong to assume that a pragmatic trial will always have greater external validity than an explanatory trial. For example, although broad eligibility criteria, limited collection of baseline data and inclusion of centers with a range of expertise and differing patient populations have many advantages, they can also make it very difficult to generalize the effect of treatment to a particular clinical setting. Moreover, no randomized trial or systematic review will ever be relevant to all patients and all settings. However, trials should be designed and reported in a way that allows clinicians to judge to whom the results can reasonably be applied. Table 18.4 lists some of the important potential determinants of external validity, each of which is reviewed briefly below.

What was the setting of the trial?

A detailed understanding of the setting in which a trial is performed, including any peculiarities of the healthcare system in particular countries, can be essential in judging external validity. The potential impact of differences between healthcare systems is illustrated by the analysis of the results of the European Carotid Surgery Trial, a randomized trial of endarterectomy versus medical treatment alone for recently symptomatic carotid stenosis (Rothwell 2005b). National differences in the speed with which patients were investigated, with a median delay from last symptoms to randomization of greater than two months in the UK (slow centers) compared with three weeks in Belgium and Holland (fast centers), resulted in very different treatment effects in these different healthcare systems – owing to the shortness of the time window for effective prevention of stroke (Fig. 18.2).

Similar differences in performance between healthcare systems will exist for other conditions, and there is, of course, the broader issue of how trials done in the developed world apply in the developing world. Moreover, other differences between countries in the methods of diagnosis and management of disease, which can be substantial, or important racial differences in pathology and natural history of disease also affect the external validity of trials. A good example is the heterogeneity of results of trials of bacille Calmette-Guérin (BCG) vaccine in prevention of tuberculosis, with a progressive loss of efficacy ($p < 0.0001$) with decreasing latitude (Fine 1995).

How were participating centers selected?

How centers and clinicians were selected to participate in trials is seldom reported, but it can also have important implications for external validity. For example, the Asymptomatic Carotid Atherosclerosis Study (ACAS) trial of endarterectomy for asymptomatic carotid stenosis only accepted surgeons with an excellent safety record, rejecting 40% of applicants initially, and subsequently barring from further participation those who had adverse operative outcomes in the trial. The benefit from surgery in the trial was a result in major

Table 18.4. Some of the factors that can affect external validity of randomized controlled trials and should be addressed in reports of the results and be considered by clinicians

	Factors
Setting of the trial	Healthcare system
	Country
	Recruitment from primary, secondary or tertiary care
	Selection of participating centers
	Selection of participating clinicians
Selection of patients	Methods of pre-randomization diagnosis and investigation
	Eligibility criteria
	Exclusion criteria
	Placebo run-in period
	Treatment run-in period
	"Enrichment" strategies
	Ratio of randomized patients to eligible non-randomized patients in participating centers
	Proportion of patients who declined randomization
Characteristics of randomized patients	Baseline clinical characteristics
	Racial group
	Uniformity of underlying pathology
	Stage in the natural history of their disease
	Severity of disease
	Comorbidity
	Absolute risks of a poor outcome in the control group
Differences between the trial protocol and routine practice	Trial intervention
	Timing of treatment
	Appropriateness/relevance of control intervention
	Adequacy of non-trial treatment: both intended and actual
	Prohibition of certain non-trial treatments
	Therapeutic or diagnostic advances since trial was performed
Outcome measures and follow-up	Clinical relevance of surrogate outcomes
	Clinical relevance, validity and reproducibility of complex scales
	Effect of intervention on most relevant components of composite outcomes
	Who measured outcome
	Use of patient-centered outcomes
	Frequency of follow-up
	Adequacy of the length of follow-up
Adverse effects of treatment	Completeness of reporting of relevant adverse effects
	Rates of discontinuation of treatment

Table 18.4. (*cont.*)

Factors
Selection of trial centers and/or clinicians on the basis of skill or experience
Exclusion of patients at risk of complications
Exclusion of patients who experienced adverse effects during a run-in period
Intensity of trial safety procedures

Source: From Rothwell (2005a).

part of the consequently low operative risk (Asymptomatic Carotid Atherosclerosis Study Group 1995). A meta-analysis of 46 surgical case series that published operative risks during the five years after the trial found operative mortality to be eight times higher and the risk of stroke and death to be about three times higher than in ACAS (Rothwell 2005a). Trials should not include centers that do not have the competence to treat patients safely, but selection should not be so exclusive that the results cannot be generalized to routine clinical practice.

How were patients selected and excluded?

Concern is often expressed about highly selective trial eligibility criteria, but there are often several earlier stages of selection that are rarely recorded or reported but can be more problematic. For example, consider a trial of a new blood pressure-lowering drug, which like most such trials is performed in a hospital clinic. Fewer than 10% of patients with hypertension are managed in hospital clinics, and this group will differ from those managed in primary care. Moreover, only one of the ten physicians who see hypertensive patients in this particular hospital is taking part in the trial, and this physician mainly sees young patients with resistant hypertension. In this way, even before any consideration of eligibility or exclusion criteria, potential recruits are already very unrepresentative of patients in the local community. It is essential, therefore, that where possible trials record and report the pathways to recruitment.

Patients are then further selected according to trial eligibility criteria. Some trials exclude women and many exclude the elderly and/or patients with common comorbidities. One review of 214 drug trials in acute myocardial infarction found that over 60% excluded patients aged over 75 years (Gurwitz *et al.* 1992), despite the fact that over 50% of myocardial infarctions occur in this older age group. A review of 41 US National Institutes of Health randomized trials found an average exclusion rate of 73% (Charleson and Horwitz 1984), but rates can be much higher. One study of an acute stroke treatment trial found that of the small proportion of patients admitted to hospital sufficiently quickly to be suitable for treatment, 96% were ineligible based on the various other exclusion criteria (Jorgensen *et al.* 1999). One center in another acute stroke trial had to screen 192 patients over two years to find one eligible patient (LaRue *et al.* 1988). Yet, highly selective recruitment is not inevitable. The Gruppo Italiano per lo Studio della Streptochinasi nell'Infarto Miocardico GISSI-1 trial of thrombolysis for acute myocardial infarction, for example, recruited 90% of patients admitted within 12 hours of the event with a definite diagnosis and no contraindications (Gruppo Italiano per lo Studio della Streptochinasi nell'Infarto Miocardico 1986).

Severe stenosis

	Surgical	Medical	ARR (%)	95% CI
Fast centers	8/162	25/106	19.9	10.7–29.1
Slow centers	25/173	25/113	7.6	−2.0 to 17.1
TOTAL	33/335	50/219	13.5	6.9–20.2
Fast centers	11/162	31/106	23.6	13.7–33.5
Slow centers	35/173	30/113	6.2	−4.3 to 16.6
TOTAL	46/335	61/219	14.7	7.4–21.9

Moderate stenosis

Ipsilateral ischemic stroke or operative stroke/death

	Surgical	Medical	ARR (%)	95% CI
Fast centers	17/174	21/127	8.3	−0.1 to 16.7
Slow centers	29/206	11/139	−5.6	−12.6 to 1.4
TOTAL	46/380	32/266	0.9	−4.5 to 6.4

Any stroke or operative death

	Surgical	Medical	ARR (%)	95% CI
Fast centers	21/174	28/127	11.8	2.4–21.2
Slow centers	38/206	25/139	0.3	−8.6 to 9.3
TOTAL	59/380	53/266	5.7	−0.8 to 12.2

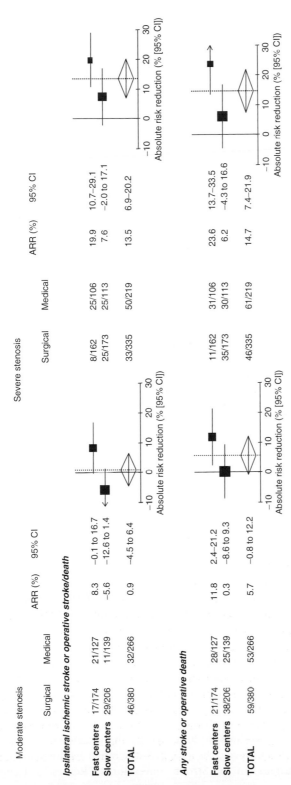

Fig. 18.2. The absolute risk reduction (ARR) at five years of ipsilateral ischemic stroke (top) and any stroke or death (bottom) with surgery in European Carotid Surgery Trial centers in which the median delay from last symptomatic event to randomization was ≤ 50 days (fast centers) compared with centers with a longer delay (slow centers) (Rothwell 2005a). Data are shown separately for patients with moderate (50–69%) and severe (70–99%) carotid stenosis. CI, confidence interval.

Strict eligibility criteria can limit the external validity of trials but physicians should at least be able to select similar patients for treatment in routine practice. Unfortunately, however, reporting of trial eligibility criteria is frequently inadequate. A review of trials leading to clinical alerts by the US National Institutes of Health revealed that, of an average of 31 eligibility criteria, only 63% were published in the main trial report and only 19% in the clinical alert (Shapiro *et al.* 2000). Inadequate reporting is also a major problem in secondary publications, such as systematic reviews and clinical guidelines, where the need for a succinct message does not usually allow detailed consideration of the eligibility and exclusion criteria or other determinants of external validity.

Was there a run-in period?

Pre-randomization run-in periods are also often used to select or exclude patients. In a placebo run-in, all eligible patients receive placebo and those who are poorly compliant are excluded. There can be good reasons for doing this, but high rates of exclusion will reduce external validity. Active treatment run-in periods in which patients who have adverse events or show signs that treatment may be ineffective are excluded are more likely to undermine external validity. For example, two trials of carvedilol, a vasodilatory beta-blocker, in chronic heart failure excluded 6% and 9% of eligible patients in treatment run-in periods, mainly because of worsening heart failure and other adverse events, some of which were fatal (Rothwell 2005a). In both trials, the complication rates in the subsequent randomized phase were much lower than in the run-in phase.

Trials also sometimes actively recruit patients who are likely to respond well to treatment (often termed "enrichment"). For example, some trials of antipsychotic drugs have selectively recruited patients who had a good response to antipsychotic drugs previously (Rothwell 2005a). Other trials have excluded non-responders in a run-in phase. One trial of a cholinesterase inhibitor, tacrine, in Alzheimer's disease recruited 632 patients to a six-week "enrichment" phase in which they were randomized to different doses of tacrine or placebo (Davis *et al.* 1992). After a washout-period, only the 215 (34%) patients who had a measured improvement on tacrine in the "enrichment" phase were randomized to tacrine (at their best dose) versus placebo in the main phase of the trial. External validity is clearly undermined here.

What were the characteristics of the randomized patients?

Even in large pragmatic trials with very few exclusion criteria, recruitment of less than 10% of potentially eligible patients in participating centers is common. Those patients who are recruited generally differ from those who are eligible but not recruited in terms of age, sex, race, severity of disease, educational status, social class and place of residence (Rothwell 2005a). The outcome in patients included in trials is also usually better than those not in trials, often markedly so, not because of better treatment but because of a better baseline prognosis. Trial reports usually include the baseline clinical characteristics of randomized patients and so it is argued that clinicians can assess external validity by comparison with their own patient(s). However, recorded baseline clinical characteristics often say very little about the real make-up of the trial population, and can be misleading. For example, Table 18.5 shows the baseline clinical characteristics of the patients randomized to warfarin in two trials of secondary prevention of stroke. In one trial, patients were in atrial fibrillation and in the other they were in sinus rhythm, but the characteristics of the two cohorts were otherwise fairly similar. However, the risk of intracranial hemorrhage on warfarin was 19 times higher ($p < 0.0001$) in the Stroke Prevention in Reversible Ischemia Trial

Table 18.5. The baseline clinical characteristics and hemorrhage outcomes of patients randomized to anticoagulation with warfarin in the European Atrial Fibrillation Trial (EAFT) and the Stroke Prevention in Reversible Ischemia Trial (SPIRIT)

	SPIRIT (n = 651)	EAFT (n = 225)
Baseline clinical characteristics (%)		
Male sex	66	55
Age > 65 years	47	81
Hypertension	39	48
Angina	9	11
Myocardial infarction	9	7
Diabetes	11	12
Leukoariosis on CT brain scan	7	14
Outcomes during trial		
Mean INR during trial (SD)	3.3 (1.1)	2.9 (0.7)
Patient-years of follow-up	735	507
Intracranial hemorrhage (No.)	27	0[a]
Extracranial hemorrhage (No.)	26	13
Adjusted hazard ratio (95% CI) for SPIRIT versus EAFT		
Intracranial hemorrhage	19.0 (2.4–250)	$p < 0.0001$
Extracranial hemorrhage	1.9 (0.8–4.7)	$p = 0.15$

Notes:
INR, international normalized ratio; SD, standard deviation; CI, confidence interval.
[a]There were no proven intracranial hemorrhages, but no CT scan was performed in two strokes. For the purpose of calculation of the adjusted hazard ratio for hemorrhage these two strokes were categorized as having been caused by intracranial hemorrhage.
Source: From Gorter (1999).

than in the European Atrial Fibrillation Trial even after adjustment for differences in baseline clinical characteristics and the intensity of anticoagulation therapy (Gorter 1999). In judging external validity, an understanding of how patients were referred, investigated and diagnosed (i.e. their pathway to recruitment) as well as how they were subsequently selected and excluded is often very much more informative than a list of baseline characteristics.

Was the intervention, control treatment and pre-trial or non-trial management appropriate?

External validity can also be affected if trials have protocols that differ from usual clinical practice. For example, prior to randomization in the trials of endarterectomy for symptomatic carotid stenosis patients had to be diagnosed by a neurologist and to have conventional arterial angiography, neither of which are routine in many centers. The trial intervention itself may also differ from that used in current practice, such as in the formulation and bioavailability of a drug, or the type of anesthetic used for an operation. The same can be true of the treatment in the control group in a trial, which may use a particularly low dose of the comparator drug or fall short of best current practice in some

Table 18.6. Examples where trials based on surrogate outcomes proved to be misleading predictors of the effect of treatment on clinical outcomes in subsequent pragmatic clinical trials

Treatment	Condition	Surrogate outcome	Clinical outcome
Fluoride	Osteoporosis	Increase in bone density	Major increase in fractures
Antiarrhythmic drugs	Post-MI	Reduction in ECG abnormalities	Increased mortality
Beta-interferon	Multiple sclerosis	70% reduction in new lesions brain MRI	No convincing effect on disability
Milrinone and epoprostanol	Heart failure	Improved exercise tolerance	Increased mortality
Ibopamine	Heart failure	Improved ejection fraction and heart rate variability	Increased mortality

Notes:
MI, myocardial infarction; ECG, electrocardiography.
Source: From Rothwell (2005a).

other way. External validity can also be undermined by too stringent limitations on the use of non-trial treatments. Any prohibition of non-trial treatments should be reported in the main trial publications along with details of relevant non-trial treatments that were used. The timing of many interventions is also critical and should be reported when relevant.

Were the outcome measures appropriate?

The external validity of a trial also depends on whether the outcomes were clinically relevant. Many trials use "surrogate" outcomes, usually biological or imaging markers that are thought to be indirect measures of the effect of treatment on clinical outcomes. Surrogate outcomes (e.g. infarct size on CT brain scan in an acute stroke trial, or MRI activity in multiple sclerosis) can be useful in explanatory trials because they may be more sensitive to the effects of the treatment than clinical outcomes, and they are readily assessed blind to treatment allocation. However, they do not measure clinical effectiveness and may sometimes be highly misleading. There are many examples of treatments that had a major beneficial effect on a surrogate outcome, which had been shown to be correlated with a relevant clinical outcome in observational studies, but where the treatments proved ineffective or harmful in subsequent large trials that used these same clinical outcomes (Table 18.6). For example, a trial of three different antiarrhythmic drugs versus placebo after acute myocardial infarction assessed the frequency of ventricular extrasystoles on 24-hour ambulatory electrocardiographic monitoring (Cardiac Arrhythmia Suppression Trial (CAST) Investigators 1989). All three drugs produced a substantial reduction in the frequency of extrasystoles, but the trial was subsequently stopped because of a major excess of deaths in the treatment group (33 versus 9 in the control group; $p = 0.0003$). Similarly, reduced bone density, which is known to be a useful marker for risk of fractures, was used as a surrogate outcome in a trial of sodium fluoride in women with osteoporosis (Riggs *et al.* 1990). Sodium fluoride produced a highly statistically significant, and apparently clinically important, increase in bone density. However, further follow-up revealed a 30% increase in vertebral fractures and a three-fold increase in non-vertebral fractures in the sodium fluoride group.

Complex scales, often made up of arbitrary combinations of symptoms and clinical signs, are also problematic. A review of 196 trials in rheumatoid arthritis identified more than 70 different outcome scales (Gøtzsche 1989). A review of 2000 trials in schizophrenia identified 640 outcome scales, many of which were devised for the particular trial and had no supporting data on validity or reliability. These unvalidated scales were more likely to show statistically significant treatment effects than established scales (Marshall *et al.* 2000). Moreover, the clinical meaning of apparent treatment effects (e.g. a 2.7 point mean reduction in a 100 point outcome scale made up of various symptoms and signs) is usually impossible to discern. Simple clinical outcomes usually have most external validity, but even then only if they reflect the priorities of patients. For example, patients with epilepsy are much more interested in the proportion of individuals rendered free of seizures in trials of anticonvulsants than they are in changes in mean seizure frequency. Who actually measured the outcome can also be important. For example, the recorded operative risk of stroke in carotid endarterectomy is highly dependent on whether patients were assessed by a surgeon or a neurologist (Rothwell and Warlow 1995).

Many trials combine events in their primary outcome measure. This can produce a useful measure of the overall effect of treatment on all the relevant outcomes, and it usually affords greater statistical power, but the outcome that is most important to a particular patient may be affected differently by treatment than the combined outcome. Composite outcomes also sometimes combine events of very different severity, and treatment effects can be driven by the least important outcome, which is often the most frequent. Equally problematic is the composite of definite clinical events and episodes of hospitalization. The fact that a patient is in a trial will probably affect the likelihood of hospitalization and it will certainly vary between different healthcare systems.

Was the follow-up sufficient?

Another major problem for the external validity of trials is an inadequate duration of treatment and/or follow-up. For example, although patients with refractory epilepsy or migraine require treatment for many years, most trials of new drugs look at the effect of treatment for only a few weeks. Whether initial response is a good predictor of long-term benefit is unknown. This problem has been identified in trials in schizophrenia, with fewer than 50% of trials having greater than six weeks of follow-up and only 20% following patients for longer than six months (Thornley and Adams 1998). The contrast between beneficial effects of treatments in short-term trials and the less-encouraging experience of long-term treatment in clinical practice has also been highlighted by clinicians treating patients with rheumatoid arthritis (Pincus 1998).

How were adverse effects of treatment assessed and reported?

Reporting of adverse effects of treatment in trials and systematic reviews is often poor. In a review of 192 pharmaceutical trials, less then a third had adequate reporting of adverse clinical events or laboratory toxicology (Ioannidis and Contopoulos-Ioannidis 1998). Treatment discontinuation rates provide some guide to tolerability but pharmaceutical trials often use eligibility criteria and run-in periods to exclude patients who might be prone to adverse effects.

Clinicians are usually most concerned about external validity of trials of potentially dangerous treatments. Complications of medical interventions are a leading cause of death in developed countries. Risks can be overestimated in trials, particularly during the introduction of new treatments when trials are often carried out with patients with very severe disease, but stringent selection of patients, confinement to specialist centers and intensive safety monitoring usually lead to lower risks than in routine clinical practice. Trials of warfarin in non-rheumatic atrial fibrillation are a good example. Prior to 2007, all trials reporting benefit with warfarin had complication rates that were much lower than in routine practice and consequent doubts about external validity were partly to blame for major underprescribing of warfarin, particularly in the elderly.

Applying the results of randomized trials to treatment decisions for individual patients

Many treatments, such as blood pressure lowering in uncontrolled hypertension, are indicated in the vast majority of patients. However, a targeted approach is useful for treatments with modest benefits (e.g. lipid lowering in primary prevention of vascular disease), for costly treatments with moderate overall benefits (e.g. beta-interferon in multiple sclerosis), if the availability of treatment is limited (e.g. organ transplantation), in developing countries with very limited healthcare budgets and, most importantly, for treatments that although of overall benefit in large trials are associated with a significant risk of harm. The crux of the problem faced by clinicians in these situations is how to use data from large randomized trials and systematic reviews, which provide the most reliable estimates of the overall average effects of treatment, to determine the likely effect of treatment in an individual.

When considering the likely effect of a treatment in an individual patient, it is important to consider the overall result of a trial or systematic review as an absolute risk reduction with treatment or the number needed to treat to prevent a poor outcome. An absolute risk reduction tells us what chance an individual has of benefiting from treatment; for example of 25% indicates that there is a 1:4 chance of benefit (four people need to be treated to ensure a good outcome in one). In contrast, a particular relative risk reduction gives absolutely no information about the likelihood of individual benefit. For example, the relative reductions in the risk of stroke were virtually identical in the Swedish Trial in Old Patients with hypertension (STOP-hypertension) trial (relative risk, 0.53; 95% confidence interval [CI], 0.33–0.86) (Dahlof et al. 1991) and the Medical Research Council Trial (relative risk, 0.55; 95% CI, 0.25–0.60) (Medical Research Council Working Party 1985) of blood pressure lowering in primary prevention, but there was a 12-fold difference in absolute risk reduction. All other things being equal, 830 of the young hypertensives in the Medical Research Council trial would have to be treated for one year to prevent one stroke compared with 69 of the elderly hypertensives in the STOP-hypertension trial.

Trials should report subgroup analyses if there are potentially large differences between groups in the risk of a poor outcome with or without treatment; if there is potential heterogeneity of treatment effect in relation to pathophysiology; if there are practical questions about when to treat (e.g. stage of disease, timing of treatment, etc.); or if there are doubts about benefit in specific groups, such as the elderly, which are likely to lead to undertreatment (Rothwell 2005b). Analyses must be predefined, carefully justified and limited to a few clinically important questions, and post-hoc observations should be treated with scepticism irrespective of their statistical significance. Concerns about heterogeneity of treatment effects will often be unfounded, but if they are not addressed they will restrict the use of treatment in routine practice. If important subgroup effects are anticipated, trials should either be powered to detect them reliably or pooled analyses of multiple trials should be undertaken.

Univariate subgroup analysis is of relatively limited value, even when done reliably, in situations where there are multiple determinants of the individual response to treatment. In this situation, targeting treatment using risk models can be useful, particularly in conditions, or for interventions, where benefit is likely to be very dependent on the absolute risk of a poor outcome with or without treatment. Stratification of trial results with independently derived and validated prognostic models can allow clinicians to systematically take into account the characteristics of an individual patient and their interactions, to consider the risks and benefits of interventions separately if required, and to provide patients with personalized estimates of their likelihood of benefit from treatment (Rothwell 2005b).

References

Anturane Reinfarction Trial Research Group (1980). Sulfinpyrazone in the prevention of sudden death after myocardial infarction. *New England Journal of Medicine* **302**:250–256

Asymptomatic Carotid Atherosclerosis Study Group (1995). Carotid endarterectomy for patients with asymptomatic internal carotid artery stenosis. *Journal of the American Medical Association* **273**:1421–1428

Barnett HJ, Taylor DW, Eliasziw M *et al.* (1998). The final results of the NASCET trial. *New England Journal of Medicine* **339**:1415–1425

Cardiac Arrhythmia Suppression Trial (CAST) Investigators (1989). Preliminary report: effect of encainide and flecainide on mortality in a randomised trial of arrhythmia suppression after myocardial infarction. *New England Journal of Medicine* **321**:406–412

Charleson ME, Horwitz RI (1984). Applying results of randomised trials to clinical practice: impact of losses before randomisation. *British Medical Journal* **289**:1281–1284

Coronary Drug Project Research Group (1980). Influence of adherence to treatment and response to cholesterol on mortality in the Coronary Drug Project. *New England Journal of Medicine* **303**:1038–1041

Dahlof B, Lindholm LH, Hansson L *et al.* (1991). Morbidity and mortality in the Swedish trial in old patients with hypertension (STOP-hypertension). *Lancet* **338**:1281–1285

Davis KL, Thal LJ, Gamzu ER *et al.* (1992). A double-blind, placebo-controlled multicenter study of tacrine for Alzheimer's disease. *New England Journal of Medicine* **321**:406–412

Farrell B, Godwin J, Richards S *et al.* (1991). The United Kingdom transient ischaemic attack (UK-TIA) aspirin trial: final results. *Journal of Neurology, Neurosurgery and Psychiatry* **54**:1044–1054

Fine PEM (1995). Variation in protection by BCG: implications of and for heterologous immunity. *Lancet* **346**:1339–1345

Gorter JW for the Stroke Prevention in Reversible Ischaemia Trial (SPIRIT) and European Atrial Fibrillation Trial (EAFT) Groups (1999). Major bleeding during anticoagulation after cerebral ischaemia: patterns and risk factors. *Neurology* **53**:1319–1327

Gøtzsche PC (1989). Methodology and overt and hidden bias in reports of 196 double-blind trials of nonsteroidal antiinflammatory drugs in rheumatoid arthritis. *Control in Clinical Trials* **10**:31–56

Gruppo Italiano per lo Studio della Streptochinasi nell'Infarto Miocardico (GISSI) (1986). Effectiveness of intravenous thrombolytic treatment in acute myocardial infarction. *Lancet* **i**:397–402

Gurwitz JH, Col NF, Avorn J (1992). The exclusion of elderly and women from clinical trials in acute myocardial infarction. *Journal of the American Medical Association* **268**:1417–1422

Ioannidis JP, Contopoulos-Ioannidis DG (1998). Reporting of safety data from randomised trials. *Lancet* **352**:1752–1753

Jorgensen HS, Nakayama H, Kammersgaard LP *et al.* (1999). Predicted impact of intravenous thrombolysis on prognosis of general population of stroke patients: simulation model. *British Medical Journal* **319**:288–289

LaRue LJ, Alter M, Traven ND *et al.* (1988). Acute stroke therapy trials: problems in patient accrual. *Stroke* **19**:950–954

Marshall M, Lockwood A, Bradley C *et al.* (2000). Unpublished rating scales: a major source of bias in randomised controlled trials of treatments for schizophrenia? *British Journal of Psychiatry* **176**:249–252

Medical Research Council Working Party (1985). MRC trial of treatment of mild hypertension: principal results. *British Medical Journal* **291**:97–104

Noseworthy JH, Ebers GC, Vandervoort MK *et al.* (1994). The impact of blinding on the results of a randomized, placebo-controlled multiple sclerosis clinical trial. *Neurology* **44**:16–20

Pincus T (1998). Rheumatoid arthritis: disappointing long-term outcomes despite successful short-term clinical trials. *Journal of Clinical Epidemiology* **41**:1037–1041

Riggs BL, Hodgson SF, O'Fallon WM *et al.* (1990). Effect of fluoride treatment on fracture rate in postmenopausal women with osteoporosis. *New England Journal of Medicine* **322**:802–809

Rothwell PM (2005a). External validity of randomised controlled trials: to whom do the results of this trial apply? *Lancet* **365**:82–93

Rothwell PM (2005b). Subgroup analysis in randomised controlled trials: importance, indications and interpretation. *Lancet* **365**:176–186

Rothwell PM, Warlow CP (1995). Is self-audit reliable? *Lancet* **346**:1623

Rothwell PM, Giles MF, Chandratheva A *et al.* (2007). Major reduction in risk of early recurrent stroke by urgent treatment of TIA and minor stroke: EXPRESS Study. *Lancet* **370**:1432–1442

Shapiro SH, Weijer C, Freedman B (2000). Reporting the study populations of clinical trials. Clear transmission or static on the line? *Journal of Clinical Epidemiology* **53**:973–979

Taylor DW, Barnett HJM, Haynes RB *et al.* (1999). Low dose and high dose acetylsalicylic acid for patients undergoing carotid endarterectomy: a randomised controlled trial. *Lancet* **353**:2179–2184

Temple R, Pledger GW (1980). The FDA's critique of the Anturane Reinfarction Trial. *New England Journal of Medicine* **303**:1488–1492

Thornley B, Adams CE (1998). Content and quality of 2000 controlled trials in schizophrenia over 50 years. *British Medical Journal* **317**:1181–1184

Chapter 19

Acute treatment of transient ischemic attack and minor stroke

Although the acute treatment of major stroke and TIA and minor stroke have many common elements, there are important differences. In the acute treatment of TIA and minor stroke, the aim is the secondary prevention of a disabling stroke, which might follow in the immediate hours and days after the initial event, as opposed to reversal of any neurological deficit caused by the stroke itself. Reduction of delays by improved public education and triage to secondary care and coordinated patient management in specialist units are vital aspects of treatment in both major stroke and TIA and minor stroke. However, there is a greater focus on urgent, effective secondary prevention for TIA and minor stroke.

Another important difference is the extent of the evidence base for treatments in major stroke compared with TIA and minor stroke. The concepts of stroke units and administration of thrombolysis have been researched, developed and implemented since the 1980s for patients with major stroke. Yet, although the concept of TIA arose in the 1950s and treatments such as carotid endarterectomy, anticoagulation, antiplatelet therapy and other risk factor management were subsequently proven effective, it was not until 2007 that the first reports were published on the feasibility and effectiveness of urgent assessment and treatment of TIA in specialist units (Rothwell *et al.* 2007; Lavallée *et al.* 2007).

This chapter will summarize the aspects of acute treatment that are specific to TIA and minor stroke.

Recognition of symptoms and delays to management

The urgent management of patients with minor stroke or TIA depends upon the correct recognition of symptoms and appropriate action by patients and their swift triage to specialist care where investigation and treatment are rapidly initiated.

Public awareness and behavior

In contrast to major stroke, where extensive studies have examined knowledge among the general public (Pancioli *et al.* 1998; Reeves *et al.* 2002; Parahoo *et al.* 2003; Carroll *et al.* 2004) and individuals' immediate behavior (Salisbury *et al.* 1998; Smith *et al.* 1998; Evenson *et al.* 2001; Lacy *et al.* 2001; Harraf *et al.* 2002), equivalent studies in minor stroke and TIA are lacking.

One study of knowledge among the general public indicated that 2.3% of a randomly selected sample of people in the USA have been told by a physician that they had a TIA, based on self-report in a telephone survey (Johnston *et al.* 2003). However an additional 3.2% of respondents recalled symptoms consistent with TIA but had not sought medical attention at all and consequently had not been diagnosed by a doctor. Of those with "diagnosed" TIA, only 64% had seen a doctor within 24-hours of the event. Only 8.2% correctly related the definition of TIA, and 8.6% were able to identify a typical symptom.

Table 19.1. Elements of early detection systems for transient ischemic attack and stroke

LAPSS	CPCC	FAST
Age > 45 years	Facial droop	Facial weakness
No previous seizure history	Arm drift	Arm and leg weakness
Onset within 24-hours	Slurred speech	Speech problems
Patient ambulant previously		
Blood glucose		
Asymmetry of:		
smile/grimace		
grip strength		
arm strength		

Notes:
LAPSS, Los Angeles Pre-hospital Stroke Scale; CPCC, Cincinatti Pre-hospital Stroke Scale; FAST, Face, Arm, Speech Test.
Sources: From Kothari et al. (1999), Kidwell et al. (2000) and Nor et al. (2004).

In a study of 422 residents of Bern, Switzerland, who were interviewed in person about their knowledge of stroke and TIA, only 8.3% recognized TIA as symptoms of stroke resolving within 24-hours, and only 2.8% identified TIA as a disease requiring immediate medical help (Nedeltchev et al. 2007). One possible explanation for this paucity of knowledge may be the lack of public education programs targeting TIA. Most public-awareness messages regarding stroke warning signs do not emphasize that the occurrence of symptoms, whether transient or permanent, demand prompt medical attention and a call to emergency medical services.

However, more relevant to delays to treatment is actual behavior in the event of a TIA or minor stroke itself as opposed to knowledge amongst the general public. Data from Oxfordshire, UK, suggest that behavior is variable and significant delays are common (Giles et al. 2006). Consecutive patients with TIA participating in the Oxford Vascular Study (OXVASC) or attending dedicated hospital clinics were interviewed. Of 241 patients, 107 (44%) sought medical attention within hours of the event and 134 (56%) did so on the same day (Giles et al. 2006). Only 24 (10%) patients immediately attended the emergency department (ED). While 101 patients (42%) correctly recognized the cause of their symptoms as a TIA or a "ministroke," this was not associated with an increased likelihood of emergency action. The main correlate with delay was the day of the week on which the TIA occurred ($p < 0.001$), with greater delays at the weekend or public holidays. These findings were supported from observations in a clinical trial of patients with asymptomatic carotid stenosis, in which only a third of those who had a TIA during follow-up reported it to medical attention within three days despite being regularly reminded to do so (Castaldo et al. 1997). These data suggest that frequent public education is required not only on the nature of a TIA but also on what to do in the event of one.

Recognition tools

Several tools have been devised to aid the correct recognition of stroke and TIA symptoms (Table 19.1). In the pre-hospital setting, FAST (Face, Arm, Speech Test; Nor et al. 2004), LAPPS (Los Angeles Pre-hospital Stroke Scale; Kidwell et al. 2000) and CPSS (Cincinatti Pre-hospital Stroke Scale; Kothari et al. 1999) have been designed for use by emergency medical services to ensure rapid transport of appropriate patients to specialist care. In the ED setting, the Recognition of Stroke in the Emergency Department (ROSIER) score has been designed to aid emergency physicians in diagnosis and, therefore, referral of stroke patients (Nor et al. 2005) (Table 19.2). These tools are based mainly on features that discriminate both positively and negatively between stroke and stroke mimics and contain symptoms and signs.

Table 19.2. The Recognition of Stroke in the Emergency Department (ROSIER) score[a]

Feature	Score for answer	
	Yes	No
If blood glucose (BM) is < 3.5 mmol/l, treat urgently and then re-assess		
Has there been loss of consciousness or syncope?	−1	0
Has there been seizure activity?	−1	0
Is there a new acute onset (or awakening from sleep)?		
Asymmetrical facial weakness	+1	0
Asymmetrical arm weakness	+1	0
Asymmetrical leg weakness	+1	0
Speech disturbance	+1	0
Visual field defect	+1	0
Total (−2 to +5)		

Note:
[a] On validation in 343 patients with suspected stroke, the optimum cut-off point for stroke diagnosis was determined to be a total score of +1 or above. Using this cut-point, the corresponding sensitivity and specificity were 92% (95% confidence interval [CI], 89–95) and 86% (95% CI, 82–90), respectively (Nor *et al.* 2005).

The primary aim of these tools has been to increase the numbers of stroke patients presenting to hospital within three hours and, therefore, increase eligibility for thrombolysis. However, with increasing emphasis on rapid management for minor stroke and TIA, their use in informing public education and correct diagnosis of minor TIA and stroke is likely to become more widespread. Indeed, the ABCD system was developed to predict the early risk of stroke following TIA and one of its main uses has been in triage between primary and secondary care (Rothwell *et al.* 2005; National Institute for Health and Clinical Excellence 2008).

Urgency and clinical setting for treatment of transient ischemic attack and minor stroke

A number of treatments have been shown to prevent stroke in the long term after a TIA or minor ischemic stroke (Ch. 24), including antiplatelet agents such as aspirin, clopidogrel, and the combination of low-dose aspirin and extended-release dipyridamole (CAPRIE Steering Committee 1996; Diener *et al.* 1996; Antithrombotic Trialists Collaboration 2002; Halkes *et al.* 2006); blood pressure-lowering drugs (PROGRESS Collaborative Group 2001); statins (Amarenco *et al.* 2006); anticoagulation for atrial fibrillation (European Atrial Fibrillation Trial Study Group 1993); and endarterectomy for symptomatic carotid stenosis ≥ 50% (Rothwell *et al.* 2003; Rothwell *et al.* 2004a). If the effects of these treatments are independent, combined use of all of these interventions in appropriate patients would be predicted to reduce the risk of recurrent stroke by 80% to 90% (Hackam and Spence 2007). However, although trials of treatment in acute stroke and acute coronary syndromes suggest that the relative benefits of several of these interventions are even greater in the acute phase, until recently there have been few if any, reliable data on the benefits of acute treatment after TIA and minor stroke.

Guidelines suggest that assessment and investigation should be completed within one week of a TIA or minor stroke (Wolfe *et al.* 1999; Johnston *et al.* 2006; National Institute for Health and Clinical Excellence 2008). However, perhaps unsurprisingly given the historical lack of evidence, there is considerable international variation in how patients with suspected TIA or minor stroke are managed in the acute phase. Some healthcare systems provide immediate emergency inpatient care, and others provide non-emergency outpatient clinic assessment (Johnston and Smith 1999; Goldstein *et al.* 2000) with little consensus on which strategy is most cost effective (Gubitz *et al.* 1999; Ovbiagele *et al.* 2004).

For example, in a Canadian study conducted in Ontario in 2000, Gladstone and colleagues (2004) found that 75% of patients with a TIA were sent home from the ED without investigation or appropriate management. Diagnostic investigations were under-used, with 58% of patients receiving CT scanning, 44% of patients receiving carotid Doppler ultrasound and 3% receiving MRI within 30 days of the event. In more than one-third of the patients, antithrombotic therapy was not prescribed at discharge. This is in contrast to France and Germany, where a policy of admission is recommended for TIA (Albucher *et al.* 2005) and the mean lengths of stay in hospital for patients with TIAs are about seven days (Weimar *et al.* 2002). In the UK, the standard means of assessment and management is a neurovascular outpatient clinic ("TIA clinic") (Intercollegiate Working Party for Stroke 2004).

The Early Use of Existing Preventive Strategies for Stroke study

The Early Use of Existing Preventive Strategies for Stroke (EXPRESS) study aimed to determine the effect of more rapid treatment after TIA and minor stroke in patients who were treated in a specialist neurovascular clinic (Rothwell *et al.* 2007) within OXVASC. In a prospective, population-based, sequential comparison study, the effect on the process of care and outcome of either urgent access and immediate treatment in a dedicated neurovascular clinic or an appointment-based access and routine treatment initiated in primary care were compared for all patients with TIA or minor stroke who did not need hospital admission. The primary outcome was the risk of stroke during the 90 days after first seeking medical attention.

The study was split into two 30-month phases lasting from April 2002 to September 2004 and from October 2004 to March 2007 (Table 19.3). Throughout the two phases, all patients in the study were ascertained and followed up in the same way, whether they were managed in the study's dedicated neurovascular clinic, admitted to hospital or were managed at home by their general practitioner (primary care physician). During the first phase, the study clinic offered appointment-based access to patients and treatment recommendations were communicated by fax or telephone to the general practitioner, who would then initiate the prescription. In the second phase, patients were sent to the clinic urgently without the need for an appointment and treatment was started immediately in the clinic. The study clinic operated at weekdays but not at weekends. Importantly, throughout the study period, the treatment regimen used and methods of assessment, imaging and follow-up did not change. If a recurrent vascular event was suspected at a follow-up visit, the patient was re-assessed and investigated by a study physician, but all potential outcome events were independently adjudicated, blinded to study period (Table 19.3).

Of the 1278 patients in the OXVASC population who presented with TIA or stroke throughout the study period, 607, predominantly with major stroke, were referred or presented directly to the hospital; 620 were referred for outpatient assessment with TIA or minor stroke; and 51 were not referred to secondary care. Of all outpatient referrals,

Table 19.3. Summary of the study design for the Early Use of Existing Preventive Strategies for Stroke (EXPRESS) study

	Phase 1	Phase 2
Period	0–30 months	30–60 months
Appointment system	Daily appointment clinic	Emergency access clinic
Treatment initiation	Advice faxed to GP	Started immediately in clinic
Treatment protocol	Similar throughout	
Patient assessment	Similar throughout	
Follow-up	Similar throughout	
Outcome adjudication	Outcomes independently audited, blind to study period	

Note:
GP, general practitioner.

Table 19.4. Delay to seeking medical attention and subsequent delay in being seen in the clinic for all patients who were referred to the study clinic in the EXPRESS study[a]

Delay	Phase 1 (n = 310)	Phase 2 (n = 281)	p-value
First call for medical attention[b]			
≤ 12 hours	128 (41.3%)	105 (37.5%)	0.35
≤ 24-hours	184 (59.4%)	160 (57.1%)	0.62
First call for attention to assessment in study clinic[c]			
≤ 6 hours	5 (1.7%)	80 (29.0%)	< 0.0001
≤ 24-hours	70 (23.4%)	163 (59.1%)	< 0.0001

Notes:
[a]See Table 19.3 for study details.
[b]Data unavailable for one patient in phase 2.
[c]Data unavailable for one patient in phase 1 and two patients in phase 2 and not applicable in a further ten patients in phase 1 and three patients in phase 2 who were referred to the EXPRESS clinic but had a stroke and were admitted to hospital prior to the clinic assessment.
Source: From Rothwell et al. (2007).

591 out of 620 (95%) were to the dedicated EXPRESS study neurovascular clinic. There were 634 events during phase 1 and 644 during phase 2.

Baseline characteristics and delays in seeking initial medical attention were similar in the two periods. However median delay to assessment in the study clinic fell from 3 days (range, 2–5) in phase 1 to < 1 (range, 0–3) in phase 2 ($p < 0.001$) (Table 19.4) and the median delay to first prescription of treatment fell from 20 days (range, 8–53) to 1 day (range, 0–3) ($p < 0.001$). Fig. 19.1 shows the cumulative proportions of patients referred to the EXPRESS clinic in phase 1 and 2 and their resulting medication. The 90-day risk of recurrent stroke in all patients referred to the study clinic was 10.3% (32/310) in phase 1 versus 2.1% (6/281) in phase 2 (hazard ratio, 0.20; 95% confidence interval [CI], 0.08–0.48; $p < 0.001$) (Fig. 19.2). There was no significant change in risk in patients treated elsewhere. The 90-day risk of recurrent stroke after all TIA or stroke presentations in the whole population fell from 9.9% (63/635) in phase 1 to 4.4% (28/644) in phase 2 ($p = 0.0002$), while that for patients with TIA alone fell from 12.4% (29/233) in phase 1 to 4.4% (11/252) in phase 2 ($p = 0.0015$). This

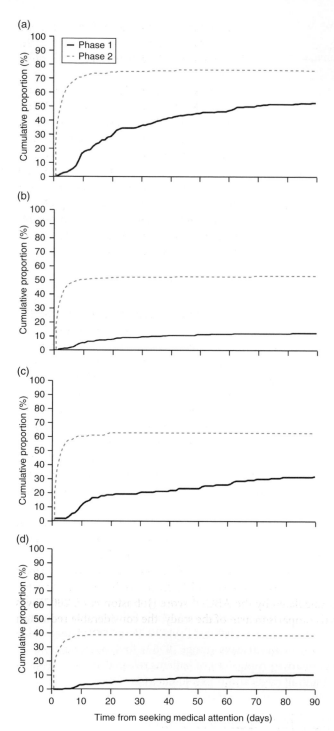

Fig. 19.1. Cumulative proportions of patients referred to the Early Use of Existing Preventive Strategies for Stroke (EXPRESS) study clinic in phases 1 — and 2 (---) prescribed new medication. (a) Any statin drug (in patients not already on a statin); (b) clopidogrel (usually in addition to aspirin); (c) initiation of a first blood pressure-lowering drug (in patients not already on such medication); (d) initiation of two blood pressure-lowering drugs (in patients previously on none or only one drug) (Rothwell *et al.* 2007).

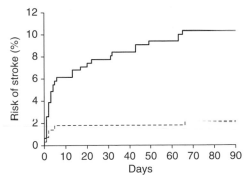

Fig. 19.2. The 90-day risk of recurrent stroke after first seeking medical attention in all patients with transient ischemic attack or stroke referred to the study clinic in the non-randomized Early Use of Existing Preventive Strategies for Stroke (EXPRESS) study (Rothwell *et al.* 2007). The continuous line represents phase 1 of the study (standard treatment) and the dotted line represents phase 2 (urgent treatment).

reduction in risk was independent of age and sex, and early treatment did not increase the risk of intracerebral hemorrhage or other bleeding.

Because the EXPRESS study was nested within OXVASC (Rothwell *et al.* 2004b), identical methods of case ascertainment, assessment and follow-up for the entire study population during both phases ensured that there were no temporal changes in referral patterns, patient characteristics or other potential sources of bias. The findings, therefore, strongly suggested that the considerable impact on outcome was a consequence of more rapid assessment and treatment.

The SOS-TIA study

The good prognosis associated with urgent and intensive treatment observed in the EXPRESS study was also highlighted by the results of the SOS-TIA study (Lavallée *et al.* 2007). In 2003, a dedicated emergency TIA clinic was set up in the Neurology Department of the Neurology and Stroke Center of Bichat Hospital in an administrative region of Paris. All 15 000 general practitioners, cardiologists, neurologists and ophthalmologists in the region were sent information about the service, which offered emergency assessment of all patients with suspected TIA via a toll-free referral telephone number. The SOS-TIA service was available and accessible 24-hours a day, seven days a week. It aimed to offer an evaluation by a vascular neurologist within four hours of referral: if a TIA was confirmed, further standardized investigations were performed including MRI, carotid Doppler and transcranial Doppler ultrasound. Medical treatment was initiated immediately. Patients were discharged home unless they fulfilled predefined criteria for admission to the hospital's stroke unit (Table 19.5).

The study recorded the medical history, medications, symptom details, examination findings, final diagnosis, treatment plans and one-year outcomes (assessed by phone calls) of all referrals. In the first report of all 629 consecutive patients with definite TIA seen from January 2003 to December 2005, there were three strokes within seven days and 12 strokes within three months of follow-up, giving risks of 0.3% and 1.9%, respectively. The expected risk of stroke at three months as calculated by the ABCD^2 score (Johnston *et al.* 2007) was 6%. Although there was no formal comparison arm of the study, the considerable reduction in observed rates of stroke compared with those expected by the ABCD^2 score was reasonably attributed to urgent access to and treatment in a dedicated specialist neurovascular unit. However, it should be noted that this study only assessed stroke risk among patients referred to the clinic and not all those within the population.

Specific treatments in transient ischemic attack and minor stroke

One potential criticism of the EXPRESS (Rothwell *et al.* 2007) and SOS-TIA (Lavallée *et al.* 2007) studies is that a "black box" intervention approach was used. All patients received

Table 19.5. Criteria for admission to the stroke unit after assessment in the SOS-TIA clinic

	Criteria
Related to TIA cause (highly suspected or identified)	High-grade stenosis of intra- or extracranial brain arteries
	Intracranial hemodynamic compromise with low flow in the middle cerebral artery
	Suspected cardiac source at high risk of recurrent embolism: prosthetic mechanical heart valve, endocarditis, aortic dissection, acute coronary syndrome, overt congestive heart failure
Related to the TIA presentation	Crescendo TIA
Cardiac monitoring over 24-hours warranted	High level of suspicion for paroxysmal atrial fibrillation

Note:
TIA, transient ischemic attack.

a standardized treatment regimen of antiplatelet agents, antihypertensives and statins plus, in selected cases, anticoagulation and carotid endarterectomy, which was administered rapidly in the context of an urgent-access dedicated neurovascular service. The relative benefit or even harm attributable to any particular part of the interventional package could not be determined.

Apart from patients with symptomatic carotid stenosis and endarterectomy, to date, only the Fast Assessment of Stroke and Transient Ischemic Attack to Prevent Early Recurrence (FASTER) trial has addressed the difference between specific treatments administered early for patients with TIA and minor stroke (Kennedy *et al.* 2007).

The Fast Assessment of Stroke and Transient Ischemic Attack to Prevent Early Recurrence (FASTER) trial

The FASTER randomized controlled pilot trial studied the benefit of clopidogrel versus placebo and simvastatin versus placebo initiated within 24-hours of symptom onset in patients with TIA or minor stroke, all of whom were treated with aspirin (Kennedy *et al.* 2007). The primary outcome was any stroke (ischemic and hemorrhagic) within 90 days. Minor stroke was defined as a score ≤ 3 on the National Institutes of Health Stroke Scale (NIHSS) at the time of randomization and TIA was defined in the usual way. In addition, patients were excluded if they did not have weakness or speech disturbance or if symptom duration was less than five minutes.

The trial was stopped early owing to a failure to recruit patients, probably because of the increased use of statins during the study period. A total of 392 patients were included (mean age 68.1 years; 185 [47.1%] female) of whom 100 received clopidogrel and simvastatin, 98 received clopidogrel and placebo, 99 received simvastatin and placebo and 95 received placebo only. In the patients taking clopidogrel, 14 (7.1%) had a stroke within 90 days, compared with 21 (10.8%) of those on placebo (risk ratio, 0.7 [95% CI, 0.3–1.2]; absolute risk reduction, -3.8% [95% CI,-9.4 to 1.9]; $p = 0.19$). Two patients on clopidogrel had intracranial hemorrhage compared with none on placebo (absolute risk increase, 1.0% [95% CI, -0.4 to 2.4]; $p = 0.5$). In the group taking simvastin, 21 (10.6%) patients had a stroke within 90 days, compared with 14 (7.3%) patients taking placebo (risk ratio taking 1.3 [95% CI, 0.7–2.4]; absolute risk increase, 3.3% [95% CI, -2.3 to 8.9]; $p = 0.25$) and there was no difference between groups for the simvastatin safety outcomes.

The study concluded that the combination of aspirin and clopidogrel started within 24-hours of symptom onset may be superior to aspirin alone in reducing the risk of stroke at 90 days after TIA or minor stroke, although at the expense of a higher rate of hemorrhage. These results form the basis of the FASTER-2 study, which will determine the risks and benefits of aspirin and clopidogrel compared with aspirin alone in larger numbers of patients. The FASTER trial did not show any benefit for simvastatin in the acute phase after TIA or minor stroke and no statin comparison is included in FASTER-2.

References

Albucher JF, Martel P, Mas JL (2005). Clinical practice guidelines: diagnosis and immediate management of transient ischemic attacks in adults. *Cerebrovascular Diseases* **20**:220–225

Amarenco P, Bogousslavsky J, Callahan A III for the Stroke Prevention by Aggressive Reduction in Cholesterol Levels (SPARCL) Investigators (2006). High-dose atorvastatin after stroke or transient ischemic attack. *New England Journal of Medicine* **355**:549–559

Antithrombotic Trialists Collaboration (2002). Collaborative meta-analysis of randomised trials of antiplatelet therapy for prevention of death, myocardial infarction, and stroke in high risk patients. *British Medical Journal* **324**:71–86

CAPRIE Steering Committee (1996). A randomised, blinded, trial of clopidogrel versus aspirin in patients at risk of ischaemic events (CAPRIE). *Lancet* **348**:1329–1339

Carroll C, Hobart J, Fox C et al. (2004). Stroke in Devon: knowledge was good, but action was poor. *Journal of Neurology, Neurosurgery and Psychiatry* **75**:567–571

Castaldo JE, Nelson JJ, Reed JF III et al. (1997). The delay in reporting symptoms of carotid artery stenosis in an at-risk population. The Asymptomatic Carotid Atherosclerosis Study experience: a statement of concern regarding watchful waiting. *Archives of Neurology* **54**:1267–1271

Diener HC, Cunha L, Forbes C et al. (1996). European secondary prevention study 2: dipyridamole and acetylsalicylic acid in the secondary prevention of stroke. *Journal of Neurology Science* **143**:1–13

European Atrial Fibrillation Trial Study Group (1993). Secondary prevention in non-rheumatic atrial fibrillation after transient ischaemic attack or minor stroke. *Lancet* **342**:1255–1262

Evenson KR, Rosamond WD, Morris DL (2001). Prehospital and in-hospital delays in acute stroke care. *Neuroepidemiology* **20**:65–76

Giles MF, Flossman E, Rothwell PM (2006). Patient behaviour immediately after transient ischemic attack according to clinical characteristics, perception of the event, and predicted risk of stroke. *Stroke* **37**:1254–1260

Gladstone DJ, Kapral MK, Fang J (2004). Management and outcomes of transient ischemic attacks in Ontario. *Canadian Medical Association Journal* **170**:1099–1104

Goldstein LB, Bian J, Samsa GP et al. (2000). New transient ischemic attack and stroke: outpatient management by primary care physicians. *Archives of International Medicine* **160**:2941–2946

Gubitz G, Phillips S, Dwyer V (1999). What is the cost of admitting patients with transient ischaemic attacks to hospital? *Cerebrovascular Diseases* **9**:210–214

Hackam DG, Spence JD (2007). Combining multiple approaches for the secondary prevention of vascular events after stroke: a quantitative modeling study. *Stroke* **38**:1881–1885

Halkes PH, van Gijn for the ESPRIT Study Group J (2006). Aspirin plus dipyridamole versus aspirin alone after cerebral ischaemia of arterial origin (ESPRIT): randomised controlled trial. *Lancet* **367**:1665–1673

Harraf F, Sharma AK, Brown MM et al. (2002). A multicentre observational study of presentation and early assessment of acute stroke. *British Medical Journal* **325**:17–22

Intercollegiate Working Party for Stroke (2004). *National Clinical Guidelines for Stroke.* London: Royal College of Physicians

Johnston SC, Smith WS (1999). Practice variability in management of transient ischemic attacks. *European Neurology* **42**:105–108

Johnston SC, Fayad PB, Gorelick PB *et al.*
(2003). Prevalence and knowledge of transient
ischemic attack among US adults. *Neurology*
60:1429–1434

Johnston SC, Nguyen-Huynh MN, Schwarz ME
et al. (2006). National Stroke Association
guidelines for the management of transient
ischemic attacks. *Annals of Neurology*
60:301–313

Johnston SC, Rothwell PM, Nguyen-Huynh MN
et al. (2007). Validation and refinement of
scores to predict very early stroke risk after
transient ischaemic attack. *Lancet*
369:283–292

Kennedy J, Hill MD, Ryckborst KJ *et al.*
FASTER Investigators (2007). Fast
Assessment of Stroke and Transient
Ischaemic Attack to Prevent Early Recurrence
(FASTER): a randomised controlled pilot
trial. *Lancet Neurology* **6**:961–969

Kidwell CS, Starkman S, Eckstein M *et al.*
(2000). Identifying stroke in the field.
Prospective validation of the Los Angeles
prehospital stroke screen (LAPSS). *Stroke*
31:71–76

Kothari RU, Pancioli A, Liu T *et al.* (1999).
Cincinnati Prehospital Stroke Scale:
reproducibility and validity. *Annals of
Emergency Medicine* **33**:373–378

Lacy CR, Suh DC, Bueno M *et al.* (2001). Delay
in presentation and evaluation for acute
stroke: Stroke Time Registry for Outcomes
Knowledge and Epidemiology (STROKE).
Stroke **32**:63–69

Lavallée PC, Meseguer E, Abboud H *et al.*
(2007). A transient ischaemic attack clinic
with round-the-clock access (SOS-TIA):
feasibility and effects. *Lancet Neurology*
6:953–960

National Institute for Health and Clinical
Excellence (2008). *Stroke: Diagnosis and
Initial Management of Acute Stroke and
Transient Ischaemic Attack (TIA). Draft
Guidance for Consultation.* London: NICE

Nedeltchev K, Fischer U, Arnold M *et al.* (2007).
Low awareness of transient ischemic attacks
and risk factors of stroke in a Swiss urban
community. *Journal of Neurology*
254:179–184

Nor A, Mc Allister C, Louw S *et al.* (2004).
Agreement between ambulance paramedic-
and physician-recorded neurological signs

using the Face Arm Speech Test (FAST) in
acute stroke patients. *Stroke* **35**:1355–1359

Nor AM, Davis J, Sen B *et al.* (2005). The
Recognition of Stroke in the Emergency
Room (ROSIER) scale: development and
validation of a stroke recognition instrument.
Lancet Neurology **4**:727–734

Ovbiagele B, Saver JL, Fredieu A *et al.* (2004).
In-hospital initiation of secondary stroke
prevention therapies yields high rates of
adherence at follow-up. *Stroke* **35**:2879–2883

Pancioli A, Broderick J, Kothari R *et al.* (1998).
Public perception of stroke warning signs and
knowledge of potential risk factors. *Journal of
the American Medical Association*
279:1288–1292

Parahoo K, Thompson K, Cooper M *et al.* (2003).
Stroke: awareness of the signs, symptoms and
risk factors – a population-based survey.
Cerebrovascular Diseases **16**:134–140

PROGRESS Collaborative Group (2001).
Randomised trial of a perindopril-based
blood-pressure-lowering regimen among
6105 individuals with previous stroke or
transient ischaemic attack. *Lancet*
358:1033–1041

Reeves MJ, Hogan JG, Rafferty AP (2002).
Knowledge of stroke risk factors and warning
signs among Michigan adults. *Neurology*
59:1547–1552

Rothwell PM, Gutnikov SA, Eliasziw M for the
Carotid Endarterectomy Trialists'
Collaboration (2003). Pooled analysis of
individual patient data from randomised
controlled trials of endarterectomy for
symptomatic carotid stenosis. *Lancet*
361:107–116

Rothwell PM, Eliasziw M, Gutnikov SA for the
Carotid Endarterectomy Trialists
Collaboration. (2004a). Effect of
endarterectomy for symptomatic carotid
stenosis in relation to clinical subgroups and
to the timing of surgery. *Lancet* **363**:915–924

Rothwell PM, Coull A, Giles MF for the Oxford
Vascular Study (2004b). Change in stroke
incidence, mortality, case-fatality, severity,
and risk factors in Oxfordshire, UK from
1981 to 2004 (Oxford Vascular Study).
Lancet **363**:1925–1933

Rothwell PM, Giles MF, Flossman E *et al.*
(2005). A simple score (ABCD) to identify
individuals at high early risk of stroke

after transient ischaemic attack. *Lancet* **366**:29–36

Rothwell PM, Giles MF, Chandratheva A *et al.* (2007). Effect of urgent treatment of transient ischaemic attack and minor stroke on early recurrent stroke (EXPRESS study): a prospective population-based sequential comparison. *Lancet* **370**:1432–1442

Salisbury HR, Banks BJ, Footitt DR *et al.* (1998). Delay in presentation of patients with acute stroke to hospital in Oxford. *Quarterly Journal of Medicine* **97**:635–640

Smith MA, Doliszny KM, Shahar E *et al.* (1998). Delayed hospital arrival for acute stroke: the Minnesota Stroke Survey. *Annals of International Medicine* **129**:190–196

Weimar C, Kraywinkel K, Rödl J *et al.* (2002). Etiology, duration, and prognosis of transient ischemic attacks: an analysis from the German Stroke Data Bank. *Archives of Neurology* **59**:1584–1588

Wolf PA, Clagett GP, Easton JD *et al.* (1999). Preventing ischemic stroke in patients with prior stroke and transient ischemic attack: a statement for healthcare professionals from the Stroke Council of the American Heart Association. *Stroke* **30**:1991–1994

Chapter 20

Acute treatment of major stroke: general principles

The general treatments described in this chapter are applicable to all patients with acute major stroke regardless of etiology. Specific treatment for ischemic and hemorrhagic stroke is discussed in Chs. 21 and 22, respectively. Therapy for acute stroke can be divided into:

- treatment of the acute event in which the aim is to minimize mortality, impairment and disability and reduce the complications of stroke
- prevention of recurrent stroke.

For patients who have suffered a major disabling stroke, emphasis is placed, at least initially, on the former whereas in patients with TIA or minor stroke, the emphasis is on the latter.

Non-neurological complications and their management

Non-neurological complications after acute stroke are more frequent with increasing age, pre-stroke disability, stroke severity and poor general nursing and other care (Box 20.1). To some extent, the site of the lesion may also be relevant; for instance, obstructive and central sleep apnea might occur more often in brainstem stroke (Davenport *et al.* 1996a; van der Worp and Kappelle 1998). Early detection and prevention of complications depends on clinical monitoring (Table 20.1).

Box 20.1. General medical complications of acute stroke

Pneumonia
  Venous thromboembolism
  Urinary incontinence and infection
  Pressure sores
  Cardiac arrhythmias, failure, myocardial infarction
  Fluid imbalance, hyponatremia
  "Mechanical" problems
- spasticity
- contractures
- malalignment/subuxation/frozen shoulder
- falls and fractures
- osteoporosis
- ankle swelling
- peripheral nerve pressure palsies
Mood disorders
Gastric ulceration and hemorrhage
Central post-stroke "thalamic" pain

Pneumonia

Pneumonia is a common complication in elderly patients confined to bed. Chest infection is particularly common after stroke because of impairment in swallow and cough reflex, poor respiratory movement and pulmonary embolism. The risks can be reduced by good nursing and chest physiotherapy. A pharyngeal airway may be required, particularly in drowsy patients or after a brainstem stroke, and ventilation may be considered in certain patients.

Venous thromboembolism

Approximately 50% of hemiparetic patients in hospital develop a deep vein thrombosis in their paralyzed leg, although this is not usually detectable clinically. However, a swollen and painful leg compromises rehabilitation. A resultant pulmonary embolism causes

Table 20.1. Routine monitoring in acute stroke

	Monitor
Vital signs	Respiratory rate and rhythmn, blood gases
	Heart rate and rhythm (often with electrocardiographic monitor)
	Blood pressure (normal arm)
	Temperature (normal axilla)
Neurological	Conscious level (Glasgow Coma Scale)
	Pupils
	Limb weakness
	Epileptic seizures
General	Fluid balance
	Electrolytes and urea
	Blood glucose
	Hematocrit

hypoxia, pneumonia, impacts on neurological recovery and may cause death (Wijdicks and Scott 1997). Evidence from clinical trials of thromboembolism prophylaxis in a variety of postoperative conditions suggests that subcutaneous heparin, graduated compression stockings and aspirin are effective in reducing the risk of deep venous thrombosis in bedridden patients (Andre *et al.* 2007). However, routine heparin prophylaxis is not recommended after stroke because of increased cerebral hemorrhage. Aspirin should be given after ischemic stroke since this reduces the risk of recurrent stroke as well as venous thromboembolism. There is no evidence that compression stockings are effective specifically after stroke, but they are the method of choice for thromboprophylaxis after primary intracerebral hemorrhage. A large multicenter randomized controlled trial of low-dose heparin versus compression stockings in ischemic stroke is currently ongoing (Dennis 2004).

Urinary incontinence

Incontinence is common after stroke and may be permanent (Brittain *et al.* 1998). Catheterization is often required to maintain skin care, at least initially. Urinary infection is common owing to immobility and the use of urinary catheters.

Pressure sores

Pressure sores may occur secondary to poor nursing, incontinence or malnourishment. They may become infected and take months to heal, thus delaying rehabilitation. Pressure sores can be avoided by attention to pressure areas, use of appropriate mattresses and supports and by regular turning of immobile patients (NHS center for Reviews and Dissemination and the Nuffield Institute for Health 1995).

Cardiac complications

Electrocardiographic ST depression, T wave flattening and inversion, U waves and a prolonged Q–T interval are common but transient occurrences after acute ischemic, and particularly after acute hemorrhagic, stroke. They seldom cause clinical problems. Some abnormalities may have preceded the stroke (Oppenheimer *et al.* 1990). It is not known whether monitoring the electrocardiogram improves the prognosis, but it is often recommended, particularly after subarachnoid hemorrhage. Some patients have a rise in blood cardiac troponin after stroke, and there is some evidence that this is more likely after involvement of the insula, particularly on the right, and may be linked to high circulating catecholamine levels (Cheshire and Saper 2006). However, it is not clear whether elevated cardiac troponin is an independent predictor of poor outcome after stroke.

Fluid imbalance
Patients unable to take sufficient fluids orally require fluid by nasogastric tube or intravenous hydration. Hyponatremia, probably reflecting salt wasting and the stress response, is particularly common after subarachnoid hemorrhage and, in general, should be treated by plasma volume expansion and not fluid restriction. Urinary tract infection and dehydration may cause renal failure.

Mechanical problems
Spasticity, muscle contractures, painful shoulder and other joints of a paralyzed limb, malalignment or subluxation of the shoulder, falls and fractures can all potentially be avoided by good nursing and physiotherapy. Osteoporosis in a paralyzed limb presumably increases the risk of fractures but may be unavoidable (Sato *et al.* 1998).

Acute gastric ulceration
Gastric ulceration, with or without hemorrhage or perforation, is a well recognized but rare complication in severe stroke and may be difficult to prevent (Davenport *et al.* 1996b).

Mood disorders
A systematic review of observational studies of post-stroke depression produced an estimated overall prevalence of 33% among all stroke survivors (Hackett *et al.* 2005). Predictors of depression include severity of stroke and cognitive impairment (Hackett and Andersen 2005). It has been postulated that left-sided brain lesions are more likely to cause depression, but this remains unproven (Bhogal *et al.* 2004). Mood disorder may impede rehabilitation and contribute to disability and handicap but usually improves with time. Treatment includes support and counseling and antidepressants.

Central post-stroke pain
Post-stroke, or "thalamic," pain is a burning, severe and paroxysmal pain exacerbated by touch and other stimuli. Such post-stroke pain is rare and usually occurs weeks or months after stroke (Nasreddine and Saver 1997; Frese *et al.* 2006). There are usually some sensory signs in the affected areas. The lesion is usually located in the contralateral thalamus but may lie elsewhere in the central sensory pathways. Treatment includes anticonvulsants, amitriptyline and various sorts of counter-stimulation but is often unsuccessful.

Generic treatment for acute stroke
Many of the interventions described below aim to prevent physiological changes such as hypotension, hyperglycemia and pyrexia. These might result in secondary ischemic injury through excacerbating the flow/metabolism mismatch in the penumbral and oligemic areas surrounding the infarcted core, resulting in extension of infarction into these areas.

> **Box 20.2.** Core features of stroke units included by Stroke Unit Trialists' Collaboration
>
> Coordinated care delivered by a multidisciplinary team
> Multidisciplinary team members interested in and specialized in stroke
> Regular training for staff provided
> Regular multidisciplinary team meetings (at least once a week)
> Involvement of carers in patient care
> Nurses have expertise in rehabilitation
> *Source:* Stroke Unit Trialists' Collaboration (1997, 2000).

Stroke units

The concept of a stroke unit as being a geographically defined service offering either acute or subacute (or both) care and rehabilitation delivered by a dedicated team is quite clear, although the exact definition of a stroke unit is less so. There is evidence that admission to an acute stroke unit providing certain core features (Box 20.2) reduces mortality and morbidity and dependency (Stroke Unit Trialists' Collaboration 2000). The benefits are seen for all ages, both sexes and across the range of stroke severity. Compared with care on general medical wards, care in a stroke unit reduces mortality and increases the chances of independence (Stroke Unit Trialists' Collaboration 1997, 2000, 2002). Stroke unit care also reduces length of stay and is cost effective in comparison with care on general wards with or without mobile specialist team input and domiciliary care (Patel *et al.* 2004; Moodie *et al.* 2006). The beneficial effects of stroke unit care are also maintained long term (Fuentes *et al.* 2006). Despite the evidence for the effectiveness of stroke units, many patients in the UK are not admitted to such a unit owing to lack of capacity, although the situation is improving (Intercollegiate Working Party on Stroke 2006).

Blood pressure

The optimal management of blood pressure in acute stroke is uncertain. Ischemic and infarcted brain cannot autoregulate and so relatively modest increases in cerebral perfusion pressure can cause hyperemia, increased cerebral blood flow, cerebral edema and hemorrhagic infarction, whereas a fall in cerebral perfusion pressure may exacerbate cerebral ischemia. Blood pressure is often elevated on admission but tends to fall spontaneously during the first few days (Bath and Bath 1997). Reliable evidence to guide blood pressure management is lacking at present (Blood Pressure in Acute Stroke Collaboration 2001) but two large ongoing randomized controlled trials should provide more reliable guidance within the next few years (Willmot *et al.* 2006; Mistri *et al.* 2006). In practice, many clinicians continue existing antihypertensive therapy but only consider active treatment of blood pressure for sustained blood pressures of around > 220/120 mmHg or > 185/105 mmHg in cerebral infarction and cerebral hemorrhage, respectively. Exceptions occur where there is coexistent hypertensive encephalopathy, aortic dissection, acute myocardial infarction or severe left ventricular failure.

Hypoxia

Damaged brain appears to have impaired responsiveness to arterial partial pressure of carbon dioxide and oxygen as well as impaired autoregulation and perfusion reserve, increasing the likelihood of further "secondary" insults such as systemic hypoxia, hypotension and raised intracranial pressure (Cormio *et al.* 1997). There are good theoretical

Box 20.3. Causes of fever after stroke

Infection:
- urinary tract
- respiratory
- pressure sores
- septicemia
- intravenous access site

Deep vein thrombosis and pulmonary embolism

Infective endocarditis

Drug reaction

reasons why routine oxygen therapy might be beneficial, but there are also potential deleterious effects (Singhal 2007) and so randomized trials are required. Oxygen should be given if saturations are less than 95%. A randomized trial of routine oxygen supplementation is ongoing (Ali *et al.* 2006).

Hyperglycemia

Hyperglycemia after acute stroke is a common finding that has consistently been associated with an increased risk of death. The hypothesis that maintenance of euglycemia post-stroke would improve outcome was tested in the UK Glucose Insulin in Stroke Trial (GIST-UK) (Gray *et al.* 2007). Infusion of glucose–potassium–insulin to maintain capillary glucose at 4–7 mmol/l showed no significant reduction in mortality or severe disability at 90 days. The authors concluded that treatment within the trial protocol was not associated with significant clinical benefit, although the study was underpowered and the difference in glycemic control between the treatment groups was small.

Fever

Fever may occur after stroke for a number of reasons (Box 20.3). Animal studies and observational data in humans suggest that pyrexia increases infarct size and is associated with poor outcome, and that the converse is true for hypothermia, but risks and benefits of active cooling in acute stroke are yet to be determined (Reith *et al.* 1996; Hemmen and Lyden 2007; Sacco *et al.* 2007). Infection should be treated promptly but there is no evidence to support the routine use of antipyretics such as paracetamol for temperatures above 37.5 °C, although they are widely used in practice.

Dehydration

Dehydration should be corrected with intravenous fluid replacement, and nasogastric feeding should be instituted in those with unsatisfactory swallow.

Impaired swallowing

Impaired swallowing with risk of aspiration and pneumonia is common in drowsy patients with severe hemispheric strokes, and those with brainstem strokes. It almost always gets better in days or weeks (Hamdy *et al.* 1997). Swallowing difficulty is tested by asking the patient to sip some water, observing any tendency to choke in the next minute or so, and for added sensitivity using simple quantification (Mari *et al.* 1997; Hinds and Wiles 1998).

Nutrition

Feeding in the first few days may not be important, but later the patient should be kept well nourished since poor nutrition may be associated with worse outcome. There is no evidence to support early initiation of percutaneous endoscopic gastrostomy feeding in patients with unsafe swallow (Dennis *et al.* 2005).

Early mobilization

Mobilization may reduce complications, including pneumonia, deep vein thrombosis, pulmonary embolism and pressure ulcers. At present, there are no reliable data to recommend the use of compression stockings or low-dose heparin for deep vein thrombosis prohylaxis (Andre *et al.* 2007) but trials are ongoing (Dennis 2004).

References

Ali K, Roffe C, Crome P (2006). What patients want: consumer involvement in the design of a randomized controlled trial of routine oxygen supplementation after acute stroke. *Stroke* 37:865–871

Andre C, de Freitas GR, Fukujima MM (2007). Prevention of deep venous thrombosis and pulmonary embolism following stroke: a systematic review of published articles. *European Journal of Neurology* 14:21–32

Bath FJ, Bath PMW (1997). What is the correct management of blood pressure in acute stroke? The Blood Pressure in Acute Stroke Collaboration. *Cerebrovascular Diseases* 7:205–213

Bhogal SK, Teasell R, Foley N *et al.* (2004). Lesion location and poststroke depression: systematic review of the methodological limitations in the literature. *Stroke* 35:794–802

Blood Pressure in Acute Stroke Collaboration (BASC) (2001). Interventions for deliberately altering blood pressure in acute stroke. *Cochrane Database of Systematic Reviews* 3:CD000039

Brittain KR, Peet SM, Castleden CM (1998). Stroke and incontinence. *Stroke* 29:524–528

Cheshire WP Jr., Saper CB (2006). The insular cortex and cardiac response to stroke. *Neurology* 66:1296–1297

Cormio M, Robertson CS, Narayan RK (1997). Secondary insults to the injured brain. *Journal of Clinical Neuroscience* 4:132–148

Davenport RJ, Dennis MS, Wellwood I *et al.* (1996a). Complications after acute stroke. *Stroke* 27:415–420

Davenport RJ, Dennis MS, Warlow CP (1996b). Gastrointestinal hemorrhage after acute stroke. *Stroke* 27:421–424

Dennis MS (2004). Effective prophylaxis for deep vein thrombosis after stroke: low-dose anticoagulation rather than stockings alone. *Stroke* 35:2912–2913

Dennis MS, Lewis SC, Warlow C *et al.* (2005). Effect of timing and method of enteral tube feeding for dysphagic stroke patients (FOOD): a multicentre randomised controlled trial. *Lancet* 365:764–772

Frese A, Husstedt IW, Ringelstein EB *et al.* (2006). Pharmacologic treatment of central post-stroke pain. *Clinical Journal of Pain* 22:252–260

Fuentes B, Diez-Tejedor E, Ortega-Casarrubios MA *et al.* (2006). Consistency of the benefits of stroke units over years of operation: an 8-year effectiveness analysis. *Cerebrovascular Diseases* 21:173–179

Gray CS, Hildreth AJ, Sandercock PA *et al.* (2007). Glucose–potassium–insulin infusions in the management of post-stroke hyperglycaemia: the UK Glucose Insulin in Stroke Trial (GIST-UK). *Lancet Neurology* 6:397–406

Hackett ML, Anderson CS (2005). Predictors of depression after stroke: a systematic review of observational studies. *Stroke* 36:2296–2301

Hackett ML, Yapa C, Parag V *et al.* (2005). Frequency of depression after stroke: a systematic review of observational studies. *Stroke* 36:1330–1340

Hamdy S, Aziz Q, Rothwell JC *et al.* (1997). Explaining oropharyngeal dysphagia after unilateral hemispheric stroke. *Lancet* 350:686–692

Hemmen TM, Lyden PD (2007). Induced hypothermia for acute stroke. *Stroke* 38:794–799

Hinds NP, Wiles CM (1998). Assessment of swallowing and referral to speech and language therapists in acute stroke. *Quarterly Journal of Medicine* 91:829–835

Intercollegiate Working Party on Stroke (2006). *National Sentinel Audit.* London: Royal College of Physicians.

Mari F, Matei M, Ceravolo MG *et al.* (1997). Predictive value of clinical indices in detecting aspiration in patients with neurological disorders. *Journal of Neurology, Neurosurgery and Psychiatry* 63:456–460

Mistri AK, Robinson TG, Potter JF (2006). Pressor therapy in acute ischemic stroke: systematic review. *Stroke* **37**:1565–1571

Moodie M, Cadilhac D, Pearce D *et al.* (2006). SCOPES Study Group. Economic evaluation of Australian stroke services: a prospective multicenter study comparing dedicated stroke units with other care modalities. *Stroke* **37**:2790–2795

Nasreddine ZS, Saver JL (1997). Pain after thalamic stroke: right diencephalic predominance and clinical features in 180 patients. *Neurology* **48**:1196–1199

NHS Centre for Reviews and Dissemination and the Nuffield Institute for Health (1995). The Prevention and Treatment of Pressure Sores. Effective Health Care **2**:1–16

Oppenheimer SM, Cechetto DF, Hachinski VC (1990). Cerebrogenic cardiac arrhythmias. Cerebral electrocardiographic influences and their role in sudden death. *Archives of Neurology* **47**:513–519

Patel A, Knapp M, Evans A *et al.* (2004). Training care givers of stroke patients: economic evaluation. *British Medical Journal* **328**:1102

Reith J, Jorgensen HS, Pedersen PM *et al.* (1996). Body temperature in acute stroke: relation to stroke severity, infarct size, mortality and outcome. *Lancet* **347**:422–425

Sacco RL, Chong JY, Prabhakaran S *et al.* (2007). Experimental treatments for acute ischemic stroke. *Lancet* **369**:331–341

Sato Y, Kuno H, Kaji M *et al.* (1998). Increased bone resorption during the first year after stroke. *Stroke* **29**:1373–1377

Singhal AB (2007). A review of oxygen therapy in ischemic stroke. *Neurology Research* **29**:173–183

Stroke Unit Trialists' Collaboration (1997). Collaborative systematic review of the randomised trials of organised inpatient (stroke unit) care after stroke. *British Medical Journal* **314**:1151–1159

Stroke Unit Trialists' Collaboration (2000). Organised inpatient (stroke unit) care for stroke. *Cochrane Database of Systematic Reviews* **2**:CD000197

Stroke Unit Trialists' Collaboration (2002). Organised inpatient (stroke unit) care for stroke: review update. *Cochrane Database of Systematic Reviews* **1**:CD000177

van der Worp HB, Kappelle LJ (1998). Complications of acute ischemic stroke. *Cerebrovascular Diseases* **8**:124–132

Wijdicks EFM, Scott JP (1997). Pulmonary embolism associated with acute stroke. *Mayo Clinic Proceedings* **72**:297–300

Willmot M, Ghadami A, Whysall B *et al.* (2006). Transdermal glyceryl trinitrate lowers blood pressure and maintains cerebral blood flow in recent stroke. *Hypertension* **47**:1209–1215

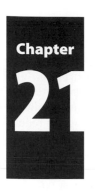

Specific treatments for major acute ischemic stroke

Many of the trials of therapy in acute stroke did not distinguish between stroke subtypes other than by division into hemorrhagic and ischemic stroke. Therefore, there is little evidence for different effectiveness for most acute ischemic stroke treatments according to stroke subtype and location. However, stroke subtype determines patient selection for specific secondary preventive strategies. Therefore, better characterization of stroke will aid overall patient management (Ch. 6).

Therapies to reduce brain damage in ischemic stroke may act by:

- prevention of thrombus extension: using antiplatelet and anticoagulant drugs
- reperfusion by restoration of blood flow; thus reducing infarction within the penumbra: thrombolysis
- limiting the extent of brain ischemia: using neuroprotective agents.

Antiplatelet therapy

Patients with acute stroke should be treated with aspirin as soon as practicable after brain imaging has excluded hemorrhage. One systematic review (Sandercock *et al.* 2003), including two very large randomized controlled trials (International Stroke Trial Collaborative Group 1997; CAST (Chinese Acute Stroke Trial) Collaborative Group 1997), has clearly established that starting aspirin therapy within the first 48 hours of acute ischemic stroke avoids death or disability at six months for approximately 10 patients per 1000 patients treated. A further 10 patients per 1000 treated will make a complete recovery. Both intracranial and extracranial hemorrhage are reported with aspirin therapy, but the rates are low, and are off-set by the benefit of extra lives saved.

There is no clear consensus about whether aspirin should be given prior to brain imaging. This applies to situations where access to imaging is delayed, or where drugs could be administered by ambulance staff. Analysis of outcome in the subgroup of patients who were randomized and who received treatment prior to brain imaging, some of whom subsequently turned out to have primary intracerebral hemorrhage, did not show any obvious difference in risk and benefit from those in the rest of the trial (International Stroke Trial Collaborative Group 1997).

There is no clear evidence that any particular dose of aspirin is more effective than others. However, the symptoms of aspirin toxicity, such as dyspepsia and constipation, are dose related, so the smallest effective dose should be used. A starting dosage of 150–300 mg per day is advised for the acute phase of ischemic stroke followed by long-term treatment with 75–150 mg per day. Patients intolerant of aspirin should be treated with clopidogrel if available, or if not with dipyridamole. These newer agents cost significantly more than aspirin. The use of combination antiplatelet therapy is discussed further in Ch. 24.

Anticoagulation

Immediate therapy with systemic anticoagulants including unfractionated heparin, low-molecular-weight heparin, heparinoids or specific thrombin inhibitors in patients with acute ischemic stroke is not associated with net short- or long-term benefit (International Stroke Trial Collaborative Group 1997; Berge 2007; Wong et al. 2007). These agents reduce the risk of deep venous thrombosis and pulmonary embolus, but they are associated with a significant risk of intracranial hemorrhage, which is dose dependent. Patients in atrial fibrillation after presumed ischemic stroke or TIA benefit from anticoagulation in the long term to prevent further stroke. However, the best time to start therapy after an ischemic stroke is unclear as the risk of hemorrhagic transformation is difficult to predict (International Stroke Trial Collaborative Group 1997; O'Donnell et al. 2006).

Intravenous thrombolysis

Thrombolysis aims to reduce the volume of infarcted brain by recanalizing the occluded vessel and restoring blood flow. Restoration of blood flow may not necessarily always be beneficial. First, studies in animals suggest that reperfusion of acutely ischemic brain may actually be harmful, through the release of free radicals and toxic products into the circulation. Second, thrombolysis will probably not be of benefit if infarction is completed or if the ischemic penumbra is small. Finally, thrombolysis may cause hemorrhagic transformation of the infarct or extracranial bleeding.

There have been a number of trials of thrombolysis in acute stroke using various thrombolytic agents, at different dosages and all the trials had strict entry criteria including age cut-offs. The relative effectiveness and the most-effective doses of the various thrombolytic agents are unclear owing to the lack of comparative data. Systematic reviews and meta-analysis (Wardlaw et al. 2003) of intravenous thrombolytic therapy using streptokinase, urokinase or recombinant tissue plasminogen activator (rt-PA) suggest some benefit from thrombolysis given within the first six hours after stroke. There was a significant reduction in combined death or dependency at the end of follow-up, with 64 fewer patients dead or dependent per 1000 patients treated. This was despite a significant increase in the number of intracranial hemorrhages and deaths, an additional 73 hemorrhages per 1000 patients treated, in other words a 3.5-fold excess, and in the numbers of deaths, amounting to an additional 46 deaths per 1000 patients treated. There was significant heterogeneity between trials, making the overall estimate difficult to interpret, but patients treated within three hours had better outcome. Some studies included only patients with middle cerebral artery territory infarction, such as the European and Australian Acute Stroke Study (ECASS; Hacke et al. 1998) whereas there was no such restriction in others, such as the National Institute of Neurological Disorders and Stroke rt-PA Study Group (NINDS 1995). Numbers were too small to examine the effect of thrombolysis on stroke subtypes.

The NINDS study of rt-PA within three hours of stroke onset in 624 patients reported a larger treatment effect (National Institute of Neurological Disorders and Stroke rt-PA Study Group 1995) than that seen overall for all studies included in the systematic reviews: 160 additional patients per 1000 patients treated were alive and independent at three months in the thrombolysis group, representing a number needed to treat of seven to prevent all death. This was despite an increase in the incidence of cerebral hemorrhage, with an excess of 58 bleeds per 1000 patients treated. The improved outcome in the thrombolysis group was maintained at one year (Kwiatkowski et al. 1999).

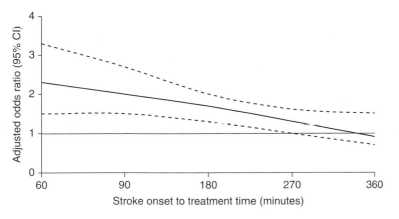

Fig. 21.1. Odds ratios of a favourable outcome at three months follow-up in patients treated with thrombolysis compared with controls by time from stroke onset to treatment, showing decrease in benefit from treatment with time based on a pooled analysis of 2776 patients from randomized controlled trials (Hacke *et al.* 2004). CI, confidence interval.

The less-striking benefit from thrombolysis indicated by the systematic reviews compared with that seen in the NINDS trial may result from methodological differences between trials. These include the fact that many of the earlier trials randomized patients up to six hours from stroke onset, and the likely pathophysiological variability in the patients studied. Further, in the NINDS trial, only carefully selected patients were included and these strict inclusion and exclusion criteria have made these trial results difficult to generalize to clinical practice. One study (Jorgensen *et al.* 1999) showed that only 5% of patients admitted to hospital in Denmark with ischemic stroke would fulfil the entry criteria for this trial and that only 45% would be eligible for thrombolysis even when the time limit was ignored.

A pooled analysis of individual patient data from the NINDS, ECASS I and II and the Alteplase Thrombolysis for Acute Noninterventional Therapy in Ischemic Stroke (ATLANTIS) trials (Hacke *et al.* 2004), which represents 99% of patients randomized in trials of rt-PA in stroke, has confirmed that benefit from thrombolysis decreases with time since stroke onset, being most beneficial if given within 90 minutes (odds ratio for favorable outcome of 2.8) (Fig. 21.1), although benefit was still present at 4.5 hours (now confirmed in ECASS III). However, it is clear that many patients will not benefit at this time point and, conversely, that other patients may benefit up to and beyond six hours in view of the fact that the ischemic penumbra may extend for much longer periods in some patients (Baron 2001). At present, only approximately 1% of UK patients receive thrombolysis (Intercollegiate Working Party on Stroke 2006) and 1–6% in North America.

Most of the data from the thrombolysis trials, together with most of the ongoing studies of diffusion-weighted imaging/perfusion-weighted imaging and CT perfusion concern embolic strokes in the middle cerebral artery territory. Consequently, there is uncertainty over whether lacunar or posterior circulation strokes should receive thrombolysis. The NINDS study found no difference in benefit for thrombolysis in lacunar compared with other stroke, but numbers were small and diagnosis of lacunar stroke was based on clinical syndrome and CT. Since lacunar stroke overall has a good prognosis and thrombolysis may be more likely to precipitate hemorrhage in the presence of small vessel disease, thrombolysis may not be beneficial, but at present there are no data to guide management. Similarly there are few data on posterior circulation stroke, although substantial diffusion-weighted/perfusion weighted imaging mismatch has been seen following basilar occlusion

Table 21.1. Absolute and relative contraindications to thrombolysis in acute major stroke used by the acute stroke team at the John Radcliffe Hospital, Oxford, UK

Contraindications
Absolute
Any intracranial hemorrhage
BP > 185/110 mmHg after two attempts to reduce BP
Surgery or trauma within the last 14 days
Active internal bleeding
Hematology abnormalities or coagulopathy
INR > 1.7, APTT > 40 seconds, platelet count < 100 × 10⁹/l
Arterial puncture at a non-compressible site within the last 7 days
Relative
Any of the following alone: hemianopia, neglect, sensory loss, dysarthria, ataxia
Pretreatment CT showing: hypodensity which could represent evolving infarct over three hours old; mass effect or edema; tumor, aneurysm or arteriovenous malformation
Intracranial or spinal surgery within two months
Any non-neurological surgery within the last six weeks
Stroke or head injury in the last three months
Gastrointestinal or urinary tract bleeding within the last three weeks
Previous history of CNS bleeding
Glucose < 2.7 or > 22 mmol/l
Seizure at stroke onset
Pregnancy
Infective endocarditis or pericarditis
Serious underlying medical illness (including dementia)
Greater than 90 minutes delay after CT scan
Decreased level of consciousness (unless caused by basilar artery occlusion)

Notes:
BP, blood pressure; INR, international normalized ratio; APTT, activated partial thromboplastin time; CT, computed tomography.

(Ostrem *et al.* 2004), and benefit of thrombolysis has been suggested as long as seven hours after stroke onset (Montavont *et al.* 2004; Lindsberg *et al.* 2004).

Several other uncertainties remain concerning thrombolysis after stroke, including the length of the treatment window, the risk–benefit ratio in older patients, the factors predicting intracranial hemorrhage and the brain imaging appearances that predict response to treatment. This, together with concern that there is a trend towards excess deaths with thrombolysis, has led to a lack of consensus regarding the use of thrombolysis and the criteria for selecting patients. Current guidelines vary but advise that thrombolysis should only be administered by a physician with expertise in stroke. Thrombolysis should be avoided in severe stroke, where there is early CT change indicating severe infarction or if more than three hours after stroke onset except as part of a randomized trial (Table 21.1).

Implementation of acute stroke imaging

The use of brain imaging to select patients for thrombolysis is discussed in detail in Ch. 11. Assuming equal access to diffusion-weighted/perfusion-weighted imaging and CT perfusion, decisions regarding optimum imaging use can be dictated by time elapsed since stroke onset and symptom severity.

At up to three hours after stroke onset

All existing trials used CT to select patients for thrombolysis. This remains the brain imaging method used in most centers for patients within the "0–3 hour" time window. Patients with hemorrhage or with signs of extensive infarction are, in general, excluded from thrombolysis. This latter exclusion remains a subject of debate since data from the NINDS trial (National Institute of Neurological Disorders and Stroke rt-PA Study Group 1995) do not support exclusion from thrombolysis on the basis of early ischemic change alone.

In view of the uncertainties surrounding thrombolysis even within the 0–3 hour time window, the ongoing Third International Stroke Trial (IST-3: www.ist3.com) is randomizing patients to alteplase (rt-PA) in the first six hours after stroke. This trial has no upper age limit in contrast to previous thrombolysis trials and aims to establish the risk–benefit ratio for thrombolysis in a broader selection of patients.

Magnetic resonance imaging takes longer than CT to perform and is less well tolerated in sick patients. However, it has been proposed that MRI may improve selection of patients for thrombolysis through greater sensitivity for excluding those likely to be harmed by treatment. At present, there are no randomized trial data, although there are studies reporting that MRI is safe and feasible in acute stroke.

At three to six hours after stroke onset

Ideally, patients presenting within the "3–6 hour" time window should be randomized to appropriate thrombolysis trials. However, some centers use diffusion-weighted/perfusion-weighted imaging and the presence of mismatch (see Ch. 11) to select patients for thrombolysis. There is some evidence that treatment with intravenous alteplase based on the presence of such a mismatch in the 3–6 hour time window produces similar functional outcomes to alteplase treatment within three hours based on CT criteria. However, it remains unclear how to identify individual patients at high risk of hemorrhagic transformation, although there is evidence that low perfusion or low apparent diffusion coefficient values (Derex *et al.* 2005) are associated with a higher risk of hemorrhage. The presence of cerebral microbleeds does not appear to be related to thrombolysis-related hemorrhage (Chs. 10 and 11).

Intra-arterial thrombolysis

Intra-arterial thrombolysis has been proposed as a treatment for acute ischemic stroke since the 1980s and may potentially overcome many of the problems associated with patient selection for intravenous therapy:

- thrombolysis only after demonstration of vessel occlusion
- higher rates of recanalization achieved
- lower dosage of thrombolytic agent required, therefore lower risks of hemorrhage
- therapeutic window for thrombolysis may be extended beyond three hours.

The first advantage is that it allows thrombolysis to be given only to those patients in whom vessel occlusion has been demonstrated. In 20% of patients presenting within six hours of stroke onset, no occlusion is identified. Second, recanalization rates appear to be higher for intra-arterial thrombolysis, approximately 70%, than for intravenous thrombolysis, approximately 34%, although there are no direct comparisons of the two techniques. Third, since intra-arterial thrombolysis involves the use of small amounts of thrombolytic agent applied directly to the site of occlusion, compared with the relatively high doses used systemically in intravenous thrombolysis, intra-arterial thrombolysis may offer the potential to treat patients at increased risk of hemorrhagic complications more safely.

Two randomized controlled trials of intra-arterial thrombolysis have been reported: the Prolyse in Acute Cerebral Thromboembolism trials PROACT I (del Zoppo *et al.* 1998) and PROACT II (Furlan *et al.* 1999). PROACT I remains the only placebo-controlled double-blind, multicenter trial of intra-arterial thrombolysis in acute ischemic stroke. Recanalization rate was 58% in the active treatment group, compared with 14% in the placebo group. Two doses of subsequent heparin were used, a high-dose 5000 U bolus followed by 100 U/hour, achieving a recanalization rate of 80% with a symptomatic intracranial hemorrhage rate of 27%. The equivalent rates in the low-dose heparin group were 47% and 6%, respectively. In PROACT II, 180 patients with a mean National Institutes of Health Stroke score of 17 were randomly assigned to receive either 9 mg of intra-arterial thrombolysis plus low-dose intravenous heparin or low-dose intravenous heparin alone. The median time from onset of symptoms to the initiation of intra-arterial thrombolysis was 5.3 hours. In the treated group, there was a 15% absolute benefit in the number of patients who achieved a modified Rankin score of ≤ 2 at 90 days ($p = 0.04$). On average, seven patients with middle cerebral artery occlusion would require intra-arterial thrombolysis for one to benefit. Symptomatic brain hemorrhage occurred in 10% of the thrombolysis group and 2% of the control group, but there was no excess mortality.

There are few data to guide intra-arterial thrombolysis in the posterior circulation. Observational studies and the one existing very small randomized controlled trial of intra-arterial thrombolysis for basilar occlusion show no evidence of benefit (Arnold *et al.* 2004, Lindsberg and Mattle 2006). However, given the poor outcome of basilar occlusion, many clinicians believe thrombolysis is justified, even many hours after the event, particularly since there is some evidence that the ischemic penumbra and thus the available window for thrombolysis may extend for many hours in the posterior circulation.

Comparisons between the different intra-arterial thrombolysis trials and between intra-arterial thrombolysis and intravenous thrombolysis is hampered by differences in methodology and type of thrombolytic therapy. In addition, within the intra-arterial thrombolysis trials, thrombolytic delivery has varied between regional into a parent vessel of the thrombosed vessel, local into the affected artery and into the thrombus itself, or combinations of these methods. In addition, the infusion process has been variable, ranging from continuous to pulsed infusion. Some studies have allowed physical clot dispersion using the tip of the microcatheter while this was prohibited in others, for instance in the PROACT trials.

It may be feasible to combine intravenous thrombolysis with intra-arterial thrombolysis. In the pilot Emergency Management of Stroke (EMS) bridging trial (Lewandowski *et al.* 1999), 70% of patients still had a clot on angiography after intravenous rt-PA. There was improved recanalization in patients who then received intra-arterial rt-PA but also an increase in bleeding complications. Other trials are ongoing. Percutaneous angioplasty of the recanalized vessel following intra-arterial thrombolysis has also been attempted, but at present there are no prospective comparisons of any of these combined techniques, making their relative merits unclear. Intra-arterial urokinase has been used to treat ischemic stroke occurring during insertion of coils for intravascular aneurysms, but since the causes of vessel occlusion secondary to arterial cannulation include intimal dissection and arterial spasm as well as local thrombosis and emboli dislodged by the catheter, thrombolysis would be unlikely to be of benefit in many such cases.

Surgical decompression for malignant middle cerebral artery infarction

Malignant middle cerebral artery territory infarction is defined as a large middle cerebral artery infarct with marked edema and swelling, leading to raised intracranial pressure and a high risk of coning (Fig. 21.2; see also Figs. 5.1 and 11.2). Malignant middle cerebral artery infarction has a mortality rate of approximately 80% with medical treatment. Non-randomized studies had suggested a reduction in mortality with decompressive surgery, consisting of hemicraniectomy and duroplasty, without a major increase in the

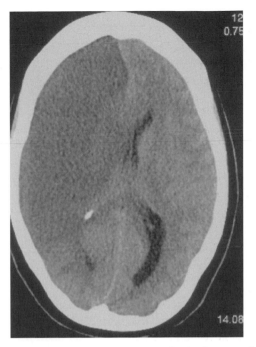

Fig. 21.2. A CT brain scan showing the development of malignant middle cerebral artery infarction in a young woman who subsequently underwent hemicraniectomy.

number of severely disabled survivors. Recently, data from three small randomized trials were pooled and showed that surgery within 48 hours of stroke onset reduced case fatality from 71% to 22%, and that 43% of survivors had a modified Rankin score of ≤ 3 at one-year follow-up (Vahedi *et al.* 2007) (Fig. 21.3). The results were highly consistent across all three trials. Since the trials excluded patients older than 60 years, and existing non-randomized data suggest poor outcome in those over 50 years, the results cannot necessarily be generalized to older patients.

Neuroprotective interventions

Potential neuroprotective agents include metalloprotease inhibitors, which reduce vascular damage, anti-inflammatory drugs and oxidative stress blockers. Several neuroprotective agents have shown promising results in animal studies but this has not, in general, translated into benefit in trials in humans (Savitz and Fisher 2007). The many possible reasons for the discrepancy in results between animals and humans include length of time to treatment, the heterogeneity of stroke in humans compared with animal stroke models and the small numbers and bias in animal studies (Muir and Teal 2005). Moreover, variation in the outcome measurements used in acute stroke trials makes comparison between studies difficult, and reanalysis of data using different methods may yield different results. The initial clinical trial of NXY-059 (SAINT-1, Lees *et al.* 2006), a free radical spin-trap agent, showed benefit in acute stroke but this was not replicated in a subsequent trial, SAINT-2 (Shuaib *et al.* 2007). Further, reanalysis of the SAINT-1 results using different methodology showed no evidence of benefit (Koziol and Feng 2006). The current consensus is that neuroprotective agents require more rigorous testing in appropriate clinically

263

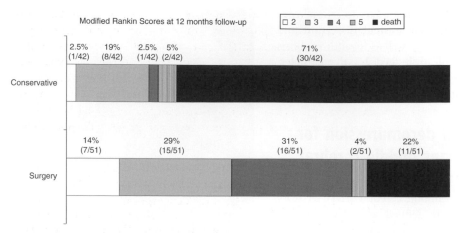

Fig. 21.3. A pooled analysis of data from three small randomized trials of hemicraniectomy versus medical treatment for malignant middle cerebral artery infarction (Vahedi *et al.* 2007). Surgery within 48 hours of stroke onset reduced case-fatality from 71% to 22% and left 43% of survivors with only mild or moderate disability (modified Rankin score of ≤ 3) at one-year follow-up.

relevant animal models before testing in humans with appropriate time windows and outcome measures (Savitz and Fisher 2007).

Newer imaging techniques may allow better patient selection for neuroprotective agents. As discussed above, initial diffusion-weighted imaging abnormality may resolve only to reappear in around 50% of patients. Although the pathological processes underlying this phenomenon are not understood, this may be an area in which neuroprotection could play a role. Further, even when lesions identified by diffusion-weighted imaging resolve without secondary reappearance, isolated necrotic neurons are seen on histological specimens in animal studies, showing that partial ischemic injury may be present even in regions with normal apparent diffusion coefficient and T_2-weighted MRI values. Therefore, neuroprotectants may also be of use in patients with fully reversible lesions on diffusion-weighted imaging.

Imaging of the ischemic penumbra has been shown to be potentially useful in selecting patients for thrombolysis. It may allow extension of the thrombolysis window in selected patients. But it has also been proposed that tissue within the ischemic penumbra represents a good target for neuroprotective agents, which are unlikely to be as effective in tissue that is already severely damaged. Neuroprotective agents might allow protection of tissue within the penumbra while perfusion is restored and, thus, extend the thrombolysis window. Alternatively, damage to the ischemic penumbral tissue could be lessened in patients who did not reperfuse with thrombolyic therapy or in whom thrombolysis was contraindicated. Finally, although salvage of penumbral tissue is possible if reperfusion occurs, neurons within this area may still be at risk of delayed injury and this may represent a further area for neuroprotectant therapy.

Hypothermia causes a variety of responses in ischemic brain that might confer neuroprotection, including significant alterations in metabolism, glutamate release and reuptake, inflammation and free radical generation (Krieger and Yenari 2004). This, together with the observation that children and adults have survived prolonged immersion in cold water without neurological sequelae, has led to the proposal that induced hypothermia may improve stroke outcome. Hypothermia may also lengthen the time window for thrombolysis. In animal models, hypothermia improves outcome in temporary cerebral vessel occlusion but effects after permanent occlusion are less consistent. In humans, two randomized trials have shown that mild hypothermia improves mortality and neurological outcome in patients who suffer cardiac arrest (Bernard *et al.* 2002; Hypothermia after Cardiac Arrest Study Group 2002). Pilot studies of hypothermia for stroke have been published but there are no large randomized trials and there is no consensus regarding timing, depth and method of induction of hypothermia: surface or endovascular (Hemmen and Lyden 2007). Anaesthetized patients have tolerated hypothermia for as long as 72 hours, but few awake patients have been treated, partly because awake patients do not tolerate deep hypothermia.

References

Arnold M, Nedeltchev K, Schroth G *et al.* (2004). Clinical and radiological predictors of recanalisation and outcome of 40 patients with acute basilar artery occlusion treated with intra-arterial thrombolysis. *Journal of Neurology, Neurosurgery and Psychiatry* 75:857–862

Baron JC (2001). Perfusion thresholds in human cerebral ischemia: historical perspective and therapeutic implications. *Cerebrovascular Diseases* 11:2–8

Berge E (2007). Heparin for acute ischemic stroke: a never-ending story? *Lancet Neurology* 6:381–382

Bernard SAGT, Buist MD, Jones BM *et al.* (2002). Treatment of comatose survivors of out-of-hospital cardiac arrest with induced hypothermia. *New England Journal of Medicine* 346:557–563

CAST (Chinese Acute Stroke Trial) Collaborative Group (1997). CAST: randomised placebo-controlled trial of early aspirin use in 20 000 patients with acute ischemic stroke. *Lancet* 349:1641–1649

del Zoppo GJ, Higashida RT, Furlan AJ *et al.* (1998). PROACT: a phase II randomized trial of recombinant pro-urokinase by direct arterial delivery in acute middle cerebral artery stroke. PROACT Investigators Prolyse in Acute Cerebral Thromboembolism. *Stroke* 29:4–11

Derex L, Hermier M, Adeleine P *et al.* (2005). Clinical and imaging predictors of intracerebral hemorrhage in stroke patients treated with intravenous tissue plasminogen activator. *Journal of Neurology, Neurosurgery and Psychiatry* 76:70–75

Furlan A, Higashida R, Wechsler L *et al.* (1999). Intra-arterial prourokinase for acute ischemic stroke. The PROACT II study: a randomized controlled trial. Prolyse in Acute Cerebral Thromboembolism. *Journal of the American Medical Association* 282:2003–2011

Hacke W, Kaste M, Fieschi C *et al.* (1998). Randomised double-blind placebo-controlled trial of thrombolytic therapy with intravenous alteplase in acute ischemic stroke (ECASS II). Second European–Australasian Acute Stroke Study Investigators. *Lancet* 352:1245–1251

Hacke W, Donnan G, Fieschi C *et al.* (2004). Association of outcome with early stroke treatment: pooled analysis of ATLANTIS ECASS and NINDS rt-PA stroke trials. *Lancet* 363:768–774

Hemmen TM, Lyden PD (2007). Induced hypothermia for acute stroke. *Stroke* 38:794–799

Hypothermia After Cardiac Arrest Study Group (2002). Mild therapeutic hypothermia to improve the neurologic outcome after cardiac arrest. *New England Journal of Medicine* 346:549–556

Intercollegiate Working Party for Stroke (2006). *National Sentinel Audit.* London: Royal College of Physicians.

International Stroke Trial Collaborative Group (1997). The International Stroke Trial (IST): a randomised trial of aspirin subcutaneous heparin both or neither among 19435 patients with acute ischemic stroke. *Lancet* 349:1569–1581

Jorgensen HS, Nakayama H, Kammersgaard LP *et al.* (1999). Predicted impact of intravenous thrombolysis on prognosis of general population of stroke patients: simulation model. *British Medical Journal* 319:288–289

Koziol JA and Feng AC (2006). On the analysis and interpretation of outcome measures in stroke clinical trials: lessons from the SAINT I study of NXY-059 for acute ischemic stroke. *Stroke* 37:2644–2647

Krieger DW, Yenari MA (2004). Therapeutic hypothermia for acute ischemic stroke: what do laboratory studies teach us? *Stroke* 35:1482–1489

Kwiatkowski TG, Libman RB, Frankel M (1999). Effects of tissue plasminogen activator for acute ischemic stroke at one year. National Institute of Neurological Disorders and Stroke Recombinant Tissue Plasminogen Activator Stroke Study Group. *New England Journal of Medicine* 340:1781–1787

Lees KR, Zivin JA, Ashwood T *et al.* (2006). Stroke–Acute Ischemic NXY Treatment (SAINT I) Trial Investigators. NXY-059 for acute ischemic stroke. *New England Journal of Medicine* 354:588–600

Lewandowski CA, Frankel M, Tomsick TA *et al.* (1999). Combined intravenous and intra-arterial r-TPA versus intra-arterial therapy of acute ischemic stroke: Emergency Management of Stroke (EMS) Bridging Trial. *Stroke* 30:2598–2605

Lindsberg PJ, Mattle HP (2006). Therapy of basilar artery occlusion: a systematic analysis comparing intra-arterial and intravenous thrombolysis. *Stroke* 37:922–928

Lindsberg PJ, Soinne L, Tatlisumak T *et al.* (2004). Long-term outcome after intravenous thrombolysis of basilar artery occlusion. *Journal of the American Medical Association* 292:1862–1866

Montavont A, Nighoghossian N, Derex L *et al.* (2004). Intravenous r-TPA in vertebrobasilar acute infarcts. *Neurology* 62:1854–1856

Muir KW and Teal PA (2005). Why have neuro-protectants failed?: lessons learned from stroke trials. *Journal of Neurology* 252:1011–1020

National Institute of Neurological Disorders and Stroke rt-PA Stroke Study Group (1995). Tissue plasminogen activator for acute ischemic stroke. *New England Journal of Medicine* 14:1581–1587

O'Donnell MJ, Berge E, Sandset PM (2006). Are there patients with acute ischemic stroke and atrial fibrillation that benefit from low molecular weight heparin? *Stroke* 37:452–455

Ostrem JL, Saver JL, Alger JR *et al.* (2004). Acute basilar artery occlusion: diffusion–perfusion MRI characterization of tissue salvage in patients receiving intra-arterial stroke therapies. *Stroke* 35:e30–e34

Sandercock P, Gubitz G, Foley P *et al.* (2003). Antiplatelet therapy for acute ischemic stroke. *Cochrane Database of Systematic Reviews* 2:CD000024

Savitz SI, Fisher M (2007). Future of neuroprotection for acute stroke: in the aftermath of the SAINT trials. *Annals of Neurology* 61:396–402

Shuaib A, Lees KR, Lyden P *et al.* (2007) SAINT II Trial Investigators. NXY-059 for the treatment of acute ischemic stroke. *New England Journal of Medicine* 357:562–571

Vahedi K, Hofmeijer J, Juettler E *et al.* (2007). Early decompressive surgery in malignant infarction of the middle cerebral artery: a pooled analysis of three randomised controlled trials. *Lancet Neurology* 6:215–222

Wardlaw JM, Zoppo G, Yamaguchi T *et al.* (2003). Thrombolysis for acute ischemic stroke. *Cochrane Database of Systematic Reviews* 3:CD000213

Wong KS, Chen C, Ng PW *et al.* (2007). Low-molecular-weight heparin compared with aspirin for the treatment of acute ischemic stroke in Asian patients with large artery occlusive disease: a randomised study. *Lancet Neurology* 6:407–413

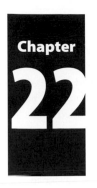

Specific treatment of acute intracerebral hemorrhage

Brain imaging using CT has a high sensitivity for intracerebral hemorrhage. The location, characteristics and number of hemorrhages can aid in the diagnosis of the underlying cause and, thus, may influence subsequent patient management. For instance, the presence of multiple lobar hemorrhages with surrounding edema should prompt a search for underlying metastatic tumor, whereas a basal ganglia hemorrhage in a hypertensive elderly person would not require further investigation. Repeat CT scanning is indicated if there is clinical deterioration, which may be caused by rebleeding or by hydrocephalus; if there are no changes, the search for systemic disorders should be intensified.

It is vital to instigate the correct management of patients with cerebellar hemorrhage as soon as possible owing to the high risk of hydrocephalus and brainstem compression.

Non-surgical treatments
Recombinant factor VIIa
Recombinant factor VIIa is known to decrease the severity of hemorrhage in certain surgical settings. Since primary intracerebral hemorrhage has a tendency to enlarge over the first few hours, it has been proposed that agents promoting hemostasis may be beneficial in treating primary intracerebral hemorrhage. A phase 2 trial of recombinant factor VIIa administered within three hours to patients with intracerebral hematoma without known structural or iatrogenic cause found that enlargement of the hematoma and poor outcome occurred significantly less often in patients treated with the active compound (Mayer *et al*. 2005). However, the confidence limits were wide, the risk of cerebral and myocardial infarction was higher in the treatment group (5% versus 0% in the placebo group) and the subsequent larger phase III trial, the Factor Seven for Acute Hemorrhagic Stroke Treatment (FAST) trial, failed to confirm benefit (Mayer *et al*. 2008).

Cerebrospinal fluid drainage
Insertion of a ventricular catheter can be life saving in patients with cerebellar hemorrhage and hydrocephalus. In patients with supratentorial hemorrhage and hydrocephalus, however, the benefits of cerebrospinal fluid (CSF) diversion are less certain. In patients with extensive intraventricular hemorrhage secondary to deep intraparenchymal or aneurysmal rupture, drainage of CSF is performed in some centers. Systematic reviews of observational studies suggest that this procedure may be helpful, especially when it is combined with instillation of fibrinolytic drugs. However, randomized trials are needed (Lee *et al*. 2003; Fountas *et al*. 2005).

Hyperventilation
Hyperventilation decreases intracranial pressure because hypocapnia, usually down to values of the order of 4 kPa, causes vasoconstriction. However, this will not necessarily be

beneficial in patients with intracerebral hemorrhage since brain ischemia caused by compression is exchanged for ischemia caused by vasoconstriction (Stocchetti *et al.* 2005). In head-injured patients, the single randomized controlled trial of prolonged hyperventilation not only failed to show any benefit but also raised concerns about potential harm (Muizelaar *et al.* 1991; Schierhout and Roberts 2000). There are no controlled trials of hyperventilation in patients with intracerebral hematomas.

Osmotic agents

Mannitol is widely used in patients with primary intracerebral hemorrhage and a depressed level of consciousness to decrease intracranial pressure and alleviate the space-occupying effect of the hematoma in a deteriorating patient, although there is a lack of randomized trials looking at clinical outcomes.

Surgical treatment
Supratentorial hemorrhage

There are four possible surgical procedures to treat intracerebral hematoma: simple aspiration, craniotomy with open surgery, endoscopic evacuation and stereotactic aspiration. Open surgery remains the technique of choice at present.

In patients with large intracerebral hemorrhages and mass effect (Fig. 22.1), it might be thought that surgical removal would improve outcome. Craniotomy with open surgery was studied in the large multicenter Surgical Trial in Intracerebral Hemorrhage (STICH; Mendelow *et al.* 2005). Nine preceding small randomized trials had produced conflicting results. The STICH trial randomized 1003 patients, all with supratentorial hemorrhages, four times as many patients as in all previous trials taken together. Patients with a hematoma of at least 2 cm in diameter and a Glasgow Coma Score of ≥ 5 were randomized to initial conservative treatment versus early surgery if the admitting surgeon was uncertain of the benefit of surgery. Patients initially randomized to medical treatment could undergo surgery at a later time point if this was felt to be indicated. Surgical technique was left to the discretion of the surgeon.

The STICH trial reported no difference in outcome between those consigned to initial conservative or surgical management. In a prespecified subgroup analysis, patients with superficial hematomas were more likely to have a favorable outcome than those with deep hematomas, and there was a non-significant relative benefit for surgery in this group. The outcome for patients with Glasgow Coma Scores of ≤ 8 was uniformly poor and there was a suggestion that surgery increased the risk of

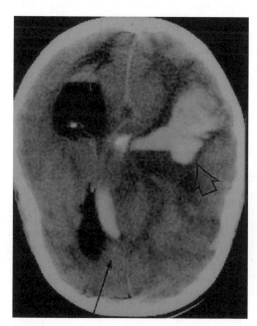

Fig. 22.1. A CT brain scan showing a primary intracerebral hemorrhage with rupture into the ventricular system (open arrow) and considerable mass effect (black arrow).

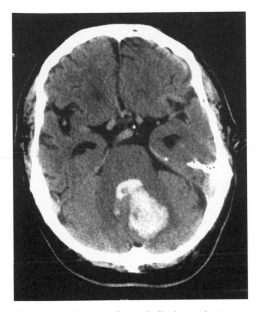

Fig. 22.2. A CT scan of a cerebellar hemorrhage.

poor outcome in these patients. It is possible that patients with deep-seated hematomas might do better with less-invasive and hence less-traumatic methods of clot evacuation, such as endoscopy. Further trials are needed to test these hypotheses.

The STICH trial did not address the question of whether operation improves outcome in patients deteriorating because of hematoma expansion. A consecutive series of 26 such patients from the Mayo Clinic, of whom 24 had lobar hemorrhage, suggested that no patient regained independence, with or without surgery, if corneal and oculocephalic reflexes had been lost. However, approximately one-quarter of the remaining group, 6 out of 21, regained independence (Rabinstein *et al.* 2002).

Cerebellar hemorrhage

Over the past few decades, surgical evacuation has been felt to be life saving and relatively complication free in patients with cerebellar hematomas who have clinical evidence of progressive brainstem compression (Fig. 22.2). Consequently, a randomized trial is unlikely to occur. Certain patients can be managed conservatively, but there is uncertainty about the selection criteria. Indications for evacuation of cerebellar hematoma include size greater than 3–4 cm and the combination of a depressed level of consciousness with signs of progressive brainstem compression (Wijdicks *et al.* 2000; Cohen *et al.* 2002; Jensen and St. Louis 2005). Where all brainstem reflexes have been lost for more than a few hours, outcome is uniformly fatal. Ventriculostomy alone may be adequate in some patients with clinical features of hydrocephalus without pontine compression, such as gradual deterioration of consciousness with sustained downward gaze and small unreactive pupils.

Other surgical approaches

Aspiration not accompanied by any other intervention was attempted mainly in the 1950s but was subsequently abandoned because only small amounts of clot could be obtained, and because the procedure could precipitate rebleeding. Since the 1990s, stereotactic aspiration of supratentorial hemorrhage without endoscopy, mostly combined with instillation of fibrinolytic agents, has been reported in several observational studies. Subsequently, two controlled trials of this technique have been performed. A Japanese trial randomized 242 patients with putaminal hemorrhage and a moderately decreased level of consciousness, involving eyes closed but opening to stimuli, between stereotactic hematoma evacuation and conservative treatment. This reported that outcome in terms of death and dependence was better in the surgical group (Hattori *et al.* 2004). A smaller trial of 70 patients in the Netherlands combined stereotactic aspiration with liquefaction by means of a plasminogen-activating substance and found no conclusive differences in outcome (Teernstra *et al.* 2003).

Treatment of specific types of intracerebral hemorrhage

Pontine hemorrhages

Pontine hemorrhages are fatal in around 50% of patients (Wijdicks and St. Louis 1997). Those caused by cavernomas or arteriovenous malformations have a better outcome (Rabinstein *et al.* 2004). The management of patients with "hypertensive" pontine hemorrhage is usually conservative, but some case reports have documented successful stereotactic aspiration. However, there is likely publication bias and the natural history of the condition is difficult to predict since patients with small hemorrhages do well with conservative management.

Lobar hemorrhage from presumed amyloid angiopathy

In patients with lobar hemorrhage from amyloid angiopathy and with an impaired level of consciousness, the prognosis is poor after surgical intervention (McCarron *et al.* 1999). It remains unclear whether the outcome would have been better without surgery (Greene *et al.* 1990; Izumihara *et al.* 1999). Given these uncertainties and the danger that the operation provokes new hemorrhages from brittle vessels at distant sites (Brisman *et al.* 1996), conservative treatment seems the best option.

Cavernous angiomas

There is little doubt that hemorrhages, which may be recurrent, from cavernous angiomas are less destructive than brainstem hemorrhages from an arterial source (Rabinstein *et al.* 2004). Also, the angioma may spontaneously regress (Yasui *et al.* 2005). Surgical treatment or stereotactic radiation is regularly performed but is not supported by controlled studies, and incomplete removal can prompt rebleeding (Kikuta *et al.* 2004). Stereotactic cobalt-generated radiation "gamma knife" therapy has been applied to a large number of patients with cavernomas, but it remains uncertain whether seizures or rebleeding are less likely to occur afterwards (Regis *et al.* 2000; Liu *et al.* 2005).

Dural arteriovenous fistulae

Arteriovenous fistulae in the dura are heterogeneous. They may or may not be secondary to occlusion of a major sinus. Abnormal venous drainage from meningeal arteries may be channelled into a dural sinus or into superficial veins of the surface of the brain, cerebellum or brainstem. Accordingly, different methods are required to occlude the fistula. Surgical techniques include selective ligation of leptomeningeal draining veins, resection of fistulous sinus tracts and a cranial base approach with extradural bone removal. Endovascular techniques may consist of an approach from the arterial or venous side, recanalization and stenting of a venous sinus, or venous embolization via a craniotomy (Tomak *et al.* 2003). Finally stereotactic cobalt-generated radiation "gamma knife" therapy is also used for obliterating arteriovenous fistulae (O'Leary *et al.* 2002; Pan *et al.* 2002), sometimes in conjunction with an endovascular approach (Friedman *et al.* 2001).

Moyamoya syndrome associated hemorrhage

Moyamoya syndrome (Ch. 6) causes gradual stenosis or occlusion of the terminal portions of the internal carotid arteries or middle cerebral arteries. This leads to formation of an abnormal collateral network of fragile vessels, which occasionally rupture. It has been proposed that constructing a bypass to relieve the pressure on the collaterals would be beneficial, for example between the superficial temporal artery and the middle cerebral artery (Kawaguchi *et al.* 2000), but whether this procedure prevents bleeding remains uncertain. In fact, an aneurysm may form and rupture at the site of the arterial bypass (Nishimoto *et al.* 2005).

Iatrogenic intracerebral hemorrhage
Anticoagulation

Anticoagulants are associated with an increased rate of intracerebral hemorrhage, and particularly high rates of hemorrhage are observed in the elderly. With increasing rates of anticoagulant use, rates of hemorrhage have risen. Observational data confirm that early normalization of clotting status is associated with a relatively low rate of hematoma enlargement (Yasaka *et al.* 2003).

It remains uncertain when to reintroduce anticoagulants in patients with a strong indication for this treatment, such as those with artificial heart valves, since only anecdotal experience is available. In the Mayo Clinic series, only one ischemic stroke occurred in 52 patients with artificial heart valves in whom anticoagulants were discontinued for a median period of 10 days (Phan *et al.* 2000). In contrast, of seven similar patients from Heidelberg, three had large ischemic strokes within a comparable period after stopping anticoagulation (Bertram *et al.* 2000). Reintroduction of anticoagulation between one and two weeks after the hemorrhage is probably reasonable (Estol and Kase 2003) and is supported by evidence of low rates of rebleeding (Wijdicks *et al.* 1998; Leker and Abramsky 1998).

Thrombolytic therapy

Thrombolytic therapy for myocardial infarction is rarely complicated by intracerebral hemorrhage, but the case-fatality is high. Treatment includes control of hypertension and the infusion of coagulation factors. However, the use of antifibrinolytic drugs is controversial. Surgical treatment is of unproven value and may be especially hazardous given that amyloid angiopathy may be a contributing factor. In patients with ischemic stroke who develop major intracerebral hemorrhage after thrombolytic treatment, treatment remains unclear.

Aspirin

Aspirin treatment is associated with a small risk of intracerebral hemorrhage. It is unclear whether prior antiplatelet therapy is associated with a worse outcome in patients with intracerebral hemorrhage. It is reasonable to stop the drug once the diagnosis is made. The antiplatelet effect lasts until several days after discontinuing the drug. In trials of aspirin for the secondary prevention of cerebral ischemia, some patients with small intracerebral hemorrhages were inadvertently included before CT scanning and did not come to obvious harm. However the number of patients was small and they were probably a rather atypical group (Keir *et al.* 2002).

References

Bertram M, Bonsanto M, Hacke W *et al.* (2000). Managing the therapeutic dilemma: patients with spontaneous intracerebral hemorrhage and urgent need for anticoagulation. *Journal of Neurology* 247:209–214

Brisman MH, Bederson JB, Sen CN *et al.* (1996). Intracerebral hemorrhage occurring remote from the craniotomy site. *Neurosurgery* 39:1114–1121

Cohen ZR, Ram Z, Knoller N *et al.* (2002). Management and outcome of non-traumatic cerebellar haemorrhage. *Cerebrovascular Diseases* 14:207–213

Estol CJ, Kase CS (2003). Need for continued use of anticoagulants after intracerebral hemorrhage. *Current Treatment Options in Cardiovascular Medicine* 5:201–209

Fountas KN, Kapsalaki EZ, Parish DC *et al.* (2005). Intraventricular administration of rt-PA in patients with intraventricular hemorrhage. *South Medical Journal* 98:767–773

Friedman JA, Pollock BE, Nichols DA *et al.* (2001). Results of combined stereotactic, radiosurgery and transarterial embolization for dural arteriovenous fistulas of the transverse and sigmoid sinuses. *Journal of Neurosurgery* 94:886–891

Greene GM, Godersky JC Biller J *et al.* (1990). Surgical experience with cerebral amyloid angiopathy. *Stroke* 21:1545–1549

Hattori N, Katayama Y, Maya Y *et al.* (2004). Impact of stereotactic hematoma evacuation on activities of daily living during the chronic period following spontaneous putaminal hemorrhage: a randomized study. *Journal of Neurosurgery* 101:417–420

Izumihara A, Ishihara T, Iwamoto N *et al.* (1999). Postoperative outcome of 37 patients with lobar intracerebral hemorrhage related to cerebral amyloid angiopathy. *Stroke* 30:29–33

Jensen MB, St. Louis EK (2005). Management of acute cerebellar stroke. *Archives of Neurology* 62:537–544

Kawaguchi S, Okuno S, Sakaki T (2000). Effect of direct arterial bypass on the prevention of future stroke in patients with the hemorrhagic variety of moyamoya disease. *Journal of Neurosurgery* 93:397–401

Keir SL, Wardlaw JM, Sandercock PAG *et al.* (2002). Antithrombotic therapy in patients with any form of intracranial haemorrhage: a systematic review of the available controlled studies. *Cerebrovascular Diseases* 14:197–206

Kikuta K, Nozaki K, Takahashi JA *et al.* (2004). Postoperative evaluation of microsurgical resection for cavernous malformations of the brainstem. *Journal of Neurosurgery* 101:607–612

Lee MW, Pang KY, Ho WW *et al.* (2003). Outcome analysis of intraventricular thrombolytic therapy for intraventricular haemorrhage. *Hong Kong Medical Journal* 9:335–340

Leker RR, Abramsky O (1998). Early anticoagulation in patients with prosthetic heart valves and intracerebral hematoma. *Neurology* 50:1489–1491

Liu KD, Chung WY, Wu HM *et al.* (2005). Gamma knife surgery for cavernous hemangiomas: an analysis of 125 patients. *Journal of Neurosurgery* 102:81–86

Mayer SA, Brun NC, Broderick J *et al.* (2005). Safety and feasibility of recombinant factor VIIa for acute intracerebral hemorrhage. *Stroke* 36:74–79

Mayer SA, Brun NC, Begtrup K *et al.* (2008). FAST Trial Investigators. Efficacy and safety of recombinant activated factor VII for acute intracerebral hemorrhage. *New England Journal of Medicine* 358:2127–2137

McCarron MO, Nicoll JA, Love S *et al.* (1999). Surgical intervention biopsy and APOE genotype in cerebral amyloid angiopathy-related haemorrhage. *British Journal of Neurosurgery* 13:462–467

Mendelow AD, Gregson BA, Fernandes HM *et al.* (2005). Early surgery versus initial conservative treatment in patients with spontaneous supratentorial intracerebral haematomas in the international Surgical Trial in Intracerebral Haemorrhage (STICH): a randomised trial. *Lancet* 365:387–397

Muizelaar JP, Marmarou A, Ward JD *et al.* (1991). Adverse effects of prolonged hyperventilation in patients with severe head injury: a randomized clinical trial. *Journal of Neurosurgery* 75:731–739

Nishimoto T, Yuki K, Sasaki T *et al.* (2005). A ruptured middle cerebral artery aneurysm originating from the site of anastomosis 20 years after extracranial-intracranial bypass for moyamoya disease: case report. *Surgical Neurology* 64:261–265

O'Leary S, Hodgson TJ, Coley SC *et al.* (2002). Intracranial dural arteriovenous malformations: results of stereotactic radiosurgery in 17 patients. *Clinical Oncology of the Royal College of Radiologists* 14:97–102

Pan DH, Chung WY, Guo WY *et al.* (2002). Stereotactic radiosurgery for the treatment of dural arteriovenous fistulas involving the transverse-sigmoid sinus. *Journal of Neurosurgery* 96:823–829

Phan TG, Koh M, Wijdicks EFM (2000). Safety of discontinuation of anticoagulation in patients with intracranial hemorrhage at high thromboembolic risk. *Archives of Neurology* 57:1710–1713

Rabinstein AA, Atkinson JL, Wijdicks EFM (2002). Emergency craniotomy in patients worsening due to expanded cerebral haematoma: to what purpose? *Neurology* 58:1367–1372

Rabinstein AA, Tisch SH, McClelland RL *et al.* (2004). Cause is the main predictor of outcome in patients with pontine hemorrhage. *Cerebrovascular Diseases* 17:66–71

Régis J, Bartolomei F, Kida Y *et al.* (2000). Radiosurgery for epilepsy associated with cavernous malformation: Retrospective study in 49 patients. *Neurosurgery* 47:1091–1097

Schierhout G and Roberts I (2000). Hyperventilation therapy for acute traumatic brain injury. *Cochrane Database of Systematic Reviews* 2:CD000566

Stocchetti N, Maas AI, Chieregato A *et al.* (2005). Hyperventilation in head injury: a review. *Chest* 127:1812–1827

Teernstra OP, Evers SM, Lodder J *et al.* (2003). Stereotactic treatment of intracerebral hematoma by means of a plasminogen activator: a multicenter randomized controlled trial (SICHPA). *Stroke* 34:968–974

Tomak PR, Cloft HJ, Kaga A *et al.* (2003). Evolution of the management of tentorial dural arteriovenous malformations. *Neurosurgery* 52:750–760

Wijdicks EF, St. Louis E (1997). Clinical profiles predictive of outcome in pontine hemorrhage. *Neurology* 49:1342–1346

Wijdicks EFM, Schievink WI, Brown RD *et al.* (1998). The dilemma of discontinuation of anticoagulation therapy for patients with intracranial hemorrhage and mechanical heart valves. *Neurosurgery* 42:769–773

Wijdicks EFM, Louis EKS, Atkinson JD *et al.* (2000). Clinician's biases toward surgery in cerebellar hematomas: An analysis of decision-making in 94 patients. *Cerebrovascular Diseases* 10:93–96

Yasaka M, Minematsu K, Naritomi H (2003). Predisposing factors for enlargement of intracerebral hemorrhage in patients treated with warfarin. *Thrombosis Haemostasis* 89:278–283

Yasui T, Komiyama M, Iwai Y *et al.* (2005). A brainstem cavernoma demonstrating a dramatic spontaneous decrease in size during follow-up: case report and review of the literature. *Surgical Neurology* 63:170–173

Chapter 23

Recovery and rehabilitation after stroke

Some degree of recovery occurs in the majority of patients after stroke, and complete recovery is possible although the prognosis is difficult to predict in an individual patient. Rehabilitation to aid recovery and enable the patient to develop strategies for coping with disability forms the mainstay of treatment after the acute stroke period.

Recovery after stroke

Approximately two-thirds of stroke survivors become independent at one year, with little difference between ischemic or hemorrhagic strokes. However, within the ischemic group, only about 5% of patients with infarction of the whole middle cerebral artery territory are alive and independent at a year post-stroke, compared with 50% of those with more restricted infarcts (Table 16.1) (Bamford *et al.* 1990). Approximately 90% of stroke survivors return home, leaving only a small proportion in institutional care, but because stroke is so common, their absolute number is large (Legh-Smith *et al.* 1986; Chuang *et al.* 2005).

The mechanisms of recovery are incompletely understood. Acute resolution of edema and recanalization of occluded vessels leading to resolution of penumbral dysfunction may contribute. In the subacute phase, changes in neuronal networks and neuronal plasticity are important (Kreisel *et al.* 2007; Nudo 2007). The mechanisms share similarities with those involved in learning and memory. The rate of recovery of all impairments is maximal in the first few weeks, slows down after two or three months and probably stops at about 6–12 months post-stroke (Pedersen *et al.* 1995; Kreisel *et al.* 2007). Later improvement in functional abilities, and particularly in social activities, is probably more to do with adaptation to disability and minimizing handicap rather than further recovery of physical impairments. Impaired quality of life is common even when patients appear to be little disabled.

Prediction of functional outcome for individuals immediately after stroke onset is difficult, and clinical features predict outcome as well or better than radiological findings (Hand *et al.* 2006). Prognostic scores have been developed but these are not particularly discriminating (German Stroke Study Collaboration 2004). About two weeks after stroke, good prognostic signs include young age, initially mild deficit, normal conscious level, good sitting balance, lack of cognitive impairment, urinary continence and rapid improvement. Independent living is often also contingent on a high level of social support.

Strategies for rehabilitation

Stroke rehabilitation attempts to restore patients to their previous physical, mental and social capability (Langton Hewer 1990; Brandstater 2005). Rehabilitation approaches include restoration of previous function, compensation by increasing function for a given impairment, environmental modification, prevention of complications such as recurrent stroke or shoulder pain, and maintenance or prevention of deterioration. Achieving optimal quality of life is the ultimate goal. Although there is good evidence that increased time undergoing therapy is beneficial (Langhorne *et al.* 1996; Kwakkel *et al.* 2004; Kwakkel 2006), in general, patients spend very little of their time awake receiving therapy, only around 5% in one study (Bernhardt *et al.* 2004). As little as five hours a week extra therapy results in clinically important improvements in walking (Blennerhassett and Dite 2004). Rehabilitation should not necessarily be confined to patients in hospital, and early discharge with multidisciplinary support achieves as good or better outcome (Langhorne and Holmqvist 2007).

The optimum time to start rehabilitation after stroke is not known, but early rehabilitation within the first week is probably beneficial given the deleterious consequences of bedrest after stroke (Langhorne *et al.* 2000) and the benefits of early mobilization following other acute medical conditions including myocardial infarction. There is some evidence from animal studies that very early intense activity may increase lesion size. Early resumption of the upright posture may compromise perfusion in the penumbral zone. Consequently, it may be reasonable to delay mobilization for the first few days after stroke (Diserens *et al.* 2006). Although improvements in mobility and activities of daily living can occur months or years after stroke (Outpatient Service Trialists 2003), benefits are greater when intervention occurs within the first six months.

There are insufficient data to determine which patient groups benefit most from rehabilitation. Although severely affected patients benefit from rehabilitation, and in fact receive the most inpatient and outpatient therapy, they have the worst functional outcomes (Alexander *et al.* 2001). Therefore, it is unclear at present how best to target the available rehabilitation resources most efficiently.

The evidence base to support particular rehabilitation strategies is limited owing to a lack of large randomized trials. Yet it is clear that multidisciplinary input facilitates recovery and reduces handicap (Bayley *et al.* 2007). Key components of inpatient rehabilitation have been identified (Stroke Unit Trialists' Collaboration 1997; Langhorne and Duncan 2001; Langhorne and Dennis 2004) as:

- coordinated, multidisciplinary care with regular team meetings
- early institution of rehabilitation within one to two weeks
- goal setting
- early assessment of impairments and function
- discharge planning with early assessment of discharge needs
- staff with a specialist interest in stroke or rehabilitation
- routine involvement of carers
- close linking of nursing with other multidisciplinary care
- regular programs of education and training for staff
- information provided about stroke, stroke recovery and available services.

A systematic review of randomized control trials of inpatient multidisciplinary stroke rehabilitation has shown the benefits of rehabilitation, beyond seven days after stroke, as distinct from the acute medical management aspects of acute stroke care in the first week after stroke (Langhorne and Duncan 2001), with a reduction in death (OR 0.66; 95% odds ratio [OR], confidence interval [CI], 0.49–0.88) and death or dependency (OR, 0.65; 95% CI, 0.50–0.85). For every 20 patients with stroke treated in a post-acute (beyond seven days) multidisciplinary rehabilitation unit, one additional person returns home independent in activities of daily living.

Table 23.1. Modified Rankin scale

Grade	Symptoms
0	No symptoms
1	Minor symptoms that do not interfere with lifestyle
2	Minor handicap; symptoms that lead to some restriction in lifestyle but do not interfere with patients' ability to look after themselves
3	Moderate handicap; symptoms that significantly restrict lifestyle and prevent totally independent existence
4	Moderately severe handicap; symptoms that clearly prevent independent existence although not needing constant care and attention
5	Severe handicap; totally dependent, requiring constant attention day and night
6	Dead

There is also evidence that outpatient (Outpatient Service Trialists 2003) and home-based (Early Supported Discharge Trialists 2005; Langhorne and Holmqvist 2007) rehabilitation are effective for patients who have returned to the community, in preventing death, deterioration and dependency and may allow earlier hospital discharge.

Assessment tools used in rehabilitation

Assessment tools identify, measure and record impairments, disabilities, handicaps and quality of life. Assessment is the first step in rehabilitation, and measurement of outcome is crucial for clinical trials, audit and comparison of different institutions. Patients' present levels of functioning must be compared with their premorbid levels, taking account of the numerous comorbidities often present in the elderly (Collen and Wade 1991).

For clinical trial and audit purposes in large samples, three simple questions group patients into those who are completely recovered, those who are still symptomatic but independent, and those who are dependent, or dead (Dennis *et al.* 1997a,b). Various more detailed assessment instruments are available that are designed to test different domains (Lyden and Hantson 1998; Warlow *et al.* 1996):

- *motricity index* and *trunk control test* (Collin and Wade 1990)
- *walking speed test* (Wade *et al.* 1987; Collen *et al.* 1990)
- *Rivermead mobility index* (Collen *et al.* 1991)
- *Frenchay Aphasia Screening Test for aphasia* (Enderby *et al.* 1986)
- *Star Cancellation Test* for neglect (Jehkonen *et al.* 1998)
- *Barthel Activities of Daily Living Index*
- *modified Rankin Scale* (Oxford Handicap Scale), may be more useful than the Barthel Index (Table 23.1) (Bamford *et al.* 1989)
- *Frenchay Activity Index* for social functioning (Wade *et al.* 1985).

It is important to try to assess mood after stroke, even though this is often difficult since the risk is high and depression contributes to poor cognitive function and outcome. The Short Form-36 is the most widely used generic instrument for assessment of 'quality of life' but the EuroQol is also used. Neither is reliable enough to monitor individuals over time but they may be used to compare groups of patients (de Haan *et al.* 1993; Dorman *et al.* 1998).

Interventions

Stroke rehabilitation teams usually consist of physiotherapists, occupational therapists, speech therapists and social workers, as well as nursing staff. The stroke rehabilitaion team provides a range of interventions and is also able to advise regarding return to work, driving, finance, benefits and sexual activity. Information about local stroke clubs and other voluntary organizations should be given to patients and carers. The latter may also need care and support since they may experience high levels of burden (van Heugten et al. 2006).

Physiotherapy improves outcome after stroke, but it is unclear which type of approach is best (Pollock et al. 2007). Physiotherapy trains patients in reaching and manipulation, sitting, sit-to-stand, standing and walking. Physiotherapists also assist with the use of foot-drop splints, sticks and wheelchairs, and they instruct carers in transferring, lifting, walking and exercises. They are also able to advise on the care of the hemiplegic arm, particularly the shoulder. There is good evidence that functional electric stimulation reduces shoulder pain, prevents shoulder subluxation, maintains range of movement and improves upper limb activity (Foley et al. 2006). Routine corticosteroid injection or ultrasound for shoulder pain have not been shown to be beneficial, and overhead arm pulleys and positional shoulder static stretches are harmful and should not be used (Gustafsson and McKenna 2006).

Occupational therapy prevents deterioration after stroke and facilitates patient independence but the exact nature of the occupational therapy intervention to achieve maximum benefit remains to be defined (Legg et al. 2006).

Speech therapy There is insufficient evidence to support or refute possible benefits of **speech therapy** after stroke for either aphasia (Greener et al. 2002) or speech apraxia (West et al. 2005), although patients and carers value such input and stroke-care guidelines recommend speech therapy. Speech therapists also have a role in the management of dysarthria and swallowing.

Neglect is one of the most disabling impairments for patients after stroke. Although individual studies of rehabilitation specifically for neglect have shown benefit, a review of 15 such studies showed no impact on disability or discharge home (Bowen et al. 2002). Visuo–spatial–motor training, in which the affected limb is moved to increase attention to that side, has been shown to be effective in a single randomized controlled trial (Kalra et al. 1997).

Spasticity, if moderate to severe, may impede rehabilitation after stroke. Botulinum toxin has been shown in small studies to reduce tone and improve range of movement but robust evidence for improvement in function is lacking (van Kuijk et al. 2002).

Secondary consequences of neurological disability include painful shoulder, shoulder–hand syndrome, contractures and falls. Physiotherapists and other members of the multi-disciplinary team should have expertise in managing these problems.

Brain imaging and recovery after stroke

The relationship between radiological findings and functional outcome has been examined in a number of studies using different imaging modalities and outcome measures. The importance of these studies from the point of view of acute stroke management is that they may allow identification of those patients who have the potential for good functional recovery. Rehabilitative and therapeutic strategies, such as neuroprotection agents, could then be targeted to those patients. The majority of studies have correlated lesion size in the acute or subacute period, using conventional CT or MRI, with outcome measured using a variety of scales of impairment or disability or combinations of these measures. Although a significant relationship between infarct size and outcome has been demonstrated in most studies, this is not invariably the case. The major reasons for a lack of correlation relate to lack of sensitivity in detection of infarcts, but, more importantly, to the fact that these studies ignore the importance of lesion location in determining outcome from stroke.

Lesion size on imaging and functional outcome

Studies using CT to measure lesion size have shown conflicting results. The largest such study (Saver *et al.* 1999) found only a modest correlation ($r=0.5$), between subacute infarct volume and the score on the National Institutes of Health Stroke Scale at three months. In addition, although patients with large infarcts tended to have a poor outcome, the functional consequences of more moderately sized infarcts were more difficult to predict: T_2-weighted MRI is more sensitive than CT at detecting infarction and thus might be expected to be somewhat better prognostically. In a study of T_2-weighted MRI and outcome, patients who were independent at three months had smaller strokes visualized by MRI than patients who were dependent or dead (Saunders *et al.* 1995). However, there was considerable overlap between infarct sizes in the three groups and the outcome measures were rather coarse. Modest but significant correlations have also been shown between acute diffusion-weighted imaging lesion volume and neurological outcome (Lovblad *et al.* 1997; Barber *et al.* 1998; Tong *et al.* 1998) although the relationship may be stronger with perfusion-weighted imaging. Subacute perfusion-weighted imaging appears to be less closely related to functional outcome, presumably because of the occurrence of spontaneous reperfusion over time.

One of the major reasons why outcome may not be correlated strongly with lesion volume is that volume measures do not take account of variations in lesion location or shape. Recently, evidence has been produced to suggest that the clinical consequences of an ischemic lesion can be predicted if damage and outcome are measured within a specific functional system (Fig. 23.1) (Binkofski *et al.* 1996; Pineiro *et al.* 2000).

Magnetic resonance spectroscopy and functional outcome

Cerebral damage following stroke has also been assessed by MR spectroscopy. This technique uses the same methods as MRI but the signal obtained is converted into chemical as opposed to spatial information. Proton MR spectroscopy allows in vivo measurement of *N*-acetyl-containing compounds, creatine, choline and lactate. The majority of the *N*-acetyl signal comes from *N*-acetyl aspartate (NAA), which is present in high concentrations in the brain. The function of NAA is unclear, but it is of particular interest in studies of the brain since it is located almost exclusively in neurons in the adult. Decreases in the NAA resonance peak in vivo indicate neuronal or axonal injury or loss.

Early studies of MR spectroscopy in stroke showed increased lactate and decreased NAA within the stroke lesion (Berkelbach van der Sprenkel *et al.* 1988; Bruhn *et al.* 1989). Subsequently, it was shown that the magnitude of neuronal damage as measured by NAA loss from the infarcted region correlated with disability and impairment in stroke patients (Ford *et al.* 1992; Federico *et al.* 1998). It remains unclear whether NAA loss is a better prognostic indicator than other factors such as infarct volume as measured on imaging or indeed simple clinical tests. However, one study (Parsons *et al.* 2000) suggested that acute lactate/choline ratios correlate better with outcome than NAA/choline ratios or infarct volume. In all the above studies, metabolite changes were measured from the center of the infarcted region and, therefore, were not representative of the total infarct damage. Also the

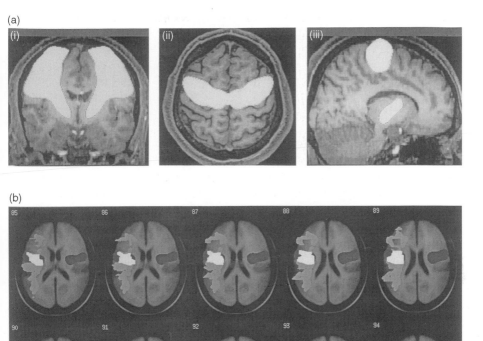

Fig. 23.1. (a) Outline or "mask" of the corticospinal tract shown in (i) coronal, (ii) axial and (iii) sagittal views (Pineiro *et al.* 2000). (b) Axial MR slices showing the intersection of a stroke with the corticospinal mask, from which the maximum proportion of the mask cross-sectional area occupied by stroke is calculated. The corticospinal mask is shown in dark gray, the stroke in light gray, and the point of intersection between the stroke and the mask in white (Pineiro *et al.* 2000).

chosen outcome measures were not necessarily relevant to the area of brain under study. These points were addressed in a study in which NAA loss was measured in the descending motor pathways and correlated to a scale designed to measure motor impairment (Fig. 23.2) (Pendlebury *et al.* 1999). This study showed that NAA loss in the descending motor pathways was significantly associated with motor deficit and with the maximum proportion of the descending motor pathway cross-sectional area occupied by stroke, as described above.

Recovery after stroke and functional imaging

Studies of brain activation patterns after stroke have used electrical or magnetic brain stimulation of pathways or imaging using positron emission tomography or functional MRI (fMRI). Functional MRI relies on the fact that deoxyhemoglobin is paramagnetic whereas oxyhemoglobin is not. During neuronal activation, the neuronal oxygen demand rises and local cerebral blood flow rises, but to a level in excess of that required to supply the increased metabolic demand. Hence activation results in a reduced concentration of deoxyhemoglobin and thus an increased signal on MRI. However, fMRI studies are

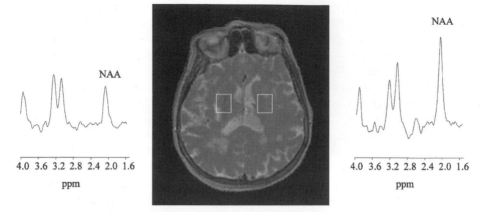

Fig. 23.2. Axial T$_2$-weighted image showing location of a spectroscopy voxel over the posterior limb of the internal capsule of each hemisphere together with the spectra obtained from the right and left internal capsules of a patient with subcortical stroke (Pendlebury *et al.* 1999). The *N*-acetyl aspartate (NAA) peak is reduced on the side of the affected right hemisphere consistent with damage to the descending motor pathways.

technically demanding to perform, require awake and cooperative subjects and assume that the normal relationship between metabolism and blood flow is maintained in normal ageing and after a stroke. In fact, there are age-related decreases in cerebral blood flow and metabolic rate, and blood flow/metabolism coupling is impaired within ischemic tissue, although blood flow increases have been reported to occur in the remaining tissue in response to brain activation (Weiller *et al.* 1992). However, this does not necessarily indicate that the blood flow/metabolism coupling is normal in non-infarcted tissue. Certainly, there are widespread changes in the resting metabolic rate and perfusion of the brain after stroke, which persist into the chronic phase and may affect areas remote from the infarct.

Despite the limitations of fMRI outlined above, fMRI studies have shown similar findings to those of positron emission tomography studies in recovery after stroke (Yozbatiran and Cramer 2006; Rijntjes 2006). Increased ipsilateral primary sensorimotor cortical activity with posterior displacement of the ipsilesional focus of activity, bilateral supplementary motor area activation and premotor cortical activation occurs after stroke with use of the affected hand in comparison with use of the unaffected hand (Weiller *et al.* 1992; Cramer *et al.* 1997; Cao *et al.* 1998; Pineiro *et al.* 2001). Specifically, in patients with capsular or other subcortical stroke, good recovery is related to enhanced recruitment of the lateral premotor cortex of the lesional hemisphere and lateral premotor and, to a lesser extent, primary sensorimotor and parietal cortex of the contralateral hemisphere (Gerloff *et al.* 2006).

The mechanisms of motor recovery vary according to location of the lesion: cortical infarcts are associated with activation of the contralateral primary sensorimotor cortex, whereas subcortical infarcts appear to activate the bilateral primary sensorimotor cortex (Kwon *et al.* 2007). Several studies indicate that worse motor performance is related to a greater amount of contralesional activation (Calautti *et al.* 2007) and that patients who activate the ipsilesional primary motor cortex early had a better recovery of hand function (Loubinoux *et al.* 2007). Repetitive peripheral magnetic stimulation increases the activation of the parieto-premotor network and thereby might have a positive conditioning effect for treatment (Struppler *et al.* 2007). In addition to changes in the activation pattern of the motor network, different activation patterns were observed in the proprioceptive system, where the initially observed blood flow increases in sensory areas I and II of the non-infarcted hemisphere vanished during successful rehabilitation and the normal activation patterns were restored, indicating an interhemispheric shift of attention associated with recovery (Thiel *et al.* 2007).

Contralateral sensorimotor cortical activation is enhanced by active rehabilitation (Cramer *et al.* 1997) and fluoxetine (Pariente *et al.* 2001): two interventions thought to improve motor recovery. It has been proposed that non-invasive functional imaging may in the future be used to select patients for specific rehabilitation therapy.

Functional imaging in recovery from aphasia supports the model of three phases of language recovery: a strongly reduced activation of remaining left language areas in the acute phase, followed (or substituted) by an upregulation of homologue language zones and finally a normalization of the activation pattern (Saur *et al.* 2006; Crinion and Leff 2007). The pattern of activation and the recruitment of regions during the rehabilitation depend on the available language-related regions, where restoration of the left hemisphere networks seems to be more effective, although in some cases right hemisphere areas are integrated successfully (Winhuisen *et al.* 2007).

References

Alexander H, Bugge C, Hagen S (2001). What is the association between the different components of stroke rehabilitation and health outcomes? *Clinical Rehabilitation* 15:207–215

Bamford J, Sandercock PAG, Warlow CP *et al.* (1989). Interobserver agreement for the assessment of handicap in stroke patients. *Stroke* 20:828

Bamford J, Sandercock PAG, Dennis M *et al.* (1990). A prospective study of acute cerebrovascular disease in the community: the Oxfordshire Community Stroke Project 1981–86. 2. Incidence, case fatality rates and overall outcome at one year of cerebral infarction, primary intracerebral and subarachnoid haemorrhage. *Journal Neurology, Neurosurgery and Psychiatry* 53:16–22

Barber PA, Darby DG, Desmond PM *et al.* (1998). Prediction of stroke outcome with echoplanar perfusion-and diffusion-weighted MRI. *Neurology* 51:418–426

Bayley MT, Hurdowar A, Teasell R *et al.* (2007). Priorities for stroke rehabilitation and research: results of a 2003 Canadian Stroke Network consensus conference. *Archives of Physical and Medical Rehabilitation* 88:526–528

Berkelbach van der Sprenkel JW, Luyten PR, van Rijen PC *et al.* (1988). Cerebral lactate detected by regional proton magnetic resonance spectroscopy in a patient with cerebral infarction. *Stroke* 19:1556–1560

Bernhardt J, Dewey H, Thrift A *et al.* (2004). Inactive and alone: physical activity within the first 14 days of acute stroke unit care. *Stroke* 35:1005–1009

Binkofski F, Seitz RJ, Arnold S *et al.* (1996). Thalamic metabolism and corticospinal tract integrity determine motor recovery in stroke. *Annals of Neurology* 39:460–470

Blennerhassett J, Dite W (2004). Additional task-related practice improves mobility and upper limb function early after stroke: A randomised controlled trial. *Australian Journal of Physiotherapy* 50:219–224

Bowen A, Lincoln NB, Dewey ME (2002). Spatial neglect: is rehabilitation effective? *Stroke* 33:2728–2729

Brandstater ME (2005). Stroke rehabilitation In *Physical Medicine and Rehabilitation: Principles and Practice*, De Lisa JA, Gans BM, Walsh NE (eds.), pp. 1165–1169. Philadelphia, PA: Lippincott Williams & Wilkins

Bruhn H, Frahm J, Gyngell ML *et al.* (1989). Cerebral metabolism in man after acute stroke: new observations using localized proton NMR spectroscopy. *Magnetic Resonance Medicine* 9:126–131

Calautti C, Naccarato M, Jones PS *et al.* (2007). The relationship between motor deficit and hemisphere activation balance after stroke: a 3T fMRI study. *Neuroimage* 34:322–331

Cao Y, D'Olhaberriague L, Vikingstad EM *et al.* (1998). Pilot study of functional MRI to assess cerebral activation of motor function after poststroke hemiparesis. *Stroke* 29:112–122

Chuang KY, Wu SC, Yeh MC *et al.* (2005). Exploring the associations between longterm care and mortality rates among stroke patients. *Journal of Nursing Research* 13:66–74

Collen FM, Wade DT (1991). Residual mobility problems after stroke. *International Disability Studies* 13:12–15

Collen FM, Wade DT, Bradshaw CM (1990). Mobility after stroke: reliability of measures of impairment and disability. *International Disability Studies* 12:6–9

Collen FM, Wade DT, Robb GF *et al.* (1991). The Rivermead Mobility Index: a further development of the Rivermead Motor Assessment. *International Disability Studies* 13:50–54

Collin C, Wade D (1990). Assessing motor impairment after stroke: a pilot reliability study. *Journal of Neurology, Neurosurgery and Psychiatry* 53:576–579

Cramer SC, Nelles G, Benson RR *et al.* (1997). A functional MRI study of subjects recovered from hemiparetic stroke. *Stroke* 28:2518–2527

Crinion JT, Leff AP (2007). Recovery and treatment of aphasia after stroke: functional imaging studies. *Current Opinions in Neurology* 20:667–673

de Haan R, Aaronson N, Limburg M *et al.* (1993). Measuring quality of life in stroke. *Stroke* 24:320–327

Dennis M, Wellwood I, Warlow C (1997a). Are simple questions a valid measure of outcome after stroke? *Cerebrovascular Diseases* 7:22–27

Dennis M, Wellwood I, O'Rourke S *et al.* (1997b). How reliable are simple questions in assessing outcome after stroke? *Cerebrovascular Diseases* 7:19–21

Diserens K, Michel P, Bogousslavsky J (2006). Early mobilisation after stroke: review of the literature. *Cerebrovascular Diseases* 22:183–190

Dorman P, Slattery J, Farrell B *et al.* (1998). Qualitative comparison of the reliability of health status assessments with the EuroQol and SF-36 questionnaires after stroke. *Stroke* 29:63–68

Early Supported Discharge Trialists (2005). Services for reducing duration of hospital care for acute stroke patients. *Cochrane Database of Systematic Reviews* 1:CD000443

Enderby PM, Wood VA, Wade DT *et al.* (1986). The Frenchay Aphasia Screening Test: a short simple test for aphasia appropriate for non-specialists. *International Rehabilitation Medicine* 8:166–170

Federico F, Simone IL, Lucivero V *et al.* (1998). Prognostic value of proton magnetic resonance spectroscopy in ischemic stroke. *Archives of Neurology* 55:489–494

Foley N, Bhogal S, Foley N (2006). Painful hemiplegic shoulder. In *Canadian Stroke Network Evidence-based Reviews of Stroke Rehabilitation* http://ebrsrcom/ index_homehtml (accessed 10 May 2007)

Ford CC, Griffey RH, Matwiyoff NA *et al.* (1992). Multivoxel 1H-MRS of stroke. *Neurology* 42:1408–1412

Gerloff C, Bushara K, Sailer A *et al.* (2006). Multimodal imaging of brain reorganization in motor areas of the contralesional hemisphere of well recovered patients after capsular stroke. *Brain* 129:791–808

German Stroke Study Collaboration (2004). Predicting outcome after acute ischemic stroke: an external validation of prognostic models. *Neurology* 62:581–585

Greener J, Enderby P, Whurr R (2002). Speech and language therapy for aphasia following stroke. *Cochrane Database of Systematic Reviews* 2:CD000425

Gustafsson L, McKenna K (2006). A programme of static positional stretches does not reduce hemiplegic shoulder pain or maintain shoulder range of motion: a randomized controlled trial. *Clinical Rehabilitation* 20:277

Hand PJ, Kwan J, Lindley RI *et al.* (2006). Distinguishing between stroke and mimic at the bedside: the brain attack study. *Stroke* 37:769–775

Jehkonen M, Ahonen JP, Dastidar P *et al.* (1998). How to detect visual neglect in acute stroke. *Lancet* 351:727–728

Kalra L, Perez I, Gupta S *et al.* (1997). The influence of visual neglect on stroke rehabilitation. *Stroke* 28:1386–1391

Kreisel SH, Hennerici MG, Bazner H (2007). Pathophysiology of stroke rehabilitation: the natural course of clinical recovery, use-dependent plasticity and rehabilitative outcome. *Cerebrovascular Diseases* **23**:243–255

Kwakkel G (2006). Impact of intensity of practice after stroke: Issues for consideration. *Disability and Rehabilitation* **28**:823–830

Kwakkel G, van Peppen R, Wagenaar RC *et al.* (2004). Effects of augmented exercise therapy time after stroke: A meta-analysis. *Stroke* **35**:2529–2536

Kwon YH, Lee MY, Park JW *et al.* (2007). Differences of cortical activation pattern between cortical and corona radiata infarct. *Neuroscience Letters* **417**:138–142

Langhorne P, Dennis MS (2004). Stroke units: The next 10 years. *Lancet* **363**:834–835

Langhorne P, Duncan P (2001). Does the organization of postacute stroke care really matter? *Stroke* **32**:268–274

Langhorne P, Holmqvist LW (2007). Early Supported Discharge Trialists. Early supported discharge after stroke. *Journal of Rehabilitation Medicine* **39**:103–108

Langhorne P, Wagenaar R, Partridge C (1996). Physiotherapy after stroke: More is better? *Physiotherapy Research International* **1**:75–88

Langhorne P, Stott D, Robertson L *et al.* (2000). Medical complications after stroke: A multicenter study. *Stroke* **31**:1223–1229

Langton Hewer R (1990). Rehabilitation after stroke. *Quarterly Journal of Medicine* **76**:659–674

Legg LA, Drummond AE, Langhorne P (2006). Occupational therapy for patients with problems in activities of daily living after stroke. *Cochrane Database of Systematic Reviews* **4**:CD0030585

Legh-Smith J, Wade DT, Langton-Hewer R (1986). Services for stroke patients one year after stroke. *Journal of Epidemiology Community Health* **40**:161–165

Loubinoux I, Dechaumont-Palacin S, Castel-Lacanal E *et al.* (2007). Prognostic value of fMRI in recovery of hand function in subcortical stroke patients. *Cerebral Cortex* **17**:2980–2987

Lovblad KO, Baird AE, Schlaug G *et al.* (1997). Ischemic lesion volumes in acute stroke by diffusion-weighted magnetic resonance imaging correlate with clinical outcome. *Annals of Neurology* **42**:164–170

Lyden PD, Hantson L (1998). Assessment scales for the evaluation of stroke patients. *Journal*

of Stroke and Cerebrovascular Diseases **7**:113–127

Nudo RJ (2007). Post infarct cortical plasticity and behavioural recovery. *Stroke* **38**:840–845

Outpatient Service Trialists (2003). Therapy-based rehabilitation services for stroke patients at home *Cochrane Database of Systematic Reviews* **1**:CD002925

Pariente J, Loubinoux I, Carel C *et al.* (2001). Fluoxetine modulates motor performance and cerebral activation of patients recovering from stroke. *Annals of Neurology* **50**:718–729

Parsons MW, Li T, Barber PA *et al.* (2000). Combined (1)H MR spectroscopy and diffusion-weighted MRI improves the prediction of stroke outcome. *Neurology* **55**:498–505

Pedersen PM, Jorgensen HS, Nakayama H *et al.* (1995). Aphasia in acute stroke: incidence determinants and recovery. *Annals of Neurology* **38**:659–666

Pendlebury ST, Blamire AM, Lee MA *et al.* (1999). Axonal injury in the internal capsule correlates with motor impairment after stroke. *Stroke* **30**: 956–962

Pineiro R, Pendlebury ST, Smith S *et al.* (2000). Relating MRI changes to motor deficit after ischemic stroke by segmentation of functional motor pathways. *Stroke* **31**:672–679

Pineiro R, Pendlebury S, Johansen-Berg H *et al.* (2001). Functional MRI detects posterior shifts in primary sensorimotor cortex activation after stroke: evidence of local adaptive reorganization? *Stroke* **32**:1134–1139

Pollock A, Baer G, Pomeroy V *et al.* (2007). Physiotherapy treatment approaches for the recovery of postural control and lower limb function following stroke. *Cochrane Database of Systematic Reviews* **1**:CD001920

Rijntjes M (2006). Mechanisms of recovery in stroke patients with hemiparesis or aphasia: new insights, old questions and the meaning of therapies. *Current Opinions in Neurology* **19**:76–83

Saunders DE, Clifton AG, Brown MM (1995). Measurement of infarct size using MRI predicts prognosis in middle cerebral artery infarction. *Stroke* **26**:2272–2276

Saur D, Lange R, Baumgacrtner A *et al.* (2006). Dynamics of language reorganization after stroke. *Brain* **129**:1371–1384

Saver JL, Johnston KC, Homer D et al. (1999). Infarct volume as a surrogate or auxiliary outcome measure in ischemic stroke clinical trials. The RANTTAS Investigators. *Stroke* **30**:293–298

Stroke Unit Trialists' Collaboration (1997). Collaborative systematic review of the randomised trials of organised inpatient (stroke unit) care after stroke. *British Medical Journal* **314**:1151–1159

Struppler A, Binkofski F, Angerer B et al. (2007). A fronto-parietal network is mediating improvement of motor function related to repetitive peripheral magnetic stimulation: A PET-H2O15 study. *Neuroimage* **36**(Suppl 2):T174–T186

Thiel A, Aleksic B, Klein J et al. (2007). Changes in proprioceptive systems activity during recovery from post-stroke hemiparesis. *Journal of Rehabilitation Medicine* **39**:520–525

Tong DC, Yenari MA, Albers GW et al. (1998). Correlation of perfusion- and diffusion-weighted MRI with NIHSS score in acute (<65 hour) ischemic stroke. *Neurology* **50**:864–870

van Heugten C, Visser-Meily A, Post M et al. (2006). Care for carers of stroke patients: evidence-based clinical practice guidelines. *Journal of Rehabilitation Medicine* **38**:153–158

van Kuijk AA, Geurts AC, Bevaart BJ et al. (2002). Treatment of upper extremity spasticity in stroke patients by focal neuronal or neuromuscular blockade: a systematic review of the literature. *Journal of Rehabilitation Medicine* **34**:51–61

Wade DT, Legh-Smith J, Langton Hewer R (1985). Social activities after stroke: measurement and natural history using the Frenchay Activities Index. *International Rehabilitation Medicine* **7**:176–181

Wade DT, Wood VA, Heller A et al. (1987). Walking after stroke. Measurement and recovery over the first 3 months. *Scandinavian Journal of Rehabilitation Medicine* **19**:25–30

Warlow CP, Dennis MS, van Gijn J et al. (1996). *Stroke: A Practical Guide to Management*, Ch. 17: What are this person's problems? A problem-based approach to the general management of stroke, pp. 477–544. Oxford: Blackwell

Weiller C, Chollet F, Friston KJ et al. (1992). Functional reorganization of the brain in recovery from striatocapsular infarction in man. *Annals of Neurology* **31**:463–472

West C, Hesketh A, Vail A et al. (2005). Interventions for apraxia of speech following stroke. *Cochrane Database of Systematic Reviews* **4**:CD004298

Winhuisen L, Thiel A, Schumacher B et al. (2007). The right inferior frontal gyrus and post stroke aphasia: a follow-up investigation. *Stroke* **38**:1286–1292

Yozbatiran N, Cramer SC (2006). Imaging motor recovery after stroke. *Neuroradiology* **3**:482–488

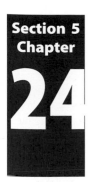

Secondary prevention
Medical therapies

As shown in Chs. 15 and 19, the early risk after TIA and minor stroke is high, but rapid treatment of TIA and minor stroke can prevent up to 80% of recurrent strokes (Rothwell *et al.* 2007). There is considerable evidence relating to the effectiveness of various treatments to reduce the medium- and long-term risk of vascular events after TIA and stroke, which is detailed in (Table 24.1).

Antiplatelet therapy

Antiplatelet therapy reduces the risk of recurrent vascular events after TIA and ischemic stroke, although few trials have distinguished between different etiological subtypes (Antithrombotic Trialists' Collaboration 2002). Most trial data concern aspirin, but other antiplatelet agents such as clopidogrel (CAPRIE Steering Committee 1996) or extended-release dipyridamole (Sivenius *et al.* 1991) have also been shown to be effective although mechanisms of action may differ (Table 24.2).

The combination of aspirin and dipyridamole is more effective than aspirin alone (Diener *et al.* 1996; Halkes *et al.* 2006). The combination results in a relative reduction in the risk of recurrent stroke of around 30% compared with aspirin alone. In contrast, the combination of clopidogrel and aspirin was not superior to clopidogrel alone in secondary prevention after stroke, TIA or other vascular disease in the Management of Atherothrombosis with Clopidogrel in High-Risk Patients with Recent Ischemic Attacks or Ischemic Strokes (MATCH) and Clopidogrel for High Athero-thrombotic Risk and Ischemic Stabilization, Management, and Avoidance (CHARISMA) trials (Diener *et al.* 2004; Bhatt *et al.* 2007). However, among patients randomized within the first week after the qualifying event, there was a non-significant trend towards benefit from combination antiplatelet treatment in the MATCH trial. The risk of life-threatening hemorrhage was significantly higher in the combination antiplatelet group at 18 months, but this difference did not become apparent until three to four months after randomization. Consequently, it is possible that a short course of clopidogrel, in addition to aspirin, might be effective in the acute phase after TIA and minor stroke.

Few trials of antiplatelet agents have distinguished between different vascular territories or mechanisms of stroke, but there are some data on antiplatelet agents in posterior circulation disease. The Canadian Cooperative Study Group (1978) showed that aspirin reduced recurrent episodes of cerebral ischemia and death in patients with vertebrobasilar events. The European Stroke Prevention Study (ESPS; Sivenius *et al.* 1991) of aspirin and immediate-release dipyridamole versus placebo appeared to show that patients with posterior circulation TIA benefited more than those with carotid disease, but the numbers of events were too small to be certain.

Table 24.1. Major trials and meta-analyses contributing to the evidence base for medical treatment in secondary prevention after TIA and ischemic stroke

Drug	Trial	Treatment
Aspirin	CAST	Aspirin versus placebo within 48 hours of major ischemic stroke
	IST	Aspirin versus placebo (and subcutaneous heparin versus placebo) acutely after major ischemic stroke
	Anti-thrombotic Trialists' Collaboration	Meta-analysis of trials studying antiplatelet agents in patients at high risk of occlusive vascular disease
Dipyridamole	ESPS II	Aspirin and modified-release dipyridamole versus placebo in a 2×2 factorial design started within three months of TIA or ischemic stroke
	ESPRIT	Aspirin versus aspirin plus dipyridamole started within six months of TIA or minor stroke
Clopidogrel	MATCH	Clopidogrel versus aspirin plus clopidogrel within six months of ischemic stroke or TIA
	CHARISMA	Aspirin versus aspirin plus clopidogrel in patients with cardiovascular disease or multiple risk factors (including ischemic stroke)
	FASTER	Aspirin versus aspirin plus clopidogrel in the acute phase after TIA or minor ischemic stroke
Antihypertensive drugs	PROGRESS	Perindopril ± indapamide versus placebo after TIA or ischemic stroke in patients with or without hypertension
Cholesterol-lowering drugs	HPS	Simvastatin versus placebo in patients with coronary disease or other occlusive vascular disease (including TIA or stroke)
	SPARCL	Atorvastatin versus placebo started within one to six months of TIA or ischemic stroke

Notes:
TIA, transient ischemic attacks, CAST, Chinese Acute Stroke Trial; IST, International Stroke Trial; ESPRIT, European/Australasian Stroke Prevention in Reversible Ischemia Trial; FASTER, Fast Assessment of Stroke and Transient Ischemic Attack to Prevent Early Recurrence; see text for other trials.

Anticoagulation

Patients in atrial fibrillation who have a TIA or stroke without other clear etiology should be given anticoagulation therapy if there are no contraindications (European Atrial Fibrillation Trial Study Group 1993, 1995). Recent studies have shown that warfarin is as safe as aspirin in elderly patients with atrial fibrillation (Rash *et al.* 2007; Mant *et al.* 2007). Patients with presumed cardioembolic TIA or stroke secondary to other causes should certainly receive antithrombotic therapy. Also they may benefit from anticoagulation in certain circumstances, such as intracardiac mural thrombosis after myocardial infarction, although there have been no randomized trials in situations other than non-valvular atrial fibrillation.

Anticoagulation is not effective in secondary prevention of stroke for patients in sinus rhythm. Warfarin treatment to a target international normalized ratio (INR) of 3–4.5 was associated with significant harm owing to a large increase in major bleeding complications, especially intracerebral hemorrhage, in patients with previous TIA or ischemic stroke in the Stroke Prevention in Reversible Ischemia Trial (SPIRIT) (Algra *et al.* 1997). The subsequent Warfarin versus Aspirin in the Secondary Prevention of Stroke (WARSS) trial of aspirin

Table 24.2. Mechanisms of action of commonly used antiplatelet agents

Agent	Mechanism of action
Antiplatelet agents in general	Prevention of propagation of arterial thrombus
	Prevent platelet aggregation in the microcirculation
	Prevent re-embolization from embolic source
	Reduce the release of eicosanoids and other neurotoxic agents
Aspirin	Inhibition of cyclooxygenase 1, reducing the breakdown of arachadonic acid to thromboxane A_2 and platelet granule release
Dipyridamole	Inhibition of phosphodiesterase, causing elevation of intracellular platelet cyclicAMP and a consequent reduction in calcium inhibitions; this platelet activation and granule releases
Clopidogrel and other thienopyridines	Blockade of platelet membrane ADP receptors, inhibiting ADP-dependent platelet activation and granule release

versus warfarin for patients in sinus rhythm and without a cardioembolic source or with > 50% carotid stenosis showed no additional benefit for warfarin at a target INR of 1.4–2.8 (Redman and Allen 2002).

There has been uncertainty as to whether anticoagulation is preferable to antiplatelet treatment for the secondary prevention of ischemia related to intracranial atherosclerosis. A retrospective analysis of 68 patients with a variety of symptomatic intracranial arterial stenoses appeared to show that warfarin was significantly better than aspirin in reducing the rate of stroke (Chimowitz *et al.* 1995). However, the subsequent randomized double-blind Warfarin–Aspirin Symptomatic Intracranial Disease (WASID) trial of warfarin, to a target INR of 2–3, versus aspirin to 1300 mg per day in patients with 50–99% stenosis of a major intracranial artery showed no significant benefit for warfarin over aspirin (Chimowitz *et al.* 2005). In fact, warfarin was associated with a significantly increased rate of adverse events, including hemorrhage; as a result of this, the study was stopped prematurely. However, patients receiving warfarin were in the therapeutic range for only about 63% of the time. Therapeutic INR appeared to be associated with a much reduced incidence of ischemic stroke and cardiac events, suggesting that anticoagulation may provide increased benefit over aspirin if therapeutic INR can be maintained consistently.

Blood pressure and cholesterol lowering

There is good evidence from randomized trials to show that both blood pressure and cholesterol lowering are effective for secondary prevention of stroke. The Perindopril Protection Against Recurrent Stroke Study (PROGRESS) of perindopril and indapamide (PROGRESS Collaborative Group 2001) showed that blood pressure reduction with an angiotensin-converting enzyme inhibitor and diuretic starting several weeks or months after TIA or stroke reduces the risk of subsequent stroke by about a third. It is likely that this result can be generalized to most etiological subtypes of TIA and ischemic stroke, although many physicians are cautious about applying the PROGRESS results to patients with bilateral severe carotid stenosis or severe basilar or bilateral vertebral artery disease. Such patients may be at risk of border-zone infarction if their existing poor cerebral blood flow is further compromised by reduction in systemic blood pressure.

There is a positive association between cholesterol and risk of ischemic stroke. Cholesterol lowering with statins reduces the risk of stroke in patients with previous stroke, coronary or peripheral vascular disease or diabetes (MRC/BHF Heart Protection Study 2002). However, this Heart Protection Study (HPS) did not show a reduction in risk of recurrent stroke on statins (Collins *et al.* 2004), possibly because patients were at low risk of stroke recurrence since the incident strokes occurred on average 4.6 years before the study onset. However, the subsequent Stroke Prevention by Aggressive Reduction in Cholesterol Levels (SPARCL) trial of atorvastatin in patients who had had a stroke or TIA within one to six months before study entry showed a reduced overall stroke risk (Amarenco *et al.* 2006). However, there was a significant concomitant increase in risk of intracerebral hemorrhage on statin treatment. Interestingly, the same increase in risk of hemorrhagic stroke had been found in the HPS in the 3280 patients with previous stroke or TIA (Collins *et al.* 2004). Statins should not, therefore, be used in patients with previous intracerebral hemorrhage unless there is a strong indication related to the risk of ischemic events.

Secondary prevention after primary intracerebral hemorrhage

Much less is known about the long-term risk of recurrence after primary intracerebral hemorrhage than after ischemic stroke. In patients with primary intracerebral hemorrhage, approximately 25–50% of recurrent strokes are further hemorrhages, depending on the underlying disease process. The absolute risk also depends on the various underlying causes, such as arteriovenous malformation, cerebral amyloid angiopathy, poorly controlled hypertension or coagulopathy. Although patients with primary intracerebral hemorrhage are at increased risk of ischemic stroke as well as further hemorrhage, most clinicians do not recommend antiplatelet therapy unless there is a particularly high risk of coronary or other ischemic vascular events. In contrast, most patients with primary intracerebral hemorrhage require blood pressure-lowering medication, with the possible exception of those elderly patients with hemorrhages secondary to amyloid angiography in whom blood pressure is sometimes already rather low.

References

Algra A, Francke CL, Koehler PJJ (1997). A randomized trial of anticoagulants versus aspirin after cerebral ischaemia of presumed arterial origin. *Annals of Neurology* **42**:857–865

Amarenco P, Bogousslavsky J, Callahan A III et al. (2006). High-dose atorvastatin after stroke or transient ischemic attack. *New England Journal of Medicine* **355**:549–559

Antithrombotic Trialists' Collaboration (2002). Collaborative meta-analysis of randomized trials of antiplatelet therapy for prevention of death, myocardial infarction and stroke in high risk patients. *British Medical Journal* **342**:71–86

Bhatt DL, Flather MD, Hacke W et al. (2007). Patients with prior myocardial infarction, stroke, or symptomatic peripheral arterial disease in the CHARISMA trial. *Journal of the American College of Cardiologists* **49**:1982–1988

Canadian Cooperative Study Group (1978). A randomized trial of aspirin and sulfinpyrazone in threatened stroke. *New England Journal of Medicine* **299**:53–59

CAPRIE Steering Committee (1996). A randomised blinded trial of clopidogrel versus aspirin in patients at risk of ischaemic events (CAPRIE). *Lancet* **348**:1329–1339

Chimowitz MI, Kokkinos J, Strong J et al. (1995). The Warfarin–Aspirin Symptomatic Intracranial Disease Study. *Neurology* **45**:1488–1493

Chimowitz MI, Lynn MJ, Howlett-Smith H et al. (2005). Comparison of warfarin and aspirin for symptomatic intracranial arterial stenosis. *New England Journal of Medicine* **352**:1305–1316

Collins R, Armitage J, Parish S et al. (2004). Effects of cholesterol-lowering with simvastatin on stroke and other major vascular events in 20 536 people with cerebrovascular disease or other high-risk conditions. *Lancet* **363**:757–767

Diener HC, Cunha L, Forbes C et al. (1996). European Stroke Prevention Study. 2. Dipyridamole and acetylsalicylic acid in the secondary prevention of stroke. *Journal of the Neurological Sciences* **143**:1–13

Diener HC, Bogousslavsky J, Brass LM et al. (2004). Aspirin and clopidogrel compared with clopidogrel alone after recent ischaemic stroke or transient ischaemic attack in high-risk patients (MATCH): randomised double-blind placebo-controlled trial. *Lancet* **364**:331–337

European Atrial Fibrillation Trial Study Group (1993). Secondary prevention in non-rheumatic atrial fibrillation after transient ischaemic attack or minor stroke. *Lancet* **342**:1255–1262

European Atrial Fibrillation Trial Study Group (1995). Optimal oral anticoagulant therapy in patients with nonrheumatic atrial fibrillation and recent cerebral ischemia. *New England Journal of Medicine* **333**:5–10

Halkes PH, van Gijn J For the ESPRIT Study Group (2006). Aspirin plus dipyridamole versus aspirin alone after cerebral ischaemia of arterial origin (ESPRIT): randomised controlled trial. *Lancet* **367**:1665–73 [Erratum in *Lancet* (2007) **369**:274]

Mant J, Hobbs FD, Fletcher K et al. (2007) Midland Research Practices Network (MidReC). Warfarin versus aspirin for stroke prevention in an elderly community population with atrial fibrillation (the Birmingham Atrial Fibrillation Treatment of the Aged Study, BAFTA): a randomised controlled trial. *Lancet* **370**:493–503

MRC/BHF Heart Protection Study Collaborative Group (2002). Heart protection study of cholesterol lowering with simvastatin in 20 536 high-risk individuals: a randomised placebo-controlled trial. *Lancet* **360**:7–22

PROGRESS Collaborative Group (2001). Randomised trial of a perindopril-based blood-pressure-lowering regimen among 6,105 individuals with previous stroke or transient ischaemic attacks. *Lancet* **358**:1033–1041

Rash A, Downes T, Portner R et al. (2007). A randomised controlled trial of warfarin versus aspirin for stroke prevention in octogenarians with atrial fibrillation (WASPO). *Age Ageing* **36**:151–156

Redman AR, Allen LC (2002). Warfarin versus aspirin in the secondary prevention of stroke: the WARSS study. *Current Atherosclerosis Reports* **4**:319–325

Rothwell PM, Giles MF, Chandratheva A et al. (2007). Effect of urgent treatment of transient ischaemic attack and minor stroke on early recurrent stroke (EXPRESS study): a prospective population-based sequential comparison. *Lancet* **370**:1432–1442

Sivenius J, Riekkinen PJ, Smets P et al. (1991). The European Stroke Prevention Study (ESPS): results by arterial distribution. *Annals of Neurology* **29**:596–600

Chapter 25

Carotid endarterectomy

The surgical removal of atheromatous plaque from within the carotid artery is termed carotid endarterectomy. The operation was first performed in an attempt to improve the flow of blood to the brain, although no systematic attempt was made to assess the risks and benefits of the procedure. Subsequently, randomized trials were performed in patients with a history of recent symptomatic stroke, and also in those with asymptomatic disease, to determine whether the operation was beneficial and, if so, what the predictors of benefit would be. As a result of these trials, carotid endarterectomy has been proven to be an effective treatment for the secondary prevention of stroke in selected patients.

History

Knowledge of the relationship between atheromatous disease of the extracranial carotid and vertebral arteries and the occurrence of ischemic stroke goes back to the nineteenth century. In 1856, Virchow described carotid thrombosis in a patient with sudden-onset ipsilateral visual loss in whom the ophthalmic and retinal arteries were patent (Gurdjian 1979). In 1888, Penzoldt reported a patient who developed sudden permanent loss of vision in the right eye and later sustained a left hemiplegia (Penzoldt 1891). At autopsy, the patient was found to have thrombotic occlusion of the right distal common carotid artery and a large area of cerebral softening in the right cerebral hemisphere. In 1905, Chiari performed a number of pathological studies that led him to suggest that emboli could break away from ulcerated carotid plaques in the neck and cause cerebral infarction. This mechanism of stroke was re-emphasized 50 years later by Miller Fisher (1951, 1954).

Several operations were developed in the 1950s and 1960s in which the aim of surgery was to restore the flow of blood to the brain in patients with stenosis or occlusion of the extracranial carotid or vertebral circulations (Thompson 1996). One of the main contributions leading up to this was the development of cerebral arteriography by Egas Moniz in 1927 and the subsequent demonstration of stenosis and occlusion of the carotid arteries in life (Moniz *et al.* 1937). The subsequent development of extracranial/intracranial bypass surgery and carotid endarterectomy are described below. Several other surgical techniques have been tried, although unlike endarterectomy and extracranial/intracranial bypass they have not been tested in randomized controlled trials. These include various bypass procedures for occlusion of the proximal neck and aortic arch vessels; vertebral artery endarterectomy, reconstruction or bypass; and various arterial transpositions involving anastomosis of the subclavian and vertebral arteries into the common carotid artery. These procedures will not be discussed further here (see Ch. 26).

The first operations on the carotid artery were ligation procedures for trauma or hemorrhage. The first report was in Benjamin Bell's *Surgery* in 1793 (Wood 1857). However, most early ligations resulted in the death of the patient. The first successful ligation was performed by a British naval surgeon, David Fleming, in 1803 (Keevil 1949).

This operation was performed for late carotid rupture following neck trauma in an attempted suicide. The first successful ligation for carotid aneurysm was performed five years later in London by Astley Cooper (Cooper 1836). By 1868, Pilz was able to collect 600 recorded cases of carotid ligation for cervical aneurysm or hemorrhage, with an overall mortality of 43% (Hamby 1952). In 1878, an American surgeon named John Wyeth reported a 41% mortality in a collected study of 898 common carotid ligations, and contrasted this with a 4.5% mortality for ligation of the external carotid artery.

There were relatively few developments for the next 70 years. However, in 1946, a Portuguese surgeon, Cid Dos Santos, introduced thromboendarterectomy for restoration of flow in peripheral vessels (Dos Santos 1976). The first successful reconstruction of the carotid artery was performed by Carrea, Molins and Murphy in Buenos Aires in 1951 (Carrea et al. 1955). However, this was not an endarterectomy. Rather they performed an end-to-end anastomosis of the left external carotid artery and the distal internal carotid artery (ICA) in a man aged 41 years with a recently symptomatic severe carotid stenosis.

In 1954, Eastcott, Pickering and Rob published a case report detailing a carotid resection performed in May 1954 on a 66-year-old woman with recurrent left carotid TIAs and a severe stenosis on angiography. The patient made an uneventful recovery and was relieved of her TIAs. In 1975, DeBakey reported that he had performed a carotid endarterectomy on a 53-year-old man in August 1953, but it was the report by Eastcott and colleagues (1954) that provided the impetus for the further development of carotid surgery. Over the next five years, there were numerous other reports of the operation being performed, and several technical improvements were suggested (Thompson 1996). Occlusion of the ICA generally came to be regarded as inoperable and surgical attempts to correct carotid coils, kinks and fibromuscular dysplasia were not generally supported.

By the early 1980s there were over 100 000 procedures per year in the USA alone (Pokras and Dyken 1988; Gillum 1995; Tu et al. 1998). However, other than innumerable surgical case series and two small inconclusive randomized trials (Fields et al. 1970; Shaw et al. 1984), there was no good evidence that the operation was of any value. This prompted several eminent clinicians in the early 1980s to question the widespread use of the operation (Barnett et al. 1984; Chambers and Norris 1984; Warlow 1984; Jonas 1987; Winslow et al. 1988), which led to a fall in the number of operations being performed and set the scene for a number of large randomized controlled trials. The first results in patients with symptomatic stenosis began to appear in the early 1990s (European Carotid Surgery Trialists' Collaborative Group 1991; Mayberg et al. 1991; North American Symptomatic Carotid Endarterectomy Trial Collaborators 1991). Surgery clearly did prevent stroke in patients with recently symptomatic severe ICA stenosis.

The operation

The carotid bifurcation is exposed, mobilized and slings placed around the internal, external and common carotid arteries. After applying clamps to these arteries, away from any atheromatous plaque, the bifurcation is opened through a longitudinal incision, the entire stenotic lesion cored out, the distal intimal margin secured, the arteriotomy closed and the clamps released to restore blood flow to the brain. Most patients should already be taking antiplatelet drugs before surgery and these should be continued afterwards because the patients are still at high risk of ischemic stroke in the territory of other arteries, and of coronary events. In addition, most surgeons give patients heparin during the procedure itself. Controlling systemic blood pressure before, during and after surgery is crucial to avoid hypotension, which will make any cerebral ischemia worse, and hypertension, which may cause cerebral edema or even intracerebral hemorrhage. Operative damage to the nerve to the carotid sinus, or changes in the carotid sinus itself, may make control of post-operative blood pressure more of a problem, but in the long term has little if any effect (Eliasziw *et al.* 1998).

One particular variation, eversion endarterectomy, is becoming increasingly popular (Loftus and Quest 1987; Darling *et al.* 1996; Cao *et al.* 1998; Brothers 2005). A systematic review of five randomized controlled trials (2590 operations) compared eversion endarterectomy versus conventional endarterectomy performed either with primary closure or patch angioplasty (Cao *et al.* 2004). Overall, there was no significant difference in the rates of perioperative stroke, stroke or death, and local complication rates, but the absolute risks were rather low (risk of stroke or death was 1.7% with eversion and 2.6% with conventional endarterectomy).

Shunting

In theory, it should be possible to prevent low cerebral blood flow during carotid clamping, and possible ischemic stroke, by inserting a temporary intralumenal shunt from the common carotid artery to the ICA distal to the operation site. Some surgeons routinely shunt for this reason, and to allow more time to teach trainees, but there are problems, including arterial dissection and transmission of emboli from thrombus in the common carotid artery, as well as an increase in the duration of surgery and possibly in local operation site complications. A compromise is to use a shunt only in selected patients who are likely to develop, or who actually are experiencing cerebral ischemia as a result of low flow. However, efforts to identify the patients who need shunts have been inconclusive (Ferguson 1986; Ojemann and Heros 1986; Naylor *et al.* 1992; Belardi *et al.* 2003) and there is considerable variation in routine practice (Bond *et al.* 2002a). Unfortunately, randomized trials of different shunting policies have been too small and too few to provide reliable answers (Bond *et al.* 2002b). As a result, there is no standard policy for either operative monitoring or the use of shunts.

Restenosis and patch angioplasty

After carotid endarterectomy, the long-term risk of ischemic stroke ipsilateral to the operated artery is so low (Cunningham *et al.* 2002) that recurrent stenosis cannot be of any great clinical concern, in the sense of causing stroke. If stenosis does recur, then a second endarterectomy is more difficult and more risky (Bond *et al.* 2003a), and angioplasty or stenting may be preferable, although there is no randomized evidence for either procedure in symptomatic or asymptomatic restenosis (Yadav *et al.* 1996). In fact, the reported rate of restenosis varies enormously depending on whether the study was pro-spective or retrospective, the completeness and length of follow-up, the sensitivity and specificity of the imaging method used, and the definition of restenosis (Frericks *et al.* 1998). Certainly, recurrent atherothrombotic stenosis can occur, but usually not for some years, while early restenosis (within a year or so) is more likely to be caused by neointimal hyperplasia (Hunter *et al.* 1987). On balance, therefore, there is little point in repeated clinical or ultrasonographic follow-up to detect asymptomatic restenosis, but if a restenosis becomes symptomatic then a repeat carotid endarterectomy or stenting is reasonable.

Many surgeons routinely use a patch of autologous vein, or synthetic material, to close the artery, enlarge the lumen and so reduce the risk of restenosis and, more importantly, of stroke. Patching increases the surgery time and there are complications, including rupture to cause a life-threatening neck hematoma, and infection if synthetic grafts are used. A meta-analysis of randomized trials of primary closure, vein patch or synthetic patch included data on 1127 patients undergoing 1307 operations in several small trials (Bond *et al.* 2004a). Carotid patch angioplasty was associated with approximately a 60% reduction in the operative risks of stroke or death during the perioperative period ($p = 0.007$) and long-term follow-up ($p = 0.004$). Patching was also associated with an 85% reduction in risk of perioperative arterial occlusion ($p = 0.00004$), and an 80% reduction in risk of restenosis during long-term follow-up in five trials ($p < 0.00001$).

Some surgeons who use carotid patching favor using a patch made from an autologous vein, while others prefer to use synthetic materials. The most recent meta-analysis of randomized trials of different types of patch included data on 1480 operations (Bond *et al.* 2004b). During follow-up for more than one year, no difference was shown between the two types of patch for the risk of stroke, death or arterial restenosis. However, the number of events was small. Based on 15 events in 776 patients in four trials, there were significantly fewer pseudoaneurysms associated with synthetic patches than vein (odds ratio [OR], 0.09; 95% confidence interval [CI], 0.02–0.49) but the clinical significance of this finding is uncertain (Bond *et al.* 2004b). Overall, it is likely that the differences between different types of patch material are small.

General versus regional anesthesia

Surgery has traditionally been performed under general rather than regional anesthesia, but surgery under locoregional anesthesia is becoming more widespread. With regional anesthesia, there is a much lower shunt rate because it is immediately obvious when a shunt is needed to restore blood flow distal to the carotid clamps; elaborate intraoperative monitoring is unnecessary, and hospital stay may be shorter. However, some patients will not tolerate the procedure and a quick change to general anesthesia may be required. A detailed systematic review and meta-analysis of randomized and non-randomized studies has provided some useful information (Rerkasem *et al.* 2004). Seven randomized trials involving 554 operations, and 41 non-randomized studies involving 25 622 operations were included. Meta-analysis of the non-randomized studies showed that the use of local anesthetic was associated with significant reductions in the odds of death (35 studies), stroke (31 studies), stroke or death (26 studies), myocardial infarction (22 studies) and pulmonary complications (7 studies) within 30 days of the operation, but these non-randomized data are potentially unreliable. Meta-analysis of the fewer and generally small randomized studies showed that the use of local anesthetic was associated with a significant reduction in local hemorrhage (OR, 0.31; 95% CI, 0.12–0.79) within 30 days of the operation, but there was only a borderline statistically significant trend towards a reduced risk of operative death and no evidence of a reduction in risk of operative stroke. A large European multicenter randomized trial (General Anaesthetic versus Local Anaesthetic for Carotid Surgery [GALA]) has now randomized over 3000 patients and is expected to report its findings in 2008 (http://www.dcn.ed.ac.uk/gala).

The risks of carotid endarterectomy

Carotid endarterectomy is associated with a variety of potential complications (Naylor and Ruckley 1996; Bond *et al.* 2002c) (Box 25.1). The most important of these are stroke and death.

Box 25.1. Potential complications of carotid endarterectomy

Death
Perioperative stroke caused by:
- temporary interruption of carotid blood flow during clamping
- embolism from operative site

Postoperative stroke caused by:
- embolism from residual atheromatous plaque
- thrombus formation on the endarterectomized surface
- thrombus formation on the on suture lines
- thrombus formation from an arterial dissection

Cerebral hyperperfusion injury and cerebral hemorrhage
Cardiovascular complications (arrhythmia, myocardial infarction)
Respiratory complications (pulmonary embolism, pneumonia)
Cranial and peripheral nerve injuries
Bleeding or infection at wound site
Headache
Facial pain

Death

Death within a few days of surgery occurs in approximately 1–2% of patients and is generally caused by stroke, myocardial infarction or some other complication of the frequently associated coronary heart disease or, rarely, by pulmonary embolism (Rothwell *et al.* 1996a). Higher rates can be found in "administrative datasets" which may be a more realistic reflection of routine practice than large randomized trials, but any comparisons are confounded by variation in case mix, particularly the proportion of patients with asymptomatic stenosis, who have a lower case-fatality (Rothwell *et al.* 1996b; Wennberg *et al.* 1998; Bond *et al.* 2003a, b).

Stroke

The main complication of surgery is perioperative stroke (Naylor and Ruckley 1996; Ferguson *et al.* 1999; Bond *et al.* 2002c) (see Ch. 27 for further discussion). The reported risk ranges from an implausibly low 1% or less to an unacceptably high 20% or more (Bond *et al.* 2004c). This variation (Campbell 1993; Rothwell *et al.* 1996b) may be explained by differences in:

- the definition of stroke
- whether all or only some strokes are included
- the accuracy of stroke diagnosis
- the completeness of the clinical details
- whether the study was retrospective or prospective
- whether the diagnosis of stroke was based on patient observation or just medical record review
- variation in case mix, surgical and anesthetic skills
- chance variation
- publication bias.

No more than 20% of perioperative strokes are likely to be fatal, and so reports of less than four times as many non-fatal as fatal strokes suggest undercounting of mild strokes, a tendency which may well be a result of surgeons reporting their own results without the "help" of any neurologists (Rothwell and Warlow 1995). Despite the obvious implications for service planning, it has been all but impossible to sort out whether there really is a systematic difference in risk between surgeons. This is largely because of problems of adjusting for case mix, as well as chance effects owing to the inevitably rather small numbers operated on by each surgeon (Rothwell *et al.* 1999). One might anticipate that surgeons with a high number of cases might have lower operative risks than those with fewer cases (Kucey *et al.* 1998, Killeen *et al.* 2007), but the data are not conclusive.

There are several causes for perioperative stroke, but these are often difficult to identify when it occurs during general anesthesia, or even afterwards. It is difficult to be sure whether any stroke is caused by embolism or low flow (Steed *et al.* 1982; Krul *et al.* 1989; Riles *et al.* 1994; Spencer 1997). Clearly, temporary reduction in ICA blood flow during carotid clamping may cause ipsilateral ischemic stroke if the collateral supply is inadequate, particularly if there is already maximal cerebral vasodilatation (i.e. cerebrovascular reserve is exhausted). However, embolism from the operation site is probably the most common cause of stroke during surgery. Atherothrombotic debris may be released while the carotid bifurcation is being mobilized, as the carotid clamps are applied, when any shunt is inserted and when the clamps are removed. Indeed, air bubbles or particulate emboli during surgery are very commonly detected by transcranial Doppler ultrasound, although most seem to be of little clinical consequence (Gaunt *et al.* 1993; Jansen *et al.* 1994a).

Postoperative ischemic stroke is usually caused by embolism from residual but disrupted atheromatous plaque; thrombus forming on the endarterectomized surface or on suture lines, or more probably on a loose distal intimal flap where the lesion has been carelessly snapped off; thrombus complicating damaged arterial wall as a result of the clamps; and thrombus complicating arterial dissection starting at a loose intimal flap of the ICA or as a result of shunt damage to the arterial wall. A high rate of postoperative microembolic signals on transcranial Doppler monitoring may predict ischemic stroke (Levi *et al.* 1997).

Cerebral hemorrhage and hyperperfusion syndrome

Intracranial hemorrhage accounts for approximately 5% of perioperative strokes (Bond *et al.* 2002c; Wilson and Ammar 2005). It can occur during surgery or up to about 1 week later, almost always ipsilateral to the operated artery. It may be a result of the increase in perfusion pressure and cerebral blood flow that occurs after removal of a severe ICA stenosis, particularly if cerebral autoregulation is defective as a consequence of a recent cerebral infarct (Ouriel *et al.* 1999). Antithrombotic drugs and uncontrolled hypertension may also play a part (Solomon *et al.* 1986; Hafner *et al.* 1987; Piepgras *et al.* 1988; Jansen *et al.* 1994b; Wilson and Ammar 2005).

Transient cerebral hyperperfusion, ipsilateral but sometimes bilateral, lasting some days is quite common after carotid endarterectomy (Adhiyaman and Alexander 2007), particularly if the lesion is severely stenosing and cerebrovascular reserve is already poor with impaired autoregulation. This may be the cause of the occasional case of ipsilateral transhemispheric cerebral edema, intracerebral hemorrhage, focal epileptic seizures and headache, which can all occur a few days after surgery. Clearly, this syndrome is different from ischemic stroke caused by low flow or embolism, and it is distinguished by the slower onset, as well as by brain and arterial imaging (Andrews *et al.* 1987; Schroeder *et al.* 1987; Naylor *et al.* 1993a; Chambers *et al.* 1994; Breen *et al.* 1996; van Mook *et al.* 2005; Adhiyaman and Alexander 2007). To complicate matters, a very similar clinical syndrome has been described as a result of cerebral vasoconstriction (Lopez-Valdes *et al.* 1997).

Cardiovascular and respiratory complications

Myocardial infarction during, or in the early days after, surgery occurs in 1–2% of patients (Bond *et al.* 2002c), more often if there is symptomatic coronary heart disease, and particularly if myocardial infarction has occurred in the previous few months or if the patient has unstable angina. Perioperative myocardial infarction can be painless so clues to the diagnosis are unexplained hypotension, tachycardia and dysrhythmias. Congestive cardiac failure, angina and cardiac dysrhythmias are also occasional concerns (Riles *et al.* 1979; North American Symptomatic Carotid Endarterectomy Trial Collaborators 1991; Urbinati *et al.* 1994; Paciaroni *et al.* 1999; Bond *et al.* 2002c). Postoperative hypertension and hypotension may be a problem, perhaps owing to operative interference with the carotid baroreceptors, but it is transient. Postoperative chest infection occurs in less than 1%.

Cranial and peripheral nerve injuries

Nerve injuries result from traction, pressure or transection and occur in up to 20% of patients, depending on how hard one looks. However, these injuries seldom have any long-term consequence (Cunningham *et al.* 2004). Damage to the recurrent and superior laryngeal branches of the vagus nerve, or more probably the vagus itself, causes change of voice quality, hoarseness, difficulty coughing and sometimes dyspnea on exertion owing to vocal cord paralysis. If a simultaneous or staged bilateral carotid endarterectomy is done, and causes bilateral vocal cord paralysis, then airway obstruction can occur. Hypoglossal nerve injury causes ipsilateral weakness of the tongue, which can lead to temporary or even permanent dysarthria, difficulty with mastication or dysphagia. Again, bilateral damage causes much more serious speech and swallowing problems, and sometimes even upper airway obstruction. Therefore, if a patient has symptoms referable to both severely stenosed carotid arteries, requiring bilateral carotid endarterectomy, it is probably safer to do the operations a few weeks apart rather than under the same anesthetic, mostly because of the dangers of bilateral hypoglossal or vagal nerve damage.

Damage to the marginal mandibular branch of the facial nerve causes rather trivial weakness at the corner of the mouth. Spinal accessory nerve injury is rare and causes pain and stiffness in the shoulder and neck, along with weakness of the sternomastoid and trapezius muscles. A high incision can cut the greater auricular nerve to cause numbness over the ear lobe and angle of the jaw, which may persist and be irritating for the patient. Damage to the transverse cervical nerves is almost inevitable and causes numbness around the scar area, which is seldom a problem. Clearly, however, permanent disability from a nerve injury can be as bad as a mild stroke and needs to be taken into account when considering the risks and benefits of surgery (Gutrecht and Jones 1988; Maniglia and Han 1991; Sweeney & Wilbourn 1992; Cunningham *et al.* 2004).

Local wound complications

Local complications are rare and include infection; hematoma or, rarely, major hemor-rhage, from leakage or rupture of the arteriotomy or patch, which can be life threatening if it causes tracheal compression; aneurysm formation weeks or years later; and malignant tumor in the scar (Graver and Mulcare 1986; Martin-Negrier *et al.* 1996; Bond *et al.* 2002c). Although surgeons often notice the hemostatic defect caused by preoperative aspirin, this probably does not increase the rate of reoperation for bleeding (Lindblad *et al.* 1993). Very rarely, the thoracic duct can be damaged and cause a chyle fistula.

Headache and facial pain

Headache ipsilateral to the operation may herald cerebral hyperperfusion (van Mook *et al.* 2005; Adhiyaman and Alexander 2007), but it may also be due to something akin to cluster headache and caused by subtle damage to the sympathetic plexus around the carotid artery

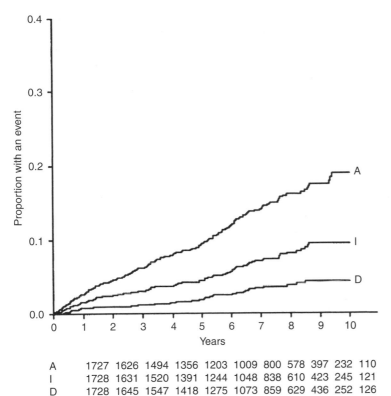

Fig. 25.1. Kaplan–Meier curves showing risks of stroke after carotid endarterectomy (excluding the 30-day immediate postoperative period). A, any stroke; I, any ipsilateral ischemic stroke; D, disabling ipsilateral ischemic stroke.

A	1727	1626	1494	1356	1203	1009	800	578	397	232	110
I	1728	1631	1520	1391	1244	1048	838	610	423	245	121
D	1728	1645	1547	1418	1275	1073	859	629	436	252	126

(De Marinis *et al.* 1991; Ille *et al.* 1995). Very rarely, focal epileptic seizures occur as well as headache (Youkey *et al.* 1984; Naylor *et al.* 2003). Facial pain ipsilateral to surgery and related to eating is unusual and may in some way be caused by disturbed innervation of the parotid gland (Truax 1989).

Potential benefits of carotid endarterectomy

As a result of the large randomized controlled trials, it is now clear that endarterectomy of recently symptomatic severe carotid stenosis almost completely abolishes the high risk of ischemic stroke ipsilateral to the operated artery over the subsequent two or three years (see Ch. 27 for detailed discussion of the selection of patients for surgery). Moreover, this effect is durable over at least 10 years (European Carotid Surgery Trialists' Collaborative Group 1991, 1998; Mayberg *et al.* 1991; North American Symptomatic Carotid Endarterectomy Trial Collaborators 1991; Barnett *et al.* 1998; Rothwell *et al.* 2003). Indeed, the ipsilateral stroke risk becomes so low that presumably both embolic and low-flow strokes are being prevented (Fig. 25.1).

On average, there is an advantage to surgery when the symptomatic stenosis exceeds 80% diameter reduction of the arterial lumen using the European Carotid Surgery Trial (ECST) method, which is about the same as 70% using the North American Symptomatic Carotid Endarterectomy Trial (NASCET) method (see Ch. 27). The risk of surgery is much the same at all degrees of stenosis and so, because the unoperated risk of stroke in patients with less than 60% stenosis (in ECST) is so low, the risk of surgery is not worthwhile for them. Because the risk of stroke in patients with moderate stenosis remains low for several years, there is no point in duplex follow-up to see if the stenosis becomes more severe. No doubt severe stenosis does sometimes develop, but, unless there are further symptoms, the stenosis by this time is essentially asymptomatic and carries such a low risk of stroke that there is no overall advantage for surgery. It is preferable to ask the patient to return if there are any further cerebrovascular symptoms and *then*, if the stenosis is 80% (ECST) or more, it is reasonable to recommend carotid endarterectomy.

Carotid endarterectomy may also improve cognitive performance, perhaps by increasing cerebral blood flow or by reducing the frequency of subclinical emboli, which declines after surgery (Markus *et al.* 1995; van Zuilen *et al.* 1995). However, subtle cognitive difficulties may complicate the procedure itself (Lloyd *et al.* 2004; Bossema *et al.* 2005; Lal 2007), and there is some evidence that previous carotid endarterectomy is associated with more rapid cognitive decline in the longer term (Bo *et al.* 2006). Unfortunately, studies addressing this issue have been beset with methodological difficulties (Lunn *et al.* 1999) and it is difficult to imagine that this balance of cognitive benefit and risk will ever be resolved because further randomized trials will probably never be done, at least not in patients with symptomatic stenosis.

It is conceivable that patients with impaired cerebral reactivity and raised oxygen extraction fraction are at particular risk of stroke without surgery, and that this impairment can be corrected by carotid endarterectomy, but the studies have been too small to be sure (Schroeder 1988; Naylor *et al.* 1993b; Yonas *et al.* 1993; Hartl *et al.* 1994; Yamauchi *et al.* 1996; Visser *et al.* 1997; Silvestrini *et al.* 2000; Markus and Cullinane 2001). Also, we do not know what proportion of strokes in patients with recently symptomatic severe carotid stenosis are actually caused by impaired cerebral reactivity, either as a direct result of low flow or perhaps indirectly as a result of an inadequate collateral circulation to compensate for acute arterial occlusion if it should occur. Nor do we know whether the risk of surgery is higher in these patients and so whether, on balance, carotid endarterectomy will indeed reduce stroke risk any more than in those without impaired reactivity.

References

Adhiyaman V, Alexander S (2007). Cerebral hyperperfusion syndrome following carotid endarterectomy. *Quarterly Journal of Medicine* 100:239–244

Andrews BT, Levy ML, Dillon W *et al.* (1987). Unilateral normal perfusion pressure breakthrough after carotid endarterectomy: case report. *Neurosurgery* 21:568–571

Barnett HJM, Plum F, Walton JN (1984). Carotid endarterectomy: an expression of concern. *Stroke* 15:941–943

Barnett HJM, Taylor DW, Eliasziw M for the North American Symptomatic Carotid Endarterectomy Trial Collaborators (1998). Benefit of carotid endarterectomy in patients with symptomatic moderate or severe stenosis. *New England Journal of Medicine* 339:1415–1425

Belardi P, Lucertini G, Ermirio D (2003). Stump pressure and transcranial Doppler for predicting shunting in carotid endarterectomy. *European Journal of Vascular Endovascular Surgery* 25:164–167

Bo M, Massaia M, Speme S *et al.* (2006). Risk of cognitive decline in older patients after carotid endarterectomy: an observational study. *Journal of the American Geriatric Society* 54:932–936

Bond R, Warlow CP, Naylor R *et al.* (2002a). Variation in surgical and anaesthetic technique and associations with operative risk in the European Carotid Surgery Trial: implications for trials of ancillary techniques. *European Journal of Vascular Endovascular Surgery* 23:117–126

Bond R, Rerkasem K, Rothwell PM (2002b). Routine or selective carotid artery shunting for carotid endarterectomy. *Cochrane Database of Systematic Reviews* 2:CD000190

Bond R, Narayan S, Rothwell PM *et al.* (2002c). Clinical and radiological risk factors for operative stroke and death in the European Carotid Surgery Trial. *European Journal of Vascular Endovascular Surgery* 23:108–116

Bond R, Rerkasem K, Rothwell PM (2003a). A systematic review of the risks of carotid endarterectomy in relation to the clinical indication and the timing of surgery. *Stroke* 34:2290–2301

Bond R, Rerkasem K, Rothwell PM (2003b). High morbidity due to endarterectomy for asymptomatic carotid stenosis. *Cerebrovascular Diseases* 16(Suppl 4):65

Bond R, Rerkasem K, Rothwell PM (2004a). Patch angioplasty versus primary closure for carotid endarterectomy. *Cochrane Database of Systemic Reviews* 2:CD000160

Bond R, Rerkasem K, Naylor R *et al.* (2004b). Patches of different types for carotid patch angioplasty. *Cochrane Database of Systemic Reviews* 2:CD000071

Bond R, Rerkasem K, Shearman CP *et al.* (2004c). Time trends in the published risks of stroke and death due to endarterectomy for symptomatic carotid stenosis. *Cerebrovascular Diseases* 18:37–46

Bossema ER, Brand N, Moll FL *et al.* (2005). Perioperative microembolism is not associated with cognitive outcome three months after carotid endarterectomy. *European Journal of Vascular Endovascular Surgery* 29:262–268

Breen JC, Caplan LR, Dewitt LD *et al.* (1996). Brain oedema after carotid surgery. *Neurology* 46:175–181

Brothers TE (2005). Initial experience with eversion carotid endarterectomy: absence of a learning curve for the first 100 patients. *Journal of Vascular Surgery* 42:429–434

Campbell WB (1993). Can reported carotid surgical results be misleading?. In *Surgery for Stroke* Greenhalgh GM and Hollier LH (eds.), pp. 331–337. London: Saunders

Cao P, Giordano G, De Rango P for the Collaborators of the EVEREST Study Group (1998). A randomised study on eversion versus standard carotid endarterectomy: study design and preliminary results: the Everest Trial. *Journal of Vascular Surgery* 27:595–605

Cao PG, De Rango P, Zannetti S *et al.* (2004). Eversion versus conventional carotid endarterectomy for preventing stroke. *Cochrane Database of Systematic Reviews*, 2:CD001921

Carrea R, Molins M, Murphy G (1955). Surgical treatment of spontaneous thrombosis of the internal carotid artery in the neck. Carotid–carotideal anastomosis. Report of a case. *Acta Neurologica Latin America* 1:71–78

Chambers BR, Norris J (1984). The case against surgery for asymptomatic carotid stenosis. *Stroke* 15:964–967

Chambers BR, Smidt V, Koh P (1994). Hyperfusion post-endarterectomy. *Cerebrovascular Diseases* 4:32–37

Chiari H (1905). Uber des verhalten des teilungswinkels der carotis communis bei der endarteritis chronica deformans. *Verhandlungen der Deutschen Gesellschaft für Pathologie* 9:326–330

Cooper A (1836). Account of the first successful operation performed on the common carotid artery for aneurysm in the year 1808 with the post-mortem examination in the year 1821. *Guy's Hospital Report* 1:53–59

Cunningham E, Bond R, Mehta Z *et al.* (2002). Long-term durability of carotid endarterectomy in the European Carotid Surgery Trial. *Stroke* 33:2658–2663

Cunningham EJ, Bond R, Mayberg MR *et al.* (2004). Risk of persistent cranial nerve injury after carotid endarterectomy. *Journal of Neurosurgery* 101:455–458

Darling RC, Paty PSK, Shah DM *et al.* (1996). Eversion endarterectomy of the internal carotid artery: technique and results in 449 procedures. *Surgery* 120:635–639

DeBakey ME (1975). Successful carotid endarterectomy for cerebrovascular insufficiency. Nineteen-year follow-up. *Journal of the American Medical Association* 233:1083–1085

De Marinis M, Zaccaria A, Faraglia V *et al.* (1991). Post-endarterectomy headache and the role of the oculosympathetic system. *Journal of Neurology, Neurosurgery and Psychiatry* 54:314–317

Dos Santos JC (1976). From embolectomy to endarterectomy or the fall of a myth. *Journal of Cardiovascular Surgery* 17:113–128

Eastcott HHG, Pickering GW, Rob CG (1954). Reconstruction of internal carotid artery in a patient with intermittent attacks of hemiplegia. *Lancet* **ii**, 994–996

Eliasziw M, Spence JD, Barnett HM for the North American Symptomatic Carotid Endarterectomy Trial (1998). Carotid endarterectomy does not affect long term blood pressure: observations from the NASCET. *Cerebrovascular Diseases* 8:20–24

European Carotid Surgery Trialists' Collaborative Group (1991). MRC European Carotid Surgery Trial: interim results for symptomatic patients with severe (70–99%) or with mild (0–29%) carotid stenosis. *Lancet* 337:1235–1243

European Carotid Surgery Trialists' Collaborative Group (1998). Randomised trial of endarterectomy for recently symptomatic carotid stenosis: final results of the MRC European Carotid Surgery Trial (ECST). *Lancet* 351:1379–1387

Ferguson GG (1986). Carotid endarterectomy. To shunt or not to shunt? *Archives of Neurology* 43:615–618

Ferguson GG, Eliasziw M, Barr HWK for the North American Symptomatic Carotid Endarterectomy Trial (NASCET) Collaborators (1999). The North American Symptomatic Carotid Endarterectomy Trial: surgical results in 1415 patients. *Stroke* **30**:1751–1758

Fields WS, Maslenikov V, Meyer JS *et al.* (1970). Joint study of extracranial arterial occlusion. V. Progress report of prognosis following surgery or nonsurgical treatment for transient cerebral ischaemic attacks and cervical carotid artery lesions. *Journal of the American Medical Association* **211**:1993–2003

Fisher M (1951). Occlusion of the internal carotid artery. *Archives of Neurology and Psychiatry* **65**:346–377

Fisher M (1954). Occlusion of the carotid arteries. *Archives of Neurology and Psychiatry* **72**:187–204

Frericks H, Kievit J, van Baalen JM *et al.* (1998). Carotid recurrent stenosis and risk of ipsilateral stroke: a systematic review of the literature. *Stroke* 29:244–250

Gaunt ME, Naylor AR, Sayers RD *et al.* (1993). Sources of air embolisation during carotid surgery: the role of transcranial Doppler ultrasonography. *British Journal of Surgery* **80**:1121

Gillum RF (1995). Epidemiology of carotid endarterectomy and cerebral arteriography in the United States. *Stroke* 26:1724–1728

Graver LM, Mulcare RJ (1986). Pseudoaneurysm after carotid endarterectomy. *Journal of Cardiovascular Surgery* 27:294–297

Gurdjian ES (1979). History of occlusive cerebrovascular disease, I: from Wepfer to Moniz. *Archives of Neurology* 36:340–343

Gutrecht JA, Jones HR (1988). Bilateral hypoglossal nerve injury after bilateral carotid endarterectomy. *Stroke* 19:261–262

Hafner DH, Smith RB, King OW *et al.* (1987). Massive intracerebral haemorrhage following carotid endarterectomy. *Archives of Surgery* **122**:305–307

Hamby WB (1952). *Intracranial Aneurysms.* Springfield, IL: Charles C Thomas

Hartl WH, Janssen I, Furst H (1994). Effect of carotid endarterectomy on patterns of cerebrovascular reactivity in patients with unilateral carotid artery stenosis. *Stroke* **25**:1952–1957

Hunter GC, Palmaz JC, Hayashi HH *et al.* (1987). The aetiology of symptoms in patients with recurrent carotid stenosis. *Archives of Surgery* **122**:311–315

Ille O, Woimant F, Pruna A *et al.* (1995). Hypertensive encephalopathy after bilateral carotid endarterectomy. *Stroke* **26**:488–491

Jansen C, Ramos LMP, van Heesewijk JPM *et al.* (1994a). Impact of microembolism and hemodynamic changes in the brain during carotid endarterectomy. *Stroke* **25**:992–997

Jansen C, Sprengers AM, Moll FL *et al.* (1994b). Prediction of intracerebral haemorrhage after carotid endarterectomy by clinical criteria and intraoperative transcranial Doppler monitoring. *European Journal of Vascular Surgery* 8:303–308

Jonas S (1987). Can carotid endarterectomy be justified? No. *Archives of Neurology* 44:652–654

Keevil JJ (1949). David Fleming and the operation for ligation of the carotid artery. *British Journal of Surgery* 37:92–95

Killeen SD, Andrews EJ, Redmond HP *et al.* (2007). Provider volume and outcomes for abdominal aortic aneurysm repair, carotid endarterectomy, and lower extremity revascularization procedures. *Journal of Vascular Surgery* **45**:615–626

Krul JMJ, van Gijn J, Ackerstaff RGA *et al.* (1989). Site and pathogenesis of infarcts associated with carotid endarterectomy. *Stroke* **20**:324–328

Kucey DS, Bowyer B, Iron K *et al.* (1998). Determinants of outcome after carotid endarterectomy. *Journal of Vascular Surgery* **28**:1051–1058

Lal BK. (2007). Cognitive function after carotid artery revascularization. *Vascular and Endovascular Surgery* **41**:5–13

Levi CR, O'Malley HM, Fell G *et al.* (1997). Transcranial Doppler detected cerebral microembolism following carotid endarterectomy. High microembolic signal loads predict postoperative cerebral ischaemia. *Brain* **120**:621–629

Lindblad B, Persson NH, Takolander R *et al.* (1993). Does low-dose acetylsalicylic acid prevent stroke after carotid surgery? A double-blind, placebo-controlled randomised trial. *Stroke* **24**:1125–1128

Lloyd AJ, Hayes PD, London NJ *et al.* (2004). Does carotid endarterectomy lead to a decline in cognitive function or health related quality of life? *Journal of Clinical and Experimental Neuropsychology* **26**:817–825

Loftus CM, Quest DO (1987). Technical controversies in carotid artery surgery. *Neurosurgery* **20**:490–495

Lopez-Valdes E, Chang HM, Pessin MS *et al.* (1997). Cerebral vasoconstriction after carotid surgery. *Neurology* **49**:303–304

Lunn S, Crawley F, Harrison MJG *et al.* (1999). Impact of carotid endarterectomy upon cognitive functioning. A systematic review of the literature. *Cerebrovascular Diseases* **9**:74–81

Maniglia AJ, Han DP (1991). Cranial nerve injuries following carotid endarterectomy: an analysis of 336 procedures. *Head and Neck* **13**:121–124

Markus H, Cullinane M (2001). Severely impaired cerebrovascular reactivity predicts stroke and TIA risk in patients with carotid artery stenosis and occlusion. *Brain* **124**:457–467

Markus HS, Thomson ND, Brown MM (1995). Asymptomatic cerebral embolic signals in symptomatic and asymptomatic carotid artery disease. *Brain* **118**:1005–1011

Martin-Negrier ML, Belleannee G, Vital C *et al.* (1996) Primitive malignant fibrous histiocytoma of the neck with carotid occlusion and multiple cerebral ischemic lesions. *Stroke* **27**:536–537

Mayberg MR, Wilson E, Yatsu F for the Veterans Affairs Cooperative Studies Programe 309 Trialist Group (1991). Carotid endarterectomy and prevention of cerebral ischaemia in symptomatic carotid stenosis. *Journal of the American Medical Association* **266**:3289–3294

Moniz E (1927). L'encephalographic arterielle: son importance dans la localisation des tumeurs cerebrales. *Revue de Neurologie* **2**:72–90

Moniz E, Lima A, de Lacerda R (1937). Hemiplegies par thrombose de la carotide interne. *Presse Medecine* **45**:977–980

Naylor AR, Ruckley CV (1996). Complications after carotid surgery. In *Complications in Arterial Surgery. A Practical Approach to Management*, Campbell (ed.), pp. 73–88. Oxford: Butterworth-Heinemann

Naylor AR, Bell PRF, Ruckley CV (1992). Monitoring and cerebral protection during carotid endarterectomy. *British Journal of Surgery* **79**:735–741

Naylor AR, Merrick MV, Sandercock PAG *et al.* (1993a). Serial imaging of the carotid bifurcation and cerebrovascular reserve after carotid endarterectomy. *British Journal of Surgery* **80**:1278–1282

Naylor AR, Whyman MR, Wildsmith JAW *et al.* (1993b). Factors influencing the hyperaemic response after carotid endarterectomy. *British Journal of Surgery* **80**:1523–1527

Naylor AR, Evans J, Thompson MM *et al.* (2003). Seizures after carotid endarterectomy: hyperperfusion, dysautoregulation or hypertensive encephalopathy? *European Journal of Vascular Endovascular Surgery* **26**:39–44

North American Symptomatic Carotid Endarterectomy Trial Collaborators (1991). Beneficial effect of carotid endarterectomy in symptomatic patients with high-grade carotid stenosis. *New England Journal of Medicine* **325**:445–453

Ojemann RG, Heros RC (1986). Carotid endarterectomy. To shunt or not to shunt? *Archives of Neurology* **43**:617–618

Ouriel K, Shortell CK, Illig KA et al. (1999). Intracerebral haemorrhage after carotid endarterectomy: incidence, contribution to neurologic morbidity, and predictive factors. *Journal of Vascular Surgery* 29:82–89

Paciaroni M, Eliasziw M, Kappelle LJ for the North American Symptomatic Carotid Endarterectomy Trial (NASCET) Collaborators (1999). Medical complications associated with carotid endarterectomy. *Stroke* 30:1759–1763

Penzoldt F (1891). Uber thrombose (autochtone oder embolische) der carotis. *Deutschen Archir Für Klinische Medizin* 28:80–93

Piepgras DG, Morgan MK, Sundt TM et al. (1988). Intracerebral haemorrhage after carotid endarterectomy. *Journal of Neurosurgery* 68:532–536

Pokras R, Dyken ML (1988). Dramatic changes in the performance of endarterectomy for diseases of the extracranial arteries of the head. *Stroke* 19:1289–1290

Rerkasem K, Bond R, Rothwell PM (2004). Local versus general anaesthetic for carotid endarterectomy. *Cochrane Database Systemic Reviews* 2:CD000126

Riles TS, Kopelman I, Imparato AM (1979). Myocardial infarction following carotid endarterectomy. A review of 683 operations. *Surgery* 85:249–252

Riles TS, Imparato AM, Jacobowitz GR et al. (1994). The cause of perioperative stroke after carotid endarterectomy. *Journal of Vascular Surgery* 19:206–216

Rothwell PM, Warlow CP (1995). Is self-audit reliable? *Lancet* 346:1623

Rothwell PM, Slattery J, Warlow CP (1996a). A systematic comparison of the risk of stroke and death due to carotid endarterectomy for symptomatic and asymptomatic stenosis. *Stroke* 27:266–269

Rothwell PM, Slattery J, Warlow CP (1996b). A systematic review of the risk of stroke and death due to carotid endarterectomy. *Stroke* 27:260–265

Rothwell PM, Warlow CP on behalf of the European Carotid Surgery Trialists' Collaborative Group (1999). Interpretation of operative risks of individual surgeons. *Lancet* 353:1325

Rothwell PM, Gutnikov SA, Warlow CP for the ECST (2003). Re-analysis of the final results of the European Carotid Surgery Trial. *Stroke* 34:514–523

Schroeder T (1988). Hemodynamic significance of internal carotid artery disease. *Acta Neurologica Scandinavica* 77:353–372

Schroeder T, Sillesen H, Sorensen O et al. (1987). Cerebral hyperfusion following carotid endarterectomy. *Journal of Neurosurgery* 66:824–829

Shaw DA, Venables GS, Cartlidge NEF et al. (1984). Carotid endarterectomy in patients with transient cerebral ischaemia. *Journal of Neurological Sciences* 64:45–53

Silvestrini M, Vernieri F, Pasqualetti P et al. (2000). Impaired cerebral vasoreactivity and risk of stroke in patients with asymptomatic carotid artery stenosis. *Journal of American Medical Association* 283:2122–2127

Solomon RA, Loftus CM, Quest DO et al. (1986). Incidence and etiology of intracerebral haemorrhage following carotid endarterectomy. *Journal of Neurosurgery* 64:29–34

Spencer MP (1997). Transcranial Doppler monitoring and causes of stroke from carotid endarterectomy. *Stroke* 28:685–691

Steed DL, Peitzman AB, Grundy BL et al. (1982). Causes of stroke in carotid endarterectomy. *Surgery* 92:634–639

Sweeney PJ Wilbourn AJ (1992). Spinal accessory (11th) nerve palsy following carotid endarterectomy. *Neurology* 42:674–675

Thompson JE (1996). The evolution of surgery for the treatment and prevention of stroke. The Willis Lecture. *Stroke* 27:1427–1434

Truax BT (1989). Gustatory pain: a complication of carotid endarterectomy. *Neurology* 39:1258–1260

Tu JV, Hannan EL, Anderson GM et al. (1998). The fall and rise of carotid endarterectomy in the United States and Canada. *New England Journal of Medicine* 339:1441–1447

Urbinati S, di Pasquale G, Andreoli A et al. (1994). Preoperative noninvasive coronary risk stratification in candidates for carotid endarterectomy. *Stroke* 25:2022–2027

van Mook WN, Rennenberg RJ, Schurink GW et al. (2005). Cerebral hyperperfusion syndrome. *Lancet Neurology* 4:877–888

van Zuilen EV, Moll FL, Vermeulen FEE et al. (1995). Detection of cerebral microemboli by means of transcranial Doppler monitoring before and after carotid endarterectomy. *Stroke* **26**:210–213

Visser GH, van Huffelen AC, Wieneke GH *et al.* (1997). Bilateral increase in CO reactivity after unilateral carotid endarterectomy. *Stroke* **28**:899–905

Warlow CP (1984). Carotid endarterectomy: does it work? *Stroke* **15**:1068–1076

Wennberg DE, Lucas FL, Birkmeyer JD *et al.* (1998). Variation in carotid endarterectomy mortality in the Medicare population: trial hospitals, volume, and patient characteristics. *Journal of the American Medical Association* **279**:1278–1281

Wilson PV, Ammar AD (2005). The incidence of ischemic stroke versus intracerebral hemorrhage after carotid endarterectomy: a review of 2452 cases. *Annals of Vascular Surgery* **19**:1–4

Winslow CM, Solomon DH, Chassin MR (1988). The appropriateness of carotid endarterectomy. *New England Journal of Medicine* **318**:721–727

Wood JR (1857). Early history of the operation of ligature of the primitive carotid artery. *New York Journal of Medicine* July:1–59

Wyeth JA (1878). Prize essay: essays upon the surgical anatomy and history of the common, external and internal carotid arteries and the surgical anatomy of the innominate and subclavian arteries. *Appendix to Transactions of the American Medical Association (AMA) Philadelphia* **29**:1–245

Yadav JS, Roubin GS, King P *et al.* (1996). Angioplasty and stenting for restenosis after carotid endarterectomy. Initial experience. *Stroke* **27**:2075–2079

Yamauchi H, Fukuyama H, Nagahama Y *et al.* (1996). Evidence of misery perfusion and risk of recurrent stroke in major cerebral arterial occlusive diseases from PET. *Journal of Neurology, Neurosurgery and Psychiatry* **61**:18–25

Yonas H, Smith HA, Durham SR *et al.* (1993). Increased stroke risk predicted by compromised cerebral blood flow reactivity. *Journal of Neurosurgery* **79**:483–489

Youkey JR, Clagett GP, Jaffin JH *et al.* (1984). Focal motor seizures complicating carotid endarterectomy. *Archives of Surgery* **119**:1080–1084

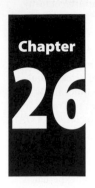

Carotid stenting and other interventions

Endovascular treatment was first used in the limbs in the 1960s and subsequently in the renal and coronary arteries (Dotter *et al*. 1967), but it was introduced more cautiously for treatment of stenosis of the cerebral, carotid and vertebral arteries because of the perception of a likely high procedural risk of stroke.

Carotid stenting

If endarterectomy of a recently symptomatic severe carotid stenosis largely abolishes the risk of ipsilateral ischemic stroke (see Chs. 25 and 27), then percutaneous translumenal balloon angioplasty, particularly with stenting to maintain arterial patency, might be expected to be similarly effective (Mathur *et al*. 1998) (Fig. 26.1 and Table 26.1). The endovascular approach is now widely used when carotid pathology makes endarterectomy difficult (e.g. high bifurcation or postradiation stenosis), although it is not always feasible because of contrast allergy, difficult vascular anatomy or lumen thrombus.

Angioplasty and stenting is usually less unpleasant and less invasive than carotid endarterectomy, and it is generally more convenient and quicker. As it is carried out under local anesthetic, there may be less perioperative hypertension, although cerebral hemorrhage and hyperperfusion have been reported (McCabe *et al*. 1999; Qureshi *et al*. 1999). It is less likely to cause nerve injuries, wound infection, venous thromboembolism or myocardial infarction, and hospital stay may be shorter. However, there are also some potential disadvantages of stenting. The angioplasty balloon may dislodge atherothrombotic debris, which then embolizes to the brain or eye, although use of protection devices might help to reduce the risk of stroke from periprocedural embolization (Reimers *et al*. 2001). The procedure may cause arterial wall dissection at the time or afterwards, and late embolization might occur from thrombus formation on the damaged plaque. The angioplasty balloon may obstruct carotid blood flow for long enough to cause low-flow ischemic stroke, and dilatation of the balloon may cause bradycardia or hypotension through carotid sinus stimulation, or aneurysm formation and even arterial rupture if the arterial wall is over-distended. Hematoma and aneurysm formation may also occur at the site of arterial cannulation in the groin. Rarely, the stent may erode through the arterial wall or fracture. In the longer term, restenosis might be more problematic after stenting than after endarterectomy.

Data on the complication rates of carotid angioplasty/stenting are available from published case series and registries but, as was demonstrated for endarterectomy (see Chs. 25 and 27), such studies tend to underestimate risks. Formal randomized comparisons of endarterectomy and angioplasty/stenting are, therefore, required for reliable determination of the overall balance of risks and benefits. Prior to 2006, only five relatively small randomized controlled trials (1269 patients) had been reported (Naylor *et al*. 1998; Alberts 2001; Brooks *et al*. 2001; CAVATAS Investigators 2001; Yadav *et al*. 2004). The largest of

Table 26.1. Potential advantages and disadvantages of carotid stenting compared with carotid endarterectomy

Advantages	Disadvantages
Faster, less-invasive procedure	Increased risk of embolization of debris from atherothrombotic plaque
Procedure carried out under local anesthetic with consequent better neurological monitoring and reduced anesthetic complications	Risk of arterial wall dissection
Reduced procedural blood pressure variability	Carotid sinus stimulation
Reduced local wound complications	Local groin injury at arterial cannulation site
Reduced local nerve damage	(Inferior long-term evidence base)
Reduced length of stay in hospital	

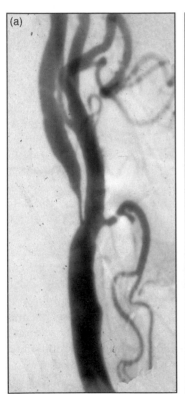 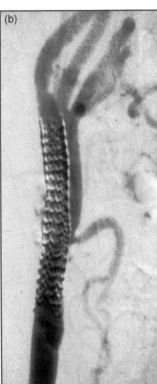

(a) (b)

Fig. 26.1. Carotid stenosis before (a) and after (b) carotid angioplasty and stenting.

these trials suggested that the procedural stroke complication rate of angioplasty and stenting was similar to that of carotid endarterectomy (albeit with wide confidence intervals [CI]) and that there are few strokes in the long term (with even wider CI values) (CAVA-TAS Investigators 2001). Taken together, the five trials suggested that angioplasty/stenting might have a higher procedural risk of stroke and death than endarterectomy (odds ratio [OR], 1.33; 95% CI, 0.86–2.04) and a higher rate of restenosis (Coward *et al.* 2005).

However, improvements in endovascular techniques and cerebral protection might have reduced the procedural risks (Reimers *et al.* 2001), and so several larger trials were initiated, two of which reported initial results in 2006. The Stent-supported Percutaneous Angioplasty of the Carotid Artery versus Endarterectomy (SPACE) trial (SPACE Collaborative Group 2006) is the largest trial of carotid stenting versus endarterectomy to date, doubling the number of randomized patients. It was intended that 1900 patients with 50–99% recently symptomatic carotid stenosis (as assessed by the North American Symptomatic Carotid Endarterectomy Trial [NASCET] method) be recruited based on a non-inferiority design, but randomization was stopped at 1200 patients, partly through a shortage of funding. The procedural 30-day risk of stroke and death was non-significantly higher in the angioplasty/stenting group (OR, 1.1; 95% CI, 0.7–1.7; $p = 0.09$), with 37 (6.3%) strokes and deaths among 584 patients (6.3%) randomized to surgery versus 41 (6.8%) in 599 patients randomized to stenting, and a similar trend for disabling ipsilateral stroke (4.01% versus 2.91%).

The Endarterectomy versus Angioplasty in Patients With Symptomatic Severe Carotid Stenosis (EVA-3S) trial also reported initial results in 2006 (Mas *et al.* 2006). This was a randomized controlled trial of angioplasty/stenting versus endarterectomy for 60–99% recently symptomatic carotid stenosis (NASCET method). The trial stopped early after a higher 30-day procedural risk of stroke and death was found after angioplasty/stenting at a planned interim analysis with 527 randomized patients: 9.6% versus 3.9%, respectively (relative risk, 2.5; 95% CI, 1.2–5.1; $p = 0.01$). There were also more local complications after angioplasty/stenting.

In both of these recent trials, participating clinicians had to demonstrate competence and a good safety record prior to joining, with a quarter of potential centers rejected by SPACE, and there was no evidence that more experienced interventionists had a lower procedural risk than average. The results of further follow-up are awaited and other large trials are currently ongoing (Featherstone *et al.* 2004; Hobson *et al.* 2004; CARESS Steering Committee 2005, Carotid Revascularization Endarterectomy versus Stenting Trial (CREST) 2006). Another important issue that is currently being addressed in a large randomized controlled trial (www.galatrial.com) is whether endarterectomy might have a lower operative risk with local versus general anesthetic, for which there is some evidence (Rerkasem *et al.* 2004). Any advantage for local anesthetic would have implications for comparisons with stenting since existing RCTs have mainly compared with endarterectomy under general anesthetic.

Taking all the currently available randomized evidence from trials comparing carotid endarterectomy and stenting, stenting appears to be associated with a higher procedural risk of stroke and death, but there is still sufficient uncertainty to justify continuation of ongoing trials. Pending the results of these trials, carotid stenting should be confined to RCTs or to patients for whom endarterectomy is technically difficult. Whichever intervention is used, early intervention and selection of patients based on predicted risk of stroke without intervention remain the keys to effective stroke prevention.

Surgery, angioplasty and stenting for vertebrobasilar ischemia

There is no good evidence (i.e. there are no large randomized trials) (Coward *et al.* 2005) that surgery improves the prognosis for patients with vertebrobasilar ischemia. There is, however, no shortage of ingenious, if technically demanding, techniques, which are far from risk free (Box 26.1).

There are no randomized trials of surgical procedures for posterior circulation disease and, therefore, data are only available from case series. For proximal vertebral reconstruction, perioperative mortality in published case series is 0–4%, with rates of stroke and death

Box 26.1. Interventional procedures for vertebrobasilar ischemia

Endarterectomy of severe carotid stenosis to improve collateral blood flow, via the circle of
  Willis, to the basilar artery distal to vertebral or basilar artery stenosis or occlusion
Resection and anastomosis
Resection and reimplantation
Bypass or endarterectomy of proximal vertebral artery stenosis
Release of the vertebral artery from compressive fibrous bands or osteophytes
Extracranial-to-intracranial procedures to bypass vertebral artery stenosis or occlusion
Angioplasty and stenting of the vertebral and basilar arteries
Sources: From Diaz et al. (1984), Harward et al. (1984), Thevenet and Ruotolo (1984), Hopkins et al.
(1987), Spetzler et al. (1987), Terada et al. (1996), and Malek et al. (1999).

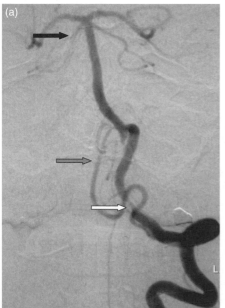 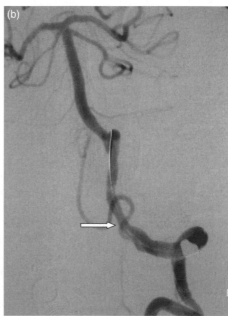

Fig. 26.2. (a) Cerebral angiogram showing proximal left vertebral stenosis (white arrow) with hypoplastic right vertebral artery (grey arrow) and poorly perfused posterior circulation owing to absence of posterior communicating arteries (black arrow). (b) Repeat angiogram after angioplasty and stenting of the left vertebral artery, showing improved perfusion of the distal posterior circulation territory (arrow).

of 2.5–25% (Eberhardt et al. 2006). For distal vertebral reconstruction, a 2–8% mortality rate has been reported.

Several case series have described angioplasty and stenting of symptomatic vertebral and basilar stenosis (Cloud et al. 2003) (Figs. 26.2 and 26.3; see also Fig. 12.4). A recent review (Eberhardt et al. 2006) of more than 600 cases published up to 2005 provides useful information on perioperative complication rates, particularly the difference in complication rates in treatment of proximal versus distal vertebrobasilar artery lesions. In early studies, proximal lesions were treated primarily with angioplasty, but this was associated with restenosis in 15–31% of patients after 15 to 30 months of follow-up. More recently, stenting has been used for the proximal vertebral system, especially ostial lesions. Several series have reported low periprocedural or post-interventional stroke rates (Eberhardt et al. 2006).

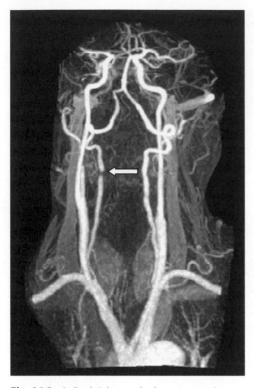

Fig. 26.3. A distal right vertebral artery stenosis (arrow) seen in MR angiography.

Pooling data from 20 reports encompassing 313 patients, there was a perioperative stroke risk of 1.3% and death rate of 0.3%. However, the rate of restenosis during a mean of 14 months of follow-up was still approximately 25%, albeit usually asymptomatic.

The complication rate for distal vertebrobasilar lesions treated with angioplasty and stenting is higher. In the review by Eberhardt *et al.* (2006), data from 170 angioplasties for distal vertebrobasilar disease were pooled. Peri-interventional complications rates were 7.1% for stroke and 3.7% for death. Data from 45 reports including 280 patients undergoing stenting, as opposed to angioplasty alone, of the distal vertebrobasilar arteries were available. This included information from the prospective multicenter Stenting of Symptomatic Atherosclerotic Lesions in the Vertebral or Intracranial Arteries (SSYLVIA) study, which included 61 vertebral and intracranial lesions (SSYLVIA Study Investigators, 2004). The pooled estimates of periprocedural risk were 3.2% for death and 10.6% for stroke, suggesting that complication rates do not differ much between angioplasty and stenting in the distal vertebrobasilar system.

One randomized trial of stenting for vertebral artery disease was started (Coward *et al.* 2005). The Carotid and Vertebral Artery Transluminal Angioplasty Study (CAVATAS) included both carotid and vertebral stenosis. However, only 16 patients were randomized between vertebral angioplasty or stenting and best medical treatment. Therefore, there are no robust data from randomized trials providing data on the safety and efficacy of vertebral artery stenting.

Subclavian steal syndome

Subclavian (and innominate) steal, although commonly detected with ultrasonography, very rarely causes neurological symptoms and does not seem to lead on to ischemic stroke. However, incapacitatingly frequent vertebrobasilar TIAs in the presence of demonstrated unilateral or bilateral retrograde vertebral artery flow distal to severe subclavian or innominate disease may sometimes be relieved by angioplasty or stenting of the subclavian artery. Other procedures that have been tried include subclavian endarterectomy, carotid-to-subclavian or femoral-to-subclavian bypass, transposition of the subclavian artery to the common carotid artery, transposition of the vertebral artery to the common carotid artery, and axillary-to-axillary artery bypass grafting. All these procedures probably carry a significant risk of complications. Irrespective of the neurological situation, some kind of interventional procedure may be needed if the hand and arm become ischemic distal to subclavian or innominate artery disease.

Extracranial-to-intracranial bypass surgery

Approximately 5–10% of patients with carotid territory TIA or minor ischemic stroke have occlusion of the internal carotid artery, stenosis of the internal carotid artery wall distal to the bifurcation, or middle cerebral artery occlusion or stenosis. Neither endarterectomy nor stenting are possible once a vessel has occluded, but many of these lesions can be bypassed by anastomosing a branch of the external carotid artery (usually the superficial temporal) via a skull burr hole to a cortical branch of the middle cerebral artery. This "surgical collateral" aims to improve the blood supply in the distal middle cerebral artery bed and so reduce the risk of stroke, and to reduce the severity of any stroke that might occur. However, there are several reasons why the procedure might not work: the artery feeding the anastomosis can take months to dilate into an effective collateral channel; many patients have good collateral flow already from orbital collaterals or via the circle of Willis; not all strokes distal to internal carotid artery/middle cerebral artery occlusion or inaccessible stenosis are caused by low flow; the risk of stroke in patients with internal carotid artery occlusion is not that high compared with severe and recently symptomatic internal carotid artery stenosis (less than 10%/year) and, anyway, not all of these strokes are ipsilateral to the occlusion; neither resting cerebral blood flow nor cerebral reactivity are necessarily depressed in these patients; and the risk of surgery may outweigh the benefit (Latchaw *et al.* 1979; Hankey and Warlow 1991; Karnik *et al.* 1992; Klijn *et al.* 1997; Powers *et al.* 2000).

The risk–benefit relationship has been evaluated in only one completed randomized trial and this failed to show any benefit from routine surgery (EC–IC Bypass Study Group 1985). However, it has been argued that patients with impaired cerebrovascular reactivity, or with maximal oxygen extraction, were not identified and perhaps it is these patients who might benefit from surgery (Warlow 1986; Derdeyn *et al.* 2005), but proof of this hypothesis would require a further randomized trial in this specific subgroup (Karnik *et al.* 1992).

In fact, a trial is now ongoing that will test the hypothesis that superficial temporal artery–middle cerebral artery anastomosis, when combined with the best medical therapy, can reduce ipsilateral ischemic stroke by 40% at two years in patients with symptomatic internal carotid artery occlusion and increased oxygen extraction fraction demonstrated by position emission tomography (Grubb *et al.* 2003). The primary endpoint will be all strokes and death occurring between randomization and the 30-day postoperative cut-off (with an equivalent period in the non-surgical group), as well as subsequent ipsilateral ischemic stroke developing within two years. It is estimated that 186 patients will be required in each group.

Other surgical procedures

Innominate or proximal common carotid artery stenosis or occlusion is quite often seen on angiograms in symptomatic patients but, unless very severe, does not influence the decision about endarterectomy for any internal carotid artery stenosis. Although it is possible to bypass such lesions, it is highly doubtful whether this reduces the risk of stroke unless, perhaps, several major neck vessels are involved and the patient has low-flow cerebral or ocular symptoms. This very rare situation can be caused by atheroma, Takayasu's disease or aortic dissection. Clearly, close consultation between physicians and vascular surgeons is needed to sort out, on an individual patient basis, what to do for the best.

Coronary artery bypass surgery (or angioplasty) may, of course, be indicated in patients presenting with cerebrovascular events who also happen to have cardiac symptoms. However, because asymptomatic coronary artery disease is so often associated with symptomatic cerebrovascular disease, would coronary intervention also be worthwhile even if there were no cardiac symptoms or signs? Given the high risk of cardiac events, which might be reduced in the long term, this is a perfectly reasonable question, but one that can only be answered by a randomized controlled trial, perhaps first in patients who are thought to be at particularly high risk of coronary events on the basis of clinical features or non-invasive cardiac investigation.

Aortic arch atheroma is now increasingly diagnosed by transesophageal echocardiography in patients with TIAs or ischemic stroke, but so far there are no surgical, or indeed medical, treatment options over and above controlling vascular risk factors and antiplatelet drugs. One trial of medical treatment has been started, the Aortic Arch Related Cerebral Hazard (ARCH) trial (MacLeod *et al.* 2004).

References

Alberts MJ for the Publications Committee of the WALLSTENT (2001). Results of a multicentre prospective randomised trial of carotid artery stenting vs. carotid endarterectomy. *Stroke* **32**:325

Brooks WH, McClure RR, Jones MR *et al.* (2001). Carotid angioplasty and stenting versus carotid endarterectomy: randomized trial in a community hospital. *Journal of the American College of Cardiologists* **38**:1589–1595

CARESS Steering Committee (2005). Carotid Revascularization Using Endarterectomy or Stenting Systems (CARESS) phase I clinical trial: 1-year results. *Journal of Vascular Surgery* **42**:213–219

Carotid Revascularization Endarterectomy versus Stenting Trial (CREST) (2006). *Stroke* **37**:e36

CAVATAS Investigators (2001) Endovascular versus surgical treatment in patents with carotid stenosis in the Carotid and Vertebral Artery Transluminal Angioplasty Study (CAVATAS): a randomised trial. *Lancet* **357**:1729–1737

Cloud GC, Crawley F, Clifton A *et al.* (2003). Vertebral artery origin angioplasty and primary stenting: safety and restenosis rates in a prospective series. *Journal of Neurology, Neurosurgery and Psychiatry* **74**:586–590

Coward LJ, Featherstone RL, Brown MM (2005). Percutaneous transluminal angioplasty and stenting for vertebral artery stenosis. *Cochrane Database of Systemic Reviews* **2**:CD000516

Derdeyn CP, Grubb RL Jr., Powers WJ (2005). Indications for cerebral revascularization for patients with atherosclerotic carotid occlusion. *Skull Base* **15**:7–14

Diaz FG, Ausman JI, de los Reyes RA *et al.* (1984). Surgical reconstruction of the proximal vertebral artery. *Journal of Neurosurgery* **61**:874–881

Dotter CT, Judkins MP, Rosch J (1967). Nonoperative treatment of arterial occlusive disease: a radiologically facilitated technique. *Radiology Clinics of North America* **5**:531–542

Eberhardt O, Naegele T, Raygrotzki S *et al.* (2006). Stenting of vertebrobasilar arteries in symptomatic atherosclerotic disease and acute occlusion: case series and review of the literature. *Journal of Vascular Surgery* **43**:1145–1154

EC–IC Bypass Study Group (1985). Failure of extracranial–intracranial arterial bypass to reduce the risk of ischaemic stroke: results of an international randomised trial. *New England Journal of Medicine* **313**:1191–1200

Featherstone RL, Brown MM, Coward LJ (2004). International carotid stenting study: protocol for a randomised clinical trial comparing carotid stenting with endarterectomy in symptomatic carotid artery stenosis. *Cerebrovascular Diseases* **18**:69–74

Grubb RL Jr., Powers WJ, Derdeyn CP *et al.* (2003). The Carotid Occlusion Surgery Study. *Neurosurgery Focus* **14**:1–7

Hankey GJ, Warlow CP (1991). Prognosis of symptomatic carotid artery occlusion. An overview. *Cerebrovascular Diseases* **1**:245–256

Harward TRS, Wickbom IG, Otis SM *et al.* (1984). Posterior communicating artery visualization in predicting results of carotid endarterectomy for vertebrobasilar insufficiency. *American Journal of Surgery* **148**:43–48

Hobson RW II, Howard VJ, Roubin GS et al. (2004). Carotid artery stenting is associated with increased complications in octogenarians: 30-day stroke and death rates in the CREST lead-in phase. Journal of Vascular Surgery 40:1106–1111

Hopkins LN, Martin NA, Hadley MN et al. (1987). Vertebrobasilar insufficiency. Part 2: microsurgical treatment of intracranial vertebrobasilar disease. Journal of Neurosurgery 66:662–674

Karnik R, Valentin A, Ammerer HP et al. (1992). Evaluation of vasomotor reactivity by transcranial Doppler and acetazolamide test before and after extracranial–intracranial bypass in patients with internal carotid artery occlusion. Stroke 23:812–817

Klijn CJM, Kappelle LJ, Tulleken CAF et al. (1997). Symptomatic carotid artery occlusion. A reappraisal of haemodynamic factors. Stroke 28:2084–2093

Latchaw RE, Ausman JI, Lee MC (1979). Superficial temporal–middle cerebral artery bypass. A detailed analysis of multiple pre- and postoperative angiograms in 40 consecutive patients. Journal of Neurosurgery 51:455–465

Macleod MR, Amarenco P, Davis SM et al. (2004). Atheroma of the aortic arch: an important and poorly recognised factor in the aetiology of stroke. Lancet Neurology 3:408–414

Malek AM, Higashida RT, Phatouros CC et al. (1999). Treatment of posterior circulation ischaemia with extracranial percutaneous balloon angioplasty and stent placement. Stroke 30:2073–2085

Mas JL, Chatellier G, Beyssen B for the EVA-3S Investigators (2006). Endarterectomy versus stenting in patients with symptomatic severe carotid stenosis. New England Journal of Medicine 355:1660–1671

Mathur A, Roubin GS, Iyer SS et al. (1998). Predictors of stroke complicating carotid artery stenting. Circulation 97:1239–1245

McCabe DJH, Brown MM, Clifton A (1999). Fatal cerebral reperfusion haemorrhage after carotid stenting. Stroke 30:2483–2486

Naylor AR, Bolia A, Abbott RJ et al. (1998). Randomized study of carotid angioplasty and stenting versus carotid endarterectomy: a stopped trial. Journal of Vascular Surgery 28:326–334

Powers WJ, Derdeyn CP, Fritsch SM et al. (2000). Benign prognosis of never-symptomatic carotid occlusion. Neurology 54:878–882

Qureshi AI, Luft AR, Sharma M et al. (1999). Frequency and determinants of postprocedural haemodynamic instability after carotid angioplasty and stenting. Stroke 30:2086–2093

Reimers B, Corvaja N, Moshiri S et al. (2001). Cerebral protection with filter devices during carotid artery stenting. Circulation 104:12–15

Rerkasem K, Bond R, Rothwell PM (2004). Local versus general anaesthetic for carotid endarterectomy. Cochrane Database of Systematic Reviews 2:CD000126

SPACE Collaborative Group (2006). 30-day results from the SPACE trial of stent-protected angioplasty versus carotid endarterectomy in symptomatic patients: a randomised non-inferiority trial. Lancet 368:1239–1247

Spetzler RF, Hadley MN, Martin NA et al. (1987). Vertebrobasilar insufficiency. Part 1: microsurgical treatment of extracranial vertebrobsilar disease. Journal of Neurosurgery 66:648–661

SSYLVIA Study Investigators (2004). Stenting of Symptomatic Atherosclerotic Lesions in the Vertebral or Intracranial Arteries (SSYLVIA): study results. Stroke 35:1388–1392

Terada T, Higashida RT, Halbach VV et al. (1996). Transluminal angioplasty for arteriosclerotic disease of the distal vertebral and basilar arteries. Journal of Neurology, Neurosurgery and Psychiatry 60:377–381

Thevenet A, Ruotolo C (1984). Surgical repair of vertebral artery stenoses. Journal of Cardiovascular Surgery 25:101–110

Warlow CP (1986). Extracranial to intracranial bypass and the prevention of stroke. Journal of Neurology 233:129–130

Yadav JS, Wholey MH, Kuntz RE et al. (2004). Protected carotid-artery stenting versus endarterectomy in high-risk patients. New England Journal of Medicine 351:1493–1501

Chapter 27

Selection of patients for carotid intervention

Although only a minority of patients with TIA or ischemic stroke are potential candidates for carotid endarterectomy (CEA) or stenting, the decision to opt for interventional treatment rather than medical treatment alone can be difficult and is, therefore, given detailed consideration in this Ch. Most of the discussion relates to CEA because far more data are available on the risks and benefits of surgery than for stenting. However, most of the issues discussed are applicable to both procedures.

If the procedural risk of stroke from endarterectomy for symptomatic stenosis is, say, 7% in routine clinical practice rather than the more optimistic estimates of some surgeons; the unoperated risk of stroke is 20% after two years, which is, on average, the case for severe stenosis; and successful surgery reduces this risk of stroke to zero, which is not far from the truth, then doing about 15 operations would cause one stroke and avoid three. The net gain would be two strokes avoided. In order to reduce the number of patients who have to undergo surgery to prevent one having a stroke and, therefore, to maximize cost effectiveness, we need to know who is at highest risk of surgical stroke, and who will survive to be at highest risk of ipsilateral ischemic stroke if surgery is not done. In other words, safe surgery should be offered to those patients who have most to gain (those at highest risk of ipsilateral ischemic stroke without surgery) and who are most likely to survive for a number of years to enjoy that gain: surgery should be targeted to the small number of patients who will have a stroke without it, not to the larger number of patients who might have a stroke, because in the latter group there will be a lot of unnecessary operations.

The cost of identifying suitable patients for carotid surgery is high, with more than 30% of the cost attributed to the initial consultation at the neurovascular clinics. The cost of preventing one stroke by CEA in the UK in 1997–1998 was in the region of £100 000 if all the costs incurred in the workup of a cohort for potential CEA are included (Benade and Warlow 2002a). Even excluding the cost of working up the very large number of patients with TIA and stroke to find the 5–10% or so suitable for surgery, surgery is not cheap: $4000 and $6000 in a private and university hospital, respectively, in the USA in 1985 (Green and McNamara 1987); US$11 602 in Sweden in 1991 (Terent et al. 1994) and approximately US$7000 in Canada in 1996 (Smurawska et al. 1998). The cost of surgery was mainly in the range (US$9500–11 500) in a recent systematic review (Benade and Warlow 2002b).

Who is at high (or low) risk of surgery?

As well as being related to the skills of the surgeon and anesthetist and aspects of the surgical technique, the operative risk of stroke and death also depends on patient age and sex; the nature of the presenting event; coexisting pathology, such as coronary heart disease; and several other factors (Table 27.1).

Table 27.1. Factors predictive of operative risk of stroke or death at endarterectomy

Related to	Factors
Presenting event	Symptomatic versus asymptomatic
	Transient ischemic attack versus stroke
	Ocular versus cerebral events
Patient	Age
	Sex
	Vascular risk factors: previous stroke, hypertension, diabetes, contralateral internal cerebral artery occlusion, peripheral vascular disease
Operation	Side of surgery
	Nature of plaque (ulcerated versus non-ulcerated)
	Timing from event to surgery

Presenting event

The operative risk of stroke and death is lower for patients with asymptomatic stenosis than for those with symptomatic stenosis (Rothwell *et al.* 1996; Bond *et al.* 2003). Not surprisingly, therefore, it also varies with the nature of the presenting symptoms. In a systematic review of all studies published from 1980 to 2000 inclusive that reported the risk of stroke and death from endartectomy (Bond *et al.* 2003), 103 of 383 studies stratified risk by the nature of the presenting symptoms (Table 27.2). As expected, the operative risk for symptomatic stenosis overall was higher than for asymptomatic stenosis (odds ratio [OR], 1.62; 95% confidence interval [CI], 1.45–1.81; $p < 0.00001$; 59 studies), but this depended on the nature of the symptoms, with the operative risk in patients with ocular events only tending to be lower than that for asymptomatic stenosis (OR, 0.75; 95% CI, 0.50–1.14; 15 studies). Operative risk was the same for stroke and cerebral TIA (OR, 1.16; 95% CI, 0.99–1.35; $p = 0.08$; 23 studies) but higher for cerebral TIA than for ocular events only (OR, 2.31; 95% CI, 1.72–3.12; $p < 0.00001$; 19 studies). Given that the operative risk of stroke is so highly dependent on the clinical indication, audits of risk should be stratified by the nature of any presenting symptoms, and patients should be informed of the risk that relates to their presenting event.

Age and sex

In the randomized trials of CEA for both symptomatic and asymptomatic carotid stenosis, benefit was decreased in women (Rothwell *et al.* 2004a; Rothwell 2004), partly because of a higher operative risk than in men, but operative risk was independent of age. However, because these trial-based observations might not be generalizable to routine clinical practice (Ch. 18), a systematic review of all publications reporting data on the association between age and/or sex and procedural risk of stroke and/or death from 1980 to 2004 was carried out (Bond *et al.* 2005). Females had a higher rate of operative stroke and death (OR, 1.31; 95% CI, 1.17–1.47; $p < 0.001$; 25 studies) than males, but no increase in operative mortality (OR, 1.05; 95% CI, 0.81–0.86; $p = 0.78$; 15 studies). Compared with younger patients, operative mortality was increased at ≥ 75 years (OR, 1.36; 95% CI, 1.07–1.68; $p = 0.02$; 20 studies), at age ≥ 80 years (OR, 1.80; 95% CI, 1.26–2.45; $p < 0.001$; 15 studies) and in older patients overall (OR, 1.50; 95% CI, 1.26–1.78; $p < 0.001$; 35 studies). In contrast, however, operative risk of non-fatal stroke alone was not increased: ≥ 75 years (OR, 1.01; 95% CI, 0.8–1.3; $p = 0.99$; 16 studies); ≥ 80 years (OR, 0.95; 95% CI, 0.61–1.20; $p = 0.43$; 15 studies). Consequently, the overall perioperative risk of stroke and death was only slightly increased at age ≥ 75 years (OR, 1.18; 95% CI, 0.94–1.44; $p - 0.06$; 21 studies), at age ≥ 80 years (OR, 1.14; 95% CI, 0.92–1.36; $p = 0.34$; 10 studies) and in older patients overall (OR, 1.17; 95% CI, 1.04–1.31; $p = 0.01$; 36 studies). Therefore, the effects of age and

Table 27.2. A systematic review of the studies reporting the operative risks of stroke or death in carotid endarterectomy according to the nature of the presenting event and stratified according to year of publication

Presenting event	Time period	Number of studies	Number of operations	Absolute risk (% [95% CI])	p value (heterogeneity)
Symptomatic	< 1995	57	17 597	5.0 (4.4–5.5)	< 0.001
	≥ 1995	38	18 885	5.1 (4.7–5.6)	< 0.001
	Total	95	36 482	5.1 (4.6–5.6)	< 0.001
Urgent	< 1995	9	143	16.8 (8.0–25.5)	< 0.001
	≥ 1995	4	65	24.6 (17.6–31.6)	< 0.001
	Total	13	208	19.2 (10.7–27.8)	< 0.001
Stroke	< 1995	27	3 071	7.3 (6.1–8.5)	< 0.001
	≥ 1995	23	4 563	7.0 (6.2–7.9)	< 0.001
	Total	50	7 634	7.1 (6.1–8.1)	< 0.001
Cerebral TIA	< 1995	11	4 279	4.6 (3.9–5.2)	< 0.001
	≥ 1995	13	3 648	6.9 (6.2–7.5)	< 0.001
	Total	24	8 138	5.5 (4.7–6.3)	< 0.001
Ocular event	< 1995	9	1 050	3.0 (2.5–3.4)	0.9
	≥ 1995	9	734	2.7 (1.9–3.3)	< 0.001
	Total	18	1 784	2.8 (2.2–3.4)	< 0.001
Non-specific	< 1995	16	1 275	4.2 (3.2–5.3)	< 0.001
	≥ 1995	8	476	4.3 (3.4–5.2)	< 0.001
	Total	24	1 751	4.2 (3.2–5.2)	< 0.001
Asymptomatic	< 1995	29	3 197	3.4 (2.5–4.4)	< 0.001
	≥ 1995	28	10 088	3.0 (2.5–3.5)	< 0.04
	Total	57	13 285	2.8 (2.4–3.2)	< 0.001
Redo surgery	< 1995	3	215	3.8 (2.7–4.9)	< 0.001
	≥ 1995	9	699	4.4 (3.1–5.8)	0.9
	Total	12	914	4.4 (2.4–6.4)	< 0.001

Notes:
CI, confidence interval; TIA, transient ischemic attack.
Source: From Bond et al. (2003).

sex on the operative risk in published case series are broadly consistent with those observed in the trials. Operative risk of stroke is increased in women, and operative mortality but the risk of stroke is not increased in patients aged ≥ 75 years.

Other patient factors

Only a few serious attempts have been made to sort out which other patient-related factors affect perioperative stroke risk, and then which factors are independent from each other so they can be used in combination to predict surgical risk in individuals (Sundt et al. 1975; McCrory et al. 1993; Goldstein et al. 1994; Riles et al. 1994; Golledge et al. 1996; Kucey et al. 1998; Ferguson et al. 1999). Risk factors almost certainly include hypertension, peripheral vascular disease, contralateral internal carotid occlusion and stenosis of the ipsilateral external carotid artery and carotid siphon (Rothwell *et al.* 1997). Operating on the left carotid artery being more risky than on the right clearly needs confirmation and, if true, might be to do with the easier detection of verbal than non-verbal cognitive deficits, or with the surgical feeling that it is more difficult operating on the left side (Barnett *et al.* 1998; Kucey *et al.* 1998; Ferguson *et al.* 1999). The independent surgical risk factors for patients in the pooled analysis of data from European Carotid Surgery Trial (ECST) and the North American Symptomatic Carotid Endarterectomy Trial (NASCET) were female sex, present-ing event, diabetes, ulcerated plaque and previous stroke (Rothwell *et al.* 2004a). Other predictors in the ECST that were not available from NASCET included systolic blood pressure and peripheral vascular disease (Bond *et al.* 2002), but the predictive model derived from the ECST patients must be validated in an independent dataset.

Timing of surgery

The optimal timing of surgery was a highly controversial topic (Pritz 1997; Eckstein *et al.* 1999). However, it is increasingly clear that surgery should be performed as soon as it is reasonably safe to do so, given the very high early risk of stroke during the first few days and weeks after the presenting TIA or stroke in patients with symptomatic carotid stenosis (Lovett *et al.* 2004; Fairhead *et al.* 2005). Any increased operative risk from early surgery must be balanced against the substantial risk of stroke occurring prior to delayed surgery (Blaser *et al.* 2002; Fairhead *et al.* 2005). If the operative risk is unrelated to the timing of surgery, then urgent surgery would, of course, be indicated. The pooled analyses of data from the randomized trials of CEA for symptomatic carotid stenosis showed that benefit from surgery was greatest in patients randomized within two weeks after their last ischemic event and fell rapidly with increasing delay (Rothwell *et al.* 2004a) For patients with $\geq 50\%$ stenosis, the number needed to undergo surgery (NNT) to prevent one ipsilateral stroke in five years was five for patients randomized within two weeks after their last ischemic event versus 125 for patients randomized > 12 weeks. This trend was a result, in part, of the fact that the operative risk of endarterectomy in the trials was not increased in patients operated on within a week of their last event (Rothwell *et al.* 2004a, b).

A systematic review of all published surgical case series that reported data on operative risk by time since presenting event also found that there was no difference between early (first three to four weeks) and later surgery in stable patients (OR, 1.13; 95% CI, 0.79–1.62; $p = 0.62$; 11 studies). For neurologically stable patients with TIA and minor stroke, benefit from endarterectomy is greatest if performed within a week of the event. However, in the same systematic review (Bond *et al.* 2003; Fairhead and Rothwell 2005), emergency CEA for patients with evolving symptoms (stroke in evolution, crescendo TIA, "urgent cases") had a high operative risk of stroke and death (19.2%; 95% CI, 10.7–27.8), which was much greater than that for surgery in patients with stable symptoms in the same studies (OR, 3.9; 95% CI, 2.7–5.7; $p < 0.001$; 13 studies). Some uncertainty does exist, therefore, in relation to the balance of risk and benefit of surgery within perhaps 24–72 hours of the presenting event, particularly in patients with stroke, and a randomized trial of early versus delayed surgery during this time scale would be ethical (Welsh *et al.* 2004; Fairhead and Rothwell 2005; Rantner *et al.* 2005). However, delays to surgery in routine clinical practice in many countries can currently be measured in months (Rodgers *et al.* 2000; Turnbull *et al.* 2000; Pell *et al.* 2003; Fairhead *et al.* 2005) and so the question of by how many hours should surgery be delayed is of somewhat theoretical interest in these healthcare systems.

Audit and monitoring of surgical results

It is very difficult to compare surgical morbidity between surgeons or institutions, in the same place at different times or before and after the introduction of a particular change in the technique without adjusting adequately for case mix: in other words, for the patient's inherent surgical risk. In addition, large enough numbers have to be collected to avoid random error (Rothwell et al. 1999a). This level of sophistication has never been achieved, and nor probably have adequate methods of routine data collection to support it, in normal clinical practice. It is clearly important, however, to have some idea of the risk of surgery in one's own hospital in the sort of patients that are usually operated on. Risks reported in the literature are irrelevant because they are not generalizable to one's own institution.

Which patients have most to gain from surgery for symptomatic carotid stenosis?

Not all patients with even extremely severe symptomatic stenosis go on to have an ipsilateral ischemic stroke: in the ECST, although approximately 30% with 90–99% stenosis had a stroke in three years, 70% did not, and these 70% could only have been harmed by surgery. Both the ECST and NASCET have shown very clearly the importance of increasing severity of carotid stenosis ipsilateral to the cerebral or ocular symptoms in the prediction of ischemic stroke in the same arterial distribution, although even this relationship is not straightforward in that if the internal carotid artery "collapses" distal to an extreme stenosis the risk of stroke is substantially reduced (Morgenstern et al. 1997; Rothwell et al. 2000a) (Fig. 27.1). Angiographically demonstrated "ulceration" or "irregularity" increases the stroke risk even more, but it is unclear whether this can be translated to the appearances on ultrasound (Eliasziw et al. 1994; Rothwell et al. 2000b). These and other determinants of benefit are reviewed below. To complicate matters further, one also must avoid offering surgery to patients unlikely to survive long enough to enjoy any benefit of stroke prevention and so for whom the immediate surgical risks would not be worthwhile. These include the very elderly and patients with advanced cancer. It would also seem sensible to avoid surgery in patients with severe symptomatic cardiac disease who are likely to die a cardiac death within a year or two.

Which range of stenosis?

To target CEA appropriately, it is first necessary to determine as precisely as possible how the overall average benefit from surgery relates to the degree of carotid stenosis. The analyses of each of the main trials of endarterectomy for symptomatic carotid stenosis were stratified by the severity of stenosis of the symptomatic carotid artery, but different methods of measurement of the degree of stenosis on pre-randomization angiograms were used, the NASCET method underestimating stenosis compared with the ECST method (Fig. 27.2) (Rothwell et al. 1994). Stenoses reported to be 70–99% in the NASCET were equivalent to 82–99% by the ECST method, and stenoses reported to be 70–99% by the ECST were 55–99% by the NASCET method (Rothwell et al. 1994).

In 1998, the ECST (European Carotid Surgery Trialists' Collaborative Group 1998) showed that there was no benefit from surgery in patients with 30–49% stenosis or 50–69% stenosis (defined by their method), but that there was major benefit in patients with 70–99% stenosis. When the results of the ECST were stratified by decile of stenosis, endarterectomy was only beneficial in patients with 80–99% stenosis. The 11.6% absolute reduction in risk of

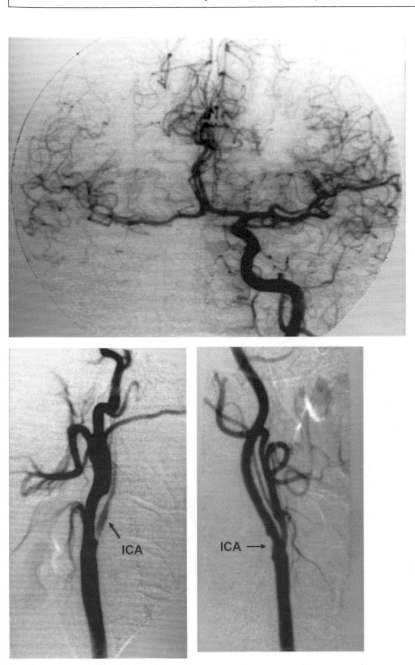

Fig. 27.1. Selective arterial angiograms of both carotid circulations in a patient with a recently symptomatic carotid "near occlusion" (lower left), and a mild stenosis at the contralateral carotid bifurcation (lower right). The near-occluded internal carotid artery (ICA) is markedly narrowed, and flow of contrast into the distal ICA is delayed. After selective injection of contrast into the contralateral carotid artery, significant collateral flow can be seen across the anterior communicating arteries with filling of the middle cerebral artery of the symptomatic hemisphere (top).

317

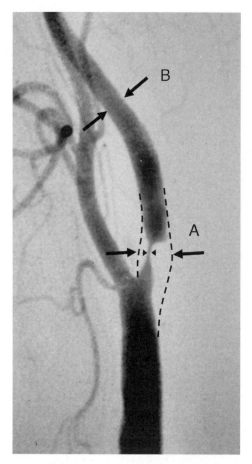

Fig. 27.2. A selective catheter angiogram of the carotid bifurcation showing a 90% stenosis. To calculate the degree of stenosis, the lumen diameter at the point of maximum stenosis (A) was measured as the numerator in both the European Carotid Surgery Trial (ECST) method and the North American Symptomatic Carotid Endarterectomy Trial (NASCET) method. However, the NASCET used the lumen diameter of the distal internal carotid artery (B) as the denominator, whereas the ECST used the estimated normal lumen diameter (dotted lines) at the point of maximum stenosis.

major stroke or death at three years was consistent with the 10.1% reduction in major stroke or death at two years reported in the NASCET (Barnett *et al.* 1998) in patients with 70–99% stenosis, as defined by NASCET. However, in contrast to the ECST, the NASCET reported a 6.9% ($p = 0.03$) absolute reduction in risk of disabling stroke or death in patients with 50–69% stenosis (equivalent to 65–82% stenosis in ECST).

Given this apparent disparity between the results of the trials, the ECST group reanalyzed their results such that they were comparable with the results of the NASCET (Rothwell *et al.* 2003a). This required that the original ECST angiograms were remeasured by the method used in the NASCET and that outcome events were redefined. Reanalysis of the ECST showed that endarterectomy had reduced the five-year risk of *any stroke or surgical death* by 5.7% (95% CI, 0–11.6) in patients with 50–69% stenosis as defined by NASCET ($n = 646$; $p = 0.05$) and by 21.2% (95% CI, 12.9–29.4) in patients with NASCET-defined 70–99% stenosis without "near occlusion" ($n = 429; p < 0.0001$). Surgery was harmful in patients with < 30% stenosis ($n = 1321$; $p = 0.007$) and of no benefit in patients with 30–49% stenosis ($n = 478$; $p = 0.6$). Therefore, the results of the two trials were consistent when analyzed in the same way. This allowed a pooled analysis of data from the ECST, NASCET and the Veterans Affairs Cooperative Study Program 309 (VA 309) trials (Mayberg *et al.* 1991), which included over 95% of patients with symptomatic carotid stenosis ever randomized to endarterectomy versus medical treatment (Rothwell *et al.* 2003b).

The pooled analysis showed that there was no statistically significant heterogeneity between the trials in the effect of the randomized treatment allocation on the relative risks of any of the main outcomes in any of the stenosis groups. Data were, therefore, merged on 6092 patients with 35 000 patient-years of follow-up (Rothwell *et al.* 2003b). The overall operative mortality was 1.1% (95% CI, 0.8–1.5), and the operative risk of stroke and death was 7.1% (95% CI, 6.3–8.1). The effect of surgery on the risks of the main trial outcomes is shown by stenosis group in Fig. 27.3. Endarterectomy reduced the five-year absolute risk of any stroke or death in patients with NASCET-defined 50–69% stenosis (absolute risk reduction [ARR], 7.8%; 95% CI, 3.1–12.5) and was highly beneficial in patients with

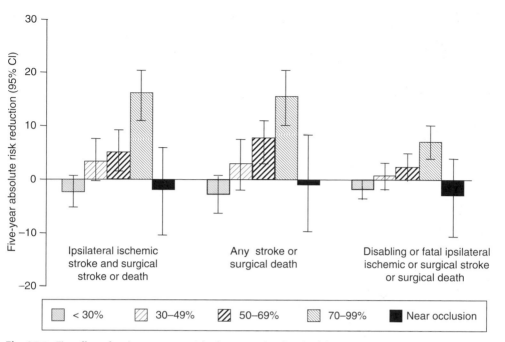

Fig. 27.3. The effect of endarterectomy on the five-year risks of each of the main trial outcomes in patients with varying degrees of stenosis (< 30%, 30–49%, ≥ 70% without near occlusion, and near occlusion) in an analysis of pooled data from the three main randomized trials of endarterectomy versus medical treatment for recently symptomatic carotid stenosis (Rothwell *et al.* 2003b).

70–99% stenosis (ARR, 15.3%; 95% CI, 9.8–20.7), but was of no benefit in patients with near occlusion. The CI values around the estimates of treatment effect in the near occlusions were wide, but the difference in the effect of surgery between this group and patients with ≥ 70% stenosis without near occlusion was statistically highly significant for each of the outcomes. Qualitatively similar results were seen for disabling stroke.

The results of these pooled analyses show that, with the exception of near occlusions, the degree of stenosis above which surgery is beneficial is 50% as defined by NASCET (equivalent to approximately 65% stenosis as defined by ECST). Given the confusion generated by the use of different methods of measurement of stenosis in the original trials, it has been suggested that the NASCET method be adopted as the standard in future (Rothwell *et al.* 2003b). There are several arguments in favor of the continued use of selective arterial angiography in the selection of patients for endarterectomy (Johnston and Goldstein 2001; Norris and Rothwell 2001). However, if non-invasive techniques are used to select patients for surgery, then they must be properly validated against catheter angiography within individual centers (Rothwell *et al.* 2000c). More work is also required to assess the accuracy of non-invasive methods of carotid imaging in detecting near occlusion (Bermann *et al.* 1995; Ascher *et al.* 2002).

What about near occlusions?

Near occlusions (Fig. 27.1) as a group were identified in the NASCET because it is not possible to measure the degree of stenosis using the NASCET method in situations where the post-stenotic internal carotid artery is narrowed or collapsed as a result of markedly reduced post-stenotic blood flow. Patients with "abnormal post-stenotic narrowing" of the internal carotid artery were also identified in the ECST (Rothwell *et al.* 2000a). In both trials, these patients had a paradoxically low risk of stroke on medical treatment. The low risk of stroke most likely reflects the presence of a good collateral circulation, which is visible on angiography in the vast majority of the patients with narrowing of the internal carotid artery distal to a severe stenosis. The benefit from surgery in the near occlusion group in the NASCET had been minimal, and both the reanalysis of the ECST (Rothwell *et al.* 2003a) and the pooled analysis (Rothwell *et al.* 2003b) suggested no benefit at all in this group in terms of preventing stroke (Fig. 27.3). Some patients with near occlusion may still wish to undergo surgery, particularly if they experience recurrent TIAs. In the reanalysis of the ECST (Rothwell *et al.* 2003a), CEA did reduce the risk of recurrent TIA in patients with near occlusion (ARR, 15%; $p = 0.007$). However, patients should be informed that endarterectomy does not prevent stroke.

Which subgroups benefit most?

The overall trial results are of only limited help to patients and clinicians in making decisions about surgery. Although endarterectomy reduces the relative risk of stroke by approximately 30% over the next three years in patients with a recently symptomatic severe stenosis, only 20% of such patients have a stroke on medical treatment alone. The operation is of no value in the other 80% of patients, who, despite having a symptomatic stenosis, are destined to remain stroke free without surgery and can only be harmed by it. It would, therefore, be useful to be able to identify in advance, and operate on, only those patients with a high risk of stroke on medical treatment alone, but a relatively low operative risk. The degree of stenosis is a major determinant of benefit from endarterectomy, but there are several other clinical and angiographic characteristics that might influence the risks and benefits of surgery.

Eleven reports of different univariate subgroup analyses were published by NASCET, which have been summarized elsewhere (Rothwell 2005). Although interesting, the results are difficult to interpret because several of the subgroups contain only a few tens of patients, with some of the estimates of the effect of surgery based on only one or two outcome events in each treatment group; the 95% CI values around the ARRs in each subgroup have generally not been given; and there have been no formal tests of the interaction between the subgroup variable and the treatment effect. It is, therefore, impossible to be certain whether differences in the effect of surgery between subgroups are real or occur by chance.

Subgroup analyses of pooled data from ECST and NASCET have greater power to determine subgroup–treatment interactions reliably, and several clinically important interactions have been reported (Rothwell *et al.* 2004a). Sex ($p = 0.003$), age ($p = 0.03$), and time from the last symptomatic event to randomization ($p = 0.009$) modify the effectiveness of surgery (Fig. 27.4). Benefit from surgery was greatest in men, patients aged ≥ 75 years, and patients randomized within two weeks after their last ischemic event, and it fell rapidly with increasing delay. For patients with $\geq 50\%$ stenosis, the number of patients needed to undergo surgery (NNT) to prevent one ipsilateral stroke in five years was 9 for men versus 36 for women, 5 for age ≥ 75 versus 18 for age < 65 years, and 5 for patients randomized within two weeks after their last ischemic event versus 125 for patients randomized > 12 weeks. The corresponding ARR values are shown separately for patients with 50–69% stenosis and 70–99% stenosis in Fig. 27.5. These observations were consistent across the 50–69% and $\geq 70\%$ stenosis groups and similar trends were present in both ECST and NASCET.

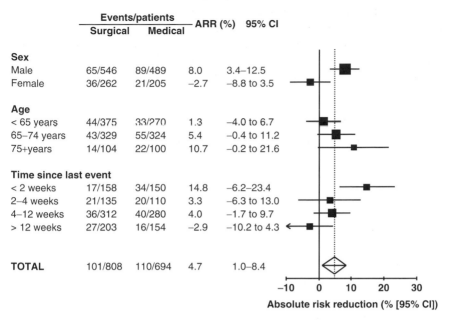

50–69% stenosis group

	Events/patients		ARR (%)	95% CI
	Surgical	Medical		
Sex				
Male	65/546	89/489	8.0	3.4–12.5
Female	36/262	21/205	−2.7	−8.8 to 3.5
Age				
< 65 years	44/375	33/270	1.3	−4.0 to 6.7
65–74 years	43/329	55/324	5.4	−0.4 to 11.2
75+years	14/104	22/100	10.7	−0.2 to 21.6
Time since last event				
< 2 weeks	17/158	34/150	14.8	−6.2–23.4
2–4 weeks	21/135	20/110	3.3	−6.3 to 13.0
4–12 weeks	36/312	40/280	4.0	−1.7 to 9.7
> 12 weeks	27/203	16/154	−2.9	−10.2 to 4.3
TOTAL	101/808	110/694	4.7	1.0–8.4

Absolute risk reduction (% [95% CI])

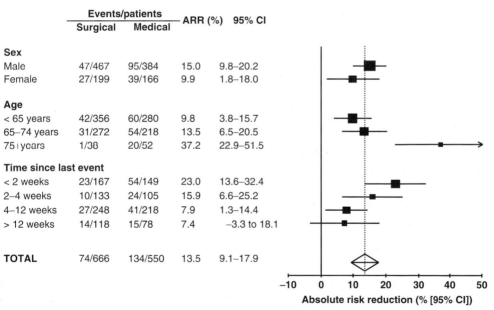

≥ 70% stenosis group

	Events/patients		ARR (%)	95% CI
	Surgical	Medical		
Sex				
Male	47/467	95/384	15.0	9.8–20.2
Female	27/199	39/166	9.9	1.8–18.0
Age				
< 65 years	42/356	60/280	9.8	3.8–15.7
65–74 years	31/272	54/218	13.5	6.5–20.5
75+years	1/38	20/52	37.2	22.9–51.5
Time since last event				
< 2 weeks	23/167	54/149	23.0	13.6–32.4
2–4 weeks	10/133	24/105	15.9	6.6–25.2
4–12 weeks	27/248	41/218	7.9	1.3–14.4
> 12 weeks	14/118	15/78	7.4	−3.3 to 18.1
TOTAL	74/666	134/550	13.5	9.1–17.9

Absolute risk reduction (% [95% CI])

Fig. 27.4. Absolute risk reduction (ARR) with surgery in the five-year risk of ipsilateral carotid territory ischemic stroke and any stroke or death within 30 days after trial surgery according to predefined subgroup variables in an analysis of pooled data from the two largest randomized trials of endarterectomy versus medical treatment for recently symptomatic carotid stenosis (Derived form Rothwell et al. 2004b). CI, confidence interval.

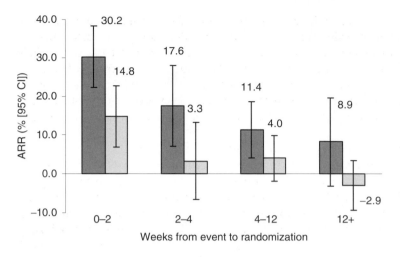

Fig. 27.5. Absolute risk reduction (ARR) with surgery in the five-year risk of ipsilateral carotid territory ischemic stroke and any stroke or death within 30 days after trial surgery in patients with 50–69% stenosis (white columns) and ≥ 70% stenosis (black columns) without near occlusion stratified by the time from last symptomatic event to randomization. This is an analysis of pooled data from the two largest randomized trials of endarterectomy versus medical treatment for recently symptomatic carotid stenosis (Rothwell *et al.* 2004a). The numbers above the bars indicate the actual absolute risk reduction. CI, confidence interval.

Women had a lower risk of ipsilateral ischemic stroke on medical treatment and a higher operative risk in comparison with men. For recently symptomatic carotid stenosis, surgery is very clearly beneficial in women with ≥ 70% stenosis, but not in women with 50–69% stenosis (Fig. 27.4). In contrast, surgery reduced the five-year absolute risk of stroke by 8.0% (95% CI, 3.4–12.5) in men with 50–69% stenosis. This sex difference was statistically significant even when the analysis of the interaction was confined to the 50–69% stenosis group. These same patterns were also shown in both of the large published trials of CEA for asymptomatic carotid stenosis (Rothwell 2004).

Benefit from CEA increased with age in the pooled analysis of trials in patients with recently symptomatic stenosis, particularly in patients aged > 75 years (Fig. 27.4). Although patients randomized in trials generally have a good prognosis and there is some evidence of an increased operative mortality in elderly patients in routine clinical practice, as discussed above, a recent systematic review of all published surgical case series reported no increase in the operative risk of stroke and death in older age groups. There is, therefore, no justification for withholding CEA in patients aged > 75 years who are deemed to be medically fit to undergo surgery. The evidence suggests that benefit is likely to be greatest in this group because of their high risk of stroke on medical treatment.

Benefit from surgery is probably also greatest in patients with stroke, intermediate in those with cerebral TIA and lowest in those with retinal events. There was also a trend in the trials towards greater benefit in patients with irregular plaque than a smooth plaque.

Which individuals benefit most?

There are some clinically useful subgroup observations in the pooled analysis of the endarterectomy trials, but the results of univariate subgroup analysis are often of only limited use in clinical practice. Individual patients frequently have several important risk factors, each of which interacts in a way that cannot be described using univariate subgroup analysis, and all of which should be taken into account in order to determine the likely balance of risk and benefit from surgery (Rothwell *et al.* 1999b). For example, what would be the likely benefit from surgery in a 78-year-old (increased benefit) female (reduced benefit) with 70% stenosis who presented within two weeks (increased benefit) of an ocular ischemic event (reduced benefit) and was found to have an ulcerated carotid plaque (increased benefit)?

One way in which clinicians can weigh the often-conflicting effects of the important characteristics of an individual patient on the likely benefit from treatment is to base decisions on the predicted absolute risks of a poor outcome with each treatment option using prognostic models (see Ch. 14). A model for prediction of the risk of stroke on medical treatment in patients with recently symptomatic carotid stenosis has been derived from the ECST (Rothwell *et al.* 1999b, 2005) (Table 27.3). The model was validated using data from the NASCET and showed very good agreement between predicted and observed medical risk (Mantel–Haenszel $\chi^2_{trend} = 41.3$ [degrees of freedom, 1]; p < 0.0001), reliably distinguishing between individuals with a 10% risk of ipsilateral ischemic stroke after five years of follow-up and individuals with a risk of over 40% (Fig. 27.6). Importantly, Fig. 27.6 also shows that the operative risk of stroke and death in patients who were randomized to surgery in NASCET was unrelated to the medical risk (Mantel–Haenszel $\chi^2_{trend} = 0.98$ [degrees of freedom, 1]; $p = 0.32$). Therefore, when the operative risk and the small additional residual risk of stroke following successful endarterectomy were taken into account, benefit from endarterectomy at five years varied significantly across the quintiles ($p = 0.001$), with no benefit in patients in the lower three quintiles of predicted medical risk (ARR, 0–2%), moderate benefit in the fourth quintile (ARR, 10.8%; 95% CI, 1.0–20.6) and substantial benefit in the highest quintile (ARR, 32.0%; 95% CI, 21.9–42.1).

Prediction of risk using models requires a computer, a pocket calculator with an exponential function or internet-access (the ECST model can be found at www.stroke. ox.ac.uk). As an alternative, a simplified risk score based on the hazard ratios derived from the relevant risk model can be derived. Table 27.3 shows a score for the five-year risk of stroke on medical treatment in patients with recently symptomatic carotid stenosis derived from the ECST model. As is shown in the example, the total risk score is the product of the scores for each risk factor. Fig. 27.7 shows a plot of the total risk score against the five-year predicted risk of ipsilateral carotid territory ischemic stroke derived from the full model and is used as a nomogram for the conversion of the score into a risk prediction.

Alternatively, risk tables allow a relatively small number of important variables to be considered and have the major advantage that they do not require the calculation of any score by the clinician or patient. Fig. 27.8 shows a risk table for the five-year risk of ipsilateral ischemic stroke in patients with recently symptomatic carotid stenosis on medical treatment, derived from the ECST model. The table is based on the five variables that were both significant predictors of risk in the ECST model (Table 27.3) and yielded clinically important subgroup–treatment effect interactions in the analysis of pooled data from the relevant trials (sex, age, time since last symptomatic event, type of presenting event(s) and carotid plaque surface morphology).

One potential problem with the ECST risk model is that it might overestimate risk in current patients because of improvements in medical treatment, such as the increased use of statins. However, such improvements in treatment pose more problems for interpretation

Table 27.3. A predictive model for five-year risk of ipsilateral ischemic stroke on medical treatment in patients with recently symptomatic carotid stenosis[a]

Model			Scoring system		
Risk factor	Hazard ratio (95% CI)	p value	Risk factor	Score	Example
Stenosis (per 10%)	1.18 (1.10–1.25)	< 0.0001	Stenosis (%)		
			50–59	2.4	2.4
			60–69	2.8	
			70–79	3.3	
			80–89	3.9	
			90–99	4.6	
Near occlusion[b]	0.49 (0.19–1.24)	0.1309	Near occlusion	0.5	No
Male sex	1.19 (0.81–1.75)	0.3687	Male sex	1.2	No
Age (per 10 years)	1.12 (0.89–1.39)	0.3343	Age (years)		
			31–40	1.1	
			41–50	1.2	
			51–60	1.3	
			61–70	1.5	1.5
			71–80	1.6	
			81–90	1.8	
Time since last event (per seven days)	0.96 (0.93–0.99)	0.0039	Time since last event (days)		
			0–13	8.7	8.7
			14–28	8.0	
			29–89	6.3	
			90–365	2.3	
Presenting event[c]		0.0067	Presenting event		
Ocular	1.000		Ocular	1.0	
Single TIA	1.41 (0.75–2.66)		Single TIA	1.4	
Multiple TIAs	2.05 (1.16–3.60)		Multiple TIAs	2.0	
Minor stroke	1.82 (0.99–3.34)		Minor stroke	1.8	
Major stroke[d]	2.54 (1.48–4.35)		Major stroke	2.5	2.5
Diabetes	1.35 (0.86–2.11)	0.1881	Diabetes	1.4	1.4
Previous MI	1.57 (1.01–2.45)	0.0471	Previous MI	1.6	No
PVD	1.18 (0.78–1.77)	0.4368	PVD	1.2	No
Treated hypertension[e]	1.24 (0.88–1.75)	0.2137	Treated hypertension	1.2	1.2

Table 27.3. (cont.)

Model			Scoring system		
Risk factor	Hazard ratio (95% CI)	p value	Risk factor	Score	Example
Irregular/ulcerated plaque	2.03 (1.31–3.14)	0.0015	Irregular/ulcerated plaque	2.0	2.0
Total risk score					263
Predicted medical risk using nomogram					37

Notes:
[a]TIA, transient ischemic attack; MI, myocardial infarction; PVD, peripheral vascular disease; CI, confidence interval. Hazard ratios derived from the model are used for the scoring system. The score for the 5-year risk of stroke is the product of the individual scores for each of the risk factors present. The score is converted into a risk using Fig. 27.6.
[b]In cases of near occlusion, enter degree of stenosis as 85%.
[c]Presenting event is coded as the most severe ipsilateral symptomatic event in the last six months (severity is as ordered above: ocular events are least severe and major stroke is most severe).
[d]Major stroke is defined as stroke with symptoms persisting for at least seven days.
[e]Treated hypertension includes previously treated or newly diagnosed hypertension.
Source: From Rothwell *et al.* (2005).

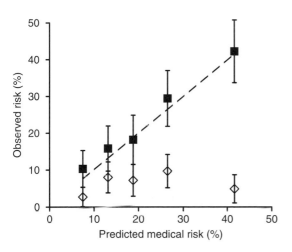

Fig. 27.6. A model derived from the data from the European Carotid Surgery Trial (ESCT) for the five-year risk of ipsilateral risk of ischemic stroke on medical treatment tested on data from the North American Symptomatic Carotid Endarterectomy Trial (NASCET). The closed squares show the risk of stroke in the medical treatment group in NASCET, stratified into quintiles on the basis of predicted risk. The open diamonds show the operative risk of stroke and death in the surgical group in NASCET stratified by their predicted medical risk.

of the overall trial results than for the risk-modeling approach. For example, it would take only a relatively modest improvement in the effectiveness of medical treatment to erode the overall benefit of endarterectomy in patients with 50–69% stenosis. In contrast, very major improvements in medical treatment would be required in order to significantly reduce the benefit from surgery in patients in the high predicted-risk quintile in Fig. 27.6. Therefore, the likelihood that ancillary treatments have improved, and are likely to continue to improve, is an argument in favor of a risk-based approach to targeting treatment. However, it would be reasonable in a patient on treatment with a statin, for example, to reduce the risks derived from the risk model by 20% in relative terms.

Other prognostic tools, such as measurements of cerebral reactivity and emboli load on transcranial Doppler (Molloy and Markus 1999; MacKinnon *et al.* 2005; Markus and

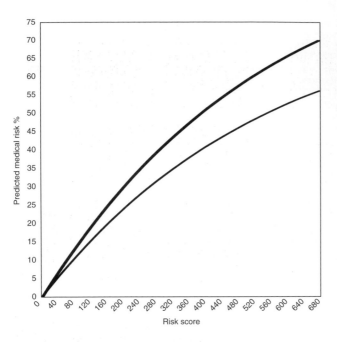

Fig. 27.7. A plot of the total risk score derived in the European Carotid Surgery Trial (ECST; see Table 27.3) against the five-year predicted risk of ipsilateral carotid territory ischemic stroke derived from the full model. This graph is used to convert the score from Table 27.3 into a risk prediction. The finer line on the graph is the predicted risk if one assumes a 20% reduction in risk with newer secondary preventive therapies compared with those available when the model was developed.

MacKinnon 2005), are not widely used in clinical practice and it is unclear to what extent they are likely to add to the predictive value of the ECST model.

Patients with multiple potential causes of stroke

Patients often have multiple possible causes for their TIA or stroke. For example, patients with a lacunar ischemic stroke or TIA may have ipsilateral severe carotid stenosis. The question then arises whether the stenosis is "symptomatic" (i.e. a small deep lacunar infarct has, unusually, been caused by artery-to-artery embolism or low flow) or "asymptomatic" (i.e. the stenosis is a coincidental bystander and the infarct was really caused by intracranial small vessel disease). Unsurprisingly, the number of such patients in the randomized trials is very small and there are only limited published data (Boiten *et al.* 1996; Inzitari *et al.* 2000), but pooled analysis of the individual patient data shows that surgery is beneficial for patients with severe stenosis ipsilateral to a lacunar TIA or stroke (PM Rothwell, unpublished data). The observational studies mostly show that severe stenosis is about equally rare in the symptomatic and contralateral carotid arteries, which supports the notion of the stenosis being coincidental (Mead *et al.* 2000), but it does not mean that surgery would not still be beneficial. In practice, most clinicians would recommend surgery, particularly if the stenosis is very severe, because even if the artery was in truth asymptomatic there is some evidence that the risk of ipsilateral ischemic stroke is high enough to justify the risk of surgery. The same arguments probably apply if there is also a major coexisting source of embolism from the heart (such as non-rheumatic atrial fibrillation), in which case the patient may reasonably be offered surgery as well as anticoagulation. With the more widespread use of diffusion-weighted imaging, it is now often possible to infer the likely etiology of stroke from the distribution of acute ischemic lesions (see Chs. 10 and 11).

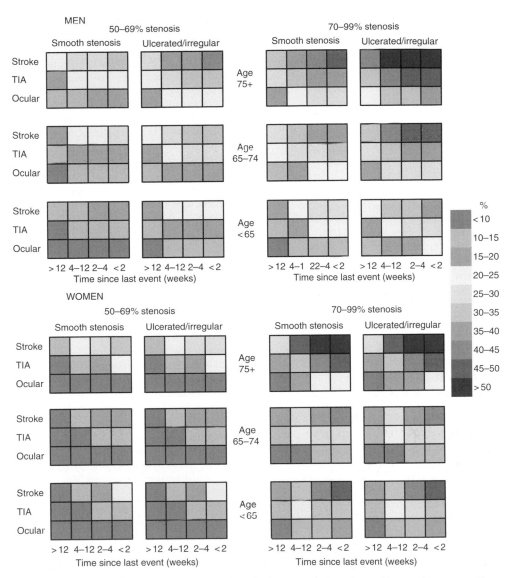

Fig. 27.8. A risk table for the five-year risk of ipsilateral ischemic stroke in patients with recently symptomatic carotid stenosis on medical treatment derived from the ECST model. European Carotid Surgery Trial (ECST) method. TIA, transient ischemic attack. (See the color plate section.)

References

Ascher E, Markevich N, Hingorani A *et al.* (2002). Pseudo-occlusions of the internal carotid artery: a rationale for treatment on the basis of a modified duplex scan protocol. *Journal of Vascular Surgery* **35**:340–350

Barnett HJM, Taylor DW, Eliasziw M for the North American Symptomatic Carotid Endarterectomy Trial Collaborators (1998).
Benefit of carotid endarterectomy in patients with symptomatic moderate or severe stenosis. *New England Journal of Medicine* **339**:1415–1425

Benade MM, Warlow CP (2002a). Cost of identifying patients for carotid endarterectomy. *Stroke* **33**:435–439

Benade MM, Warlow CP (2002b). Costs and benefits of carotid endarterectomy and associated preoperative arterial imaging: a systematic review of health economic literature. *Stroke* **33**:629–638

Bermann SS, Devine JJ, Erdos LS *et al.* (1995). Distinguishing carotid artery pseudo-occlusion with colour-flow Doppler. *Stroke* **26**:434–438

Blaser T, Hofmann K, Buerger T *et al.* (2002). Risk of stroke, transient ischaemic attack, and vessel occlusion before endarterectomy in patients with symptomatic severe carotid stenosis. *Stroke* **33**:1057–1062

Boiten J, Rothwell PM, Slattery J for the European Carotid Surgery Trialists' Collaborative Group (1996). Lacunar stroke in the European Carotid Surgery Trial: risk factors, distribution of carotid stenosis, effect of surgery and type of recurrent stroke. *Cerebrovascular Diseases* **6**:281–287

Bond R, Narayan S, Rothwell PM *et al.* (2002). Clinical and radiological risk factors for operative stroke and death in the European Carotid Surgery Trial. *European Journal of Vascular Endovascular Surgery* **23**:108–116

Bond R, Rerkasem K, Rothwell PM (2003). A systematic review of the risks of carotid endarterectomy in relation to the clinical indication and the timing of surgery. *Stroke* **34**:2290–2301

Bond R, Rerkasem K, Cuffe R *et al.* (2005). A systematic review of the associations between age and sex and the operative risks of carotid endarterectomy. *Cerebrovascular Diseases* **20**:69–77

Eckstein H, Schumacher H, Klemm K *et al.* (1999). Emergency carotid endarterectomy. *Cerebrovascular Diseases* **9**:270–281

Eliasziw M, Streifler JY, Fox AJ for the North American Symptomatic Carotid Endarterectomy Trial (1994). Significance of plaque ulceration in symptomatic patients with high-grade carotid stenosis. *Stroke* **25**:304–308

European Carotid Surgery Trialists' Collaborative Group (1998). Randomised trial of endarterectomy for recently symptomatic carotid stenosis: final results of the MRC European Carotid Surgery Trial (ECST). *Lancet* 351:1379–1387

Fairhead JF, Rothwell PM (2005). The need for urgency in identification and treatment of

symptomatic carotid stenosis is already established. *Cerebrovascular Diseases* **19**:355–358

Ferguson GG, Eliasziw M, Barr HWK for the North American Symptomatic Carotid Endarterectomy Trial (NASCET) Collaborators (1999). The North American Symptomatic Carotid Endarterectomy Trial: surgical results in 1415 patients. *Stroke* **30**:1751–1758

Goldstein LB, McCrory DC, Landsman PB *et al.* (1994). Multicenter review of preoperative risk factors for carotid endarterectomy in patients with ipsilateral symptoms. *Stroke* **25**:1116–1121

Golledge J, Cuming R, Beattie DK *et al.* (1996). Influence of patient-related variables on the outcome of carotid endarterectomy. *Journal of Vascular Surgery* **24**:120–126

Green RM, McNamara J (1987). Optimal resources for carotid endarterectomy. *Surgery* **102**:743–748

Inzitari D, Eliasziw M, Gates P for the North American Symptomatic Carotid Endarterectomy Trial Group (2000). The causes and risk of stroke in patients with asymptomatic internal-carotid-artery stenosis. *New England Journal of Medicine* **342**:1693–1700

Johnston DC, Goldstein LB (2001). Clinical carotid endarterectomy decision making: non-invasive vascular imaging versus angiography. *Neurology* **56**: 1009–1015

Kucey DS, Bowyer B, Iron K *et al.* (1998). Determinants of outcome after carotid endarterectomy. *Journal of Vascular Surgery* **28**:1051–1058

Lovett JK, Coull A, Rothwell PM on behalf of the Oxford Vascular Study (2004). Early risk of recurrent stroke by aetiological subtype: implications for stroke prevention. *Neurology* **62**:569–574

MacKinnon AD, Aaslid R, Markus HS (2005). Ambulatory transcranial Doppler cerebral embolic signal detection in symptomatic and asymptomatic carotid stenosis. *Stroke* **36**:1726–1730

Markus HS, MacKinnon A (2005). Asymptomatic embolization detected by Doppler ultrasound predicts stroke risk in symptomatic carotid artery stenosis. *Stroke* **36**:971–975

Mayberg MR, Wilson E, Yatsu F for the Veterans Affairs Cooperative Studies Program 309 Trialist Group (1991). Carotid endarterectomy and prevention of cerebral ischaemia in symptomatic carotid stenosis. *Journal of the American Medical Association* **266**:3289–3294

Mccrory DC, Goldstein LB, Samsa GP *et al.* (1993). Predicting complications of carotid endarterectomy. *Stroke* **24**:1285–1291

Mead GE, Lewis SC, Wardlaw JM, Dennis MS, Warlow CP (2000). Severe ipsilateral carotid stenosis in lacunar ischaemic stroke: innocent bystanders? *Journal of Neurology* **249**:266–271

Molloy J, Markus HS (1999). Asymptomatic embolization predicts stroke and TIA risk in patients with carotid artery stenosis. *Stroke* **30**:1440–1443

Morgenstern LB, Fox AJ, Sharpe BL *et al.* for the North American Symptomatic Carotid Endarterectomy Trial (NASCET) Group (1997). The risks and benefits of carotid endarterectomy in patients with near occlusion of the carotid artery. *Neurology* **48**:911–915

Norris J, Rothwell PM (2001). Noninvasive carotid imaging to select patients for endarterectomy: Is it really safer than conventional angiography? *Neurology* **56**:990–991

Pell JP, Slack R, Dennis M *et al.* (2003). Improvements in carotid endarterectomy in Scotland: results of a national prospective survey. *Scottish Medical Journal* **49**:53–56

Pritz MB (1997). Timing of carotid endarterectomy after stroke. *Stroke* **28**:2563–2567

Rantner B, Pavelka M, Posch L, Schmidauer C, Fraedrich G (2005). Carotid endarterectomy after ischemic stroke: is there a justification for delayed surgery? *European Journal of Vascular Endovascular Surgery* **30**:36–40

Riles TS, Imparato AM, Jacobowitz GR *et al.* (1994). The cause of perioperative stroke after carotid endarterectomy. *Journal of Vascular Surgery* **19**:206–216

Rodgers H, Oliver SE, Dobson R *et al.* (2000). A regional collaborative audit of the practice and outcome of carotid endarterectomy in the United Kingdom. Northern Regional Carotid Endarterectomy Audit Group. *European Journal of Vascular Endovascular Surgery* **19**:362–369

Rothwell PM (2004). ACST: which subgroups will benefit most from carotid endarterectomy? *Lancet* **364**:1122–1123

Rothwell PM (2005). Risk modelling to identify patients with symptomatic carotid stenosis most at risk of stroke. *Neurology Research* **27**(Suppl 1):S18–S28

Rothwell PM, Gibson RJ, Slattery J *et al.* (1994). Equivalence of measurements of carotid stenosis: A comparison of three methods on 1001 angiograms. *Stroke* **25**:2435–2439

Rothwell PM, Slattery J, Warlow CP (1996). A systematic comparison of the risk of stroke and death due to carotid endarterectomy for symptomatic and asymptomatic stenosis. *Stroke* **27**:266–269

Rothwell PM, Slattery J, Warlow CP (1997). Clinical and angiographic predictors of stroke and death from carotid endarterectomy: systematic review. *British Medical Journal* **315**:1571–1577

Rothwell PM, Warlow CP on behalf of the European Carotid Surgery Trialists' Collaborative Group (1999a). Interpretation of operative risks of individual surgeons. *Lancet* **353**:1325

Rothwell PM, Warlow CP on behalf of the European Carotid Surgery Trialists' Collaborative Group (1999b). Prediction of benefit from carotid endarterectomy in individual patients: a risk modelling study. *Lancet* **353**:2105–2110

Rothwell PM, Warlow CP on behalf of the European Carotid Surgery Trialists' Collaborative Group (2000a). Low risk of ischaemic stroke in patients with reduced internal carotid artery lumen diameter distal to severe symptomatic carotid stenosis. *Stroke* **31**:622–630

Rothwell PM, Gibson R, Warlow CP on behalf of the European Carotid Surgery Trialists' Collaborative Group (2000b). Interrelation between plaque surface morphology and degree of stenosis on carotid angiograms and the risk of ischaemic stroke in patients with symptomatic carotid stenosis. *Stroke* **31**:615–621

Rothwell PM, Pendlebury ST, Wardlaw J *et al.* (2000c). Critical appraisal of the design and reporting of studies of imaging and measurement of carotid stenosis. *Stroke* **31**:1444–1450

Rothwell PM, Gutnikov SA, Warlow CP for the ECST (2003a). Re-analysis of the final results of the European Carotid Surgery Trial. *Stroke* **34**:514–523

Rothwell PM, Gutnikov SA, Eliasziw M *et al.* for the Carotid Endarterectomy Trialists' Collaboration (2003b). Pooled analysis of individual patient data from randomised controlled trials of endarterectomy for symptomatic carotid stenosis. *Lancet* **361**:107–116

Rothwell PM, Eliasziw M, Gutnikov SA for the Carotid Endarterectomy Trialists Collaboration (2004a). Effect of endarterectomy for symptomatic carotid stenosis in relation to clinical subgroups and to the timing of surgery. *Lancet* **363**:915–924

Rothwell PM, Gutnikov SA, Eliasziw M *et al.* (2004b). Sex difference in effect of time from symptoms to surgery on benefit from endarterectomy for transient ischaemic attack and non-disabling stroke. *Stroke* **35**:2855–2861

Rothwell PM, Mehta Z, Howard SC *et al.* (2005). From subgroups to individuals: general principles and the example of carotid endartectomy. *Lancet* **365**:256–265

Smurawska LT, Bowyer B, Rowed D *et al.* (1998). Changing practice and costs of carotid endarterectomy in Toronto, Canada. *Stroke* **29**:2014–2017

Sundt TM, Sandok BA, Whisnant JP (1975). Carotid endarterectomy. Complications and preoperative assessment of risk. *Mayo Clinic Proceedings* **50**:301–306

Terent A, Marke LA, Asplund K *et al.* (1994). Costs of stroke in Sweden. A national perspective. *Stroke* **25**:2363–2369

Turnbull RG, Taylor DC, Hsiang YN *et al.* (2000). Assessment of patient waiting times for vascular surgery. *Canadian Journal of Surgery* **43**:105–111

Welsh S, Mead G, Chant H *et al.* (2004). Early carotid surgery in acute stroke: a multicentre randomized pilot study. *Cerebrovascular Disease* **18**:200–205

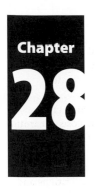
28 Intervention for asymptomatic carotid stenosis

Although asymptomatic carotid stenosis can be identified during screening programs of apparently healthy people (i.e. in a primary prevention setting), it is also often identified in a secondary prevention setting, such as when a carotid bruit is heard in patients with angina, claudication or non-focal neurological symptoms; when bilateral carotid imaging is done in patients with unilateral carotid symptoms (i.e. the patient is symptomatic but one carotid artery is asymptomatic); and when patients are being assessed for major surgery below the neck.

When asymptomatic carotid stenosis is discovered, four questions arise.

- What is the risk of operating?
- What is the risk (of stroke) if the stenosis is left unoperated?
- Does surgery reduce the risk of stroke?
- What is the balance of immediate surgical risk versus long-term benefit?

The answers to these questions are different for asymptomatic carotid stenosis than for symptomatic stenosis, because the risk of stroke on medical treatment alone is lower distal to an asymptomatic stenosis (Fig. 28.1).

Is there evidence of benefit from sugery?

Whether the benefits of carotid endarterectomy or stenting in patients with asymptomatic stenosis justify the risks and cost is still unclear (Chaturvedi *et al.* 2005; Chambers and Donnan 2005), particularly in an era of improved medical treatments. Until relatively recently, guidelines on endarterectomy for asymptomatic stenosis were largely based on the results of the Asymptomatic Carotid Atherosclerosis Study (ACAS) (Executive Committee for the Asymptomatic Carotid Atherosclerosis Study 1995) and a few other smaller trials (Chambers and Donnan 2005). The ACAS reported a 47% relative reduction in the risk of ipsilateral stroke and perioperative death in the surgical arm despite a five-year risk of ipsilateral stroke without the operation of only 11%. However, even in this optimal trial environment, the absolute reduction in risk of stroke with endarterectomy was only about 1% per year. In addition, the very low operative risks in ACAS may not be matched in routine clinical practice. This study only accepted surgeons with an excellent safety record, rejecting 40% of initial applicants and subsequently barring from further participation some surgeons who had adverse operative outcomes during the trial (Moore *et al.* 1996).

The more pragmatic Medical Research Council Asymptomatic Carotid Surgery Trial (ACST) has probably produced more widely generalizable results (Halliday *et al.* 2004). Between 1993 and 2003, ACST randomized 3120 patients with > 60% mainly asymptomatic carotid stenosis (12% had symptoms at least six months previously) to immediate endarterectomy plus medical treatment versus medical treatment alone or until the operation became necessary. Surgeons were required to provide evidence of an operative risk of 6%

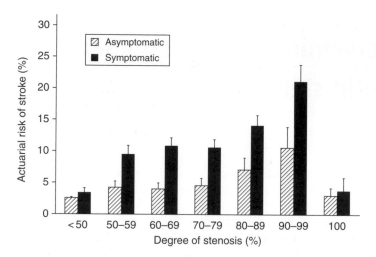

Fig. 28.1. The three-year risk of carotid territory ipsilateral ischemic stroke distal to symptomatic carotid stenosis versus that distal to contralateral asymptomatic carotid stenosis in patients with a recent transient ischemic attack or ischemic stroke in the Carotid Endarterectomy Trialists' Collaboration (PM Rothwell, unpublished data).

or less for their last 50 patients having an endarterectomy for asymptomatic stenosis, but none was excluded on the basis of his/her operative risk during the trial. Selection of patients was based on the "uncertainty principle," with very few exclusion criteria.

Despite the differences in methods of ACST and ACAS, the absolute reductions in five-year risk of stroke with surgery were similar: 5.3% (95% confidence interval [CI], 3.0–7.8 and 5.1% (95% CI, 0.9–9.1), respectively. In addition, whereas ACAS had reported only a non-significant 2.7% reduction ($p = 0.26$) in the absolute risk of disabling or fatal stroke with surgery, ACST reported a significant 2.5% (95% CI, 0.8–4.3; $p = 0.004$) absolute reduction, although the number needed to treat to prevent one disabling or fatal stroke after five years remained about 40. The main differences between the trials were in the 30-day operative risks of death (0.14% [95% CI, 0–0.4] in ACAS and 1.11% [95% CI, 0.6–1.8] in ACST; $p = 0.02$) and in the combined operative risk of stroke and death (1.5% [95% CI, 0.6–2.4] in ACAS and 3.0% [95% CI, 2.1–4.0] in ACST; $p = 0.04$).

Selection of patients for endarterectomy for asymptomatic stenosis

The decision to perform carotid endarterectomy or stenting for asymptomatic stenosis should not be taken lightly, given the inevitable anxiety and procedural risks faced by the patient. If the procedural risk of stroke is, say, 4% in routine clinical practice, the risk of stroke on intensive medical treatment alone is 10% after 5 years, and successful surgery reduces this risk of stroke to almost zero, then doing about 100 operations would cause 4 strokes and avoid up to 10. To maximize cost effectiveness, it is essential that we know who is at highest risk of surgical stroke, and who will survive to be at highest risk of ipsilateral ischemic stroke if surgery is not done. Furthermore, given the high cost of intervention for symptomatic carotid stenosis (Benade and Warlow 2002a, b), we need to be aware of the health-economic and public health issues related to intervention for asymptomatic stenosis.

Risk of carotid endarterectomy for asymptomatic carotid stenosis

There are a large number of case series with very different reported surgical stroke risks, for the same reasons as in symptomatic carotid stenosis (Ch. 27). Overall, the risk is about

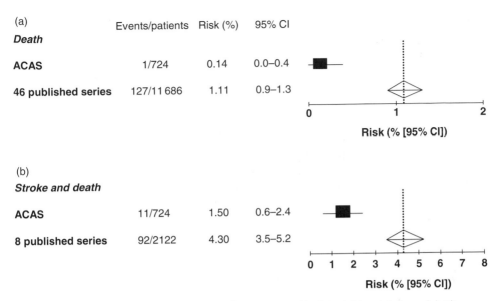

(a)
Death

	Events/patients	Risk (%)	95% CI
ACAS	1/724	0.14	0.0–0.4
46 published series	127/11 686	1.11	0.9–1.3

Risk (% [95% CI])

(b)
Stroke and death

	Events/patients	Risk (%)	95% CI
ACAS	11/724	1.50	0.6–2.4
8 published series	92/2122	4.30	3.5–5.2

Risk (% [95% CI])

Fig. 28.2. The overall results of a meta-analysis of the operative risk of death (a) and stroke and death (b) from all studies published between 1990 and 2000 inclusive that reported risks from carotid endarterectomy for asymptomatic stenosis (Bond *et al.* 2003a) compared with the same risks in the ACAS Trial (Executive Committee for the Asymptomatic Carotid Atherosclerosis Study 1995). Studies in the analysis of risk of stroke and death are confined to those in which patients were assessed by neurologists. CI, confidence interval.

half that for symptomatic carotid stenosis (Rothwell *et al.* 1996; Bond *et al.* 2003a), but the risk may not necessarily be low in all patients, for example patients with angina whose carotid stenosis was discovered during preparation for coronary artery surgery, or patients who have already had an endarterectomy on one side and are at risk of bilateral vagal or hypoglossal nerve palsies if both sides are operated on.

As for symptomatic stenosis, the risk of surgery cannot be generalized from the literature to one's own institution, a risk that should be known locally. For example, ACAS reported an operative mortality of 0.14% and a risk of stroke and death of 1.5%. However, a systematic review of all studies published during 1990–2000 inclusive that reported the risks of stroke and death from endarterectomy for asymptomatic stenosis found much higher risks (Bond *et al.* 2003b). The overall risk of stroke and death was 3.0% (95% CI, 2.5–3.5) in 28 studies published post-ACAS (1995–2000). The risk in 12 studies in which outcome was assessed by a neurologist (4.6%; 95% CI, 3.6–5.7) was three times higher than in ACAS (odds ratio [OR], 3.1; 95% CI, 1.7–5.6; $p = 0.0001$). Operative mortality during 1995–2000 (1.1% 95% CI, 0.9–1.4) was eight times higher than in ACAS OR, 8.1; 95% CI, 1.3–58; $p = 0.01$; Fig. 28.2). In studies that reported outcome after endarterectomy for symptomatic and asymptomatic stenosis in the same institution, operative mortality was no lower for asymptomatic stenosis (OR, 0.80; 95% CI, 0.6–1.1). The proportion of patients operated for asymptomatic stenosis in these studies increased from 16% during 1990–1994 to 45% during 1995–2000. Therefore, published risks of stroke and death from surgery for asymptomatic stenosis are considerably higher than in ACAS, particularly if outcome was assessed by a neurologist. If operative mortality is eight times higher than in ACAS, then endarterectomy for asymptomatic carotid stenosis in routine clinical practice might even increase population mortality through stroke. Even after community-wide performance measurement and feedback, the overall risk for stroke or death after endarterectomy performed for asymptomatic stenosis in 10 US states was 3.8% (including 1% mortality) (Kresowik *et al.* 2004).

Who benefits most from surgery for asymptomatic carotid stenosis?

Given the surgical risk (which depends on the type of patient under consideration as well as surgical skill), the added risk of any preceding catheter angiography, and what appears to be a remarkably low risk of stroke in unoperated patients, there is clearly no reason to recommend routine carotid endarterectomy for asymptomatic stenosis. It follows that deliberately screening apparently healthy people for carotid stenosis is unwarranted. A prognostic model (Ch. 14) is required to identify those very few patients whose asymptomatic stenosis is particularly likely to cause stroke, to whom surgery may be offered.

Which range of stenosis?

Although there is evidence that the risk of ipsilateral ischemic stroke on medical treatment increases with degree of angiographic asymptomatic carotid stenosis (Fig. 28.1), in contrast to trials of endarterectomy in patients with symptomatic carotid stenosis (Ch. 27), neither ACST nor ACAS showed increasing benefit from surgery with increasing degree of stenosis within the 60–99% range. There are several possible explanations for this.

First, ultrasound may be less accurate than catheter angiography in measuring the degree of stenosis. In ACAS, only patients randomized to surgery underwent catheter angiography, and in ACST all imaging was by Doppler ultrasound without any centralized audit (Halliday *et al.* 1994). The importance of the precise methods used to measure stenosis was highlighted in a study of patients randomized to the medical arm of the ECST, which demonstrated that angiographic measures of stenosis were most reliable in predicting recurrent stroke when selective carotid contrast injections had been given, biplane views were available and when the mean of measurements made by two independent observers was used (Cuffe and Rothwell 2006).

Second, patients with carotid near occlusion, which is not readily detectable on ultrasound, were not identified in the randomized trials of endarterectomy for asymptomatic stenosis. In the European Carotid Surgery Trial (ECST), for example, the proportion of near occlusions was 0.6% at 60–69% stenosis, 2.3% at 70–79% stenosis, 9.2% at 80–89% stenosis and 29.5% at 90–99% stenosis (Rothwell *et al.* 2000), and only when near occlusions were removed was the increased benefit of endarterectomy with increasing stenosis between 70% and 99% clearly apparent (Rothwell *et al.* 2003). This issue is further complicated by the findings of a recent study of 1115 patients with asymptomatic stenosis, in which increasing stenosis on ultrasound was positively associated with risk of ipsilateral hemispheric ischemic events at a mean of 38 months of follow-up when stenosis was measured using ECST criteria, but not when North American Symptomatic Carotid Endarterectomy Trial (NASCET) criteria were used (Nicolaides *et al.* 2005a).

Third, the rate of stenosis progression may determine the risk of stroke in patients with asymptomatic stenosis, which is potentially very important considering the longer time-frame over which strokes occur in patients with asymptomatic compared with symptomatic stenosis. In the ECST, a strong association between the risk of ipsilateral stroke and the degree of carotid stenosis was only seen for strokes that occurred during the first year after randomization, and no relationship was seen between initial stenosis and strokes occurring more than two years later (European Carotid Surgery Trialists' Collaborative Group 1998;

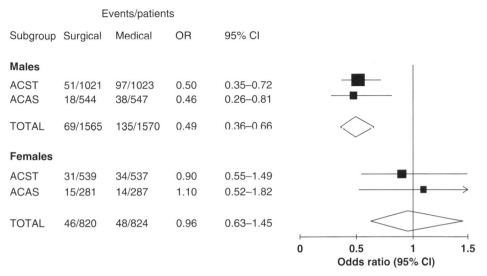

Events/patients

Subgroup	Surgical	Medical	OR	95% CI
Males				
ACST	51/1021	97/1023	0.50	0.35–0.72
ACAS	18/544	38/547	0.46	0.26–0.81
TOTAL	69/1565	135/1570	0.49	0.36–0.66
Females				
ACST	31/539	34/537	0.90	0.55–1.49
ACAS	15/281	14/287	1.10	0.52–1.82
TOTAL	46/820	48/824	0.96	0.63–1.45

Fig. 28.3. The effect of endarterectomy for asymptomatic carotid stenosis on the risk of any stroke and operative death by sex (Rothwell 2004) in the Asymptomatic Carotid Surgery Trial (ACST; Halliday *et al.* 2004) and the ACAS Trial (Executive Committee for the Asymptomatic Carotid Atherosclerosis Study 1995). CI, confidence interval.

Rothwell *et al.* 2000). While this could have been partly a consequence of plaque "healing," it is conceivable that in some patients the degree of stenosis had progressed and the rate of this progression, rather than the degree of stenosis at baseline, was the important determinant of stroke risk.

Which subgroups benefit most?

Although some subgroup analyses were reported in ACAS, the trial had insufficient power to analyze subgroup–treatment effect interactions reliably. Because of its larger sample size, ACST had greater power to evaluate subgroups, although no analyses were prespecified in the trial protocol (Halliday *et al.* 1994). Although ACST did perform some subgroup analyses, the trial only reported results separately for the reduction in risk of non-perioperative stroke (i.e. the benefit) and the perioperative risk (i.e. the harm) (Halliday *et al.* 2004). The overall balance of hazard and benefit, which is of most importance to patients and clinicians, was not reported, although the data could be extracted from the web tables that accompanied the ACST report (Halliday *et al.* 2004).

The ACAS reported a statistically borderline sex–treatment effect interaction, with no benefit from endarterectomy in women (Executive Committee for the Asymptomatic Carotid Atherosclerosis Study 1995). The same trend was seen in ACST (Halliday *et al.* 2004). A meta-analysis of the effect of endarterectomy on the five-year risk of any stroke and perioperative death in ACAS and ACST (Rothwell 2004) (Fig. 28.3) showed that benefit from surgery was greater in men than in women (pooled interaction, $p = 0.01$), and that it remained uncertain whether there is any worthwhile benefit in women at five years of follow-up, although some benefit may accrue with longer follow-up in ACST.

In patients with symptomatic 70–99% carotid stenosis, the surgical complication rate is higher in the presence of contralateral occlusion, although the evidence still favors endarterectomy in these patients (Rothwell *et al.* 2004). However, a post-hoc analysis from

ACAS found that patients with contralateral occlusion derived no long-term benefit from endarterectomy, largely because of the lower long-term risk on medical treatment (Baker *et al.* 2000), but this analysis was under-powered (163 patients) and there was no significant heterogeneity according to presence of contralateral occlusion in ACST (Halliday *et al.* 2004).

Which individuals benefit most?

Given the small absolute reductions in the risk of stroke with endarterectomy in ACST and ACAS, there is an urgent need to identify which individual patients are at highest risk of stroke and which individuals are at such low risk of stroke that the risks of surgery cannot be justified. A risk-modeling approach similar to that used in symptomatic carotid stenosis is required (Chs. 14 and 27), perhaps combining patient clinical features with the results of potentially prognostic investigations, such as transcranial Doppler-detected emboli, impaired cerebral reactivity, the nature of the stenotic plaque on imaging and the rate of plaque progression.

Rates of microembolic signals detected on transcranial Doppler ultrasound scanning might well provide prognostically useful information. A study of 200 patients with recently symptomatic carotid stenosis ≥ 50% found that microembolic signals detected on a one-hour transcranial Doppler recording predicted the 90-day risk of recurrent stroke (Markus *et al.* 2005). In another study of 319 patients with asymptomatic stenosis ≥ 60% (19% had symptoms > 18 months previously), patients with microembolic signals on two one-hour transcranial Doppler recordings were more likely to have a stroke within the first year of follow-up than patients with no such signals (adjusted OR for stroke and TIA combined, 4.72; (95% CI, 1.99–11.19; $p < 0.001$) (Spence *et al.* 2005). However, a multicenter study of 202 patients with asymptomatic stenosis, in which a variable number (mean 4.3) of one-hour transcranial Doppler recordings were made, found only a non-significant trend for more ipsilateral events in arteries positive for microembolic signals (Abbott *et al.* 2005) Further data will soon be available from the ongoing ACES study (Markus and Cullinane 2000).

Several observational studies have suggested that increased plaque echolucency (a marker of plaque lipid and hemorrhage content) on ultrasound is associated with higher risks of stroke and TIA distal to a carotid stenosis. However, most of these studies were in patients with symptomatic stenosis and included TIA in the primary endpoint. In a recent analysis of imaging data from a cohort study of 1115 patients with asymptomatic stenosis, with a mean of 37 months of follow-up, patients were grouped according to the presence of echolucency on baseline ultrasound (Nicolaides *et al.* 2005b). The cumulative stroke rate was 2% per year in patients with plaques that were uniformly or partly echolucent and 0.14% per year in the remaining patients. However, plaque echolucency on ultrasound was not associated with benefit from endarterectomy in ACST (Halliday *et al.* 2004) and further research is required to clarify the significance of plaque lipid content in patients with asymptomatic stenosis.

Other methods of plaque imaging might also be of prognostic value. In a study of 154 patients with asymptomatic carotid stenosis imaged with multi-contrast-weighted MRI and followed up for a mean of 38 months, thin or ruptured fibrous cap, intraplaque hemorrhage and large lipid core on MRI were all associated with ipsilateral TIA and stroke on follow-up (Takaya *et al.* 2006). With gadolinium enhancement, the fibrous cap can be visualized more easily on MRI, which may allow accurate quantification of fibrous cap thickness (Cai *et al.* 2005).

There is also good evidence that inflammation has a causal role in carotid plaque instability (van der Wal *et al.* 1994; Redgrave *et al.* 2006). Visualization of plaque macrophages by MRI after their uptake of ultra-small particles of iron oxide is now possible (Trivedi *et al.* 2004; Tang *et al.* 2006). However, large prospective studies are required to determine whether these imaging characteristics predict the risk of stroke.

Carotid intervention before or during coronary artery surgery

If patients with recently symptomatic carotid stenosis also have symptomatic coronary heart disease requiring surgery, it is unclear whether coronary artery bypass (CABG) should be done before the carotid endarterectomy (and risk a stroke during the procedure), after the carotid endarterectomy (and risk cardiac complications during carotid endarterectomy) or simultaneously under the same general anesthetic (and risk both stroke and cardiac complications all at once) (Graor and Hertzer 1988; Akins 1995; Davenport *et al.* 1995). The apparently high risk of the last option may well be unacceptable, although a small quasi-randomized trial suggests otherwise (Hertzer *et al.* 1989; Borger *et al.* 1999).

Although carotid endarterectomy or stenting are increasingly recommended before coronary surgery, there is little evidence to support this practice. In an attempt to determine the role of carotid artery disease in the etiology of stroke after CABG, Naylor *et al.* (2002) performed a systematic review of published case series. The risk of stroke during the first few weeks after CABG was approximately 2% and remained unchanged from 1970 to 2000. Two-thirds of strokes occurred after day one and 23% died. There was no significant carotid disease in 91% of screened CABG patients. Stroke risk was approximately 3% in predominantly asymptomatic patients with a unilateral 50–99% stenosis, 5% in those with bilateral 50–99% stenoses and 7–11% in patients with carotid occlusion. Significant predictive factors for post-CABG stroke included carotid bruit (OR, 3.6; 95% CI, 2.8–4.6), prior stroke/TIA (OR, 3.6; 95% CI, 2.7–4.9) and severe carotid stenosis/occlusion (OR, 4.3; 95% CI, 3.2–5.7). However, the systematic review indicated that 50% of stroke sufferers did not have significant carotid disease and 60% of territorial infarctions on CT scan/autopsy could not be attributed to carotid disease alone. Therefore, although carotid disease is an important etiological factor in the pathophysiology of post-CABG stroke, carotid endarterectomy could only ever prevent approximately 40% of procedural strokes at most, even assuming that prophylactic carotid endarterectomy carried no additional risk.

In a subsequent systematic review, Naylor *et al.* (2003) aimed to determine the overall cardiovascular risk for patients with coronary and carotid artery disease undergoing synchronous CABG and carotid endarterectomy, staged endarterectomy then CABG and reverse staged CABG then endarterectomy. In a systematic review of 97 published studies following 8972 staged or synchronous operations, mortality was highest in patients undergoing synchronous endarterectomy plus CABG (4.6%; 95% CI, 4.1–5.2). The risk of death or stroke was also highest in patients undergoing this approach (8.7%; 95% CI, 7.7–9.8) and lowest following staged endarterectomy then CABG (6.1%; 95% CI, 2.9–9.3). The risk of death/stroke or myocardial infarction was 11.5% (95% CI, 10.1–12.9) following synchronous procedures. Therefore, approximately 10–12% of patients undergoing staged or synchronous procedures suffer death or major cardiovascular morbidity (stroke, myocardial infarction) within 30 days of surgery.

In summary, the available data suggest that only approximately 40% of strokes complicating CABG could be attributable to ipsilateral carotid artery disease. The rate of death and stroke following staged or synchronous carotid surgery in published series is high, but a large randomized trial is necessary to determine whether a policy of prophylactic carotid endarterectomy reduces the risk of stroke after cardiac surgery. However, in the absence of any randomized evidence of benefit, the available data do not support a policy of routine intervention for carotid stenosis in patients undergoing CABG (Naylor, 2004).

References

Abbott AL, Chambers BR, Stork JL et al. (2005). Embolic signals and prediction of ipsilateral stroke or transient ischemic attack in asymptomatic carotid stenosis: a multicenter prospective cohort study. Stroke 36:1128–1133

Akins CW (1995). The case for concomitant carotid and coronary artery surgery. British Heart Journal 74:97–98

Baker WH, Howard VJ, Howard G et al. (2000). Effect of contralateral occlusion on long-term efficacy of endarterectomy in the asymptomatic carotid atherosclerosis study (ACAS). ACAS Investigators. Stroke 31:2330–2334

Benade MM, Warlow CP (2002a). Cost of identifying patients for carotid endarterectomy. Stroke 33:435–439

Benade MM, Warlow CP (2002b). Costs and benefits of carotid endarterectomy and associated preoperative arterial imaging: a systematic review of health economic literature. Stroke 33:629–638

Bond R, Rerkasem K, Rothwell PM (2003a). A systematic review of the risks of carotid endarterectomy in relation to the clinical indication and the timing of surgery. Stroke 34:2290–2301

Bond R, Rerkasem K, Rothwell PM (2003b). High morbidity due to endarterectomy for asymptomatic carotid stenosis. Cerebrovascular Diseases 16(Suppl 4):65

Borger MA, Fremes SE, Weisel RD et al. (1999). Coronary bypass and carotid endartertomy: a combined approach increases risk? A meta-analysis. Annals of Thoracic Surgery 68:14–21

Cai J, Hatsukami TS, Ferguson MS et al. (2005). In vivo quantitative measurement of intact fibrous cap and lipid-rich necrotic core size in atherosclerotic carotid plaque: comparison of high-resolution, contrast-enhanced magnetic resonance imaging and histology. Circulation 112:3437–3444

Chambers BR, Donnan GA (2005). Carotid endarterectomy for asymptomatic carotid stenosis. Cochrane Database of Systemic Reviews; 4:CD001923

Chaturvedi S, Bruno A, Feasby T et al. (2005). Carotid endarterectomy-an evidence-based review: report of the Therapeutics and Technology Assessment Subcommittee of the American Academy of Neurology. Neurology 65:794–801

Cuffe RL, Rothwell PM (2006). Effect of non-optimal imaging on the relationship between the measured degree of symptomatic carotid stenosis and risk of ischemic stroke. Stroke 37:1785–1791

Davenport RJ, Dennis MS, Sandercock PA et al. (1995). How should a patient presenting with unstable angina and a recent stroke be managed? British Medical Journal 310:1449–1452

European Carotid Surgery Trialists' Collaborative Group (1998). Randomised trial of endarterectomy for recently symptomatic carotid stenosis: final results of the MRC European Carotid Surgery Trial (ECST). Lancet 351:1379–1387

Executive Committee for the Asymptomatic Carotid Atherosclerosis Study (1995). Endarterectomy for asymptomatic carotid artery stenosis. Journal of the American Medical Association 273:1421–1428

Graor RA, Hertzer NR (1988). Management of coexistent carotid artery and coronary artery disease. Stroke 19:1441–1443

Halliday AW, Thomas D, Mansfield A (1994). The Asymptomatic Carotid Surgery Trial (ACST). Rationale and design. Steering Committee. European Journal of Vascular Surgery 8:703–710

Halliday A, Mansfield A, Marro J et al. (2004). Prevention of disabling and fatal strokes by successful carotid endarterectomy in patients without recent neurological symptoms: randomised controlled trial. Lancet 363:1491–1502

Hertzer NR, Loop FD, Beven EG et al. (1989). Surgical staging for simultaneous coronary and carotid disease: a study including prospective randomisation. Journal of Vascular Surgery 9:455–463

Kresowik TF, Bratzler DW, Kresowik RA *et al.* (2004). Multistate improvement in process and outcomes of carotid endarterectomy. *Journal of Vascular Surgery* **39**:372–380

Markus HS, Cullinane M (2000). Asymptomatic Carotid Emboli (ACES) Study. *Cerebrovascular Diseases* **10**(Suppl 1):3

Markus HS, MacKinnon A (2005). Asymptomatic embolization detected by Doppler ultrasound predicts stroke risk in symptomatic carotid artery stenosis. *Stroke* **36**:971–975

Moore WS, Young B, Baker WH *et al.* (1996). Surgical results: a justification of the surgeon selection process for the ACAS trial. The ACAS Investigators. *Journal of Vascular Surgery* **23**:323–328

Naylor AR (2004). A critical review of the role of carotid disease and the outcomes of staged and synchronous carotid surgery. *Seminars in Cardiothoracic Vascular Anesthesia* **8**:37–42

Naylor AR, Mehta Z, Rothwell PM *et al.* (2002). Carotid artery disease and stroke during coronary artery bypass: a critical review of the literature. *European Journal of Vascular Endovascular Surgery* **23**:283–294

Naylor AR, Cuffe RL, Rothwell PM *et al.* (2003). A systematic review of outcomes following staged and synchronous carotid endarterectomy and coronary artery bypass. *European Journal of Vascular Endovascular Surgery* **25**:380–389

Nicolaides AN, Kakkos SK, Griffin M *et al.* (2005a). Severity of asymptomatic carotid stenosis and risk of ipsilateral hemispheric ischaemic events: results from the ACSRS study. *European Journal of Vascular Endovascular Surgery* **30**:275–284

Nicolaides AN, Kakkos SK, Griffin M *et al.* (2005b). Effect of image normalization on carotid plaque classification and the risk of ipsilateral hemispheric ischemic events: results from the asymptomatic carotid stenosis and risk of stroke study. *Vascular* **13**:211–221

Redgrave JN, Lovett JK, Gallagher PJ *et al.* (2006). Histological assessment of 526 symptomatic carotid plaques in relation to the nature and timing of ischemic symptoms: the Oxford plaque study. *Circulation* **113**:2320–2328

Rothwell PM (2004). ACST: which subgroups will benefit most from carotid endarterectomy? *Lancet* **364**:1122–1123

Rothwell PM, Slattery J, Warlow CP (1996). A systematic review of the risk of stroke and death due to carotid endarterectomy. *Stroke* **27**:260–265

Rothwell PM, Warlow CP on behalf of the European Carotid Surgery Trialists' Collaborative Group (2000). Low risk of ischaemic stroke in patients with reduced internal carotid artery lumen diameter distal to severe symptomatic carotid stenosis. *Stroke* **31**:622–630

Rothwell PM, Gutnikov SA, Eliasziw M for the Carotid Endarterectomy Trialists' Collaboration. (2003). Pooled analysis of individual patient data from randomised controlled trials of endarterectomy for symptomatic carotid stenosis. *Lancet* **361**:107–116

Rothwell PM, Eliasziw M, Gutnikov SA *et al.* for the Carotid Endarterectomy Trialists Collaboration. (2004). Effect of endarterectomy for symptomatic carotid stenosis in relation to clinical subgroups and to the timing of surgery. *Lancet* **363**:915–924

Spence JD, Tamayo A, Lownie SP *et al.* (2005). Absence of microemboli on transcranial Doppler identifies low-risk patients with asymptomatic carotid stenosis. *Stroke* **36**:2373–2378

Takaya N, Yuan C, Chu B *et al.* (2006). Association between carotid plaque characteristics and subsequent ischemic cerebrovascular events: a prospective assessment with MRI-initial results. *Stroke* **37**:818–823

Tang T, Howarth SP, Miller SR *et al.* (2006). Assessment of inflammatory burden contralateral to the symptomatic carotid stenosis using high-resolution ultrasmall, superparamagnetic iron oxide-enhanced MRI. *Stroke* **37**:2266–2270

Trivedi RA, King-Im JM, Graves MJ *et al.* (2004). In vivo detection of macrophages in human carotid atheroma: temporal dependence of ultrasmall superparamagnetic particles of iron oxide-enhanced MRI. *Stroke* **35**:1631–1635

van der Wal AC, Becker AE, van der Loos CM *et al.* (1994). Site of intimal rupture or erosion of thrombosed coronary atherosclerotic plaques is characterized by an inflammatory process irrespective of the dominant plaque morphology. *Circulation* **89**:36–44

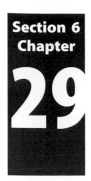

Miscellaneous disorders
Cerebral venous thrombosis

Thrombosis in the dural sinuses or cerebral veins is much less common than cerebral arterial thromboembolism. It causes a variety of clinical syndromes, which often do not resemble stroke (Bousser and Ross Russell 1997). While ischemic arterial stroke and cerebral venous thrombosis share some causes (Southwick *et al.* 1986), others are specific to cerebral venous thrombosis (Table 29.1). A particularly high index of suspicion is required in women on the oral contraceptive pill (Saadatnia and Tajmirriahi 2007) and in the puerperium. In the past, cerebral venous thrombosis was strongly associated with otitis media and mastoiditis, "lateral sinus thrombosis" or "otitic hydrocephalus," but the most common causes are now pregnancy and the puerperium, which cause 5–20% of the cerebral venous thrombosis in the developed world, the oral contraceptive pill, malignancy, dehydration, inflammatory disorders and hereditary coagulation disorders. No cause is found in around 20% of cases.

Clinical features

In cerebral venous thrombosis, the superior sagittal sinus (Fig. 29.1) and the lateral sinuses are those most commonly affected. These are followed by the straight sinuses and the cavernous sinuses (Stam 2005; Girot *et al.* 2007) (see Fig. 4.4 [p. 44] for anatomy). Thrombosis of the galenic system or isolated involvement of the cortical veins is infrequent. Cerebral venous thrombosis causes a rise in venous pressure, leading to venous distension and edema. This may be accompanied by raised intracranial pressure since the dural sinuses contain most of the arachnoid villi and granulations in which cerebrospinal fluid absorption takes place. Occlusion of one of the larger venous sinuses is not likely to cause localized tissue damage unless there is involvement of cortical veins or the galenic venous system, since alternative drainage routes will suffice. Thrombosis in cerebral veins, with or without dural sinus thrombosis, causes multiple "venous" infarcts, which are congested, edematous and often hemorrhagic. Subarachnoid bleeding may occur. Transient neurological deficits may be caused by temporary ischemia and edema.

The incidence of cerebral venous thrombosis is uncertain since it has a wide range of clinical manifestations (Bousser 2000), which may sometimes be obscured by the underlying disease process, such as meningitis. It may be asymptomatic, and diagnosis depends on access to cerebral imaging. Cerebral venous thrombosis should be suspected when a patient develops signs of raised intracranial pressure with or without focal neurological deficits, papilloedema and seizures, particularly when the CT brain scan is normal (Box 29.1). Headache, which is often the presenting complaint, is present in 75% of those affected and has no specific characteristics: it may be acute or chronic, localized or diffuse (Agostoni 2004). Papilloedema occurs in approximately 50%. Focal deficits, seizures and alterations in conscious level occur in approximately 30%. Isolated cranial nerve palsies have been

Table 29.1. Causes of intracranial venous thrombosis

Disorder	Examples
Conditions affecting the cerebral veins and sinuses directly	Head injury (with or without fracture)
	Intracranial surgery
	Local sepsis (sinuses, ears, mastoids, scalp, nasopharynx)
	Subdural empyema
	Bacterial meningitis
	Dural arteriovenous fistula
	Tumor invasion of dural sinus (malignant meningitis, lymphoma, skull base secondary, etc.)
	Catheterization of jugular vein
	Lumbar puncture
Systemic disorders	Dehydration
	Septicemia
	Pregnancy and the puerperium
	Oral contraceptives/hormone replacement therapy
	Hematological disorders
	Prothrombotic states
	Inflammatory vascular disorders
	Homocysteinuria
	Congestive cardiac failure
	Inflammatory bowel disease
	Androgen therapy
	Antifibrinolytic drugs
	Non-metastatic effect of extracranial malignancy
	Nephrotic syndrome

described with transverse sinus thrombosis (Kuehnen *et al.* 1998). Cerebral venous thrombosis may be the underlying cause in patients with features suggestive of diffuse encephalopathy, stroke and, rarely, subarachnoid hemorrhage (de Bruijn *et al.* 1996), psychosis or migraine (Jacobs *et al.* 1996). It should be considered in all cases of apparent idiopathic intracranial hypertension, particularly when the patient is male or a non-obese female (Tehindrazanarivelo *et al.* 1992).

The progression of symptoms and signs in cerebral venous thrombosis is highly variable, ranging from less than 48 hours to greater than 30 days. A gradual onset over days or weeks of headache; papilloedema and, less frequently, cranial nerve VI palsy, tinnitus and transient visual obscuration may occur. The prognosis of cerebral venous thrombosis is also variable and difficult to predict for an individual patient: a comatose patient may go on to make a complete recovery whereas a patient with few signs may gradually deteriorate and die. The current case-fatality rate appears to be 10–20%, with a further 10–20% surviving with persistent deficits (Bousser 2000; Girot *et al.* 2007). Independent predictors of death in one study were coma, mental disturbance, deep thrombosis,

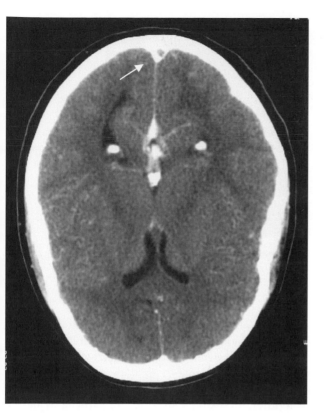

Fig. 29.1. A CT brain scan from a young woman with superior sagittal sinus thrombosis showing the "empty delta sign" – a triangular pattern of enhancement surrounding a central relatively hypodense area of thrombosis (arrow).

intracerebral hemorrhage and posterior fossa lesions (Canhao *et al.* 2005). In the International Study on Cerebral Vein and Dural Sinus Thrombosis (Girot *et al.* 2007), independent predictors of a poor outcome, as defined by death or disability at six months, were older age, male gender, having a deep cerebral venous system thrombosis or a right lateral sinus thrombosis, and having a motor deficit. The prognosis for thrombosis of the deep cerebral veins is particularly poor.

Box 29.1. Clinical features of cerebral venous thrombosis
Headache
Seizure
Reduced conscious level
Focal neurological deficit
• Cranial nerve palsies
Features of raised intracranial pressure:
• papilloedema
• vomiting

Cavernous sinus thrombosis is a restricted form of cerebral venous thrombosis, usually associated with sepsis spreading from the veins in the face, nose, orbits or sinuses (Ebright *et al.* 2001). In diabetics and immunocompromised hosts, fungal infection can be responsible, particularly mucormycosis. The presentation is with unilateral orbital pain, periorbital edema, chemosis, proptosis, reduced visual acuity and papilloedema. Cranial nerves III, IV, VI and the upper two divisions of V may be involved. Thrombus may propagate to the other cavernous sinus to cause bilateral signs. Septic meningitis and epidural empyema are occasional complications. The patients are generally severely toxic and ill. The differential diagnosis includes severe facial and orbital infection, and caroticocavernous fistula.

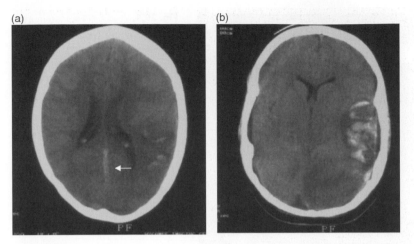

Fig. 29.2. Non-contrast CT brain scans showing fresh thrombus in the straight sinus ("cord sign") (a; arrow) and a hemorrhagic left temporal lobe infarct (b).

Diagnosis

Headache, papilloedema and a normal CT scan should raise the possibility of cerebral venous thrombosis. Often cerebral venous thrombosis is not considered until other diagnoses have been excluded, particularly when the presentation is atypical. However, it is not a diagnosis of exclusion – it must be confirmed on imaging.

Although brain CT with contrast is normal in up to 25% of patients with proven cerebral venous thrombosis, it is an appropriate first-line investigation particularly in sick patients in whom MRI is difficult to undertake. Hemorrhagic and non-hemorrhagic infarcts outwith the usual arterial territories, edema and intense contrast enhancement of the falx and tentorium may be seen. Sometimes there is subarachnoid blood, which is most unusual following either arterial infarcts or primary intracerebral hemorrhage (Bakac and Wardlaw 1997). Specific but less-common changes include the "empty delta sign," a triangular pattern of enhancement from dilated venous collateral channels surrounding a central relatively hypodense area of thrombosis, indicating superior sagittal sinus thrombosis (Fig. 29.1). Another is the "cord sign" seen on a single slice only on non-contrast-enhanced CT scans, in which fresh thrombus appears as increased density relative to gray matter in structures parallel to the scanning plane such as the straight sinus (Fig. 29.2).

Magnetic resonance imaging has greater sensitivity than CT for the changes of cerebral venous thrombosis (Bousser and Ross Russell 1997; Ferro *et al.* 2007). In the acute phase, at less than three to five days, the thrombus is isointense on both T_1- and T_2-weighted sequences. Subsequently, the thrombus becomes hyperintense (Fig. 29.3). After two to three weeks, findings depend on whether or not the sinus remains occluded or whether it is partly or completely recanalized.

The imaging changes in patients with deep cerebral venous thrombosis are particularly striking, with bilateral deep hemorrhagic infarction (Fig. 29.4). Magnetic resonance imaging and venography can now provide a definitive diagnosis in most patients, although care must be taken to exclude artefacts.

Cerebral angiography with late venous views is the "gold standard" for the diagnosis of cerebral venous thrombosis. Nowadays, this should only be performed in those cases where the diagnosis remains in doubt after MRI. There should be total or partial occlusion of

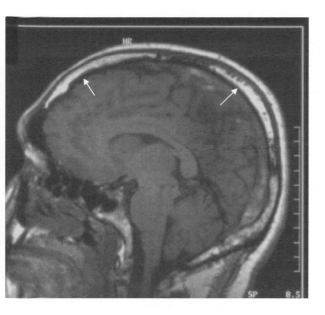

Fig. 29.3. Saggital T$_1$-weighted MRI showing hyperintensity in the saggital sinus indicating subacute thrombosis (arrows).

(a)

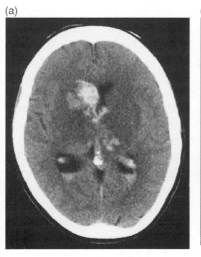

(b)

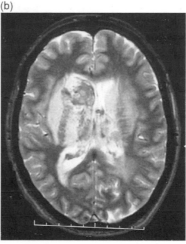

Fig. 29.4. Axial CT (a) and T$_2$-weighted MR brain (b) slices in a patient with deep cerebral venous thrombosis with bilateral deep hemorrhagic infarction.

at least one dural sinus on two projections. Often, there is also occlusion of cerebral veins, late venous emptying and evidence of venous collateral circulation. In subacute encephalopathies of uncertain cause, cerebral angiography or MR venography should always be carried out to exclude cerebral venous thrombosis before resorting to brain biopsy.

Cerebrospinal fluid is often abnormal in cerebral venous thrombosis: the pressure is usually raised and there may be elevated protein and pleocytosis, especially in patients with focal signs. Lumbar puncture may be indicated in patients with isolated intracranial hypertension in order to lower cerebrospinal fluid pressure when vision is threatened and to exclude meningeal infection.

The electroencephalogram is abnormal in approximately 75% of patients with cerebral venous thrombosis, but changes are non-specific, with generalized slowing, often asymmetric, with superimposed epileptic activity.

Treatment

The general principles of stroke treatment apply. There is little evidence for specific treatments in cerebral venous thrombosis. Despite this, most clinicians advocate anticoagulant therapy in line with guidelines for venous thromboembolism. This may prevent extension of the clot into neighboring sinuses and veins, which is often accompanied by rapid deterioration (Einhaupl *et al.* 2006). Heparin has been reported to be safe and to improve prognosis in one small trial (Einhaupl *et al.* 1991), but this was not confirmed in a larger trial (de Bruijn *et al.* 1999). Anticoagulant therapy is associated with hemorrhage into venous infarcts, but it is currently not possible to identify patients at high risk of this complication. Thrombolytic infusion has been used in patients with cerebral venous thrombosis, but there are no randomized data (Kasner *et al.* 1998) and it should be reserved for patients who continue to deteriorate despite anticoagulation and supportive measures.

The European Federation of Neurological Societies guidelines (Einhaupl *et al.* 2006) advise as follows

> Patients with cerebral venous thrombosis without contraindications to anticoagulation should be treated either with body weight-adjusted subcutaneous low molecular weight or dose-adjusted intravenous heparins. Concomitant intracranial hemorrhage related to cerebral venous thrombosis is not a contraindication for heparin therapy. The optimal duration of oral anticoagulation after the acute phase is unclear. Oral anticoagulation may be given for 3 months if cerebral venous thrombosis was secondary to a transient risk factor, for 6–12 months in patients with idiopathic cerebral venous thrombosis and in those with "mild" hereditary thrombophilia. Indefinite anticoagulation should be considered in patients with two or more episodes of cerebral venous thrombosis or in those with one episode of cerebral venous thrombosis and "severe" hereditary thrombophilia. There is insufficient evidence to support the use of either systemic or local thrombolysis in patients with cerebral venous thrombosis. If patients deteriorate despite adequate anticoagulation and other causes of deterioration have been ruled out, thrombolysis may be a therapeutic option in selected cases, possibly in those without intracranial hemorrhage. There are no controlled data about the risks and benefits of certain therapeutic measures to reduce an elevated intracranial pressure with brain displacement in patients with severe cerebral venous thrombosis. Antioedema treatment, including hyperventilation, osmotic diuretics and craniectomy, should be used as life saving interventions.

Any underlying cause should be addressed: for example, patients with a definite thrombophilia should probably take anticoagulation drugs for life; oral contraceptives should never be used again, but a further pregnancy may be safe (Preter *et al.* 1996).

References

Agostoni E (2004). Headache in cerebral venous thrombosis. *Neurology Science* 25:S206–S210

Bakac G, Wardlaw JM (1997). Problems in the diagnosis of intracranial venous infarction. *Neuroradiology* 39:566–570

Bousser MG (2000). Cerebral venous thrombosis: diagnosis and management. *Journal of Neurology* 247:252–258

Bousser MG, Ross Russell R (1997). *Cerebral venous thrombosis*. London: Saunders

Canhao P, Ferro JM, Lindgren AG *et al.* (2005). Causes and predictors of death in cerebral venous thrombosis. *Stroke* 36:1720–1725

de Bruijn SFTM, Stam J (1999). Randomised placebo controlled trial of anticoagulant treatment with low molecular weight heparin for cerebral sinus thrombosis. *Stroke* 30:484–488

de Bruijn SFTM, Stam J, Kappelle LJ (1996). Thunderclap headache as first symptom of cerebral venous sinus thrombosis. *Lancet* 348:1623–1625

Ebright JR, Pace MT, Niazi AF (2001). Septic thrombosis of the cavernous sinuses. *Archives of Internal Medicine* **161**:2671–2676

Einhaupl KM, Villringer A, Meister W *et al.* (1991). Heparin treatment in sinus venous thrombosis. *Lancet* **338**:597–600

Einhaupl K, Bousser MG, de Bruijn SF *et al.* (2006). EFNS guideline on the treatment of cerebral venous and sinus thrombosis. *European Journal of Neurology* **13**:553–559

Ferro JM, Morgado C, Sousa R *et al.* (2007). Interobserver agreement in the magnetic resonance location of cerebral vein and dural sinus thrombosis. *European Journal of Neurology* **14**:353–356

Girot M, Ferro JM, Canhao P *et al.* (2007). Predictors of outcome in patients with cerebral venous thrombosis and intracerebral hemorrhage. *Stroke* **38**:337–342

Jacobs K, Moulin T, Bogousslavsky J *et al.* (1996). The stroke syndrome of cortical vein thrombosis. *Neurology* **47**:376–382

Kasner SE, Gurian JH, Grotta JC (1998). Urokinase treatment of sagittal sinus thrombosis with venous haemorrhagic infarction. *Journal of Stroke and Cerebrovascular Diseases* **7**:421–425

Kuehnen J, Schwartz A, Neff W *et al.* (1998). Cranial nerve syndrome in thrombosis of the transverse/sigmoid sinuses. *Brain* **121**:381–388

Preter M, Tzourio C, Ameri A *et al.* (1996). Long-term prognosis in cerebral venous thrombosis: follow-up of 77 patients. *Stroke* **27**:243–246

Saadatnia M, Tajmirriahi M (2007). Hormonal contraceptives as a risk factor for cerebral venous and sinus thrombosis. *Acta Neurology Scandinavica* **115**:295–300

Southwick FS, Richardson EP, Swartz MN (1986). Septic thrombosis of the dural venous sinuses. *Medicine (Baltimore)* **65**:82–106

Stam J (2005). Thrombosis of the cerebral veins and sinuses. *New England Journal of Medicine* **352**:1791–1798

Tehindrazanarivelo A, Evrard S, Schaison M *et al.* (1992). Prospective study of cerebral sinus venous thrombosis in patients presenting with benign intracranial hypertension. *Cerebrovascular Diseases* **2**:22–27

Chapter 30

Spontaneous subarachnoid hemorrhage

Subarachnoid hemorrhage (SAH) is a fairly rare condition but it is relatively more common in younger people than other forms of cerebrovascular disease. Although the prognosis is grave, there has been a fall in mortality over recent decades, which suggests improvements in management of the condition. The presentation is usually dramatic, with sudden-onset severe headache, but diagnostic difficulty may arise in atypical cases or with other conditions that can mimic SAH.

Epidemiology

The incidence of subarachnoid hemorrhage increases with age and is approximately 5–10 per 100 000 population/annum. Nonetheless, half of cases occur in those younger than 55 years (Linn *et al.* 1996; Rothwell *et al.* 2004). Data from the Oxford Community Stroke Project (OCSP) and Oxford Vascular Study (OXVASC) show that there has been no change in the incidence of SAH since the late 1980s but there has been a fall in mortality, suggesting improved management of the condition. Risk factors for SAH include hypertension, smoking, alcohol, oral contraceptives and possibly coronary heart disease (Feigin *et al.* 2005a).The overall prognosis is poor: half of patients die and around one-third of survivors are left dependent (Hop *et al.* 1997; van Gijn *et al.* 2007). Coma on admission, old age and a large amount of blood on the initial CT scan all are associated with a worse prognosis (Kassell *et al.* 1990a, b). Focal neurological deficits and, more commonly, cognitive deficits, behavioral disorders, seizures, anxiety, depression and poor quality of life are frequent long-term sequelae (Hop *et al.* 1999). Chronic or repeated subarachnoid bleeding can produce the rare syndrome of superficial hemosiderosis of the central nervous system (CNS), with sensorineural deafness, cerebellar ataxia, pyramidal signs, dementia and bladder disturbance (Fearnley *et al.* 1995).

Causes

Approximately 85% of spontaneous SAHs are caused by ruptured aneurysm; 10% are perimesencephalic and the remainder are caused by rare disorders (van Gijn and Rinkel 2001). The pattern of bleeding on CT is a clue to the underlying cause. Blood in the interhemispheric fissure suggests an anterior communicating artery aneurysm and in the sylvian fissure suggests internal carotid artery or middle cerebral artery aneurysm (Fig. 30.1).

Intracranial aneurysms are not congenital but develop over the course of life. Approximately 10% of aneurysms are familial, and candidate genes identified thus far include those coding for the extracellular matrix. Saccular aneurysms tend to occur at branching points on the circle of Willis and proximal cerebral arteries: approximately 40% on the anterior communicating artery complex, 30% on the posterior communicating artery or distal internal carotid artery, 20% on the middle cerebral artery and 10% in the posterior

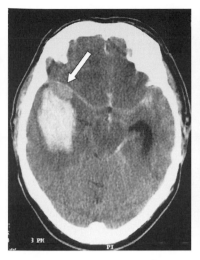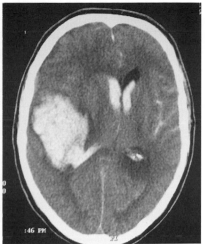

Fig. 30.1. These CT brain scans from a patient with a burst right middle cerebral artery aneurysm (arrow) show widespread subarachnoid blood, and rupture into the right cerebral hemisphere and the ventricular system.

circulation (Fig. 30.2). Approximately 25% occur at multiple sites. Aneurysms vary from a few millimeters to several centimeters in diameter, can enlarge with time and are an incidental finding in about 6% of cerebral angiograms. This is almost certainly an over-estimate of the true rate, which may be around 2% (Rinkel *et al.* 1998).

Aneurysms may present with various clinical features:

- most commonly in middle life with subarachnoid hemorrhage
- with primary intracerebral hemorrhage
- with compression of adjacent structures, such as the optic nerve by an anterior communicating artery aneurysm, III, IV, V cranial nerves by a distal internal carotid artery or posterior communicating artery aneurysm, or brainstem by a basilar artery aneurysm
- with seizures
- with TIA or ischemic stroke through embolism of intra-aneurysmal thrombus (Chs. 6, 8 and 9)
- with caroticocavernous fistula from rupture of an intracavernous internal carotid artery aneurysm (Raps *et al.* 1993).

Clinical features

Subarachnoid hemorrhage may be provoked by exertion and rarely occurs during sleep (Ferro and Pinto 1994; Vermeer *et al.* 1997). The cardinal symptom is sudden severe headache, usually generalized, but other modes of presentation are possible. It is described as of instantaneous onset in around 50% of patients but it may develop subacutely over five minutes or more (Linn *et al.* 1998), and may persist for weeks (Vermeulen *et al.* 1992; Warlow *et al.* 1996a; Schievink 1997). Headaches preceding SAH, thought to be caused by so-called "warning leaks" or "sentinel bleeds," are rare and overestimation of their import-ance is likely to have resulted from recall bias in hospital studies. Therefore, the presence or absence of previous headache has no bearing on the diagnosis of SAH. About a quarter of patients presenting with sudden severe headache will have SAH; a further 40% will have

349

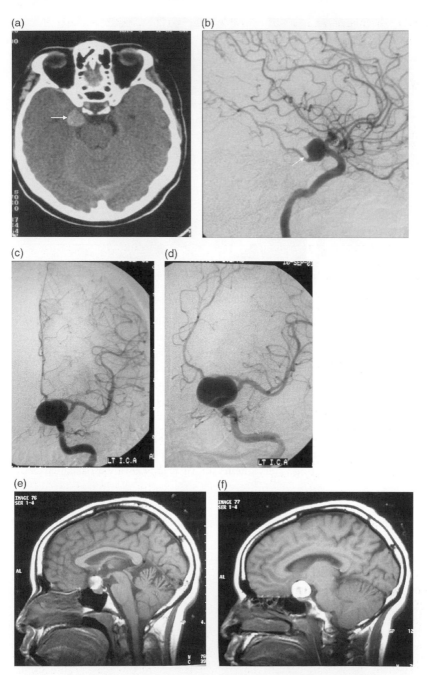

Fig. 30.2. (a, b) Unruptured aneurysm of posterior communicating artery on CT brain imaging (a) and catheter angiography (b). (c, d) Cerebral angiogram showing a large aneurysm at the origin of the left internal carotid artery. (e, f) Sagittal T1-weighted MRI showing a large thrombosed aneurysm.

benign thunderclap headache and about an eighth have some other serious neurological disorder. The remainder have other headache syndromes (Linn *et al.* 1998).

Headache may be the only symptom in SAH or there may be accompanying symptoms that may also be seen with other causes of sudden-onset headache and so are not diagnostic. Patients are often irritable and photophobic. Loss of consciousness occurs in around half the patients but may only be brief. Nausea and vomiting are less common. Partial or generalized seizures occasionally occur at the onset period; since these do not occur in perimesencephalic hemorrhage or in thunderclap headache, their presence is a strong indicator of aneurysmal rupture (Pinto *et al.* 1996). Early development of focal symptoms and signs suggest:

- an associated intracerebral hematoma
- local pressure from an aneurysm, such as posterior communicating artery aneurysm causing a third nerve palsy.

Later on, focal symptoms are more likely to result from delayed cerebral ischemia. Meningism develops over a few hours, and pain may radiate down the legs, mimicking sciatica, but neck stiffness may be absent in unconscious patients. Preretinal and subhyaloid hemorrhages occur in a seventh of patients. There may be a mild fever and raised blood pressure and electrocardiographic changes that may be mistaken for myocardial infarction. Cardiac arrest occurs at onset of hemorrhage in approximately 3% of patients, half of whom survive to independent existence with resuscitation (Toussaint *et al.* 2005). Approximately 10% of SAHs results in sudden death and approximately 15% of patients die before receiving medical attention (Huang and van Gelder 2002). The patient's state can be graded using the World Federation of Neurological Surgeons Scale (Table 30.1).

Table 30.1. World Federation of Neurological Surgeons' Scale for grading subarachnoid hemorrhage

Grade	Glasgow Coma Scale	Motor or language deficit
I	15	Absent
II	14–13	Absent
III	14–13	Present
IV	12–7	Present or absent
V	6–3	Present or absent

Table 30.2. Differential diagnosis of sudden unexpected headache

Neck rigidity	Subarachnoid hemorrhage
	Acute painful neck conditions
	Meningitis/encephalitis
	Cerebellar/brainstem stroke
	Intraventricular hemorrhage
	Recent head injury
Without neck rigidity	Migraine
	Thunderclap headache
	Sex headache
	Benign exertional headache
	Pituitary apoplexy
	Pheochromocytoma
	Expanding intracranial aneurysm
	Carotid or vertebral artery dissection
	Intracranial venous thrombosis
	Occipital neuralgia
	Acute obstructive hydrocephalus

Diagnosis

Since no clinical feature is specific to SAH, the diagnosis must be excluded in anyone presenting with sudden-onset severe headache lasting more than an hour and for which there is no alternative explanation. However, the differential diagnosis is wide (Table 30.2).

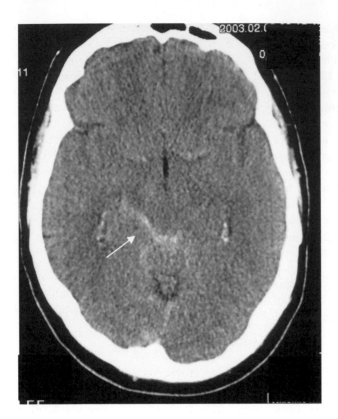

Fig. 30.3. A CT brain scan showing a perimesencephalic subarachnoid hemorrhage with blood in the basal cisterns only (arrow).

Brain imaging

Unenhanced CT scan is the quickest, most informative and cost-effective confirmatory investigation to detect blood in the subarachnoid space (Warlow *et al.* 1996b). The sensitivity of CT for detecting subarachnoid blood depends on the amount of subarachnoid blood, the interval after symptom onset, the resolution of the scanner and the skills of the radiologist. Scanning with CT misses approximately 2% of SAHs within 12 hours and this rises to 7% at 24-hours. Blood is almost completely reabsorbed within 10 days, and probably sooner with very mild SAHs (Brouwers *et al.* 1992). A false-positive diagnosis of SAH may be made in diffuse brain swelling when congested subarachnoid blood vessels cause a hyperdense appearance in the subarachnoid space.

Use of CT provides a baseline for the diagnosis of later rebleeding, reveals any intra-cerebral, ventricular or subdural hematoma or complicating hydrocephalus and may show calcification in the rim of an aneurysm. The pattern of bleeding may indicate the culprit aneurysm if multiple aneurysms are found on later angiography (Adams *et al.* 1983; Vermeulen and van Gijn 1990), or it may show benign perimesencephalic hemorrhage (Rinkel *et al.* 1991) (Fig. 30.3). Evidence of primary or secondary head injury, including brain contusion, soft tissue swelling of the scalp and skull fracture, may be present.

Lumbar puncture

All patients with suspected SAH and a normal CT brain require lumbar puncture (van der Wee *et al.* 1995). The lumbar puncture should be delayed until at least 12 hours after the onset of the headache, unless CNS infection is suspected, to allow hemoglobin to degrade into oxyhemoglobin and bilirubin (van Gijn and Rinkel 2001). Bilirubin signifies SAH since it is only synthesized in vivo, whereas oxyhemoglobin may result from a traumatic spinal tap. Acutely, the cerebrospinal fluid (CSF) glucose may be low, and the protein slightly raised with mild pleocytosis. The presence of "xanthochromia," the yellow bilirubin pigment present in CSF following SAH, may be seen when the CSF is examined with the naked eye against a white background (Linn *et al.* 2005). However samples of CSF should also be sent for spectrophotometry to detect bilirubin (UK National External Quality Assessment Scheme for Immunochemistry Working Group 2003). The least blood-stained sample of CSF should be taken to the laboratory and centrifuged immediately. The sample should be protected from light to prevent degradation of bilirubin. The estimation of red blood cell counts in serial samples does not reliably distinguish SAH from traumatic tap (van Gijn and Rinkel 2001).

Subarachnoid hemorrhage presenting more than two weeks after onset

If CT and CSF examination are normal within two weeks of headache onset, then SAH has been excluded. However, since xanthochromia is only detected in 70% of patients after three weeks and only 40% after four weeks, patients presenting beyond two weeks require investigation with CT or MR angiography or by catheter angiography.

Angiography

The chosen method of imaging of the cerebral circulation depends on the available technology. Multislice CT angiography is becoming more widespread because of its speed, tolerability, safety and potential for three-dimensional reconstructions. The sensitivity of CT angiography for aneurysms > 3 mm diameter is approximately 96% but it is less for smaller aneurysms. The sensitivity for detecting ruptured aneurysms with conventional angiography as the gold standard is currently around 95% (Villablanca *et al.* 2002; Chappell *et al.* 2003; Wintermark *et al.* 2003). Angiography using MR has similar resolution to CT angiography but is less convenient and easy to use, especially in sick patients. Four-vessel catheter angiography may be required when non-invasive imaging is negative or unavailable.

Perimesencephalic subarachnoid hemorrhage

Idiopathic perimesencephalic SAH is restricted to the perimesencephalic cistern anterior to the midbrain (Fig. 30.3) (Schwartz and Solomon 1996). Patients present with acute headache, which may be more gradual in onset than in aneurysmal rupture (Linn *et al.* 1998) but loss of consciousness, focal symptoms and seizures are rare. The cause of perimesencephalic SAH is usually unknown but it has an extremely good prognosis since rebleeding and vasospasm are unlikely (Rinkel *et al.* 1993). Aneurysms of the basilar and vertebral arteries may occasionally cause extravasation of blood into the midbrain cisterns in 2.5–5% of cases of perimesencephalitic SAH (Pinto *et al.* 1993). Such aneurysms may be excluded by performing high-quality CT angiography (Ruigrok *et al.* 2000).

Angiogram-negative subarachnoid hemorrhage

In up to 20% of CT- or CSF-positive SAH, the cerebral angiogram shows no aneurysm, so-called "angiogram negative SAH." It should be noted that a traumatic lumbar puncture may be misdiagnosed as xanthochromic. Angiogram-negative SAH results when there is a false-negative angiogram (in 2–23%) or when the SAH was caused by something other than an intracerebral aneurysm (Rinkel *et al.* 1993). The pattern of subarachnoid bleeding is an important clue as to whether the bleed is likely to have been caused by an underlying aneurysm. In two-thirds of patients with angiogram-negative SAH, the CT shows perimesencephalic blood (Fig. 30.3). Patients with diffuse or anteriorly located blood on CT that represents an aneurysmal pattern of hemorrhage are at risk of rebleeding, and repeat angiography should be performed. Repeat angiography is also required where the previous angiogram was technically inadequate, or if views of the cerebral vasculature were incomplete owing to vasospasm or hemorrhage.

Spinal subarachnoid hemorrhage

Spinal subarachnoid hemorrhage is very rare. It is caused by a vascular malformation, hemostatic failure, coarctation of the aorta, inflammatory vascular disease, mycotic aneurysm or a vascular tumor such as ependymoma. Accumulating hematoma may compress the spinal cord. Suspicion is aroused if the cerebral angiogram is negative and the patient develops spinal cord signs.

Treatment

The aims of management are to identify the cause of the SAH, to treat the source of the bleeding to prevent recurrence, to prevent the general complications of stroke and to manage the complications of SAH (Vermeulen *et al.* 1992; Wijdicks 1995). Close monitoring using the Glasgow Coma Score and pupillary responses as well as for the development of focal deficits is required.

General measures and medical treatment

The patient should be nursed in a quiet, darkened room. As with other stroke types, the management of raised blood pressure is controversial.

Secondary ischemia is a frequent complication after SAH and is responsible for a substantial proportion of patients with poor outcome. The cause of secondary ischemia is unknown, but hypovolemia and fluid restriction are important risk factors. Hypovolemia should be avoided and intravenous fluids given, at least 3 liters per day, to reduce the likelihood of delayed ischemia. Indeed, volume expansion therapy is frequently used in patients with SAH to prevent or treat secondary ischemia. However, the risks and benefits of volume expansion therapy have been studied properly in only two trials of patients with aneurysmal SAH, with very small numbers (Rinkel *et al.* 2004). At present, there is no good evidence for the use of volume expansion therapy in patients with aneurysmal SAH.

The risk of delayed cerebral ischemia is also thought to be reduced and the overall outcome improved by prophylactic calcium blockers, specifically nimodipine, 60 mg every four hours, administered orally or by nasogastric tube for 21 days (Rinkel *et al.* 2005). If this causes hypotension, then the dose should be reduced. There is no good evidence to support intravenous nimodipine, which is particularly likely to cause hypotension. Evidence is inconclusive for other potentially neuroprotective drugs, such as nicardipine and magnesium (Rinkel *et al.* 2005). There is also no evidence of benefit from corticosteroids in patients with either SAH or primary intracerebral hemorrhage (Feigin *et al.* 2005b).

Cardiac arrhythmias are common in the first few days but seldom need treatment (Andreoli *et al.* 1987; Brouwers *et al.* 1989), although electrocardiographic monitoring is advisable. Neurogenic pulmonary edema is rare but can occur very early, causing diagnostic confusion. The mechanism is unclear but intensive cardiovascular monitoring and treatment are required (Parr *et al.* 1996). The patient can be mobilized when the headache has resolved (Warlow *et al.* 1996b).

Surgical treatments for certain patients

Intracerebral extension of the hemorrhage occurs in at least a third of patients. Patients with a large hematoma and depressed consciousness might require immediate evacuation of the hematoma, preferably preceded by occlusion of the aneurysm (Niemann *et al.* 2003). Alternatively, extensive craniectomy can be employed to allow expansion of the brain, as for malignant middle cerebral artery infarction (Smith *et al.* 2002). Subdural hematomas are rare but life threatening and should be removed.

Rebleeding risk

Approximately 10% of untreated saccular aneurysms rebleed within hours and another 30% within a few weeks (Brilstra *et al.* 2002). Subsequently, the rebleeding rate is approximately 2–3% per annum. Deterioration is usually sudden, with reduced conscious level or fixed dilatation of the pupils in ventilated patients.

Ruptured arteriovenous malformations have a lower mortality than aneurysmal SAH and are less likely to rebleed, certainly in the early period after the initial hemorrhage (Mast *et al.* 1997). It is unclear how to identify lesions at particularly high risk of bleeding or epilepsy (Duong *et al.* 1998).

Endovascular and surgical treatment

The purpose of occluding the source of SAH is to prevent rebleeding. Occlusion may not be appropriate in severe cases or where there is significant comorbidity. Neurosurgical "clipping" was used routinely for ruptured saccular aneurysms, but endovascular occlusion using detachable electrically released thrombogenic platinum coils ("coiling") is now the method of choice (Fig. 30.4). For aneurysms suitable for either treatment, the International Subarachnoid Aneurysm Trial (ISAT) indicated that coiling confers an absolute risk reduction over clipping of approximately 7%, with 25% relative risk reduction for dependency or death at one year (Molyneux *et al.* 2002). The risk of rebleeding from the ruptured aneurysm after one year was 2 per 1276 and 0 per 1081 patient-years for patients allocated endovascular and neurosurgical treatment, respectively (Molyneux *et al.* 2002). The risk of epilepsy was also substantially lower in patients allocated to endovascular treatment (Molyneux *et al.* 2005).

The survival benefit in patients randomized to endovascular treatment in ISAT was still evident after seven years of follow-up. Although the risk of late rebleeding was low, it was more common after endovascular coiling than after neurosurgical clipping. Further follow-up is ongoing to determine the long-term risks of rebleeding, but the early benefits of endovascular treatment have convinced most centers to adopt this approach if feasible. Patients randomized in the trial were mostly young, had good grades on the World Federation of Neurology Score and small anterior circulation aneurysms, thus representing half to three quarters of those with aneurysmal SAH. The configuration of aneurysms of the middle cerebral artery is often less favorable for coiling. Aneurysm occlusion should be attempted as soon as practicable, preferably within three to four days after onset of the SAH to prevent rebleeding.

Treatment of arteriovenous malformations and cavernomas is discussed in Ch. 22.

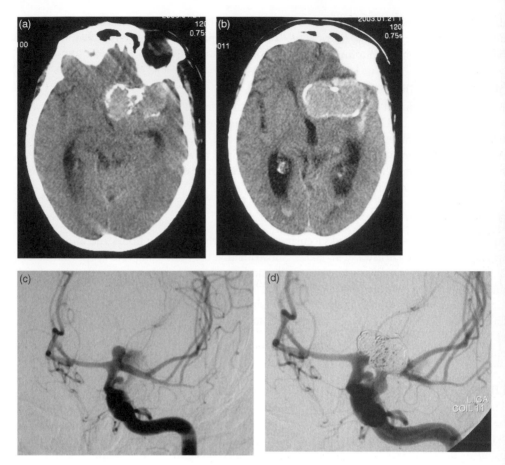

Fig. 30.4. (a,b) Brain CT images showing a large calcified aneurysm in the frontal region. (c,d) Cerebral angiograms show a small area of filling within the aneurysm owing to occlusion of a large part of the aneurysm with thrombus, making the aneurysm appear relatively small (c); this is then completely occluded by endovascular coiling (d).

Complications
Hydrocephalus

Hydrocephalus is caused by blood obstructing CSF flow and it occurs within days of onset in approximately 20% of patients. It may cause clinical deterioration, including a gradual reduction in conscious level. Patients with intraventricular blood or with extensive hemorrhage in the perimesencephalic cisterns are particularly predisposed to developing acute hydrocephalus. The diagnosis is confirmed with CT scanning. Temporary external ventricular drainage may lead to dramatic improvement, but complications may occur, including ventriculitis, and the risk of rebleeding of an untreated aneurysm may be slightly increased (Hellingman *et al.* 2007). Lumbar puncture may be performed in patients without a space-occupying lesion or gross intraventricular hemorrhage, but this requires certainty that the site of obstruction is in the subarachnoid space and not the ventricular system. In addition, it is not clear whether lumbar puncture increases the risk of rebleeding (Ruijs *et al.* 2005). Months or years after SAH, organized thrombus and fibrosis in the CSF pathways can lead to the syndrome of normal pressure hydrocephalus.

Delayed cerebral ischemia

Delayed ischemia secondary to vasospasm appears 4–14 days after onset in approximately 25% of patients and has a bad prognosis. Loss of consciousness at onset, large quantities of subarachnoid or intraventricular blood on CT, hyponatremia and the use of antifibrinolytic drugs are all risk factors (Brouwers *et al.* 1992; Hop *et al.* 1999). Clinical onset is usually gradual, with deteriorating conscious level and evolving focal neurological signs.

Hyponatremia

Hyponatremia occurs in approximately a third of patients in the first week or two after SAH and is related to the severity of the initial presentation. It is not usually caused by inappropriate antidiuretic hormone secretion but by "salt wasting," in which there is excessive loss of salt and water by the kidneys with a decrease in plasma volume. Below a plasma sodium of approximately 125 mmol/l, correction is necessary by plasma volume expansion (Berendes *et al.* 1997).

Intracerebral hematoma

Intracerebral hematoma may cause a focal deficit and should be considered for removal if there is associated coma, clinical deterioration and brain shift.

Long-term complications

Late rebleeding occurs in 2–3% of patients in the first 10 years after clipping of an aneurysm, half of such bleeds being caused by newly developed aneurysms. After endovascular coiling, the long-term risks are unclear, being recorded at 0.7% between one month and one year in ISAT (Molyneaux *et al.* 2005) and at 2–3% in one month to four years in a Dutch cohort (Sluzewski *et al.* 2005).

Epilepsy develops in 14–20% of patients, and putative risk factors include subdural hematoma, cerebral infarction, disability on discharge, ventricular drain insertion and surgical treatment (Olafsson *et al.* 2000; Claassen *et al.* 2003).

Anosmia is a sequela in almost 30% of patients, particularly after surgery and anterior communicating artery aneurysms.

Cognitive deficits and psychosocial dysfunction are common in the first year in patients who otherwise make a good recovery. They persist for years. In one study, a quarter of previously employed patients had stopped working, and another quarter worked shorter hours or in a position with reduced responsibility (Wermer *et al.* 2007). Changes in personality included increased irritability and emotionality. Overall, only 25% of those living independently reported a complete absence of psychosocial problems.

Unruptured aneurysms

Unruptured aneurysms in patients surviving a SAH should be treated unless they are very small or difficult to reach. There is an assumed high risk of rupture in such aneurysms, based on limited data (Wiebers *et al.* 2003). The adverse psychological impact of untreated aneurysms in patients who have survived a previous life-threatening aneurismal rupture is an equally important factor in determining optimal treatment.

Unruptured aneurysms not associated with SAH should normally be clipped or coiled if they are symptomatic, for instance if there is a third nerve palsy caused by a posterior communicating artery aneurysm (Fig. 30.2) (Raps *et al.* 1993). The optimal management of incidental unruptured asymptomatic aneurysms is unclear because the risk of rupture is low: up to 4% per annum if $> 10\,$mm in diameter, and $< 1\%$ per annum for smaller aneurysms (International Study of Unruptured Aneurysm Investigators 1998; Rinkel *et al.* 1998; Wermer *et al.* 2007). The risk of clipping or coiling is not insignificant (Raaymakers *et al.* 1998). The risks of rupture are higher with older age, female gender, increasing aneurysm size, posterior circulation aneurysm and geography, with patients from Japan and Finland seemingly at higher risk (Wermer *et al.* 2007).

Individuals with an affected first-degree relative have a 5–12 times greater lifetime risk of SAH than the general population, representing a lifetime risk of 2–5%. However, the chances of finding an aneurysm by screening in an individual with a single affected relative is only 1.7 times higher than in the general population. This suggests that familial aneurysms have a higher rupture rate or grow faster than others. The indications for screening in those perceived to be at increased risk of SAH are at present unclear (Teasdale *et al.* 2005). It could be argued that screening is not effective in those with only one affected relative but should be considered in those with two or more affected relatives, or those with polycystic kidney disease (Raaymakers 1999) or some of the other conditions associated with intracranial aneurysms (Box 30.1). Repeat screening should be discussed since the risk of finding an aneurysm after five years is around 7% (Wermer *et al.* 2007). Patients should be referred to specialist clinics where an informed decision can be made on the basis of that individual's risks and benefits and their preferences. Screening for new aneurysms in those who have survived SAH is not thought to be beneficial except in those with multiple aneurysms or who are very young at presentation.

> **Box 30.1.** Associations of intracranial saccular aneurysms
>
> Polycystic kidney disease[a]
> Fibromuscular dysplasia
> Cervical artery dissection[a]
> Coarctation of the aorta
> Intracranial arteriovenous malformations[a]
> Marfan's syndrome[a]
> Ehlers–Danlos syndrome[a]
> Pseudoxanthoma elasticum[a]
> Neurofibromatosis type I[a]
> α_1-Antitrypsin deficiency[a]
> Hereditary hemorrhagic telangiectasia[a]
> Moyamoya syndrome
> Klinefelter's syndrome
> Progeria
>
> *Note:*
> [a]These can be familial.

References

Adams HP, Kassell NF, Torner JC *et al.* (1983). CT and clinical correlations in recent aneurysmal subarachnoid haemorrhage: a preliminary report of the Cooperative Aneurysm Study. *Neurology* **33**:981–988

Andreoli A, di Pasquale G, Pinelli G *et al.* (1987). Subarachnoid haemorrhage: frequency and severity of cardiac arrhythmias. A survey of 70 cases studied in the acute phase. *Stroke* **18**:558–564

Berendes E, Walter M, Cullen P *et al.* (1997). Secretion of brain natriuretic peptide in patients with aneurysmal subarachnoid haemorrhage. *Lancet* **349**:245–249

Brilstra EH, Algra A, Rinkel GJ *et al.* (2002). Effectiveness of neurosurgical clip application in patients with aneurismal subarachnoid hemorrhage. *Journal of Neurosurgery* **97**:1036–1041

Brouwers JAM, Wijdicks EFM, Hasan D *et al.* (1989). Serial electrocardiographic recording in aneurysmal subarachnoid haemorrhage. *Stroke* **20**:1162–1167

Brouwers JAM, Wijdicks EFM, van Gijn J (1992). Infarction after aneurysm rupture does not depend on distribution or clearance rate of blood. *Stroke* **23**:374–379

Chappell ET, Moure FC, Good MC (2003). Comparison of computed tomographic angiography with digital subtraction angiography in the diagnosis of cerebral aneurysms: a meta-analysis. *Neurosurgery* **52**:624–631

Claassen J, Peery S, Kreiter KT *et al.* (2003). Predictors and clinical impact of epilepsy after subarachnoid hemorrhage. *Neurology* **60**:208–214

Duong DH, Young WL, Vang MC *et al.* (1998). Feeding artery pressure and venous drainage pattern are primary determinants of haemorrhage from cerebral arteriovenous malformations. *Stroke* **29**:1167–1176

Fearnley JM, Stevens JM, Rudge P (1995). Superficial siderosis of the central nervous system. *Brain* **118**:1051–1066

Feigin VL, Rinkel GJ, Lawes CM *et al.* (2005a). Risk factors for subarachnoid hemorrhage: an updated systematic review of epidemiological studies. *Stroke* **36**:2773–2780

Feigin VL, Anderson N, Rinkel GJ (2005b). Corticosteroids for aneurysmal subarachnoid haemorrhage and primary intracerebral haemorrhage. *Cochrane Database of Systematic Reviews* **3**:CD004583

Ferro JM, Pinto AN (1994). Sexual activity is a common precipitant of subarachnoid haemorrhage. *Cerebrovascular Diseases* **4**:375

Hellingman CA, van den Bergh WM, Beijer IS *et al.* (2007). Risk of rebleeding after treatment of acute hydrocephalus in patients with aneurysmal subarachnoid hemorrhage. *Stroke* **38**:96–99

Hop JW, Rinkel GJE, Algra A *et al.* (1997). Case-fatality rates and functional outcome after subarachnoid haemorrhage: a systematic review. *Stroke* **28**:660–664

Hop JW, Rinkel GJ, Algra A *et al.* (1999). Initial loss of consciousness and risk of delayed cerebral ischemia after aneurysmal subarachnoid hemorrhage. *Stroke* **30**:2268–2271

Huang J, van Gelder JM (2002). The probability of sudden death from rupture of intracranial aneurysms: a meta-analysis. *Neurosurgery* **51**:1101–1107

International Study of Unruptured Intracranial Aneurysms Investigators (1998). Unruptured intracranial aneurysms: risk of rupture and risks of surgical intervention. *New England Journal of Medicine* **339**:1725–1733

Kassell NF, Torner JC, Haley EC *et al.* (1990a). The International Cooperative Study on the Timing of Aneurysm Surgery Part 1: Overall management results. *Journal of Neurosurgery* **73**:18–36

Kassell NF, Torner JC, Jane JA *et al.* (1990b). The International Cooperative Study on the Timing of Aneurysm Surgery. Part 2: Surgical results. *Journal of Neurosurgery* **73**:37–47

Linn FHH, Rinkel GJE, Algra A *et al.* (1996). Incidence of subarachnoid haemorrhage. Role of region, year and rate of computed tomography: a meta-analysis. *Stroke* **27**:625–629

Linn FH, Rinkel GJ, Algra A *et al.* (1998). Headache characteristics in subarachnoid haemorrhage and benign thunderclap headache. *Journal of Neurology, Neurosurgery and Psychiatry* **65**:791–793

Linn FH, Voorbij HA, Rinkel GJ *et al.* (2005). Visual inspection versus spectrophotometry in detecting bilirubin in cerebrospinal fluid. *Journal of Neurology, Neurosurgery and Psychiatry.* **76**:1452–1454

Mast H, Young WL, Koennecke HC *et al.* (1997). Risk of spontaneous haemorrhage after diagnosis of cerebral arteriovenous malformation. *Lancet* **350**:1065–1068

Molyneux A, Kerr R, Stratton I *et al.* (2002). International Subarachnoid Aneurysm Trial (ISAT) of neurosurgical clipping versus endovascular coiling in 2143 patients with ruptured intracranial aneurysms: a randomised trial. *Lancet* **360**:1267–1274

Molyneux AJ, Kerr RS, Yu LM *et al.* (2005). International subarachnoid aneurysm trial (ISAT) of neurosurgical clipping versus endovascular coiling in 2143 patients with ruptured intracranial aneurysms: a randomised comparison of effects on survival, dependency, seizures, rebleeding subgroups and aneurysm occlusion. *Lancet* **366**:809–817

Niemann DB, Wills AD, Maartens NF *et al.* (2003). Treatment of intracerebral hematomas caused by aneurysm rupture: coil placement followed by clot evacuation. *Journal of Neurosurgery* **99**:843–847

Olafsson E, Gudmundsson G, Hauser WA (2000). Risk of epilepsy in long-term survivors of surgery for aneurysmal subarachnoid hemorrhage: a population-based study in Iceland. *Epilepsia* **41**:1201–1205

Parr MJA, Finfer SR, Morgan MK (1996). Reversible cardiogenic shock complicating subarachnoid haemorrhage. *British Medical Journal* **313**:681–683

359

Pinto AN, Ferro JM, Canhao P et al. (1993). How often is a perimesencephalic subarachnoid haemorrhage CT pattern caused by ruptured aneurysms? *Acta Neurochirurgie* 124:79–81

Pinto AN, Canhao P, Ferro JM (1996). Seizures at the onset of subarachnoid haemorrhage. *Journal of Neurology* 243:161–164

Raaymakers TW (1999). Aneurysms in relatives of patients with subarachnoid hemorrhage: frequency and risk factors. MARS Study Group. Magnetic Resonance Angiography in Relatives of patients with subarachnoid hemorrhage. *Neurology* 53:982–988

Raaymakers TWM, Rinkel GJE, Limburg M et al. (1998). Mortality and morbidity of surgery for unruptured intracranial aneurysms: a meta-analysis. *Stroke* 29:1531–1538

Raps EC, Rogers JD, Galetta SL et al. (1993). The clinical spectrum of unruptured intracranial aneurysms. *Archives of Neurology* 50:265–268

Rinkel GJE, Wijdicks EFM, Hasan D et al. (1991). Outcome in patients with subarachnoid haemorrhage and negative angiography according to pattern of haemorrhage on computed tomography. *Lancet* 338:964–968

Rinkel GJE, van Gijn J, Wijdicks EFM (1993). Subarachnoid haemorrhage without detectable aneurysm. A review of the causes. *Stroke* 24:1403–1409

Rinkel GJE, Djibuti M, Algra A et al. (1998). Prevalence and risk of rupture of intracranial aneurysms: a systematic review. *Stroke* 29:251–256

Rinkel GJ, Feigin VL, Algra A et al. (2004). Circulatory volume expansion therapy for aneurysmal subarachnoid haemorrhage. *Cochrane Database of Systematic Reviews* 4:CD000483

Rinkel GJ, Feigin VL, Algra A et al. (2005). Calcium antagonists for aneurysmal subarachnoid haemorrhage. *Cochrane Database of Systematic Reviews* 1:CD000277

Rothwell PM, Coull AJ, Giles MF et al. (2004). Change in stroke incidence, mortality, case-fatality, severity and risk factors in Oxfordshire, UK from 1981 to 2004 (Oxford Vascular Study). *Lancet* 363:1925–1933

Ruigrok YM, Rinkel GJ, Buskens E (2000). Perimesencephalic hemorrhage and CT angiography: a decision analysis. *Stroke* 31:2976–2983

Ruijs AC, Dirven CM, Algra A et al. (2005). The risk of rebleeding after external lumbar drainage in patients with untreated ruptured cerebral aneurysms. *Acta Neurochirurgie* 147:1157–1161

Schievink WI (1997). Intracranial aneurysms. *New England Journal of Medicine* 336:28–40

Schwartz TH, Solomon RA (1996). Perimesencephalic nonaneurysmal subarachnoid hemorrhage: review of the literature. *Neurosurgery* 39:433–440

Sluzewski M, van Rooij WJ, Beute GN et al. (2005). Late rebleeding of ruptured intracranial aneurysms treated with detachable coils. *American Journal of Neuroradiology* 26:2542–2549

Smith ER, Carter BS, Ogilvy CS (2002). Proposed use of prophylactic decompressive craniectomy in poor-grade aneurismal subarachnoid hemorrhage patients presenting with associated large sylvian haematomas. *Neurosurgery* 51:117–124

Teasdale GM, Wardlaw JM, White PM et al. (2005). The familial risk of subarachnoid haemorrhage. *Brain* 128:1677–1685

Toussaint LG III, Friedman JA, Wijdicks EF et al. (2005). Survival of cardiac arrest after aneurysmal subarachnoid hemorrhage. *Neurosurgery* 57:25–31

UK National External Quality Assessment Scheme for Immunochemistry Working Group (2003). National guidelines for analysis of cerebrospinal fluid for bilirubin in suspected subarachnoid haemorrhage. *Annals of Clinical Biochemistry* 40:481–488

van der Wee N, Rinkel GJE, Hasan D et al. (1995). Detection of subarachnoid haemorrhage on early CT: is lumbar puncture still needed after a negative scan? *Journal of Neurology Neurosurgery and Psychiatry* 58:357–359

van Gijn J, Rinkel GJ (2001). Subarachnoid haemorrhage: diagnosis, causes and management. *Brain* 124:249–278

van Gijn J, Kerr RS, Rinkel GJ (2007). Subarachnoid haemorrhage. *Lancet* 369:306–318

Vermeer SE, Rinkel GJE, Algra A (1997). Circadian fluctuations in onset of subarachnoid haemorrhage. New data on aneurysmal and perimesencephalic haemorrhage and a systematic review. *Stroke* **28**:805–808

Vermeulen M, van Gijn J (1990). The diagnosis of subarachnoid haemorrhage. *Journal of Neurology, Neurosurgery and Psychiatry* **53**:365–372

Vermeulen M, Lindsay KW, van Gijn J (1992). *Subarachnoid Haemorrhage*. London: Saunders

Villablanca JP, Hooshi P, Martin N *et al.* (2002). Three-dimensional helical computerized tomography angiography in the diagnosis, characterization and management of middle cerebral artery aneurysms: comparison with conventional angiography and intraoperative findings. *Journal of Neurosurgery* **97**:1322–1332

Warlow CP, Dennis MS, van Gijn J *et al.* (1996a). *Stroke: A Practical Guide to Management*, Ch. 5: What pathological type of stroke is it? pp. 146–189. Oxford: Blackwell Scientific

Warlow CP, Dennis MS, van Gijn J *et al.* (1996b). *Stroke: A Practical Guide to Management*, Ch. 13: Specific treatment of aneurysmal subarachnoid haemorrhage, pp. 438–468. Oxford: Blackwell Scientific

Wermer MJ, Kool H, Albrecht KW *et al.* (2007). Aneurysm Screening after Treatment for Ruptured Aneurysms Study Group. Subarachnoid hemorrhage treated with clipping: long-term effects on employment, relationships, personality and mood. *Neurosurgery* **60**:91–97

Wiebers DO, Whisnant JP, Huston J III *et al.* (2003). Unruptured intracranial aneurysms: natural history, clinical outcome and risks of surgical and endovascular treatment. *Lancet* **362**:103–110

Wijdicks EFM (1995). Worse-case scenario: management in poor-grade aneurysmal subarachnoid haemorrhage. *Cerebrovascular Diseases* **5**:163–169

Wintermark M, Uske A, Chalaron M *et al.* (2003). Multislice computerized tomography angiography in the evaluation of intracranial aneurysms: a comparison with intraarterial digital subtraction angiography. *Journal of Neurosurgery* **98**:828–836

Chapter 31

Vascular cognitive impairment: definitions and clinical diagnosis

Stroke is associated with a high risk of future dementia. Dementia with an underlying vascular etiology, "vascular dementia," may also occur in patients without a history of clinically eloquent stroke when it is in association with silent large or small vessel disease and/or widespread white matter disease. Vascular dementia may also coexist with Alzheimer's disease. The incidence of all types of dementia including vascular dementia rises rapidly with age and, therefore, cognitive impairment is likely to become an increasing problem as the numbers of people surviving into old age increases. At present, it is unclear to what extent aggressive treatment of vascular risk factors will influence the development and progression of vascular cognitive impairment, but there is much research interest in defining the predictors and thus possible therapeutic strategies in vascular dementia.

Epidemiology

Vascular dementia is the second most common cause of dementia in later life in white populations and the most common cause in Far Eastern countries (Jorm 1991; Jorm and Jolley 1998; Neuropathology Group of the Medical Research Council Cognitive Function and Ageing Study 2001). The overall incidence of dementia rises exponentially up to the age of 90 years, with no sign of leveling off, and although the incidence rates for vascular dementia vary greatly from study to study, the trend is also for an exponential rise with age (Jorm and Jolley 1998). There is no overall sex difference in dementia incidence, but women tend to have a higher incidence of Alzheimer's disease in very old age, and men tend to have a higher incidence of vascular dementia at younger ages. Rates of vascular dementia double approximately every five years (Alzheimer's disease rates double approximately every four years) (Jorm et al. 1987; Jorm and Jolley 1998).

Given the high prevalence of stroke and dementia disorders, they will often coexist, particularly since epidemiological studies have shown an association between stroke and dementia: individuals with stroke are more likely to be demented and individuals with dementia are at increased risk of stroke compared with age-matched controls. Population-based cohort studies have shown that vascular risk factors in midlife, particularly hypertension but also high cholesterol, are associated with increased risk of the development of dementia in later life (Skoog et al. 1996; Freitag et al. 2006; Solomon et al. 2007) both vascular cognitive impairment and Alzheimer's disease. Consistent with this, neuropathological data show the frequent coexistence of Alzheimer's pathology with cerebrovascular disease, and it has been proposed that the development of neurofibrillary tangles and amyloid plaques may, in part, be secondary to ischemia (de la Torre 2002). The overlap of risk factors and the coexistence of vascular and Alzheimer's type pathology means that vascular cognitive impairment cannot be considered in isolation and there may be important synergistic relationships between the two syndromes.

Studies of the natural history of vascular dementia show a significantly shorter survival time compared with Alzheimer's disease owing to increased vascular death, but speed of cognitive progression is much the same (Chui and Gonthier 1999). Similarly, rates of serial atrophy on MRI over a one-year period in patients with Alzheimer's disease and vascular dementia are not significantly different (O'Brien *et al.* 2001). In contrast, patients selected for clinical trials with probable vascular dementia appear to have a more stable course than those with Alzheimer's disease (Erkinjuntti *et al.* 2002, Black *et al.* 2003; Wilkinson *et al.* 2003). It is unclear whether the discrepancy between rates of progression of cognitive impairment seen in trials and in observational studies is because of better control of vascular risk factors, the selection of stable subjects or other selection bias owing to use of highly specific clinical criteria.

Definitions and clinical features of vascular cognitive impairment

There is no universally accepted definition for the clinical diagnosis of dementia, and the various definitions available (e.g. the *International Classification of Diseases*, 10th revision [ICD-10; World Health Organization 1987] and the Diagnostic and *Statistical Manual of Mental Disorders*, 3rd edition [DSM-III] and 4th edition [DSM-IV; American Psychiatric Association 1989, 1994]) use different diagnostic criteria: both DSM-IV and ICD-10 require the presence of memory impairment together with one or more (DSM-IV) or two or more (ICD-10) other cognitive domains to be affected. Patients with vascular cognitive impairment may have severe impairment of cognitive function but relatively well preserved memory, and will not, therefore, be classified as demented by the DSM-IV and ICD-10 criteria. This is likely to lead to an underestimate of the true prevalence of vascular cognitive impairment. Further, it is likely that a number of patients fulfilling the criteria for vascular dementia by criteria that include memory impairment are likely to have coexistent Alzheimer's disease (i.e. have mixed dementia), because memory impairment will be more common in this group.

The term vascular cognitive impairment is used here to include both dementia and cognitive impairment not severe enough to cause dementia (cognitive impairment, no dementia [CIND]): a syndrome defined as cognitive decline greater than expected for an individual's age and education level that does not interfere notably with activities of daily living. Vascular cognitive impairment is a heterogeneous syndrome encompassing cognitive impairment associated with large cortical infarcts, single strategically sited infarcts, multiple small infarcts, cerebral hemorrhage, and vasculopathies including cerebral autosomal dominant arteriopathy with silent infarcts and leukoaraiosis (CADSIL), lipohyalinosis and cerebral amyloid angiopathy (Table 31.1).

Different subtypes of vascular pathology may coexist in an individual patient. The earliest attempt to improve the definition of vascular dementia as a distinct subtype of dementia was made by Hachinski and colleagues (1975), who proposed an ischemic score derived from the multi-infarct model of dementia. The Hachinski score requires a history of stroke and the presence of focal neurological signs, and it separates vascular dementia secondary to multi-infarct dementia from Alzheimer's disease effectively. However, it is rather insensitive for other subtypes of vascular dementia. Both ICD-10 and DSM-IV contain diagnostic criteria for vascular dementia, but most clinicians and researchers use the Neuroepidemiology Branch of the National Institute of Neurological Disorders and Stroke–Association Internationale pour la Recherche et l'Enseignement en Neurosciences (NINDS/AIREN) consensus criteria based on ICD-10 (Román *et al.* 1993).

Table 31.1. Subtypes of vascular cognitive impairment

Type	Causes
Multi-infarct dementia (cortical vascular dementia)	Primarily from cortical infarcts
Small vessel dementia (subcortical vascular dementia)	Primarily from subcortical lacunes, white and/or deep gray matter lesions
Strategic infarct dementia	Unilateral or bilateral infarction in a strategic area (e.g. thalamus, hippocampus)
Hypoperfusion dementia	Hypoperfusion-induced brain damage, e.g. caused by systemic hypotension or cardiac arrest
Hemorrhagic dementia	Intracerebral hemorrhage
Alzheimer's disease with cerebrovascular disease (mixed)	Coexistent degenerative and vascular pathology, on the basis of the clinical picture and brain imaging, both of which contribute to the dementia
Hereditary vascular dementia (CADASIL)	Autosomal dominant arteriopathy (with silent infarcts and leukoaraiosis)

Table 31.2. NINDS/AIREN imaging criteria for vascular cognitive impairment

Criterion	Features
Topography	Large vessel strokes
	Extensive white matter changes
	Lacunes (frontal/basal ganglia)
	Bilateral thalamic lesions
Severity	Large vessel lesion of dominant hemisphere
	Bilateral strokes
	White matter lesion affecting > 25% white matter

Note:
NINDS/AIREN, Neuroepidemiology Branch of the National Institute of Neurological Disorders and Stroke–Association Internationale pour la Recherche et l'Enseignement en Neurosciences

The NINDS/AIREN criteria divide cases into probable and possible vascular dementia along the lines of the NINCDS/ADRDA criteria for Alzheimer's disease (McKhann *et al.* 1984). Probable vascular dementia requires the presence of dementia, defined as memory and at least one other cognitive domain being affected, and the presence of cerebrovascular disease (focal neurological signs and evidence of relevant cerebrovascular disease on brain imaging). The onset of cognitive impairment must occur within three months of the cerebrovascular disease or must be abrupt with a stepwise/fluctuating course. The less-certain diagnosis of possible vascular dementia can be made if brain imaging criteria are not met or if the relationship between cerebrovascular disease and dementia is not clear. The NINDS/AIREN criteria were among the first to propose clear neuroimaging criteria for the diagnosis of vascular dementia, requiring a combination of topography (lesion location) and severity. These criteria are shown in Table 31.2.

Unlike in Alzheimer's disease, autopsy confirmation of the diagnostic accuracy of the NINDS/AIREN and other criteria for vascular dementia is not well established. There is no agreed universal gold standard by which vascular dementia can be diagnosed pathologically and few prospective neuropathological studies. Neuropathological criteria include the relative absence of Alzheimer-type pathology and the presence of some vascular change, both of which are subjective and remain areas of controversy. Despite these drawbacks, initial validation studies suggest reasonable specificity for the NINDS/AIREN criteria for probable (sensitivity 20%; specificity 93%) and possible (sensitivity 55%; specificity 84%) vascular dementia (Gold *et al.* 2002), although it has also been shown that different criteria sets for vascular dementia identify different subsets of subjects (Lopez *et al.* 2005). Diagnostic criteria have been proposed for subtypes of vascular dementia, including subcortical ischemic vascular dementia (Erkinjuntti *et al.* 2002).

The term cognitive impairment no dementia of the vascular type (CIND-V) has been used to describe the group of patients with cognitive impairment secondary to cerebrovascular disease not meeting the criteria for dementia. This mirrors the use of the term CIND to describe patients with mild Alzheimer's type cognitive deficits (principally memory deficit). Patients with CIND of Alzheimer's type have a high rate of progression to frank Alzheimer's disease. The prognosis of patients with CIND-V is less clear, although as many as half may progress to dementia (Wentzel *et al.* 2001).

Not withstanding the problems in defining vascular cognitive impairment and dementia, the neuropsychological deficits seen in cognitive impairment associated with cerebrovascular disease are, in general, qualitatively different from those seen in Alzheimer's disease, certainly in the early stages. The different underlying pathologies causing vascular cognitive impairment have different disease mechanisms and cognitive profiles (Bastos-Leite *et al.* 2007). The cognitive deficits seen in strategic infarct dementia and multi-infarct dementia are variable, depending to a greater or lesser degree on lesion location. Medial temporal lobe atrophy and large vessel disease contribute to global cognitive dysfunction, whereas small vessel disease appears to be more specifically related to deficits predominantly in attentional, motivational and executive domains (Desmond 2004; Prins *et al.* 2005; Bastos-Leite *et al.* 2007). This is in contrast to Alzheimer's disease, in which memory deficits are prominent.

Commonly used screening instruments for dementia such as the Mini-Mental State Examination (Folstein *et al.* 1983) and the ADAS-cog (Rosen *et al.* 1984), which were primarily developed for assessing cognition in Alzheimer's disease, are relatively insensitive to executive and attentional function. Additional tests such as verbal fluency, trail making or maze tests, clock drawing, and reversed digit span are required to document deficits in fronto-subcortical circuits (Royall and Román 1999) and such tests have been incorporated into the ADAS-cog to create the VADAS-cog, for use in vascular cognitive impairment (Mohs *et al.* 1997). However, the presence of frontal lobe dysfunction on neuropsychological testing is not diagnostic of vascular cognitive impairment and cannot be used in isolation to distinguish between Alzheimer's disease and vascular dementia (Reed *et al.* 2007).

Further support for a distinctive pattern of cognitive deficits in vascular disease comes from studies of patients with CADASIL (Ch. 3) in which multiple subcortical infarcts occur at a young age when neurodegenerative changes would not be expected to be important (Buffon *et al.* 2006). Patients with CADASIL show early impairment of executive function that is frequently associated with a decline in attention and memory performance compatible with some degree of dysfunction in subcortico-frontal networks (Buffon *et al.* 2006). Later in the course of the disease, there is extension of cognitive deficits to involve multiple cognitive domains. However, even late in the disease, memory impairment does not involve the encoding process in that retrieval is significantly improved with cues. This is in stark contrast to what is seen in Alzheimer's disease, in which early impairment of memory encoding is characteristic. Cholinergic neuronal impairment occurs in CADASIL and provides a rationale for therapies to enhance cholinergic function in subcortical vascular cognitive impairment (Mesulam *et al.* 2003).

Non-cognitive disturbances are common in patients with vascular cognitive impairment, with high rates of depression and apathy, particularly in those with small vessel disease. For example, in the Cache County Study, significantly more participants with vascular dementia (32%) than Alzheimer's disease (20%) suffered from depression, the reverse being true for the presence of delusions (Lyketsos *et al.* 2000). It has been suggested that the high depression rate is related to preserved insight, but the location of infarction in the deep white matter is also likely to be important. Other non-cognitive disturbances such as agitation, disinhibition, aggression, aberrant motor behavior and hallucinations appear to be equally frequent in Alzheimer's disease and vascular cognitive impairment (Lyketsos *et al.* 2000). In a prospective population-based study, depression was associated with increased risk of developing CIND (Barnes *et al.* 2006).

Overlap between vascular cognitive impairment and Alzheimer's disease

In clinical practice, distinguishing between Alzheimer's disease and vascular cognitive impairment is often difficult, and many patients are likely to have coexistent pathology. In a large community-based study of unselected older people who were followed longitudinally and underwent autopsy, mixed Alzheimer's and vascular pathology was found to be the most common cause of cognitive impairment (Neuropathology Group of the Medical Research Council Cognitive Function and Aging Study 2001). This is consistent with other studies showing mixed pathology to be at least as common as "pure" vascular dementia (Knopman *et al.* 2003). There is also poor correlation between clinical diagnosis of dementia subtype and neuropathological findings: up to 30% of patients diagnosed with Alzheimer's disease have evidence of vascular pathology at autopsy. Further, there are no defined criteria for the vascular pathological changes required for a neuropathological diagnosis of vascular or mixed dementia. Deep white matter lesions can also be demonstrated on MRI in approximately 50% of those with Alzheimer's disease, with periventricular lesions found in over 90%.

However, despite the problems associated with defining vascular cognitive impairment and its associated neuropathological changes, it is clear that there is an interaction between cerebral infarcts and Alzheimer's pathology: patients with Alzheimer's pathology and cerebrovascular disease have a greater severity of cognitive impairment than those with similar severity of either pathology (Snowdon *et al.* 1997; Esiri *et al.* 1999; Schneider *et al.* 2007). After controlling for cortical infarcts and Alzheimer's pathology, subcortical infarcts increase the risk of dementia by almost four times (Schneider *et al.* 2007). However, the synergistic effect between cerebrovascular disease and Alzheimer's pathology is only seen in those with mild neurodegenerative change: in patients with severe neurodegenerative disease, associated vascular pathology becomes irrelevant.

Vascular mechanisms may be important in the expression and development of Alzheimer's pathology. Vascular risk factors are risk factors for Alzheimer's disease, and cerebral hypoperfusion and microcirculatory changes may precede the neuropathological and clinical changes of Alzheimer's disease, making it, in effect, a vascular disorder (Kalaria 2000; de la Torre 2002). Further evidence for a vascular mechanism comes from the observation that biochemical and structural changes occur in cerebral vessel walls in patients with early Alzheimer's disease, leading to altered vasoreactivity, impaired autoregulation and a greater degree of arterial pressure transmittal to the capillary circulation, thus predisposing to microvessel damage (Stopa *et al.* 2008).

Post-stroke cognitive impairment and dementia

Dementia occurring as a result of stroke is a subtype of vascular dementia.

Most studies of post-stroke dementia are of hospital series and tend to focus on major strokes; very few include patients with TIA. Prevalence rates in hospital-based series vary from

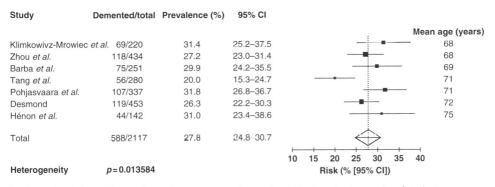

Study	Demented/total	Prevalence (%)	95% CI		Mean age (years)
Klimkowivz-Mrowiec *et al.*	69/220	31.4	25.2–37.5		68
Zhou *et al.*	118/434	27.2	23.0–31.4		68
Barba *et al.*	75/251	29.9	24.2–35.5		69
Tang *et al.*	56/280	20.0	15.3–24.7		71
Pohjasvaara *et al.*	107/337	31.8	26.8–36.7		71
Desmond	119/453	26.3	22.2–30.3		72
Hénon *et al.*	44/142	31.0	23.4–38.6		75
Total	588/2117	27.8	24.8–30.7		
Heterogeneity	*p*=0.013584			Risk (% [95% CI])	

Fig. 31.1. Pooled prevalence of rates for post-stroke dementia within three to six months of stroke in hospital-based studies that did not exclude pre-stroke dementia. CI, confidence interval. Study sources: Klimkowicz-Mrowiec *et al.* (2006); Zhou *et al.* (2004); Barba *et al.* (2001); Tang *et al.* (2004a,b); Pohjasvaara *et al.* (1999); Desmond (2004); Hénon *et al.* (1997, 2001).

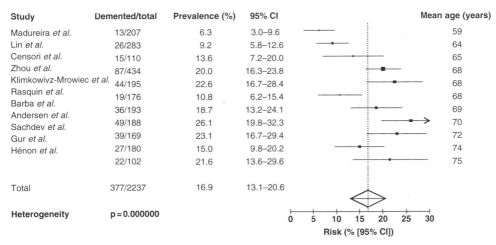

Study	Demented/total	Prevalence (%)	95% CI		Mean age (years)
Madureira *et al.*	13/207	6.3	3.0–9.6		59
Lin *et al.*	26/283	9.2	5.8–12.6		64
Censori *et al.*	15/110	13.6	7.2–20.0		65
Zhou *et al.*	87/434	20.0	16.3–23.8		68
Klimkowivz-Mrowiec *et al.*	44/195	22.6	16.7–28.4		68
Rasquin *et al.*	19/176	10.8	6.2–15.4		68
Barba *et al.*	36/193	18.7	13.2–24.1		69
Andersen *et al.*	49/188	26.1	19.8–32.3		70
Sachdev *et al.*	39/169	23.1	16.7–29.4		72
Gur *et al.*	27/180	15.0	9.8–20.2		74
Hénon *et al.*	22/102	21.6	13.6–29.6		75
Total	377/2237	16.9	13.1–20.6		
Heterogeneity	p = 0.000000			Risk (% [95% CI])	

Fig. 31.2. Pooled prevalence of rates for post-stroke dementia within three to six months in hospital-based studies that did exclude pre-stroke dementia. CI, confidence interval. Study sources: Madureira *et al.* (2001); Lin *et al.* (2003); Censori *et al.* (1996); Zhou *et al.* (2004); Klimkowicz-Mrowiec *et al.* (2006); Rasquin *et al.* (2004, 2005); Barba *et al.* (2000); Andersen *et al.* (1999); Sachdev *et al.* (2006); Gur *et al.* (1994); Hénon *et al.* (1997, 2001).

30% at three months in those studies that did not exclude pre-stroke dementia (Fig. 31.1), to 10–20% at six months in studies where pre-stroke dementia was excluded (Fig. 31.2) with overall prevalence rates of 27.8% (95% CI, 24.8–30.7) and 16.9% (95% CI, 13.1–20.6), respectively (Pendlebury and Rothwell 2008). Dementia rates are lower in population-based studies probably because of the inclusion of more patients with mild strokes (Fig. 31.3) with overall prevalence rates of 14.9% (95% CI, 7.3–22.4) when patients with pre-stroke dementia were not excluded (Pendlebury and Rothwell 2008). Factors that increase the risk of post-stroke dementia include increasing age, prior or recurrent stroke, prior cognitive impairment and low educational attainment. Vascular risk factors seem not to be important with the possible exception of diabetes and atrial fibrillation.

The risk of new-incident dementia following stroke is non-linear, being particularly high within the first six months after stroke. However, the increased risk of dementia persists in the long term: there was a 10-fold increased risk of dementia with stroke at five years after stroke onset (Kokmen *et al.* 1996). Significant numbers of patients presenting with stroke

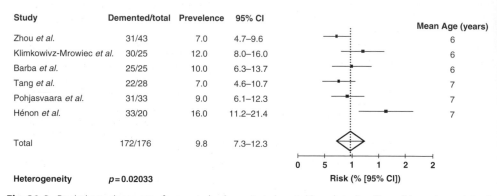

Study	Demented/total	Prevalence (%)	95% CI
Srikanth *et al.*	11/88	12.5	5.6–19.4
House *et al.*	24/115	20.9	13.4–28.3
Kokmen *et al.*	107/971	11.0	9.0–13.0
Appelros *et al.*	67/232	28.9	23.0–34.7
Total	209/1406	14.9	7.3–22.4
Heterogeneity	*p*=0.000000		

Fig. 31.3. Pooled prevalence rates for post-stroke dementia within one year in community-based studies not excluding pre-stroke dementia. CI, confidence interval. Study sources: Srikanth *et al.* (2003, 2006); House *et al.* (1990); Kokmen *et al.* (1996); Appelros (2005).

Study	Demented/total	Prevelence	95% CI	Mean Age (years)
Zhou *et al.*	31/43	7.0	4.7–9.6	6
Klimkowivz-Mrowiec *et al.*	30/25	12.0	8.0–16.0	6
Barba *et al.*	25/25	10.0	6.3–13.7	6
Tang *et al.*	22/28	7.0	4.6–10.7	7
Pohjasvaara *et al.*	31/33	9.0	6.1–12.3	7
Hénon *et al.*	33/20	16.0	11.2–21.4	7
Total	172/176	9.8	7.3–12.3	
Heterogeneity	*p*=0.02033			

Fig. 31.4. Pooled prevalence rates for pre-stroke dementia in hospital-based studies. CI, confidence interval. Study sources: Zhou *et al.* (2004); Klimkowicz-Mrowiec *et al.* (2006); Barba *et al.* (2001); Tang *et al.* (2004a,b); Pohjasvaara *et al.* (1999); Hénon *et al.* (1997, 2001).

have prior dementia, with overall rates of 9.8% (95% CI, 7.3–12.3) and 4.1% (95% CI, 1.9–6.2) in hospital-based (Fig. 31.4) and population-based studies, respectively (Pendlebury and Rothwell 2008). Many of these patients have Alzheimer's disease either alone or in combination with cerebrovascular disease, and this Alzheimer's disease may be 'unmasked' by a stroke.

A few studies have looked at cognitive impairment, no dementia (CIND-V) post-stroke although problems exist regarding varying criteria for diagnosis, and many commonly used tests of cognitive function, including the Mini-Mental Status Examination, have limited sensitivity for vascular cognitive impairment. However, it is clear from these studies that not all patients who show early cognitive impairment after stroke will decline: many patients improve (del Ser *et al.* 2005; Rasquin *et al.* 2005a; Srikanth *et al.* 2006). There is a suggestion that diabetic patients are less likely to improve than other patients and that initial attentional and executive deficits are less likely to get better than memory deficits. The incidence of CIND-V may be particularly high in those with lacunar infarction. In a study of 40 patients one month after stroke with lacunar infarction, CIND-V was found in 22 patients (Grau-Olivares *et al.* 2007). This may even have been an underestimate, since the diagnosis of CIND-V in this study required the presence of memory impairment.

The exact etiology of post-stroke dementia is unclear. A stroke may cause decompensation of a brain with pre-existing reduced cognitive reserve, as suggested by the increased risk of dementia after stroke in those with prior CIND. In addition, factors such as hypertension that cause the vascular changes predisposing to stroke may also contribute to neuronal and other cellular abnormalities, resulting in cognitive decline. Lastly, stroke may combine with the existing degenerative changes of incipient Alzheimer's disease to cause post-stroke dementia. While both primary and secondary prevention of stroke will reduce the overall burden of cognitive impairment, it is unclear to what extent treatment of vascular risk factors in the secondary prevention of stroke will reduce post-stroke cognitive decline beyond preventing recurrent events. Treatment of vascular dementia as a whole is discussed in Ch. 32.

References

American Psychiatric Association (1989). *Diagnostic and Statistical Manual of Mental Disorders*, 3rd edn. Washington, DC: American Psychiatric Press.

American Psychiatric Association (1994). *Diagnostic and Statistical Manual of Mental Disorders*, 4th edn. Washington, DC: American Psychiatric Press.

Andersen G, Vestergaard K, Ostergaard Riis J, Ingemen-Nielsen M (1996). Intellectual impairment in the first year following stroke compared to an age-matched population sample. *Cerebrovascular Diseases* 6:363–369

Appelros P (2005). Characteristics of Mini-Mental State Examination 1 year after stroke. *Acta Neurologica Scandinavica* 112:88–92

Barba R, Martínez-Espinosa S, Rodríguez-García E *et al.* (2000). Poststroke dementia: clinical features and risk factors. *Stroke* 31:1494–1501

Barba R, Castro MD, del Mar Morín M *et al.* (2001). Prestroke dementia. *Cerebrovascular Diseases* 11:216–224

Barnes DE, Alexopoulos GS, Lopez OL *et al.* (2006). Depressive symptoms, vascular disease, and mild cognitive impairment: findings from the Cardiovascular Health Study. *Archives of General Psychiatry* 63:273–279

Bastos-Leite AJ, van der Flier WM, van Straaten EC *et al.* (2007). The contribution of medial temporal lobe atrophy and vascular pathology to cognitive impairment in vascular dementia. *Stroke* 38:3182–3185

Black S, Roman GC, Geldmacher DS *et al.* (2003). Efficacy and tolerability of donepezil in vascular dementia: positive results of a 24-week, multicenter, international, randomized, placebo-controlled clinical trial. *Stroke* 34:2323–2330

Buffon F, Porcher R, Hernandez K *et al.* (2006). Cognitive profile in CADASIL. *Journal of Neurology, Neurosurgery and Psychiatry* 77:175–180

Censori B, Manara O, Agostinis C *et al.* (1996). Dementia after first stroke. *Stroke* 27:1205–1210

Chui H, Gonthier R (1999). Natural history of vascular dementia. *Alzheimer Disease Association Disorders* 13(Suppl 3):S124–S130

de la Torre JC (2002). Alzheimer disease as a vascular disorder: nosological evidence. *Stroke* 33:1152–1162

del Ser T, Barba R, Morin MM *et al.* (2005). Evolution of cognitive impairment after stroke and risk factors for delayed progression. *Stroke* 36:2670–2675

Desmond DW (2004). The neuropsychology of vascular cognitive impairment: is there a specific cognitive deficit? *Journal of Neurology Science* 226:3–7

Erkinjuntti T, Kurz A, Gauthier S *et al.* (2002). Efficacy of galanthamine in probable vascular dementia and Alzheimer's disease combined with cerebrovascular disease: a randomised trial. *Lancet* 359:1283–1290

Esiri MM, Nagy Z, Smith MZ *et al.* (1999). Cerebrovascular disease and threshold for dementia in the early stages of Alzheimer's disease. *Lancet* 354:919–920

Folstein MF, Robins LN, Helzer JE (1983). The Mini-Mental State Examination. *Archives of General Psychiatry* 40:812

Freitag MH, Peila R, Masaki K *et al.* (2006). Midlife pulse pressure and incidence of dementia: the Honolulu–Asia Aging Study. *Stroke* 37:33–37

Gold G, Bouras C, Canuto A *et al.* (2002). Clinicopathological validation study of four sets of clinical criteria for vascular dementia. *American Journal of Psychiatry* 159:82–87

Grau-Olivares M, Bartrés-Faz D, Arboix A *et al.* (2007). Mild cognitive impairment after lacunar infarction: voxel-based morphometry and neuropsychological assessment. *Cerebrovascular Diseases* 23:353–361

Gur AY, Neufeld MY, Treves TA *et al.* (1994). EEG as predictor of dementia following first ischemic stroke. *Acta Neurologica Scandinavica* **90**:263–265

Hachinski VC, Iliff LD, Zilhka E *et al.* (1975). Cerebral blood flow in dementia. *Archives of Neurology* **32**:632–637

Hénon H, Pasquier F, Durieu I (1997). Preexisting dementia in stroke patients. Baseline frequency, associated factors, and outcome. *Stroke* **28**:2429–2436

Hénon H, Durieu I, Guerouaou D *et al.* (2001). Poststroke dementia: incidence and relationship to prestroke cognitive decline. *Neurology* **57**:1216–1222

Hénon H, Pasquier F, Leys D (2006). Poststroke dementia. *Cerebrovascular Diseases* **22**:61–70

House A, Dennis M, Warlow C, Hawton K, Molyneux A (1990). The relationship between intellectual impairment and mood disorder in the first year after stroke. *Psychological Medicine* **20**:805–814

Jorm AF (1991). Cross-national comparisons of the occurrence of Alzheimer's and vascular dementias. *European Archives of Psychiatry and Clinical Neuroscience* **240**:218–222

Jorm AF, Jolley D (1998). The incidence of dementia: a meta-analysis. *Neurology* **51**:728–733

Jorm AF, Korten AE, Henderson AS (1987). The prevalence of dementia: a quantitative integration of the literature. *Acta Psychiatrica Scandinavica* **76**:465–479

Kalaria RN (2000). The role of cerebral ischemia in Alzheimer's disease. *Neurobiology Aging* **21**:321–330

Klimkowicz A, Dziedzic T, Slowik A *et al.* (2002). Incidence of pre- and poststroke dementia: cracow stroke registry. *Dementia and Geriatric Cognitive Disorders* **14**:137–140

Klimkowicz-Mrowiec A, Dziedzic T, Słowik A, Szczudlik A (2006). Predictors of poststroke dementia: results of a hospital-based study in Poland. *Dementia and Geriatric Cognitive Disorders* **21**:328–334

Knopman DS, Parisi JE, Boeve BF *et al.* (2003). Vascular dementia in a population-based autopsy study. *Archives of Neurology* **60**:569–575

Kokmen E, Whisnant JP, O'Fallon WM *et al.* (1996). Dementia after ischemic stroke: a population-based study in Rochester, Minnesota (1960–1984). *Neurology.* **46**:154–159

Lin JH, Lin RT, Tai CT *et al.* (2003). Prediction of poststroke dementia. *Neurology* **61**:343–348

Lopez OL, Kuller LH, Becker JT *et al.* (2005). Classification of vascular dementia in the Cardiovascular Health Study Cognition Study. *Neurology* **64**:1539–1547

Lyketsos CG, Steinberg M, Tschanz JT *et al.* (2000). Mental and behavioral disturbances in dementia: findings from the Cache County Study on Memory in Aging. *American Journal of Psychiatry* **157**:708–714

Madureira S, Guerreiro M, Ferro JM (2001). Dementia and cognitive impairment three months after stroke. *European Journal of Neurology* **8**:621–627

McKhann G, Drachman D, Folstein M *et al.* (1984). Clinical diagnosis of Alzheimer's disease: report of the NINCDS–ADRDA Work Group under the auspices of Department of Health and Human Services Task Force on Alzheimer's Disease. *Neurology* **34**:939–944

Mesulam M, Siddique T, Cohen B (2003). Cholinergic denervation in a pure multi-infarct state: observations on CADASIL. *Neurology* **60**:1183–1185

Mohs RC, Knopman D, Petersen RC *et al.* (1997). Development of cognitive instruments for use in clinical trials of antidementia drugs: additions to the Alzheimer's Disease Assessment Scale that broaden its scope. The Alzheimer's Disease Cooperative Study. *Alzheimer Disease Association Disorders* **11**(Suppl 2):S13–S21

Neuropathology Group Medical Research Council Cognitive Function and Aging Study (2001). Pathological correlates of late-onset dementia in a multicentre, community-based population in England and Wales. *Lancet* **357**:169–175

O'Brien JT, Paling S, Barber R *et al.* (2001). Progressive brain atrophy on serial MRI in dementia with Lewy bodies, AD, and vascular dementia. *Neurology* **56**:1386–1388

Pasquini M, Leys D, Rousseaux M *et al.* (2007). Influence of cognitive impairment on the institutionalisation rate 3 years after a stroke. *Journal Neurology, Neurosurgery and Psychiatry* **78**:56–59

Pendlebury ST, Rothwell PM (2007). Understanding heterogeneity in studies of post-stroke dementia. *Cerebrovascular Diseases* **25**(Suppl 2):1–20

Pohjasvaara T, Mäntylä R, Aronen HJ *et al.* (1999). Clinical and radiological determinants of prestroke cognitive decline in a stroke cohort. *Journal Neurology, Neurosurgery and Psychiatry* 67:742–748

Prins ND, van Dijk EJ, den Heijer T *et al.* (2005). Cerebral small-vessel disease and decline in information processing speed, executive function and memory. *Brain* 128:2034–2041

Rasquin SM, Lodder J, Ponds RW *et al.* (2004). Cognitive functioning after stroke: a one-year follow-up study. *Dementia and Geriatric Cognitive Disorders* 18:138–144

Rasquin SM, Lodder J, Verhey FR (2005a). Predictors of reversible mild cognitive impairment after stroke: a 2-year follow-up study. *Journal of Neurology Science* 15:21–25

Rasquin SM, Lodder J, Verhey FR (2005b). The effect of different diagnostic criteria on the prevalence and incidence of post-stroke dementia. *Neuroepidemiology* 24:189–195

Reed BR, Mungas DM, Kramer JH *et al.* (2007). Profiles of neuropsychological impairment in autopsy-defined Alzheimer's disease and cerebrovascular disease. *Brain* 130:731–739

Román GC, Tatemichi TK, Erkinjuntti T *et al.* (1993). Vascular dementia: diagnostic criteria for research studies. Report of the NINDS–AIREN International Workshop. *Neurology* 43:250–260

Rosen WG, Mohs RC, Davis KL (1984). A new rating scale for Alzheimer's disease. *American Journal of Psychiatry* 141:1356–1364

Royall DR, Román GC (1999). [On "Proposal for the application and scoring of the clock drawing test in Alzheimer's disease."] *Revista de Neurología* 29:1348–1349

Sachdev PS, Brodaty H, Valenzuela MJ *et al.* (2006). Clinical determinants of dementia and mild cognitive impairment following ischaemic stroke: the Sydney Stroke Study. *Dementia and Geriatric Cognitive Disorders* 21:275–283

Schneider JA, Boyle PA, Arvanitakis Z *et al.* (2007). Subcortical infarcts, Alzheimer's disease pathology, and memory function in older persons. *Annals of Neurology* 62:59–66

Skoog I, Lernfelt B, Landahl S *et al.* (1996). 15-year longitudinal study of blood pressure and dementia. *Lancet* 27:1141–1145

Snowdon DA, Greiner LH, Mortimer JA *et al.* (1997). Brain infarction and the clinical expression of Alzheimer disease. The Nun Study. *Journal of American Medical Association* 277:813–817

Solomon A, Kåreholt I, Ngandu T *et al.* (2007). Serum cholesterol changes after midlife and late-life cognition: twenty-one-year follow-up study. *Neurology* 68:751–756

Srikanth VK, Thrift AG, Saling MM *et al.* (2003). Community-Based Prospective Study of Nonaphasic English-Speaking Survivors. Increased risk of cognitive impairment 3 months after mild to moderate first-ever stroke: a Community-Based Prospective Study of Nonaphasic English-Speaking Survivors. *Stroke* 34:1136–1143

Srikanth VK, Quinn SJ, Donnan GA *et al.* (2006). Long-term cognitive transitions, rates of cognitive change, and predictors of incident dementia in a population-based first-ever stroke cohort. *Stroke* 37:2479–2483

Stopa EG, Butala P, Salloway S *et al.* (2008). Cerebral cortical arteriolar angiopathy, vascular [beta]-amyloid, smooth muscle actin, Braak stage and *APOE* genotype. *Stroke* 39:814–821

Tang WK, Chan SS, Chiu HF *et al.* (2004a). Frequency and determinants of prestroke dementia in a Chinese cohort. *Journal of Neurology* 251:604–608

Tang WK, Chan SS, Chiu HF *et al.* (2004b). Frequency and determinants of poststroke dementia in Chinese. *Stroke* 35:930–935

Tatemichi TK, Paik M, Bagiella E *et al.* (1994). Dementia after stroke is a predictor of long-term survival. *Stroke* 25:1915–1919

Wentzel C, Rockwood K, MacKnight C *et al.* (2001). Progression of impairment in patients with vascular cognitive impairment without dementia. *Neurology* 57:714–716

Wilkinson D, Doody R, Helme R *et al.* (2003). Donepezil in vascular dementia: a randomized, placebo-controlled study. *Neurology* 61:479–486

Woo J, Kay R, Yuen YK *et al.* (1992). Factors influencing long-term survival and disability among three-month stroke survivors. *Neuroepidemiology* 11:143–150

World Health Organization (1987). *International Classification of Diseases*, 10th revision. Geneva: World Health Organization

Zhou DHD, Wang JYJ, Li J *et al.* (2004). Study on frequency and predictors of dementia after ischemic stroke. The Chongqing Stroke Study. *Journal of Neurology* 251:421–427

Chapter 32

Vascular cognitive impairment: investigation and treatment

For any patient with cognitive impairment, it is important to rule out reversible causes and to exclude alternative diagnoses that may present with similar symptoms. Once cognitive impairment is confirmed, the underlying cause should be determined; that is, the subtype of cognitive impairment should be defined since this will influence prognosis and treatment.

Routine investigations

In elderly patients, depression may mimic dementia, and in the elderly confused patient in hospital, it may be difficult to distinguish between dementia and delirium in which there is fluctuating confusion, poor attention and changes in arousal secondary to underlying physiological disturbance. Factors distinguishing between dementia and delirium are shown in Table 32.1.

Routine blood tests that should be requested in the investigation of cognitive impairment are shown in Table 32.2. Current UK guidelines state that all patients undergoing investigation for cognitive impairment should receive structural brain imaging to exclude pathologies such as space-occupying lesion or subdural hematoma and to aid in dementia subtype identification. There is a preference for MRI over CT owing to its better special resolution and sensitivity.

Perfusion hexamethylpropyleneamine oxime (HMPAO) single-photon emission computed tomography (SPECT) or 2-[^{18}F]fluoro-2-deoxy-D-glucose positron emission tomography (FDG PET) can be used to help to differentiate between Alzheimer's disease, vascular dementia and frontotemporal dementia if the diagnosis is in doubt.

Cerebrospinal fluid examination and electroencephalography are not required routinely in the investigation of dementia. Lumbar puncture is indicated in suspected Creutzfeldt–Jakob disease or other forms of rapidly progressive dementia. Electroencephalography should be considered if delirium, frontotemporal dementia or Creutzfeldt–Jakob disease are possibilities. Electroencephalography may also be required in the assessment of associated seizure disorder in those with dementia.

Once it has been established that a patient has dementia, it is necessary to try and define the subtype of dementia in order to enable prognostication and treatment. There is no diagnostic finding on brain imaging for vascular cognitive impairment but imaging abnormalities are used together with clinical features to aid diagnosis. As outlined in Ch. 31, it is often difficult to distinguish between vascular dementia and Alzheimer's disease. The brain imaging changes that impact on the understanding of vascular cognitive impairment are outlined below.

Silent infarcts, white matter changes and microbleeds

As stated in Ch. 31, vascular changes on brain imaging are required for a diagnosis of vascular dementia using the Neuroepidemiology Branch of the National Institute of Neurological

Table 32.1. Distinguishing between dementia and delirium

Feature	Delirium	Dementia
Onset	Acute, often at night	Insidious
Course	Fluctuating, lucid times	Stable
Duration	Hours/weeks	Months/years
Awareness	Reduced	Clear
Alertness	Abnormal (low/high)	Usually normal
Attention	Impaired, distractible	Usually unaffected
Orientation	Impaired	Impaired in later stages
Short-term memory	Always impaired	Normal at first
Episodic memory	Impaired	Impaired
Thinking	Disorganized, delusions	Impoverished
Perception	Illusions/hallucinations	Absent early, common later
Sleep cycle	Always disrupted	Usually normal

Table 32.2. Routine tests for the investigation of cognitive impairment

Test	Comments
Full blood count	
Electrolytes, creatinine	
Glucose	
Calcium	
Liver function	
Vitamin B$_{12}$	Cognitive impairment may occur in the absence of other symptoms
Folate	
Erythrocyte sedimentation rate	Temporal arteritis may cause strokes and cognitive impairment
Midstream urine	If delirium suspected
Syphilis serology	Only if clinical picture is suggestive
Human immunodeficiency virus	Only if clinical picture is suggestive

Disorders and Stroke–Association Internationale pour la Recheiche et l'Enseignement en Neurosciences (NINDS/AIREN) criteria (Roman *et al.* 1993). However, uncertainties exist regarding the significance of some abnormalities and the effect on cognition. Frequent findings on brain imaging in patients with cognitive impairment include silent infarcts, white matter changes and microbleeds (Chs. 7 and 10) and these are discussed below.

The exact effect of silent infarcts and white matter change on cognition is uncertain. Studies of normal elderly people (Smith *et al.* 2000) have shown that such lesions may exist in the presence of normal cognition. However, clinical, epidemiological and pathological studies suggest that, in general, people with white matter change and silent infarcts are more likely to have cognitive impairment than those with normal brains (Frisoni *et al.* 2007; Vermeer *et al.* 2007). Severity of white matter change, brain atrophy and the presence of infarction are associated with decline in information-processing speed and executive function (Prins *et al.* 2005). Presence of subcortical hyperintensities is associated with cognitive impairment following clinical stroke secondary to lacunar infarction (Mok *et al.* 2005; Grau-Olivares *et al.* 2007).

The neuropathology of white matter changes seen on brain imaging is variable and includes partial neuronal loss, axonal loss, demyelination and gliosis (Jagust *et al.* 2008). The mechanisms underlying such changes are uncertain but there are associations with age, hypertension and diabetes. It is not known how white matter changes may contribute to cognitive impairment, but there is some evidence that interruption of fronto-subcortical circuits linking the frontal lobes to the striatum, globus pallidus and ventral anterior and mediodorsal thalamus may be important (Castaigne *et al.* 1981). Interruption of specific parts of the fronto-subcortical circuit causes specific deficits: executive dysfunction and impaired recall (dorsolateral circuit), behavioral and emotional change (orbitofrontal circuit), and abulia and akinetic mutism (anterior cingulate circuit) (Cummings 1993; Tekin and Cummings 2002). The extent and location of white matter changes determine the neuropsychological profile in healthy individuals, patients with stroke and patients with cognitive impairment and dementia (Delano-Wood *et al.* 2008; Libon *et al.* 2008; Swartz *et al.* 2008; Wright *et al.* 2008). Several studies highlight the critical role of the thalamus in cognitive function: patients with thalamic dysfunction secondary to thalamic lesions or to subcortical diaschisis perform poorly in cognitive tests involving frontal and temporal lobe function (Stebbins *et al.* 2008; Swartz *et al.* 2008; Wright *et al.* 2008).

It should be noted that the abnormalities on brain imaging described above are not exclusive to or diagnostic of vascular cognitive impairment: deep white matter lesions and periventricular lesions have been shown in 50% and 90%, respectively, of patients with Alzheimer's disease and are also often present in patients with Lewy body disease (Barber *et al.* 1999).

Cerebral microbleeds seen on T_2^*-weighted MRI (see Ch. 7) are associated with lacunar infarcts, hemorrhages, white matter changes, hypertension and cognitive impairment. The number of microbleeds may be independent predictors of cognitive impairment in multiple domains and severity of dementia (Won Seo *et al.* 2007). Cerebral microbleeds are associated with cerebral amyloid angiopathy (Ch. 7) in which there is often coexisting leukoaraiosis and cognitive impairment.

Brain atrophy and temporal lobe atrophy

Generalized brain atrophy is associated with cognitive impairment in small vessel disease (Mungas *et al.* 2001; O'Sullivan *et al.* 2004; Mok *et al.* 2005). This may be related to white matter tract degeneration and disconnection (Fein *et al.* 2000), a process supported by recent diffusion tensor imaging studies (O'Sullivan *et al.* 2005) (see below). However, a primary mechanism cannot be excluded. Loss of brain volume in the syndrome of cerebral autosomal dominant arteriopathy with silent infarcts and leukoaraiosis (CADASIL) is predicted by age, apparent diffusion coefficient and volume of lacunar lesion, suggesting that brain atrophy is related to both the consequences of lacunar lesions and the widespread microstructural changes beyond the lacunar lesions (Jouvent *et al.* 2007).

Temporal lobe atrophy is a well-recognized association of Alzheimer's disease, and early loss of temporal lobe volume occurs in people who are cognitively intact but who go on to develop Alzheimer's disease (Jobst *et al.* 1992; de Leon *et al.* 1993). Neuropathological studies have confirmed that the medial temporal lobes are affected very early on in the course of the disease and the resultant impairment of temporal lobe function causes early memory loss. Medial temporal lobe atrophy is also associated with vascular cognitive impairment defined by various different criteria including the *Diagnostic and Statistical Manual of Mental Disorders,* 3rd edition (DSM-III) and NINDS/AIREN (Laakso *et al.* 1996; O'Brien *et al.* 2000; Fein *et al.* 2000; Gainotti *et al.* 2004; Bastos-Leite *et al.* 2007; Grau-Olivares *et al.* 2007). This may partly be an artefact of the requirement for the presence of memory impairment in the diagnosis of vascular cognitive impairment.

However, neuropathological examination in three patients with temporal lobe atrophy and vascular dementia found no evidence of Alzheimer's type pathology in the cortex (Fein *et al.* 2000). Therefore, medial temporal lobe atrophy is not specific to Alzheimer's dementia. However, it may be of some discriminatory value in early disease (Jobst *et al.* 1998; O'Brien *et al.* 2000), although this may be less so in elderly patients in whom medial temporal lobe atrophy may simply reflect age-related cerebral atrophy.

Medial temporal lobe atrophy is associated with a greater risk of developing post-stroke dementia in patients who were not demented prior to stroke (Cordoliani-Mackowiak *et al.* 2003; Firbank *et al.* 2007). Of the patients who become demented post-stroke, medial temporal lobe atrophy appears to be a near universal finding in those felt to have Alzheimer's disease but is seen in only half of those with vascular dementia. In a study of delayed cognitive impairment after stroke, medial temporal lobe atrophy, but not white matter hyperintensity volume, was associated with delayed (more than three months after stroke) cognitive decline (Firbank *et al.* 2007). The authors suggested that this indicated a greater role for Alzheimer's rather than vascular pathology in delayed post-stroke cognitive impairment. However, given the lack of specificity of medial temporal lobe atrophy for Alzheimer's disease this may be oversimplistic.

Diffusion tensor imaging

As stated above, there is poor correlation between lesion volume and cognitive deficit. This mirrors the poor correlation seen between lesion volume and motor function (Ch. 24) and is not surprising given the fact that lesion volume alone does not take into account the importance of lesion location. While the effect of a lesion on well-defined white matter tracts such as the descending motor pathways can be estimated with some accuracy (Pendlebury *et al.* 1999; Pineiro *et al.* 2000) (Ch. 23), it is almost impossible to do this for tracts passing through the deep white matter since the anatomy and connections of these tracts are not well known. Even if the anatomy of the deep white matter tracts was better understood, it would be impossible to define the exact intersections between multiple such tracts and multiple white matter lesions, which in any case are neuropathologically heterogeneous using standard structural imaging.

Recently, diffusion tensor imaging has been used to perform tractography (the imaging of defined fiber tracts), including of the thalamocortical projections and the limbic network. Tractography has been used quantitatively to correlate stroke severity and outcome from lenticulostriate infarcts with damage to the corticospinal tract (Konishi *et al.* 2005). Studies of cognitive change and tractography are few, but greater understanding of the anatomy of the deep white matter tracts may aid in defining the prognosis and response to treatment in patients with vascular cognitive impairment.

Diffusion tensor imaging may also be used to measure fractional anisotropy, a marker of the degree of disruption of fiber tracts. Decreased fractional anisotropy has been shown in leukoaraiosis and also in normal-appearing white matter in patients with leukoraiosis, the latter correlating with the degree of executive impairment (O'Sullivan *et al.* 2001). Reductions in fractional anisotropy have also been reported from elderly people with normal brain imaging (Taylor *et al.* 2007). Therefore, fractional anisotropy appears to be a more sensitive tool for the detection of white matter damage than standard structural MRI, including FLAIR. Changes in fractional anisotropy correlate with N-acetyl aspartate measured using MR spectroscopy (Charlton *et al.* 2006). Since decreased fractional anisotropy is seen in normal-appearing white matter, it may prove useful in identifying those at risk of subsequent cognitive decline. Patients with Alzheimer's disease also exhibit reduced fractional anisotropy, and this correlates with cortical atrophy, lending further support to the idea that there may be an early vascular component to Alzheimer's disease.

Therapeutic approaches for vascular cognitive impairment

Therapy can be divided into primary prevention (preventing cerebrovascular disease and its related cognitive decline), secondary prevention (preventing worsening or recurrence of cerebrovascular disease), symptomatic treatments and disease-modifying treatments. Effective primary prevention of vascular disease, particularly of stroke, will reduce vascular cognitive impairment secondary to stroke. However, the degree to which primary prevention affects vascular change in the absence of clinical stroke, in particular small vessel disease and white matter lesions, remains unclear. It is likely that prevention of progression of such lesions will reduce cognitive decline.

Regarding specific primary preventive therapies and prevention of cognitive impairment and dementia, there is some evidence that antihypertensive drugs may influence cognitive decline: a meta-analysis of four randomized, controlled trials of antihypertensive drugs included over 20 000 subjects and found a non-significant trend (relative risk, 0.80; 95% confidence interval, 0.63–1.02; $p = 0.07$) towards reduction in cognitive decline with blood pressure-lowering treatment (Feigin et al. 2005). One observational study of statin use and cognitive function in the elderly found a slight reduction in cognitive decline in those using statins that could not be completely explained by the effect of statins on lowering of serum cholesterol (Bernick et al. 2005). However, no favorable effect of statins was seen in two large randomized trials (Heart Protection Study Collaborative Group 2002; Shepherd et al. 2002).

Preventing recurrent stroke is likely to reduce the incidence of dementia, although dementia might still be related to the common underlying risk factors, such as hypertension. In the Perindopril Protection Against Recurrent Stroke Study (PROGRESS) of blood pressure lowering after stroke (PROGRESS Collaborative Group 2001), the incidence of dementia was less in the treatment group in those who suffered a recurrent stroke than in the placebo group. Further studies are needed to determine whether the incidence of dementia post-stroke falls with more aggressive secondary preventive therapy. Data on the effectiveness of antiplatelet therapy in preventing stroke-associated dementia are also lacking.

Regarding symptomatic treatment, several randomized, double-blind, placebo-controlled trials have been undertaken in vascular dementia, although they have been criticized for using design and outcomes designed for Alzheimer's disease. Early studies concentrated on agents such as vasodilators and antioxidants but were disappointing. Only one study of aspirin in 70 people with multi-infarct dementia has been undertaken (Meyer et al. 1989), which showed that those taking 325 mg aspirin (compared with no treatment) had significantly higher cognitive performance at the end of three years, although dropout rates were high (61% by three years).

There have been two studies of memantine, an NMDA receptor antagonist, in vascular dementia, both of which showed significant effects on cognition compared with placebo over a six-month period. However, there was no effect on global outcome measure, making the results of uncertain clinical relevance (Orgogozo et al. 2002; Wilcock et al. 2002). Similar improvement in cognition without consistent changes in activities of daily living, behavior and global assessment were seen in studies of cholinesterase inhibitors: three studies of donepezil and two of galanthamine, of which two remain unpublished (Erkinjuntti *et al.* 2002; Black *et al.* 2003; Wilkinson *et al.* 2003). Therefore, the use of cholinesterase inhibitors in patients with probable vascular dementia is not recommended, although they may be effective in patients with mixed Alzheimer's disease and vascular dementia.

As stated above, there is a high incidence of depression in patients with vascular cognitive impairment, and depression may precede the onset of cognitive change. Treatment of depression may improve function as well as improving the patient's quality of life. There is no evidence to support the use of any particular type of antidepressant. Behavioral disturbance is as common in vascular cognitive impairment as it is in Alzheimer's disease and should be managed with non-pharmacological interventions in the first instance. Non-pharmacological interventions include stimulating activity, increased carer attention, cognitive behavioral therapy and nursing in a calm and quiet environment. If drug therapy is required to alleviate patient distress or for reasons of patient or carer safety, then benzodiazepines should be used first. If neuroleptic therapy is required, careful assessment of risks and benefits is needed since such drugs may increase the risk of stroke. Cholinesterase inhibitors are not recommended for behavioral disturbance in vascular cognitive impairment but may be used in Lewy body disease and Alzheimer's disease.

References

Barber R, Scheltens P, Gholkar A *et al.* (1999). White matter lesions on magnetic resonance imaging in dementia with Lewy bodies, Alzheimer's disease, vascular dementia, and normal aging. *Journal of Neurology, Neurosurgery and Psychiatry* **67**:66–72

Bastos-Leite AJ, van der Flier WM, van Straaten EC *et al.* (2007). The contribution of medial temporal lobe atrophy and vascular pathology to cognitive impairment in vascular dementia. *Stroke* **38**:3182–3185

Bernick C, Katz R, Smith NL *et al.* (2005). Statins and cognitive function in the elderly: the Cardiovascular Health Study. *Neurology* **65**:1388–1394

Black S, Roman GC, Geldmacher DS *et al.* (2003). Efficacy and tolerability of donepezil in vascular dementia: positive results of a 24-week, multicenter, international, randomized, placebo-controlled clinical trial. *Stroke* **34**:2323–2330

Castaigne P, Lhermitte F, Buge A *et al.* (1981). Paramedian thalamic and midbrain infarct: clinical and neuropathological study. *Annals of Neurology* **10**:127–148

Charlton RA, Barrick TR, McIntyre DJ *et al.* (2006). White matter damage on diffusion tensor imaging correlates with age-related cognitive decline. *Neurology* **66**:217–222

Cordoliani-Mackowiak M, Hénon H, Pruvo J *et al.* (2003). Post stroke dementia: influence of hippocampal atrophy. *Archives of Neurology* **60**:585–590

Cummings JL (1993). Frontal-subcortical circuits and human behavior. *Archives of Neurology* **50**:873–880

Delano-Wood L, Abeles N, Sacco JM *et al.* (2008). Regional white matter pathology in mild cognitive impairment: differential influence of lesion type on neuropsychological functioning. *Stroke* **39**:794–799

de Leon MJ, Golomb J, George AE *et al.* (1993). The radiologic prediction of Alzheimer disease: the atrophic hippocampal formation. *American Journal of Neuroradiology* **14**:897–906

Erkinjuntti T, Kurz A, Gauthier S *et al.* (2002). Efficacy of galanthamine in probable vascular dementia and Alzheimer's disease combined with cerebrovascular disease: a randomised trial. *Lancet* **359**:1283–1290

Feigin V, Ratnasabapathy Y, Anderson C (2005). Does blood pressure lowering treatment prevent dementia or cognitive decline in patients with cardiovascular and cerebrovascular disease? *Journal of Neurology Science* **15**:151–155

Fein G, Di Sclafani V, Tanabe J *et al.* (2000). Hippocampal and cortical atrophy predict dementia in subcortical ischemic vascular disease. *Neurology* 55:1626–1635

Firbank MJ, Burton EJ, Barber R *et al.* (2007). Medial temporal atrophy rather than white matter hyperintensities predict cognitive decline in stroke survivors. *Neurobiology Aging* 28:1664–1669

Frisoni GB, Galluzzi S, Pantoni L *et al.* (2007). The effect of white matter lesions on cognition in the elderly–small but detectable. *Nature Clinical and Practical Neurology* 3:620–627

Gainotti G, Acciarri A, Bizzarro A *et al.* (2004). The role of brain infarcts and hippocampal atrophy in subcortical ischaemic vascular dementia. *Neurology Science* 25:192–197

Grau-Olivares M, Bartrés-Faz D, Arboix A *et al.* (2007). Mild cognitive impairment after lacunar infarction: voxel-based morphometry and neuropsychological assessment. *Cerebrovascular Diseases* 23:353–361

Heart Protection Study Collaborative Group (2002). MRC/BHF Heart Protection Study of cholesterol lowering with simvastatin in 20 536 high-risk individuals: a randomised placebo-controlled trial. *Lancet* 360:7–22

Jagust WJ, Zheng L, Harvey DJ (2008). Neuropathological basis of magnetic resonance images in aging and dementia. *Annals of Neurology* 63: 72–82

Jobst KA, Smith AD, Szatmari M *et al.* (1992). Detection in life of confirmed Alzheimer's disease using a simple measurement of medial temporal lobe atrophy by computed tomography. *Lancet* 340:1179–1183

Jobst KA, Barnetson LP, Shepstone BJ (1998). Accurate prediction of histologically confirmed Alzheimer's disease and the differential diagnosis of dementia: the use of NINCDS–ADRDA and DSM-III-R criteria, SPECT, X-ray CT, and Apo E4 in medial temporal lobe dementias. Oxford Project to Investigate Memory and Aging. *International Psychogeriatrics* 10:271–302

Jouvent E, Viswanathan A, Mangin JF *et al.* (2007). Brain atrophy is related to lacunar lesions and tissue microstructural changes in CADASIL. *Stroke* 38:1786–1790

Konishi J, Yamada K, Kizu O *et al.* (2005). MR tractography for the evaluation of functional recovery from lenticulostriate infarcts. *Neurology* 64:108–113

Laakso MP, Partanen K, Riekkinen P *et al.* (1996). Hippocampal volumes in Alzheimer's disease, Parkinson's disease with and without dementia, and in vascular dementia: An MRI study. *Neurology* 46:678–681

Libon DJ, Price CC, Giovannetti T *et al.* (2008). Linking MRI hyperintensities with patterns of neuropsychological impairment: evidence for a threshold effect. *Stroke* 39:806–813

Meyer JS, Rogers RL, McClintic K *et al.* (1989). Randomized clinical trial of daily aspirin therapy in multi-infarct dementia. A pilot study. *Journal of the American Geriatric Society* 37:549–555

Mok V, Wong A, Tang WK *et al.* (2005). Determinants of post stroke cognitive impairment in small vessel disease. *Dementia and Geriatric Cognitive Disorders* 20: 225–230

Mungas D, Jagust WJ, Reed BR *et al.* (2001). MRI predictors of cognition in subcortical ischemic vascular disease and Alzheimer's disease. *Neurology* 57:2229–2235

O'Brien JT, Metcalfe S, Swann A (2000). Medial temporal lobe width on CT scanning in Alzheimer's disease: comparison with vascular dementia, depression and dementia with Lewy bodies. *Dementia and Geriatric Cognitive Disorders* 11:114–118

Orgogozo JM, Rigaud AS, Stoffler A *et al.* (2002). Efficacy and safety of memantine in patients with mild to moderate vascular dementia: a randomized, placebo-controlled trial (MMM 300). *Stroke* 33:1834–1839

O'Sullivan M, Summers PE, Jones DK *et al.* (2001). Normal-appearing white matter in ischemic leukoaraiosis: a diffusion tensor MRI study. *Neurology* 57:2307–2310

O'Sullivan M, Morris RG, Huckstep B *et al.* (2004). Diffusion tensor MRI correlates with executive dysfunction in patients with ischaemic leukoaraiosis. *Journal of Neurology, Neurosurgery and Psychiatry* 75:441–447

O'Sullivan M, Barrick TR, Morris RG *et al.* (2005). Damage within a network of white matter regions underlies executive dysfunction in CADASIL. *Neurology* 65:1584–1590

Pendlebury ST, Blamire AM, Lee MA *et al.* (1999). Axonal injury in the internal capsule correlates with motor impairment after stroke. *Stroke* 30:956–962

Pineiro R, Pendlebury ST, Smith S *et al.* (2000). Relating MRI changes to motor deficit after ischemic stroke by segmentation of functional motor pathways. *Stroke* **31**:672–679

Prins ND, van Dijk EJ, den Heijer T *et al.* (2005). Cerebral small-vessel disease and decline in information processing speed, executive function and memory. *Brain* **128**:2034–2041

PROGRESS Collaborative Group (2001). Randomised trial of a perindopril-based blood-pressure-lowering regimen among 6105 individuals with previous stroke or transient ischaemic attack. *Lancet* 358:1033–1041

Roman GC, Tatemichi TK, Erkinjuntti T *et al.* (1993). Vascular dementia: diagnostic criteria for research studies. Report of the NINDS–AIREN International Workshop. *Neurology* 43:250–260

Shepherd J, Blauw GJ, Murphy MB *et al.* (2002). PROspective Study of Pravastatin in the Elderly at Risk. Pravastatin in elderly individuals at risk of vascular disease (PROSPER): a randomised controlled trial. *Lancet* **360**:1623–1630

Smith CD, Snowdon DA, Wang H *et al.* (2000). White matter volumes and periventricular white matter hyperintensities in aging and dementia. *Neurology* **54**:838–842

Stebbins GT, Nyenhuis DL, Wang C *et al.* (2008). Gray matter atrophy in patients with ischemic stroke with cognitive impairment. *Stroke* **39**:785–793

Swartz RH, Stuss DT, Gao F *et al.* (2008). Independent cognitive effects of atrophy, diffuse subcortical and thalamo-cortical cerebrovascular disease in dementia. *Stroke* **39**:822–830

Taylor WD, Bae JN, MacFall JR *et al.* (2007). Widespread effects of hyperintense lesions on cerebral white matter structure. *American Journal of Roentgenology* **188**:1695–1704

Tekin S, Cummings JL (2002). Frontal-subcortical neuronal circuits and clinical neuropsychiatry: an update. *Journal of Psychosomatic Research* **53**:647–654

Vermeer SE, Longstreth WT Jr., Koudstaal PJ (2007). Silent brain infarcts: a systematic review. *Lancet Neurology* **6**:611–619

Wilcock G, Mobius HJ, Stoffler A *et al.* (2002). A double-blind, placebo-controlled multicentre study of memantine in mild to moderate vascular dementia (MMM500). *International Clinical Psychopharmacology* **17**:297–305

Wilkinson D, Doody R, Helme R *et al.* (2003). Donepezil in vascular dementia: a randomized placebo-controlled study. *Neurology* **61**:479–486

Won Seo S, Hwa Lee B, Kim EJ *et al.* (2007). Clinical significance of microbleeds in subcortical vascular dementia. *Stroke* **38**:1949–1951

Wright CB, Festa JR, Paik MC *et al.* (2008). White matter hyperintensities and subclinical infarction: associations with psychomotor speed and cognitive flexibility. *Stroke* **39**:800–805

Index